Ethical Issues in Neurology

THIRD EDITION

Ethical Issues in Neurology

THIRD EDITION

James L. Bernat, M.D.

Professor of Medicine (Neurology)
Dartmouth Medical School
Hanover, New Hampshire

Attending Neurologist
Director, Program in Clinical Ethics
Dartmouth-Hitchcock Medical Center
Lebanon, New Hampshire

Wolters Kluwer | Lippincott Williams & Wilkins
Health

Philadelphia · Baltimore · New York · London
Buenos Aires · Hong Kong · Sydney · Tokyo

Acquisitions Editor: Frances DeStefano
Managing Editor: Leanne McMillan
Project Manager: Alicia Jackson
Manufacturing Coordinator: Kathleen Brown
Marketing Manager: Kimberly Schonberger
Design Coordinator: Holly McLaughlin
Cover Designer: Carol Tippet Woolworth
Production Service: GGS Book Services

Library of Congress Cataloging-in-Publication Data
Bernat, James L.
 Ethical issues in neurology / James L. Bernat. — 3rd ed.
  p. ; cm.
 Includes bibliographical references and index.
 ISBN-13: 978-0-7817-9060-4
 ISBN-10: 0-7817-9060-3
 1. Neurology—Moral and ethical aspects. I. Title.
 [DNLM: 1. Nervous System Diseases—therapy. 2. Bioethical Issues. 3. Ethics, Medical. WL 140 B524e
2008]
 RC346.B479 2008
 174.2—dc22

                                                                 2007044264

978-0-7817-9060-4
0-7817-9060-3

                                                        10 9 8 7 6 5 4 3 2 1

To my father
Mitchell Joseph Bernat (1916–1999)

Preface

My goal in writing this monograph is to provide neurologists, neurosurgeons, and other clinicians who treat neurological patients with a current, comprehensive, reasoned, and balanced account of the important ethical problems they face in their practices. Although clinicians are well aware of these ethical problems, many are unfamiliar with the empirical data, insightful analyses, and thoughtful commentaries that constitute the burgeoning literature of clinical ethics. In this book, I attempt to analyze and discuss what others have written and to synthesize the best of these ideas and a few of my own into a rigorous and coherent approach to resolve these dilemmas.

The internal organization of the book proceeds from the general to the specific. In the first section, I present the fundamental vocabulary of ethical theory and practice, discuss the requirements of professional ethics, highlight the relationship of clinical ethics to the law, review the workings of the hospital ethics committee, and outline systematic approaches to resolving ethical dilemmas. In the next section, I discuss several important ethical issues that converge in the care of the dying patient, including in the provision of palliative care, withholding and withdrawing life-sustaining treatment, addressing requests for physician-assisted suicide or euthanasia, and physicians' use of the "medical futility" justification for unilaterally withholding or withdrawing therapy. In the third section, I analyze ethical and philosophical issues arising in specific disorders of the nervous system, including brain death, the vegetative state, the minimally conscious state, neurologically ill newborns, severe paralysis, dementia, mental retardation, neurogenetic disorders, and HIV/AIDS. I conclude with chapters reviewing the ethical issues arising in the conduct of clinical research and the ethical questions raised by neuroscience research, which comprise the emerging field called "neuroethics."

Unlike the customary format of most medical texts in which references are cited individually, I employ the endnotes format used more commonly in scholarly works. Using endnotes permits me to digress on particular points of interest without interrupting the flow of the discussion and to cite and briefly discuss related articles for the reader who wishes additional background information or more detailed discussion.

In each chapter, I review what, in my judgment, are the important published works in clinical ethics and related fields, especially those reporting valid empirical data. After each review, I offer my personal approach to solving the dilemma. I justify my conclusions and recommendations by citing ethical principles, accepted guidelines, empirical data, and by using reasoned arguments. This work is not simply a survey of the findings and opinions of others; my personal opinions and prejudices are exposed for criticism.

Accompanying many ethics discussions, I include a brief consideration of relevant statutory, case, and administrative law in the United States and occasionally elsewhere. Although this selective citation does not purport to be a comprehensive summary of the law, I have chosen cases that represent important judicial precedents and that illustrate some of the similarities and differences between law and ethics.

I am pleased that the publication of this edition by Lippincott Williams & Wilkins has been coordinated with the publication of the new edition of the American Academy of Neurology Ethics, Law & Humanities Committee's neurology resident ethics teaching casebook entitled *Practical Ethics in Clinical Neurology* and edited by Tyler E. Reimschisel and Michael A. Williams. We hope that the synergy of the two works can optimize neurology resident and staff education in clinical ethics.

The six years since the second edition of this book was published have witnessed a continued growth of interest in ethical problems in medicine in general and neurology in particular. Thousands of scholarly articles have been published in journals and hundreds of books have been written on ethics topics relevant to the care of neurological patients. But many of these works have been published in ethics, law, or humanities journals that lie outside the usual reading lists of practicing clinicians. For the third edition, in addition to updating and rewriting the chapters in the second edition to incorporate these new works and in response to the suggestions of several readers, I added two new chapters on the topics of resolving ethical dilemmas and neuroethics.

The topics I discuss in *Ethical Issues in Neurology* will become only more important in the future with continued advances in technology that offer new medical tests and treatments, and with market-driven changes in the provision of medical care that jeopardize the patient-physician relationship. I hope this book will serve as an ethical map for clinicians caring for neurological patients to assist them in defining right actions as they navigate the rough seas of technologic and social change.

J.L.B.

Acknowledgments

Authors do not write books *ex vacuo* and this one is no exception. I am fortunate to have been taught by skilled teachers and to have worked with generous colleagues. It is my pleasure to acknowledge and thank these teachers and colleagues.

My interest in this area began nearly 40 years ago as a Cornell medical student studying cases of coma, vegetative state, and brain death under the direction of Drs. Fred Plum and Jerome Posner, and studying medical jurisprudence under Dr. H. Richard Beresford. Thereafter at Dartmouth, I have benefited immensely from a 30-year collaboration with philosophy professor Bernard Gert as we have pursued ethical and philosophical questions in medicine. Bernie has been a generous and patient teacher and mentor.

My published writings in ethical issues in neurology began in 1981 with the first of a series of biophilosophical papers on the definition and criterion of death written with Bernard Gert and Charles M. Culver. Thereafter my interest broadened to encompass other ethical and philosophical issues in neurological practice. To stimulate the interest of other neurologists in this field, I edited two collections of articles on ethical issues in neurology that were published in the *Seminars in Neurology* in 1984 and in the *Neurologic*

Clinics in 1989. I am indebted to the authors of those articles for teaching me about these topics.

I again offer gratitude to Dr. Robert J. Joynt of the University of Rochester for encouraging me to write a monograph on ethical issues in neurology for his loose-leaf textbook *Clinical Neurology*, published in 1987 and 1991, and updated again in 1997, 2000, and 2003 in collaboration with Robert M. Taylor. Writing that chapter and its updates gave me the opportunity to collect and systematize much of the literature I present here in greater depth.

The first two editions of this book were published in 1994 and 2002 by Butterworth-Heinemann, prior to its purchase by Elsevier. I especially thank Susan F. Pioli for initially suggesting that I write a book-size monograph on this subject and for providing assistance and encouragement during my writing of the first and second editions.

My colleagues on the Dartmouth-Hitchcock Medical Center Bioethics Committee have been a constant springboard for ideas. I particularly acknowledge committee members Drs. Marie Bakitas, William H. Edwards, Richard B. Ferrell, Timothy P. Lahey, Diane M. Palac, Lynn M. Peterson, Thomas J. Prendergast, and John H. Sanders, and Kate Clay, Rev. Patrick McCoy, Margaret Minnock, Fr. Roland S. Nadeau,

Margaret Plunkett, Elizabeth R. Stanton, Esq. and Ryan Walther. I also thank my local and regional clinical ethics colleagues: Dean Stephen P. Spielberg of Dartmouth Medical School, Prof. Ronald M. Green of the Dartmouth Institute for Applied and Professional Ethics, Rev. William Nelson of the Dartmouth Rural Ethics Initiative, Drs. Robert D. Orr and Robert C. Macauley of Fletcher-Allen Health Care, and Dr. Arnold Golodetz of the Vermont Ethics Network. I am especially grateful for critiques of my thinking to Dr. David Steinberg of the Lahey Clinic Medical Center with whom I have collaborated for over a decade editing our newsletter *Medical Ethics.*

I also gratefully acknowledge the contributions of colleagues with whom I have co-authored articles or chapters I discuss here: Drs. John A. Baron, H. Richard Beresford, Alan C. Carver, Michael T. Claessens, Ronald E. Cranford, Charles M. Culver, Kathleen M. Foley, Bernard Gert, Michael L. Goldstein, Robert I. Grossman, Robert G. Holloway, Christopher M. Keran, R. Peter Mogielnicki, Lynn M. Peterson, Steven P. Ringel, David A. Rottenberg, Matthew P. Sweet, Robert M. Taylor, Barbara G. Vickrey, and H. Gilbert Welch.

I fondly acknowledge the guidance of Dr. Ronald E. Cranford (1940–2006) who, in 1983 as chairman, invited me to serve on the American Academy of Neurology Ethics and Humanities Subcommittee (now the Ethics, Law and Humanities Committee). My 25-year service on that committee has been one of the highlights of my professional life. I acknowledge other colleagues who have served with me on this committee during portions of the past quarter-century and who have taught me, contributed ideas, and coauthored papers cited here: Drs. H. Richard Beresford, Gastone G. Celesia, Maynard M. Cohen, John P. Conomy, John R. Delfs, Richard P. Foa, Kathleen M. Foley, David Goldblatt (1930–2007), James Gordon, David L. Jackson, Peter L. Jacobson, Daniel Larriviere, Glenn D. Mackin, Michael P. McQuillen, Robert F. Nelson, Lois M. Nora, Thomas R. Pellegrino, Tyler E. Reimschisel, Matthew Rizzo, Murray G. Sagsveen, Russell D. Snyder, Jr., Robert M. Taylor, Alison Wichman, Michael A. Williams, and Professor John C. Fletcher (1932–2004).

Several colleagues kindly read drafts of chapters and made valuable suggestions in this or in previous editions. I am grateful to Drs. Stephen Ashwal, H. Richard Beresford, Paula R. Clemens, Timothy P. Lahey, Daniel Larriviere, Robert D. Orr, James E. Reagan, Tyler E. Reimschisel, Lawrence J. Schneiderman, Michael I. Shevell, Robert M. Taylor, and C. Fordham von Reyn for their many valuable suggestions.

I especially acknowledge and thank the late Dr. David Goldblatt of the University of Rochester. David painstakingly edited every chapter of this book with his careful editorial eye, his broad knowledge of the subject material, and his lifetime experience as a compassionate neurologist and master teacher. He contrasted the difference between his life as an academic neurologist and as a medical editor (Editor of the *Seminars of Neurology* and Associate Editor of the *Archives of Neurology*) by remarking, "I saved more sentences than lives." He certainly saved many sentences in this volume. David died on September 1, 2007, shortly after his editing work was completed.

I am grateful to the following publishers for permissions to use copyrighted material as cited in the text: Oxford University Press for the Appendix to chapter 3; Cambridge University Press for the Appendix to chapter 5; the American Medical Association for a passage quoted in chapter 12; and the AMA and my co-authors for selections from our 1993 paper in the *Archives of Internal Medicine* cited in chapter 9.

I thank the reference librarians of the Matthews-Fuller Health Sciences Library at Dartmouth-Hitchcock Medical Center and the Dana Biomedical Library at Dartmouth Medical School for numerous kindnesses.

I thank Murray G. Sagsveen, Esq, and Tami R. Boehne, Esq. of the American Academy of Neurology and Bruce Polsky of AAN Enterprises, Inc. for assistance in suggesting and coordinating the "bundling" of this edition with the new edition of the neurology resident ethics teaching casebook *Practical Ethics in Clinical Neurology,* edited by Drs. Tyler E. Reimschisel and Michael A. Williams, and also published by Lippincott Williams & Wilkins.

I lovingly acknowledge the levelheaded advice and counsel of my wife Judy with whom

I have discussed many of the issues I consider in this book during 38 years of married life together. She has helped me formulate ideas and concepts, and gently told me when my thinking was off base.

Finally, I express my gratitude to the editorial and publishing staffs at Lippincott Williams & Wilkins who helped make this edition possible, particularly Frances DeStefano, Leanne McMillan, Alicia Jackson, and Kimberly Schonberger, and to Andrea Shearer at GGS Book Services.

J.L.B.

Table of Contents

Ethical Issues in Neurology

THIRD EDITION

THE THEORY AND PRACTICE OF CLINICAL ETHICS

I

Ethical Theory

1

Neurologists routinely encounter ethical problems in everyday clinical practice. To resolve these clinical-ethical problems, usually they draw on their medical experience, clinical judgment, and moral intuitions rather than on knowledge of sophisticated formal systems of moral analysis. Indeed, most neurologists have not received formal education in moral philosophy and likely would regard such a course requirement as unnecessary and irrelevant to clinical practice.[1] Then of what value to clinicians is a general working knowledge of ethical theory?

A working knowledge of ethical theory provides clinicians with the foundation for a coherent and comprehensive framework of morality. Possessing this knowledge-construct confers three benefits. First, neurologists are able to better understand the theoretical basis of the essential concepts of ethical medical practice, such as valid consent, rationality, and paternalism, as well as how they should respond to patients' treatment decisions (discussed in chapter 2). Second, knowledge of ethical theory permits neurologists to apply abstract moral concepts and rules to tangible clinical situations in a consistent and clear manner, in much the same way that knowledge of basic pathology and physiology permits clinicians to understand disease and thereby to prescribe rational treatment. Third, familiarity with ethical theory helps neurologists distinguish ethical "dilemmas" amidst more mundane ethical "issues."

Most ethical issues can be resolved satisfactorily. An ethical dilemma is an ethical issue that seems to elude satisfactory resolution because, on diligent examination, there is no obvious singular right, good, or desirable action to take. Rather, all plausible alternatives present elements of benefits and burdens (good and evil). In medicine, dilemmas of competing goods usually are not problematic. Those of competing evils are more challenging, and it may be discouraging to discover that the best choice one can make or recommend is that which is the "least bad." I say more about the specific ethical dilemmas in neurological practice in the following chapters.

The unwary neurologist may hastily and mistakenly identify an ethical issue as a dilemma and make it more complicated than it actually is. In fact, true dilemmas are uncommon, in part because a comprehensive ethical theory provides the analytical tools for neurologists to resolve most ethical issues. A working knowledge of ethical theory helps neurologists disarm falsely claimed dilemmas and, perhaps more importantly, identify and competently face real ones. The frontier between ethical issues and dilemmas is constantly moving as consensus grows about the solution of the latter.

In this chapter, I outline the principal ethical theories, highlighting the concepts and rules derived from them. I briefly discuss alternative ethical considerations that complement and add richness to the analytical approaches. I distinguish secular and religious ethical requirements and briefly discuss the ethical systems of the principal religions as they apply to the common clinical example of end-of-life care. I present the ethical concepts that derive from these theories in chapter 2, and I discuss the methods clinicians can use to recognize, analyze, and resolve ethical dilemmas in neurological practice in chapter 6.

DEFINITIONS AND DISTINCTIONS

A number of terms used in ethical theory require definitions and distinctions. In this section, I delineate several simplified distinctions that I use throughout this book.

Morality vs. Ethics

Bernard Gert, a leading moral philosopher, has rigorously defined morality: it is "an informal public system applying to all rational persons, governing behavior that affects others, and includes what are commonly known as the moral rules, ideals and virtues, and has the lessening of evil or harm as its goal."[2] Ethics was defined by a neuroscientist as "a group of moral principles or set of values ... governing the behavior of an individual or profession."[3] Some authors use the terms "morality" and "ethics" synonymously; others make subtle distinctions between the two. Still others prefer to use the word "ethics" for all clinical contexts because they consider the word "morality" to have religious connotations because it was used originally in religious traditions. Because the similarities in the meanings of both terms far exceed their differences for the purposes of clinical medicine, they are sufficiently synonymous for me to use them interchangeably in this book.

Normative Ethics vs. Non-normative Ethics

The study of ethics can be divided into normative and non-normative divisions. Normative ethics refers to the substance and content of ethical living, including ethical theories, concepts, and rules, and their application in solving specific ethical problems. All discussions of ethical concepts and practices in this book and, indeed, almost all writings on clinical ethics concern claims of normative ethics.

By contrast, non-normative ethics does not concern itself with the content of an ethical life but rather with a description of the process of ethical deliberation. Descriptive ethics, the largest branch of non-normative ethics, defines the anthropological, sociological, psychological, and historical study of why and how people reason and make moral judgments as they do. Another branch, metaethics, provides a philosophical analysis of ethical discourse, including what is meant by moral judgments. Metaethics attempts to define precisely such terms as "right," "good," "wrong," and "bad."[4]

Religious Ethics vs. Secular Ethics

Each of the world's major religions is bound by a sacred body of scriptural writings on morality that comprise an essential component of its teachings and beliefs. The biblical Ten Commandments of Judaism and Christianity, and the volumes of associated commentary, exemplify the sophisticated moral systems of organized religions. In general, these systems are based on theological and religious beliefs in which moral laws represent the direct words of God revealed and communicated to humankind. Morality in these terms is not merely the product of human effort. That said, some religious thinkers have employed tenets of secular, rational ethics to flesh out the claims of their faiths. For example, "natural law," as taught by Thomas Aquinas, recommended for all persons a morality similar to that of his religion. But knowledge of this morality did not require revelation from God and could be acquired and understood by all rational persons who put their minds to it.

By contrast, secular ethics is solely the product of human rational discourse. Secular ethics assumes that humankind can devise a complete and universal system of morality without necessarily invoking a foundation of theological beliefs.[5] The clinical ethics discussed in this book are secular. Later in this chapter I briefly summarize the morality systems of several major religions. In subsequent chapters, I discuss the religious dimensions of specific problems in clinical ethics.

Theoretical Ethics vs. Applied Ethics

Theoretical ethics is to applied ethics as physics is to engineering. Theoretical ethics consists of the systems of morality and their derivative abstract concepts. The field of applied ethics attempts to solve specific clinical-ethical problems through an analytical process using abstract concepts. Medical ethics, clinical ethics, and bioethics all are examples of applied ethics.

Medical Ethics vs. Clinical Ethics

Clinical ethics has been defined in a leading textbook as "the identification, analysis and resolution of moral problems that arise in the care of a particular patient."[6] I define clinical ethics somewhat differently as "the identification of morally correct actions and the resolution of ethical dilemmas in medical decision-making through the application of moral concepts and rules to medical situations."[7] Clinical ethics comprises medical and nursing ethics as well as ethics of other professionals in clinical healing practices.

Clinical Ethics vs. Bioethics

Bioethics, having a broader scope than clinical ethics, embraces the intersection of biology with ethics; therefore, bioethics encompasses all clinical ethics but not vice versa. The major field of bioethical inquiry outside the strict purview of clinical ethics is the ethics of research. Research specifically involving human subjects also may be considered within the realm of clinical ethics, however. Because they enroll their patients in research studies and supervise them during such protocols, physicians retain ethical responsibilities toward these patients.

SYSTEMS OF ETHICAL THEORY

Ethical theory has been a subject of scholarly writing in Western and other cultures since antiquity. The Greek philosophers of Western civilization, particularly Plato and Aristotle, devoted several volumes to profound considerations of the essential questions of morality including the definition of a good life and how to live it, questions that continue to stimulate discussion today.[8] In the seventeenth century, Thomas Hobbes ushered in the modern era of Western ethical theory, which developed into the deontological and utilitarian writings in Europe during the mid-eighteenth and nineteenth centuries. The major contemporary schools of Western ethical theory are derived from these great traditions.[9]

Utilitarianism

The founders of the utilitarian (or consequentialist) school of morality were David Hume (1711–1776), Jeremy Bentham (1748–1832), and most notably John Stuart Mill (1806–1873). Utilitarian philosophy determines the morality of an act solely by an analysis of its consequences. The greater the extent to which an act leads to nonmoral goods, such as happiness, pleasure, or health, the more it is likely to be morally right. The tendency of an act to yield such nonmoral goods is its "utility." Conversely, the greater the tendency of an act not to produce nonmoral goods, the greater is its "disutility." Mill wrote: "Actions are right in proportion as they tend to promote happiness, wrong as they tend to produce the reverse of happiness."[10]

Commonly, a given act will have complex effects, producing both harms and benefits for one person, or combinations of benefits for one person and harms for another. In this situation, the degree of moral rightness of an act is directly proportional to its net utility, defined as the difference between its overall utility and disutility. The principle of utility is not a sophisticated philosophical concept. It is a common, intuitive process that judges, legislators, policymakers, and other responsible public officials in our society use to reach complex and difficult decisions that simultaneously help and hurt others.

The utilitarian school can be divided into those who believe that the principle of utility should be applied directly to individual acts on a case-by-case basis and those who believe that the principle should be applied to classes of acts indirectly through rules derived from the principle. The former are known as act-utilitarians and the latter as rule-utilitarians. Act-utilitarians examine the net utility resulting from a single act and thereby determine the morality of the act. In clinical practice, this process involves a comparison between the benefits accrued and the burdens borne from the performance of a given act. Rule-utilitarians apply a general rule derived from the principle of utility, such as "do not kill," and render a moral judgment independent of the details of a particular act.

Deontology

The founder of the most important modern school of deontology was Immanuel Kant (1724–1804). The term deontology is derived from the Greek *deon*, meaning "duty" or "that which is binding." Unlike utilitarians, who determine the morality of an act solely on the basis of its consequences, deontologists determine the morality of an act on the basis of the intent of an act, the sense of duty that motivates an act, the intention to do one's duty, and the other factors that determine why and how a person acts. Kantian deontologists are concerned more with the moral rightness of intentions that drive acts than with the results of acts. Kant criticized utilitarianism because it failed to account for our complete set of moral intuitions. He pointed out that if an act performed with the intent of helping another person that ordinarily would be expected to help the person ends up—through no fault of the actor—producing a net harm to the other person, it should not be considered immoral, as it would be from a purely utilitarian perspective. Kant argued that the actor's intention to do his duty should outweigh the bad consequences and thereby make it a moral act.

Kant's test for the moral rightness of an act was his "categorical imperative": "I ought never to act except in such a way that I can also will that my maxim should become a universal law."[11] This imperative means that in everyday living, persons should always act in ways that they can rationally and rightly expect others to act. Consider "telling the truth," a duty universally expected of physicians. Kant believed truth-telling to be universally rational and right because the contrary default mode, deception, is so obviously irrational. It would be impossible to know how to act rationally if deception were the default mode of behavior. The universal rightness of truth-telling follows from its rationality: because one can legitimately

expect the truth from others (in order to have the best chance at acting rationally), one must always tell the truth to others to give them the same chance at rationality that one claims for oneself. Kant believed in the universality of morality and in its scope as a public system. The rightness of ethical action is independent of the observer and should be universally accepted by all impartial persons.

Deontologists can be divided into those who apply the categorical imperative directly to acts and those who apply it indirectly through rules to classes of acts. Act-deontologists examine the intentions and sense of duty behind a given act to assess its moral rightness, whereas rule-deontologists develop a set of moral rules based on intrinsic features of acts that they subsequently apply to classes of cases.

Contemporary Moral Philosophers

Most contemporary philosophers are rooted in both utilitarianism and deontology because neither approach alone can fully account for the richness and completeness of our body of moral intuitions.[12] They recognize that we can determine the moral correctness of an act only by understanding its intentions and other intrinsic characteristics as well as its consequences. Contemporary moral theories differ on the extent to which they emphasize the intentions or consequences of an act in assessing its morality and their systems of moral justification. Interestingly, a comparison of the lists of moral rules devised by rule-utilitarians and rule-deontologists reveals a remarkable similarity. It is the derivation of the rules and their justification processes that differ more than the content of the rules themselves.

Bernard Gert is a leading contemporary moral philosopher with roots both in rule-deontology and in rule-utilitarianism. In his *Morality: Its Nature and Justification*, (revised edition, 2005), a work in evolution and refinement for four decades, Gert has formulated a complete public system of morality composed of moral rules, moral attitudes, and moral ideals that provides a rigorous process to analyze and justify the morality of actions. Gert explains that morality has two features as a public system: "(1) everyone who is subject to moral judgment must know what kind of behavior morality prohibits, requires, discourages, encourages, and allows, and (2) it is not irrational for any of them to use morality as a guide for their own conduct."[13]

Ten moral rules form the backbone of Gert's account of our moral system. Gert formulated these rules to summarize the essential universal guidelines for ethical behavior. All impartial, rational persons would publicly advocate that everyone obey the ten moral rules at all times, unless there exists adequate justification for breaking them, because obeying them protects a person and those for whom the person cares from suffering unnecessary evil.

Gert's moral rules are delineated in two groups that rank their importance. The first group of five usually has the highest priority. When these rules are violated, serious evils such as death, pain, disability, and loss of freedom, opportunity, or pleasure are inflicted directly on people. The first set of rules is:

1. Do not kill.
2. Do not cause pain.
3. Do not disable.
4. Do not deprive of freedom.
5. Do not deprive of pleasure.[14]

The second group of rules generally has a lower priority. If they are violated, the probability that someone will suffer an evil increases, although this effect is neither as direct nor as certain as that resulting from a violation of a moral rule from the first set. As was true for the first set, all rational, impartial persons should advocate universal and public adherence to these rules, unless there is adequate justification for not doing so, because obeying the rules prevents evils from occurring to persons and those for whom they care. The second five rules are:

1. Do not deceive.
2. Keep your promises.
3. Do not cheat.
4. Obey the law.
5. Do your duty.[15]

Nonetheless, all rational persons would not want these moral rules to be followed mindlessly at all times without exception. Gert devoted considerable attention to analyzing the justifiable violations of the rules. There exist justifications for violating the moral rules that all rational persons should advocate publicly. Consider, for example, the second moral rule "Do not cause pain." Clinicians are morally justified in producing a temporary and small degree of pain as they diagnose and treat a patient's serious disease, because they have the patient's consent and because the pain they inflict is a prerequisite for initiating effective treatment that can prevent the patient from suffering much more serious evils, such as death, disability, or more severe pain. Gert's system of morality provides a rigorous analytical process to test violations of moral rules for their adequate justification. Acts violating moral rules that fail the justification test are immoral.

Gert has defined the "moral attitude" as the attitude that a person should take when considering whether or not to violate a moral rule. A person taking this attitude makes it clear that no one should violate a moral rule unless "a fully informed, rational person can publicly allow violating it." That is, a person should be willing for everyone to know that this kind of violation is acceptable.[16] No impartial, rational person would be willing to allow any kind of violation publicly unless he believed that less harm would result if everyone knew that this violation was allowed than would result if everyone knew that this kind of violation was not allowed. Willingness to adopt the moral attitude, with the accompanying risk that one might be mistaken, is the strongest indication that the rule violation has been made rationally, impartially, and justifiably. Gert has identified 10 questions whose answers determine what constitutes the morally relevant features that are necessary to justify violating a moral rule.

1. What moral rules are being violated?
2. What harms are being avoided, prevented, or caused?
3. What are the relevant desires and beliefs of the person toward whom the rule is being violated?

4. Is the relationship between the person violating the rule and the person toward whom the rule is being violated such that the former has a duty to violate moral rules with regard to the latter independent of the person's consent?

5. What goods (including kind, degree, probability, duration, and distribution) are being promoted by the violation?

6. Is the rule being violated toward a person in order to prevent the person from violating a moral rule when the violation would be unjustified or weakly justified?

7. Is the rule being violated toward a person because he has violated a moral rule unjustifiably or with weak justification?

8. Are there any alternative actions or policies that would be preferable?

9. Is the violation being done intentionally or only knowingly?

10. Is the situation an emergency such that no person is likely to plan to be in that kind of situation?[17]

When considering the harms being avoided, prevented, or caused and the benefits being promoted, one must consider not only the kind of benefit or harm involved but also its seriousness, duration, and probability. If more than one person is affected, one must consider the number of affected people as well as the distribution of harms and benefits. If two violations are the same in all their morally relevant features, they count as the same kind of violation. Anyone who claims to be acting or judging as an impartial, rational person in allowing one violation publicly must hold that the other also be publicly allowed. This follows from the account of impartiality. However, this does not mean that two people, both impartial and rational, who agree that two actions count as the same kind of violation, must always agree on whether or not to advocate that this kind of violation be publicly allowed. Both parties may differ in their estimate of the consequences of allowing this kind of violation publicly, or they may rank the benefits and harms involved differently.

In our case of the physician causing the patient mild, temporary pain, violating the moral rule not to cause pain is justified because: (1) with testing and treatment, the physician can prevent the patient from suffering the evils of death, disability, and severe pain; (2) the patient wants to be treated and has given consent; and (3) the evils of temporary pain are very much less than those probably avoided. Physicians should be willing to defend this position publicly, and, in fact, they do so commonly, in their practices and in formal clinical practice guidelines. Gert has explained why a theoretically coherent and practically trustworthy public ethics requires a combination of utilitarian and deontological features. The deontologist is correct in that a moral system requires rules, and the utilitarian is correct in that a system of morality must have a purpose. The pure deontologist errs in not understanding that all rules have exceptions and therefore require interpretation in light of the goal that the rules achieve. The pure utilitarian errs in not understanding that a public system, available to all rational persons, must have rules to provide guidance. A complete public system of morality must include moral rules for guidance and moral attitudes that interpret and offer the means to justify violations of the rules, it must give them moral direction, and it must explain how and why the rules should be obeyed.[18] Gert recently defended his system against the criticism that it was not useful to resolve moral dilemmas in medicine.[19]

ETHICAL CONCEPTS AND PRINCIPLES

Other moral philosophers have configured their moral systems differently and generally less rigorously. Presently, the most popular system of bioethics in the United States is that developed by Tom Beauchamp and James Childress and taught at the Kennedy Institute of Ethics at Georgetown University. The Beauchamp-Childress system is based on four essential ethical "principles": (1) respect for autonomy, (2) nonmaleficence, (3) beneficence, and (4) justice. In their morality hierarchy, Beauchamp and Childress rank their four ethical principles just below the level of ethical theories but above the level of moral rules.[20]

Because of the intuitive appeal of these "principles," many subsequent writers and commentators in clinical ethics have accepted them as dogma: completely and without criticism. Indeed, the four principles have been recited so frequently in bioethical discourse that they have become known in clinical ethics circles as the "Georgetown mantra." Most impressively, the four principles have become the basis of a large textbook of bioethics in which they have been elevated to axiomatic status with all chapters devoted to their analysis in various ethical, philosophical, legal, and medical contexts.[21]

In several penetrating articles criticizing "principlism," Danner Clouser and Bernard Gert pointed out that these alleged principles of medical ethics are not true principles but rather are category headings of four complex moral subjects that, if considered as principles, would "obscure and confuse moral reasoning by their failure to be guidelines and by their eclectic and unsystematic use of moral theory."[22] Clouser and Gert point out that the four principles do not comprise, in and of themselves, a complete system of morality. Indeed, the principles frequently conflict with each other but contain no process that permits users to analyze and resolve these conflicts, such as in the common situation in which the duty to respect personal autonomy conflicts with the duty to promote beneficence.

Yet, despite their lack of analytical rigor, coherence, and completeness, the intuitive appeal of these principles is undeniable. Their widespread acceptance by clinicians is evidence of their usefulness. They encompass four broad concepts of ethical discourse that are highly relevant clinically, whose elements can be grasped and applied quickly, albeit superficially, by clinicians. They are most useful as easy-to-recall mental reminders of clinically relevant ethical concepts. Because the Beauchamp-Childress ethical principles are obviously useful in clinical practice, I believe that they should be retained as categories but renamed "concepts" to acknowledge that they are titles summarizing complex concepts embodying important moral ideas. But alone, these concepts neither constitute fundamental moral principles nor jointly comprise a coherent and complete framework of morality.

The Concept of Respect for Autonomy

The concept of respect for personal autonomy or self-rule is derived from the moral rules not to deprive of freedom and not to disable. Respect for autonomy implies a respect for persons and for the decisions they make for themselves unconstrained by others.[23] Some authors prefer to talk of "autonomous choices" rather than "autonomous persons," emphasizing that it is only the freedom to choose and the breadth of available choices that permit a person to have self-rule. Other authors emphasize that it is the requirement to obtain the permission of the individual for any act affecting the person that is paramount in a concept of autonomy.[24]

Beauchamp and Childress have outlined the criteria that make an action autonomous: the action is made intentionally, with understanding and without influences that determine it.[25] In the common clinical situation in which patients are asked to give their consent for treatment, for example, the patient cannot make a truly autonomous treatment choice unless he has the capacity to decide, has received adequate information necessary to make his decision, and has not been coerced into this decision.[26]

Respect for patients' autonomy resonates with American tradition. In American law, respect for personal autonomy is embodied in the doctrine of "self-determination." This concept of law arises from the American Constitution and its amendments, which provide inalienable liberty rights for all citizens based on innate human dignity, freedom, and respect for persons. The concept of personal autonomy in the clinical context was epitomized by future U.S. Supreme Court Justice Benjamin Cardozo in a landmark decision in a medical malpractice case in which a surgeon neglected to seek a patient's consent before an elective operation. Justice Cardozo famously wrote, "Every human being of adult years and sound mind has a right to determine what shall be done with his own body."[27]

Daniel Brock explained why autonomy is such an important objective in any system of morality. Autonomy, or self-determination, encompasses a person's interest to make decisions for himself, according to his own concept of what constitutes the good life, and to be free to act on those decisions. Respecting self-determination is important because it permits persons to live in accordance with their concept of the good life within the constraints of justice and with the responsibility to respect the rights of the self-determination of others. When we respect our right of self-determination, we take full responsibility for our lives and our actions, and for respecting the possibility of the same by all others. The major component of human dignity is found in the capacity of persons to direct their lives by self-determination and to respect this capacity in all others.[28]

One of the defining trends of Western medical ethics in the early 21st century is a growing emphasis on respect for patients' autonomy, with a concomitant lessening influence of medical paternalism.[29] Today, more patients are asserting their right to make their own medical decisions and are not accepting their doctor's recommendation unquestionably. The trend to grant primacy to the patient's treatment preferences and values over those of the physician has been called "patient-centered medicine."[30] In the United States, the growing emphasis on respect for personal autonomy parallels the growing authority of the civil rights and human rights movements.[31] Concomitantly, the reduced professional authority of physicians parallels the diminished influence and respect for all authority figures in contemporary society.

Strengthening of respect for autonomy and weakening of paternalism has costs, one of which is that the traditional medical value of promoting the patients' best and most beneficial interests has been put on the defensive.[32] Further, growth of respect for autonomy may diminish the physician's role as medical advisor to the patient's detriment. Making autonomy absolute is undesirable because autonomy is only one of many competing goods in the total sphere of morality.[33] If autonomy alone were paramount, society would disintegrate as

individuals pursued their own personally valid goals and ignored the rights of others. Complete and unbridled autonomy would signal the end of professional beneficence because there would be no way of justifying the special powers that professionals possess, powers that they may use to provide sound counsel and sometimes must use to prevent autonomous persons from making terrible mistakes.[34]

Childress has argued that respect for autonomy is a *prima facie* principle of morality (see my previous disclaimer of "principle"), but one that can be overridden by four conditions: (1) proportionality, that is, when other more binding moral factors take precedence; (2) effectiveness, that is, when there is a high likelihood that another moral consideration would take precedence; (3) last resort, that is, when compromising respect for autonomy is necessary to protect the more important moral factor; and (4) least infringement, that is, when compromising respect for autonomy is the least intrusive or restrictive condition consistent with upholding the competing moral factor.[35] This method of hierarchical analysis is similar to but less systematic than the process embodied in Bernard Gert's account in which it is necessary to rigorously justify violations of moral rules by appealing to an understanding of their impact and purpose.

Several scholars have pointed out other categorical limitations on relying on respect for autonomy as a guiding concept in bioethics. First, the idea that sick patients typically function as autonomous agents is a "hyper-rationalistic" formulation that does not correlate with empirical studies of how ill patients actually make clinical decisions.[36] Studies show that patients often make clinical decisions affecting themselves badly because of the effects of illness, inadequate or poorly communicated information from physicians, misunderstanding, and irrational thinking.[37] Second, patients' values and preferences may be unstable over time leading one to question the existence of a stable autonomous agent.[38] Third, respecting autonomy as the highest ethic is a quintessential American concept whose cultural bias is not universal.[39] Finally, because patients rarely make decisions based only on the impact on themselves, and most often after considering how others, particularly family members, will be affected, some scholars have advocated replacing the individualistic concept of autonomy with a family-centered relational model.[40]

The Concept of Nonmaleficence

The ethical duty of nonmaleficence requires that we not inflict evil or harm on another person. It is a summary of the first five moral rules that proscribe killing, causing pain and disability, and depriving freedom and pleasure. Therefore, nonmaleficence is the one Beauchamp-Childress principle that is closest to a moral rule. Medical-ethical concepts of nonmaleficence originated in antiquity and are embodied in the Latin motto of unknown authorship: *Primum non nocere* (above all, do no harm).[41] From the writings of Hippocrates we also derive the phrase "at least, do no harm."

Nonmaleficence-based ethical duties have both utilitarian and deontological roots. The rule-deontological origin of nonmaleficence is obvious in its derivation from the first five moral rules. From a utilitarian perspective, acts of physicians must be graded by their consequences. It is common for a medical act, such as prescribing a therapy, to have multiple effects, some of which are beneficial and others of which are harmful. Therapies known to exert net effects that are harmful should be avoided because of nonmaleficence-based ethical duties.

Scholars have long studied the moral justification of acts that simultaneously and unavoidably produce both beneficial and harmful effects. In Roman Catholic moral writings, the principle of double effect was proposed to justify the morality of a single act known to have two morally opposite effects, beneficial and harmful, one intended and the other foreseen but unintended. Over the past generation, discussions of the principle of double effect have entered secular medical ethics with some scholars strongly endorsing the principle, especially as it applies to palliative medicine, and others opposing it.[42]

Clinical examples of the principle of double effect are common. Consider the case in which a physician prescribes an appropriate dose of morphine to relieve a dying patient's pain and shortness of breath, but the patient dies sooner than he would have without the morphine because of respiratory depression. (The acceleration of death in this setting occurs only rarely in practice.[43]) The intent of the physician was to relieve the patient's pain and shortness of breath and the choice of drug and the dosage were appropriate for palliative purposes. The acceleration of death was a foreseen but unavoidable and unintended consequence. The physician therefore, has performed an act with a double effect. Is the prevention or palliation of pain and air hunger morally justifiable despite the simultaneous acceleration of the moment of death?

Roman Catholic theologians have generated criteria to morally justify acts that produce double effects: (1) the act must not be intrinsically wrong; (2) the intended effect must be the good effect, even though the bad effect may have been anticipated; (3) the bad effect must not be a means to the end of creating the good effect; (4) the act is undertaken for a proportionately serious reason; and (5) the good result must exceed the evil produced by the bad effect.[44] The physician's act in our example satisfies the principle of double effect because: (1) giving morphine in the dosage administered to relive suffering is not intrinsically wrong; (2) relieving suffering was the desired effect even though the risk of death was foreseen; (3) death was not the means for providing the desired effect; (4) prevention of suffering during dying is an important goal; and (5) prevention of suffering exceeds the evil of dying slightly sooner in a dying patient.

Once the principle of double effect has established that the act is morally acceptable, patient consent is also necessary. The patient or surrogate should be adequately informed that a palliative dosage of morphine possibly may accelerate the moment of death. If she has consented to receiving a palliative dosage of morphine with this knowledge and if the criteria for double effect have been satisfied, the act is morally justified.

The Concept of Beneficence

Beneficence is the moral duty to promote good. Unlike nonmaleficence, a concept that summarizes Gert's first five moral rules, beneficence encompasses the moral ideals. Gert has explained that moral ideals differ from moral rules in that the ideals help *prevent* evils from occurring. Thus, for example, for the moral rule "do not cause pain," the concomitant moral ideal is "prevent pain."[45] Following moral ideals usually demands more of a person than following moral rules and therefore is not required.

Beneficence includes nonmaleficence in some classifications because the first step in the duty to promote good is to avoid causing harm. Beneficence has a hallowed tradition in medicine, at least since the time of Hippocrates. The Hippocratic oath articulates a duty of beneficence by stating: "I will apply measures to benefit the sick according to my ability and judgment; I will keep them from harm and injustice.... In whatever houses I may visit I will come for the benefit of the sick, remaining free of all intentional injustice."[46]

In an influential book, Edmund Pellegrino and David Thomasma argued that the duty of beneficence forms the primary ethical foundation for the relationship between physician and patient. They point out that the goal of the practice of medicine is beneficent because the patient's problems and needs should take precedence over all other considerations in the medical encounter. The physician must avoid harms in order to help the patient, and his respect for the patient's autonomy should be superseded by the concern for what can most help the patient. Clinicians have a special ethical duty in guiding patients to the right treatment choice because patients are inherently vulnerable as the result of illness. To be able to act in this capacity, physicians must have moral integrity and must not abandon the search for the morally right solution in cases of moral ambiguity.[47]

The tension between respecting autonomy and promoting beneficence is a subject of widespread discourse. I agree with Thomasma and Pellegrino that respect for autonomy has been falsely and sometimes harmfully elevated to the highest ethic in contemporary Western medical practice. This over-emphasis on patient autonomy and de-emphasis on physician beneficence is harmful because it can damage the relationship between the patient and the physician. If autonomy were paramount, patients simply would tell physicians what they wanted and physicians would comply like technicians or automatons. Such a relationship ignores the fundamental nature of illness in which patients often are vulnerable and ignorant, and cannot always make rational choices. An attitude of physician beneficence helps provide good and prevent harms to patients.

But over-emphasis on beneficence with de-emphasis on autonomy is not ideal either because it can lead to unjustified paternalistic acts. However, there are certain beneficent physician behaviors that can be justified readily. Physicians can make minor and inconsequential decisions for patients without consent. They can accept the "doctor knows best" mandates when they assess that patients really mean it. They may make recommendations on major decisions and vigorously recommend certain courses of action to patients that clearly will benefit them. They may refuse certain requests from patients because they are medically inappropriate. Further analysis of the topics of consent, refusal, and justified and unjustified paternalism is presented in chapter 2.

In a provocative article, Robert Veatch predicted that the 21st century will see a reduction in physician beneficence because society will increasingly recognize that physicians cannot know what is best for patients. He believes that physicians cannot be experts in deciding which treatment strategy will predictably benefit a patient. Veatch believes that physicians will have a progressively limited authority to determine patient well-being and will be reduced to advisors to "the consumer of health care" to whom they should remain loyal without dictating what course of action is best.[48]

The concept of beneficence also encompasses morally desirable but unrequired forms of human behavior, including supererogatory acts. Supererogatory acts are those acts of goodness that are "above and beyond the call of duty," and thus they represent a moral ideal. However, there is a transitional type of beneficent duty relevant to medical practice that falls just short of a truly supererogatory act. This is the moral duty to rescue.

Consider the case in which a passerby encounters a swimmer drowning in a lake. What is the passerby's moral duty to save the drowning person? One's moral intuition holds that if the passerby can help at all, it would be wrong of him not to attempt to save the swimmer. But at what risk to his personal safety does the passerby continue to have a moral duty to rescue? Clearly, if the rescue can be accomplished with minimal risk to the passerby, the duty to rescue is greater than it is if the attempted rescue may result in death or serious injury to the passerby. In the latter case, attempting a rescue would count as a heroic or supererogatory act.[49]

Beauchamp and Childress provide a cogent analysis of a person's obligation to attempt an act of rescue that I will translate into a medical context. A physician has a beneficence-based obligation to attempt to rescue an imperiled patient if and only if: 1) the patient is at risk to suffer significant loss or damage; 2) the physician's action is needed, singly or in concert with others, to prevent or minimize the loss; 3) the physician is capable, alone or with others, of attempting the necessary action; 4) there is a high probability that individual or group action will be successful; 5) in acting, the physician will not incur significant risks, costs or burdens; and 6) the patient's expected benefits outweigh the possible harms, costs, or burdens that the physician could incur.[50]

A clinical example of the moral duty to attempt rescue is the physician's obligation to encourage organ donations from a brain-dead patient for needy recipients who will die without a transplanted organ. As can he seen clearly, this situation fulfills Beauchamp and Childress' criteria, producing a moral duty to attempt rescue. Thus, clinicians have beneficence-based ethical duties under the rule of rescue to encourage families of their brain-dead patients to donate organs for dying transplantation recipients.[51]

The Concept of Justice

A discussion of the concept of justice in a treatise on bioethical topics at first seems misplaced. However, it has become obvious that the totality of health-care resources within all health-care systems is finite; therefore, it is axiomatic that resources devoted to one person necessarily are not available to others, an entity economists call an "opportunity cost."[52] This reality forces society on a "macro" scale and physicians on a "micro" scale to address issues allocation and rationing of these finite resources. Questions of allocation and rationing ultimately pose ethical issues because decisions of where and how to devote health-care dollars turn largely on the values and objectives of our heath-care system, as well as on the concept of justice. It is with in this context that justice, particularly distributive justice, becomes relevant as a bioethical concept.[53]

Generally speaking, justice refers to society's system for the social distribution of resources and rewards based on concepts of fairness and desert. Justice in the bioethical context (distributive justice) can be defined as the distribution of societal resources such that each person gets an equal share according to one or more of the following criteria: (1) individual need, (2) individual effort, (3) societal contribution, (4) merit or desert, and (5) personal contribution that satisfies whatever is desired by others in free-market exchanges. The fact that these criteria commonly conflict with each other produces ongoing scholarly debates in the philosophy of justice.[54] Justice can be exercised in clinical practice by the development of just clinical protocols, guidelines, and policies.

Philosophical theories of justice have separate roots in utilitarianism, libertarianism, egalitarianism, and other political philosophies.[55] Utilitarians such as John Stuart Mill view justice as simply the application of the principle of utility to the allocation of resources. Society establishes rules to apportion resources in order to provide the greatest good for the greatest number. In general, disadvantaged people fare well under utilitarian theories of justice because society creates rules to confer compensatory benefits on them. Utilitarian rules to redistribute wealth are designed to promote the greatest net utility.

Libertarians, such as Robert Nozick, hold that people are equal in their most fundamental moral rights; but thereafter, the libertarian interests of citizens become unjustifiably compromised when society requires them to sacrifice their personal goods for the benefit of others. In Nozick's libertarian view, people's rights are respected most when they are permitted to keep and control that which they have acquired legitimately without violating the rights of others. Forced redistribution is evil in a libertarian system because it treats the private property of citizens as if it were public property. Libertarians believe that utilitarian or egalitarian rules for social distribution are acceptable only if they are agreed on freely by a group of citizens.[56]

The egalitarian school, led by John Rawls, holds that the quintessence of justice is fairness and impartiality. Society must devise a way of fundamentally respecting the equality of all citizens despite obvious differences of birth, luck, ability, and accomplishment that create powerful inequalities. Although we cannot eliminate inequality we can try to make it fair. The Rawlsian doctrine of fairness requires that society first design rules to assure that all citizens have equal opportunity to succeed, and only on that basis permit substantive inequalities based on differences of birth, luck, abilities, and accomplishments. Conversely, inequalities that develop because of unequal opportunity are unfair. For example, citizens who have advantages only because of better birth, luck, ability, or accomplishment do not deserve them, and citizens who are disadvantaged only because of deficits of the same deserve better. To create justice, society should develop rules to guarantee fair and equal opportunity for all citizens.[57]

ALTERNATIVE ETHICAL THEORIES

In addition to the traditional analytical models of ethical theory, several newer theories have been proposed that stress factors other than rationality. In many ways, these theories are complementary to the more traditional theories rather than substitutes for them because they represent perspectives and viewpoints. They do not claim to be complete, formal systems of morality. Alternative ethical theories include virtue-based ethics, care-based ethics, narrative ethics, and feminist ethics.

Virtue-based ethics dates back to the writings of Plato and Aristotle on the virtues man should cultivate to lead the good life. In the medical context, the argument for virtue-based ethics has been made most persuasively by Edmund Pellegrino and David Thomasma.[58] They argued that the patient-physician relationship is covenantal. They pointed out if all physicians could cultivate and practice ideal virtues and could make medical decisions based on virtuous behavior, there would be no need to propose elaborate systems of ethical theory to govern their actions; patients could simply trust their physicians to do the right thing. The virtues physicians should cultivate include *phronesis* (intuitive sound judgment to make the right decision), compassion, honesty, justice, fortitude, temperance, integrity, trustworthiness, tact, self-awareness, prudence, reverence, courage, humility, and self-effacement.[59] Because medicine is fundamentally a moral enterprise, physicians have a fiduciary duty always to do the right actions for their patients and thus to be virtuous practitioners. A recent survey of patients showed that the ideal physician possesses seven characteristics: she is confident, empathetic, humane, personal, forthright, respectful, and thorough.[60]

Care-based ethics stresses that the fundamental partnership between the patient and caregiver is predicated on a caring relationship. It has roots in nursing and relational ethics, and emphasizes that the relationship between the patient and the caregiver is one of partnership, not one of power inequality causing paternalism.[61] Care-based ethics is a holistic concept, in which medical care is only one dimension of the totality of care for sick persons. It underscores the importance of the patient's family, community, other caregivers, and the patient in insuring the patient's continued health. The emotional feelings that result from the interpersonal relationships generate moral duties of caring. Care-based ethics de-emphasizes patient autonomy and views the impact and meaning of the patient's illness in the context of personal relationships to family and friends. As such it is more of a perspective than a freestanding moral theory.[62]

Narrative ethics focuses on the story of the patient's life and the meaning of the patient's illness in the context of this story. Narrative ethics emphasizes that the patient's interpretation of the meaning of her illness within the context of her life is the best starting point of diagnosis and care.[63] Like care-based ethics, narrative ethics attempts to change the patient-physician interaction from treating an illness to caring for a person, a perspective Arthur Frank calls "illness outside patienthood."[64] Only by understanding the patient's life story and the resultant meanings attached to the illness (thereby achieving "narrative competence"[65]) can a physician hope to provide appropriate and successful care. The meaning of illness is determined personally and culturally. Anne Fadiman best illustrated this phenomenon in her poignant and haunting story of how the failure to understand the personal and cultural narrative of illness in a Hmong immigrant girl led otherwise excellent physicians to treat her unsuccessfully with a tragic outcome.[66] Studying literature can help physicians develop more complex perspectives on moral problems and better understand patients' personal narratives.[67]

Feminist ethics views the relationship between patient and physician from a perspective of societal hierarchies of power and analyzes how inequalities based on gender act to disempower women in particular and all patients in general.[68] Feminist ethics also considers specific issues of systematic, institutionalized discrimination against women such as the way in which male stereotypes of females harm women both as patients and clinicians.[69] The psychoanalytic concept of hysteria and its original application to women exemplifies the negative effect of stereotypes on medical diagnosis and treatment. In some accounts, feminist theory incorporates care-based ethics and nursing ethics because of the intrinsic feminine and nursing emphasis on caring and human relationships. Feminist ethics also considers harms resulting from treating women's bodies as objects. The institutionalized discrimination against women entering the medical profession that was widespread in the United States until the past generation, and

the remaining discrimination against women entering certain specialty training areas, also is a concern of feminist ethics.

RELIGIOUS DOCTRINE AND MEDICAL ETHICS

Organized religions produced the first detailed accounts of morality, with doctrines that include moral rules and attitudes that are intrinsic and essential to the belief systems of each religion and that form the moral basis for the community of believers. Some commentators have argued that religious belief is a prerequisite for any system of ethics because the absolute authoritarianism of religion provides a necessary anchor to stabilize the unavoidable relativistic swaying of secularized ethics.

For example, in an influential book, Tristram Englehardt argued that "a canonical, content-full secular morality cannot be discovered" because people encounter "moral strangers" with whom they do not share moral values and principles. Englehardt cites the intractable disagreement on the morality of abortion or euthanasia to exemplify his concept of moral estrangement and to conclude that rational discourse alone, without a commonality of religious beliefs, never can permit the creation of a universal, secular morality. However, his project to justify a "moral framework by which individuals who belong to diverse moral communities, who do not share a content-full moral vision, can still regard themselves bound by a common moral fabric and can appeal to a common bioethics" is similar in intent to Gert's project to make explicit the intuitions of our common morality.[70]

The universality of secular morality was emphasized by Kant and more recently and clearly in the work of Gert. These philosophers appealed to rationality as the basis of the universality of morality and asserted that the moral system applies equally and impartially to all rational persons. I concur with Gert that a secular morality such as he has explicated has the capacity to comprise a universal code of human conduct acceptable to all rational, impartial persons without first requiring them to adhere to any particular religious moral doctrine.

Danner Clouser outlined three criteria that separate religion from ethics.[71] First, ethics must have universal appeal to all rational persons. Each rational person wishes that everyone would agree to obey a set of moral rules, the adherence to which furthers the welfare of all members of society. Religion, by contrast, never can be acceptable to all because its theological doctrines, belief systems, and practices attract only certain populations and must lack universal appeal. Second, requirements of religious ethics are both too strong and too weak to do the work of secular ethics. For example, some religious ethics demand supererogatory acts of individuals not necessitated by secular ethics, and some permit prejudice against groups that secular ethics does not allow. Both supererogatory requirements and unjust discriminations limit the extent to which all persons could be reasonably expected to subscribe to religious ethics. Finally, although the punishment and rewards systems of organized religions effectively elicit motivation from some believers to act morally, these systems of motivation are not indispensable components of a universal secular code of ethics.

Nevertheless, religions have made seminal contributions to morality, and their religious beliefs and motives remain a real and important part of the moral intuitions of most people. Particularly at the end of their lives, patients' religious beliefs may be awakened or intensified.[72] Religious patients who believe in eternal life may approach medical decisions differently from humanist patients who do not.[73] Physicians need to understand the basic elements of religious doctrines, at least insofar as they apply to consenting to or refusing life-sustaining therapies.[74] In some cases, patients will incorrectly cite their religious doctrinal requirements as grounds for certain clinical decisions that conflict with the clinician's judgment.[75] Clinicians can consider requesting expert assistance from relevant clergy to clarify religious requirements in such cases.

The following is a brief and necessarily oversimplified summary in historical order of some moral doctrines relevant to medical ethics that arise from the ancient, rich traditions of Judaism, Christianity, Islam, Hinduism, and Buddhism. Interested readers can refer to the end notes as cited for more detailed discussions of how the moral insights embedded in these religious teachings can be applied to specific contemporary bioethical problems.[76]

Judaism

Judaism has been epitomized as "ethical monotheism." Its law is derived from the Torah, the first five books of the Hebrew scriptures known in Christianity as the Old Testament. The Torah contains a wealth of ethical rules in addition to the Ten Commandments in Exodus for living a good Jewish life. Additionally, rabbinic scholars over three millennia have produced many volumes of commentary on the Torah, the most important of which is the Talmud. These learned commentaries expand on the laws and pronouncements of the Torah by explaining how they should be applied to specific examples in life. The scripture of the Torah, along with Talmudic and other commentaries, have been encoded into the Halachah, the ancient code of Jewish common law and ethics.

Louis Newman identified five essential principles of Jewish bioethics.[77] Human life is sacred and possesses intrinsic and infinite value. Preservation of life is the highest moral imperative. All lives are equal. All lives are really not our own. The sacredness of human life inheres within the human being as a whole, both body and soul.

Elliot Dorff recently summarized the Jewish perspective on end-of-life care.[78] He pointed out that because the human body belongs to God, Jews have a duty to seek preventive and curative treatment, and generally to follow their physicians' treatment recommendations. The rabbi has a greater role for advising Orthodox and Conservative Jews than among Reform believers, because of Reform's emphasis on individual autonomy. Suicide and assisted suicide are prohibited but physicians should not prolong the dying process. Once patients are terminally ill, they and their physicians are permitted to withdraw and withhold therapies if doing so is in the patient's interest, although there remains a debate about artificial hydration and nutrition. Palliative care is desirable but the principle of double effect is debatable.

Much of the commentary on Jewish ethical duties emphasizes the essential concepts of respect for life and health, nonmaleficence, beneficence, performing *mitzvot* (commandments), and *tzedakah*, a unique concept of justice in which the more fortunate have a moral duty to help the less fortunate. There is a wealth of contemporary writings on Jewish bioethics that apply Halakhic laws to current bioethical controversies.[79]

Christianity

Christians use the Hebrew scripture as the first half of their bible because Christianity initially was derived from Judaism. The latter half of the Christian Bible is the New Testament, which concerns the life, teachings, death, resurrection, and divinity of Jesus Christ. Christian ethics, therefore, is a product of both Hebrew and Christian scriptural sources. Like Jews, Christians respect the sacred nature of the Ten Commandments, accept the same biblically given duties of nonmaleficence, and believe in the sacredness, preservation, and transcendent value of life. Christians have imposed additional duties of beneficence and virtue from the New Testament recordings of the teachings of Jesus. The practice of casuistry (discussed in chapter 6) originated in early Christian moral writings. The covenantal relationship between God and humankind, introduced in the Old Testament, is presently an important area of emphasis in Protestant Christian ethics.[80]

Tristram Englehardt and Ana Smith Iltis recently pointed out that understanding Christian teachings about end-of-life decisions is complicated by three factors: (1) the dominance of Christian culture in Western civilization has greatly influenced secular culture and public policy making it difficult to separate Christianity's secularized cultural influence from its spiritual commitments; (3) Christianity encompasses a large cluster of diverse religious groups ranging from Unitarians to Seventh-Day Adventists, Mormons, Lutherans, Anglicans, Roman Catholics, and Orthodox Christians, whose reliance on traditional Christian beliefs ranges from strict to loose, making it difficult to find uniformly shared beliefs in specific bioethical areas; (3) many Christian communities are in disarray about particular areas of moral theology.[81] Although there are areas of commonality, it is desirable for physicians to understand the specific teachings of individual Christian religious groups and the extent to which patients are strict believers.

Of the branches of Christianity, Roman Catholicism has the most unified and distinctly explicated tradition of medical ethics. Papal encyclicals over several centuries have distilled the mass of Catholic thought, incorporating the writings of St. Augustine and Thomas Aquinas, among others, into clearly articulated principles and proscriptions. Catholic doctrine prohibits abortion, unnatural forms of contraception, euthanasia, and suicide because these acts cause death or interfere with the generation of life. Catholic writings on morality have pioneered the principle of double effect, the concepts of proportionality, and the dialectic of extraordinary versus ordinary medical care.[82]

Hazel Markwell recently summarized Catholic perspectives on end-of-life care.[83] Life is a sacred gift from God and has intrinsic worth and dignity. Bodily life is not an absolute good to be preserved at all costs. God participates in the human condition. Attempts must be made to alleviate sickness and suffering, although these experiences can have a positive meaning. The values of human dignity and interconnectedness of all people ground all other values. We are accountable to God for our lives. The value of the common good calls us to promote a just social order. Charity demands us to respond to others in need, particularly the poor. Covenant best describes the ideal relationship between physician and patient. Medicine is a sacrament.[84]

Islam

Islam, the third and youngest principal monotheistic religion, regards Judaism and Christianity as its progenitors; Islamic believers consider their religion to be the final step in the evolution of monotheistic religions; therefore, they retain a special place for Jews and Christians as "people of the book." Islam honors Abraham, Moses, and Jesus as prophets but denies the divinity of Jesus. In addition to their respect for the Jewish and Christian bibles, they revere the Qur'an as the Book of Islam. The Qur'an is sacred because it represents the direct words of God (*Allah*) as conveyed to the Prophet Mohammed by the angel Gabriel. The Qur'an and Mohammed's exemplary life are the foundations of Islamic religious life to which Moslems must submit. (*Islam* means submission.) A large body of commentary supplements the text of the Qur'an. Much of the Qur'an and its Qur'anic commentary convey Islamic moral duties.

There are five pillars of Islamic faith and religious practice: the declaration of faith in God (*shadadah*) and the mission of the Prophet Mohammed; undertaking of canonical worship (*salat*) and fasting (*saum*) during the month of Ramadan; supporting the underprivileged through charity (*zakat*); and completion of the pilgrimage to Mecca (*hajj*) at least once in one's lifetime, money and health permitting.[85]

Islam has a sacred code of laws and ethics known as the *Shari'ia*.[86] The Shari'ia provides for the indispensable needs of the people, which include the preservation of self, mind, religion, ownership, and honor, as well as for the ordinary and complementary needs of the people. In general, separation of church and state is not a characteristic of Islamic belief. The Shari'ia permits justified exceptions to its rules of nonmaleficence, adopts a utilitarian perspective on choosing the lesser of two harms, and considers the law of Allah to follow that which is in the best interest of the nation.

In end-of-life care, physicians are expected to do everything possible to prevent premature death because life is a divine trust and a sacred gift from Allah. Active euthanasia and assisted suicide are forbidden but palliative care and withholding or withholding life support to treat intractable suffering may be permitted if the intent is not to have the patient die. Based on sources in the Qur'an. Shari'ia, and their commentaries, the Islamic Code of Medical Ethics was published in 1981.[87] The Islamic Juridical Council as an organ of the Organization of Islamic Conferences formulates responses to bioethical dilemmas and publishes rulings in their quarterly journal *Majallah Majma'al-Fiqh al-l-Islami*.[88]

Hinduism

Hindus refer to their religion as *sanatanad-harma*, the eternal religion or law. Hindus are born into one of four castes or *varnas*. Each *varna* has its own social and ethical code of virtuous behavior and morality (*dharma*). Each dharma has a unique *karma*, in which all acts, moral and immoral, have consequences in the next life. Thus, good *karma* yields good rebirth and bad *karma* bad rebirth. Suffering now may be the result of bad *karma* in a previous life. There are four stages of life, the *ashrama*. There are several gods of Hinduism. Many Hindus are devoted to Krishna and believe that a virtuous life is rewarded with heaven and escape from the cycle of birth and death (*samsara*).[89]

Hindu beliefs about end-of life care are complicated because they depend on education, class, and religious condition. Most Hindus believe that good deaths occur in old age, at the right astrological time, and in the right place (at home or on the banks of the sacred Ganges River). Bad deaths are violent, premature, uncontrolled, and occur at the wrong time in the wrong place. In general, Hindu beliefs include reincarnation, *karma* is the meaning of suffering, a family has a sacred duty to assist the dying patient to reach the next life after a good death, there may be tension between allowing a person to know she is dying to prepare for death and the family's desire to protect the patient, suicide is banned but voluntary euthanasia may be permitted on strict religious grounds, and withdrawing and withholding of treatment sometimes can be justified to prevent extreme suffering.[90]

Buddhism

Buddhism, a major Eastern religion, is based in the life and teaching of the Buddha (The Enlightened One). The Buddha taught that the self or soul does not exist, that humans are caught in the cycle of births and deaths and that position and well being in this life are the result of behavior in previous lives, that the body is impermanent, and subject to misery resulting from seeking pleasure and an attachment to worldly things. The path to reach peace and happiness (*nirvana*) is by breaking the attachment to pleasure and worldly things and by following the "Middle Way" in life, avoiding a preoccupation with both satisfying human desires and extremes of self-denial. The noble Eightfold Path to *nirvana* includes knowing truth, resisting evil, not hurting others, respecting life, morality, and property, working that does not harm others, freeing one's mind from evil thoughts, controlling one's thoughts and feelings, and practicing concentration and meditation.[91]

Buddhist end-of-life values derive from no central authority but rather from individuals applying Buddhist teaching to medical situations. In general, Buddhist teaching imposes no special requirements on the patient-physician relationship or on the dying patient, other than that the dying patient have a clear mind, if possible, to permit meditation and reflection and to lead to a better rebirth. Palliative and hospice care are particularly compatible with Buddhist teaching because of the high value placed by the Buddha on compassion. There is not a moral imperative to preserve life at all costs but euthanasia is prohibited. Patients who are obviously dying are not required to maintain life-sustaining therapy.[92]

NOTES

1. Loretta Kopelman explained the value to physicians of learning philosophy and developing philosophical skills. See Kopelman LM. Philosophy and medical education. *Acad Med* 1995;70:795–805.

2. Gert B. *Morality: Its Nature and Justification,* revised edition. New York: Oxford University Press, 2005:14. In his current revision, Bernard Gert has provided a rigorous and complete account of morality with refinements to his earlier account in response to critics. For those interested in reading his shorter, more accessible account that contains a helpful glossary of terms and a morality flow chart, see Gert B. *Common Morality: Deciding What to Do.* New York: Oxford University Press, 2004.

3. Pfaff DW, ed. *Ethical Questions in Brain and Behavior.* New York: Springer-Verlag, 1983:1.

4. Beauchamp TL, Childress JF. *Principles of Biomedical Ethics.* 4th ed. New York: Oxford University Press, 1994:4–5.

5. Religious believers, atheists, and agnostic "secular humanists" can share this position.

6. Jonsen AR, Siegler M, Winslade WJ. *Clinical Ethics.* 2nd ed. New York: Macmillan, 1986:3.

7. Bernat JL, Taylor RM. Ethical issues in neurology. In Joynt RJ, Griggs RC, eds. *Baker's Clinical Neurology.* Philadelphia: Lippincott Williams & Wilkins, 2000:2.

8. See Carrick P. *Medical Ethics in Antiquity.* Dordrecht, Netherlands: D Reidel Publishing Co, 1985.

9. The following discussion of utilitarianism and deontology was abstracted from Beauchamp TL, Childress JF. *Principles of Biomedical Ethics,* 1994:44–62: and from Hunt R. Arras J, eds. *Ethical Issues in Modern Medicine.* Palo Alto, CA: Mayfield Publishing Co, 1977:12–38. See these sources for a more detailed discussion of and references on utilitarianism and deontology.

10. Mill JS. *Utilitarianism.* New York: Liberal Arts Press, 1957:10.

11. Kant I. *Groundwork of the Metaphysics of Morals.* New York: Harper & Row, 1964:70.

12. See, for example, McIntyre A. *After Virue,* 2nd ed. Notre Dame, IN: University of Notre Dame Press, 1984; Baier K. *The Moral Point of View.* Ithaca, NY: Cornell University Press, 1958; and Sidgwick H. *The Methods of Ethics,* 7th ed. Indianapolis: Hackett Publishing Co, 1981.

13. Gert B. *Morality: Its Nature and Justification,* revised edition. New York: Oxford University Press, 2005:11.

14. Gert B. *Morality: Its Nature and Justification,* revised edition, 2005:159–186.

15. Gert B. *Morality: Its Nature and Justification,* revised edition, 2005:187–219.

16. Gert B. *Morality: Its Nature and Justification,* revised edition, 2005:222–223.

17. Gert B. *Morality: Its Nature and Justification,* revised edition, 2005:226–236.

18. Gert B. *Morality: A New Justification of the Moral Rules,* 1988:159.

19. Carson Strong recently criticized Bernard Gert's account of morality as clinically not useful in Strong C. Gert's moral theory and its application to bioethics cases. *Kennedy Inst Ethics J* 2006;16: 39–58. Gert responded by pointing out Strong's misunderstanding in Gert B. Making the morally relevant features explicit: a response to Carson Strong. *Kennedy Inst Ethics J* 2006;16:59–71.

20. Beauchamp TL, Childress JF. *Principles of Biomedical Ethics*, 5th ed. New York: Oxford University Press, 2001.

21. Gillon R, ed. *Principles of Health Care Ethics*. Chichester: John Wiley & Sons, 1994.

22. Clouser KD, Gert B. A critique of principlism. *J Med Philosophy* 1990; 15:219–236. For a useful historical perspective on the rise and fall of principlism in medical ethics, see Pellegrino ED. The metamorphosis of medical ethics: A 30-year retrospective. *JAMA* 1993;269:1158–1162. For the most recent dialogue in the ongoing philosophical debate about principlism, see Green RM, Gert B, Clouser DK. The method of public morality versus the method of principlism. *J Med Philosophy* 1993;18:477–489; Lustig BA. Perseverations on a critical theme. *J Med Philosophy* 1993;18:491–502; and Gert B, Culver CM, Clouser KD. *Bioethics: A Systematic Approach*, 2nd edition. New York: Oxford University Press, 2006: 99–127.

23. Gauthier CC. Philosophical foundations of respect for autonomy. *Kennedy Inst Ethics J* 1993;3:21–37.

24. Engelhardt HT Jr. *The Foundations of Bioethics*, 2nd ed. New York: Oxford University Press, 1996.

25. Beauchamp TL, Childress JF. *Principles of Biomedical Ethics*, 2001:120–124.

26. Childress JF. The place of autonomy in bioethics. *Hastings Cent Rep* 1990;20(1):12–17. These three criteria are the same as the Culver-Gert criteria for valid consent, which are discussed further in chapter 2. See also Yeide H Jr. The many faces of autonomy. *J Clin Ethics* 1992;3:269–274.

27. *Schloendorff v Society of New York Hospital*, 211 NY 125, 129–130; 105 NE 92, 92 (1914). See the interesting recent historical analysis of this famous case in Lombardo PA. Phantom tumors and hysterical women: revising our view of the Schloendorff case. *J Law Med Ethics* 2005;33:791–801.

28. Brock DW. Voluntary active euthanasia. *Hastings Cent Rep* 1992;22(2):10–22.

29. See Veatch RM. *A Theory of Medical Ethics*. New York: Basic Books, 1981 and Veatch RM. Autonomy's temporary triumph. *Hastings Cent Rep* 1984;14(5):38–40. Paternalism is defined and discussed further in chapter 2.

30. Laine C, Davidoff F. Patient-centered medicine: a professional evolution. *JAMA* 1996;275:152–156.

31. See, for example, Annas GJ. Human rights and health—The Universal Declaration of Human Rights at 50. *N Engl J Med* 1998;339:1778–1782; General Assembly of the United Nations. Universal Declaration of Human Rights. *JAMA* 1998;280:469–470; and Thomasma DC. Bioethics and international human rights. *J Law Med Ethics* 1997;25:295–306.

32. See Clements CD, Sider RC. Medical ethics' assault upon medical values. *JAMA* 1983;250:2011–2015. This issue is considered also in Engelhardt HT Jr. *The Foundations of Bioethics*. New York: Oxford University Press, 1986:66–68, 82–84.

33. See the discussion of this point in the symposium: Can the moral commons survive autonomy? *Hastings Cent Rep* 1996;26(6):41–47.

34. See Callahan D. Autonomy: A moral good, not a moral obsession. *Hastings Cent Rep* 1984; 14(5):40–42; Morison RS. The biological limits on autonomy. *Hastings Cent Rep* 1984;14(5):43–49; and Pellegrino ED, Thomasma DC. *For the Patient's Good. The Restoration of Beneficence in Health Care*. New York: Oxford University Press, 1988:11–36. For a theoretical discussion of autonomy and its moral and political limitations, see Dworkin G. *The Theory and Practice of Autonomy*. Cambridge: Cambridge University Press, 1988.

35. Childress JF. *Hastings Cent Rep* 1990:15.

36. Schneider CE. *The Practice of Autonomy* and the practice of bioethics. *J Clin Ethics* 2002;13:72–77.

37. Schneider CE. *The Practice of Autonomy: Patients, Doctors and Medical Decisions*. New York: Oxford University Press, 1998. Also see several critical commentaries on Schneider's conclusions in *J Clin Ethics* 2002;13:57–71.

38. Kohut N, Sam M, O'Rourke K, MacFadden DK, Salit I, Singer PA. Stability of treatment preferences: although most preferences do not change, most people change some of their preferences. *J Clin Ethics* 1997;8:124–135.

39. Glick SM. Unlimited human autonomy—a cultural bias. *N Engl J Med* 1997;336: 954–956.

40. Breslin JM. Autonomy and the role of the family in making medical decisions at the end of life. *J Clin Ethics* 2005;16:11–19.

41. See the discussion of the good and bad points of this ancient motto in Brewin T. Primum non nocere? *Lancet* 1994;344:1487–1488. The "Tavistock group" effort to develop "ethical principles for everybody in health care" cited the principle "do no harm" as one of seven principles. The others were: (1) people have a right to health care; (2) care of individual patients is central, but the health of populations is also our concern; (3) in addition to treating illness, we have an obligation to ease suffering, minimize disability, prevent disease, and promote health; (4) health care succeeds only if we cooperate with those we serve, each other,

and those in other sectors; (5) improving health care is a serious and continuing responsibility; and (6) being open, honest, and trustworthy is vital in health care. See Smith R, Hiatt H, Berwick D. A shared statement of ethical principles for those who shape and give health care: a working draft from the Tavistock group. *Ann Intern Med* 1999;130:143–147 and Davidoff F. Changing the subject: ethical principles for everyone in health care. *Ann Intern Med* 2000;133:386–389.

42. Several scholars have written arguments attacking the validity of the principle of double effect. For example, see Quill TE, Dresser R, Brock DW. The rule of double effect—a critique of its role in end-of-life decision making. *N Engl J Med* 1997;337:1768–1771; and Nuccetelli S, Seay G. Relieving pain and foreseeing death: a paradox about accountability and blame. *J Law Med Ethics* 2000;28:19–25. Other scholars have defended the principle contending that the detractors do not understand it. See Sulmasy DP, Pellegrino ED. The rule of double effect: clearing up the double talk. *Arch Intern Med* 1999;159:545–550; and Sulmasy DP. Commentary: double effect—intention is the solution, not the problem. *J Law Med Ethics* 2000;28:26–29.

43. A large study found no correlation between opioid dosage and survival in hospice patients. See Portenoy RK, Sibirceva U, Smout R, et al. Opioid use and survival at the end of life: a survey of a hospice population. *J Pain Symptom Manage* 2006;32:532–540. A recent study showed no respiratory suppression in cancer patients receiving parenteral opioid therapy. See Estfan B, Mahmoud F, Shaheen P, et al. Respiratory function during parenteral opioid titration for cancer pain. *Palliative Med* 2007;21:81–86.

44. For a balanced and well-referenced discussion of the principle of double effect, see Beauchamp TL, Childress JF. Principles of Biomedical Ethics, 1989:127–134. See, also, Griese ON. The principle of double effect. In, *Catholic Identity in Health Care: Principles and Practice*. Braintree, MA: The Pope John Center, 1987:246–299.

45. Gert B. *Morality: A New Justification of the Moral Rules*, 1988:160–162.

46. Edelstein L. Hippocratic oath. In Temkin O, Temkin CL, eds. *Ancient Medicine: Selected Papers of Ludwig Edelstein*. Baltimore: Johns Hopkins University Press, 1967.

47. Pellegrino ED, Thomasma DC. *For the Patient's Good. The Restoration of Beneficence in Health Care*. New York: Oxford University Press, 1988:25–36.

48. Veatch RM. Doctor does not know best: why in the new century physicians must stop trying to benefit patients. *J Med Philosophy* 2000;25:701–721.

49. This example is from Beauchamp TL, Childress JE. *Principles of Biomedical Ethics*, 1989:200–201.

50. Beauchamp TL, Childress JF. *Principles of Biomedical Ethics*, 1989:201. See a similar example and discussion in Gert B. *Morality: A New Justification of the Moral Rules*, 1988:155.

51. The ethics of organ donation is considered further in chapter 11.

52. Palmer S, Raftery J. Economic notes: opportunity cost. *BMJ* 1999;318:1551–1552.

53. The ethics of health-care rationing and its place in the determination of medical futility are considered further in chapter 10.

54. This definition was culled from Outka G. Social justice and equal access to health care. *J Religious Ethics*. 1974;2:11–32; and Beauchamp TL, Childress JF. *Principles of Biomedical Ethics*. 1989:261. The following three paragraphs were abstracted from Beauchamp TL, Childress JF. *Principles of Biomedical Ethics*, 1989:265–270.

55. For general readings on theories of justice, see Solomon RC, Murphy MC. *What is Justice? Classic and Contemporary Readings*. New York: Oxford University Press, 1990. For a debate of theories of justice in the bioethics context, see the symposium: Is justice enough? Ends and means in bioethics. *Hastings Cent Rep* 1996;26(6):9–37.

56. See Nozick R. *Anarchy, State, and Utopia*. New York: Basic Books, 1974 and Nozick R. *Philosophical Explanations*. Cambridge, Mass: Belknap Press, 1981.

57. See Rawls J. *A Theory of Justice*. Cambridge, MA: Harvard University Press, 1971.

58. Pellegrino ED, Thomasma DC. *The Virtues in Medical Practice*. New York: Oxford University Press, 1993 and Pellegrino ED. Toward a virtue-based, normative ethics for the health professions. *Kennedy Inst Ethics J* 1995;5:253–277.

59. These ideal virtues are discussed in Pellegrino ED, Thomasma DC. *The Virtues in Medical Practice* and in Walker FO. Cultivating simple virtues in medicine. *Neurology* 2005;65:1678–1680.

60. Bendapudi NM, Berry LL, Frey KA, Parish JT, Rayburn WL. Patients' perspectives on ideal physician behaviors. *Mayo Clin Proc* 2006;81:338–344.

61. Wilson-Barnett J. The nurse-patient relationship. In, Gillon R (ed). *Principles of Health Care Ethics*. Chichester: John Wiley & Sons, 1994:367–376.

62. Carse AL, Nelson HL. Rehabilitating care. *Kennedy Inst Ethics J* 1995;5:253–277.

63. For examples of narrative ethics, see Kleinman A. *The Illness Narratives: Suffering, Healing & the Human Condition*. New York: Basic Books, 1988; Hunter KM. Narrative, literature, and the clinical exercise of practical reason. *J Med Philosophy* 1996;21:303–320; Charon R. Narrative medicine: form, function, and ethics. *Ann Intern Med* 2001;134:83–87; and Charon R. *Narrative Medicine: Honoring the Stories of Illness*. New York: Oxford University Press, 2006.

64. Frank AW. *The Wounded Storyteller: Body, Illness, and Ethics*. Chicago: University of Chicago Press, 1995.

65. The concept of narrative competence is discussed in Charon R. Narrative medicine: a model for empathy, reflection, profession, and trust. *JAMA* 2001;286:1897–1902.

66. Fadiman A. *The Spirit Catches You and You Fall Down: A Hmong Child, Her American Doctors, and the Collision of Two Cultures*. New York: Farrar, Straus and Giroux, 1997.

67. Montgomery K. Literature, literary studies, and medical ethics: the interdisciplinary question. *Hastings Cent Rep* 2001;31(3):36–43.

68. For example, see Sherwin S. *No Longer Patient: Feminist Ethics and Health Care*. Philadelphia: Temple University Press, 1992; the symposium in several issues of the *Journal of Clinical Ethics* summarized in Tong R. An introduction to feminist approaches to bioethics. *J Clin Ethics* 1996;7:13–19; and the special issue Feminist Perspectives on Bioethics. *Kennedy Inst Ethics J* 1996;6:1–103.

69. Howe EG. Implementing feminist perspectives in clinical care. *J Clin Ethics* 1996;7:2–12.

70. Engelhardt HT Jr. *The Foundations of Bioethics*, 2nd ed, 1996:ix, 8, 32–101.

71. Clouser KD. Some things medical ethics is not. *JAMA* 1973;223:787–789.

72. Lo B, Ruston D, Kates LW, et al. Discussing religious and spiritual issues at the end of life: a practical guide for physicians. *JAMA* 2002;287:749–754.

73. Baggini J, Pym M. End-of-life: the humanist view. *Lancet* 2006;366:1235–1237.

74. Orr RD, Genesen LB. Requests for "inappropriate" treatment based on religious beliefs. *J Med Ethics* 1997;23:142–147.

75. Brett AS, Jersild P. "Inappropriate" treatment near the end of life: conflict between religious convictions and clinical judgment. *Arch Intern Med* 2003;163:1645–1649.

76. For general discussions of the interface of religion and bioethics, see Lammers SE, Verhey A, eds. On Moral Medicine. *Theological Perspectives in Medical Ethics*. Grand Rapids, Mich: William B. Eerdmans Publishing Co, 1987; Pellegrino E, Mazzarella P, Corsi P, eds. *Transcultural Dimensions in Medical Ethics*. Frederick, Md: University Publishing Group, 1992; Cahill LS, ed. Theology and bioethics. *J Med Philosophy* 1992;17:263–364; and Shelp EE, ed. *Theology and Bioethics*. New York: D Reidel Publishing Co, 1985.

77. Newman LE. Jewish theology and bioethics. *J Med Philosophy* 1992;17:309–327.

78. Dorff EN. End-of-life: Jewish perspectives. *Lancet* 2006;366:862–865.

79. For sources on Jewish bioethics, see Rosner F, Bleich JD, eds. *Jewish Bioethics*. New York: Sanhedrin Press; 1979; Tendler MD, ed. *Medical Ethics: A Compendium of Jewish Moral, Ethical and Religious Principles in Medical Practice*. 5th ed. New York: Federation of Jewish Philanthropies, 1975; Novak D. Judaism and contemporary bioethics. *J Med Philosophy* 1979;4:347–366; and Rosner F. *Modern Medicine and Jewish Ethics*. New York: Ktav and Yeshiva University; 1986. Jewish physician-scholars also have contributed specific analyses of contemporary clinical-ethical dilemmas using Jewish law. For example, see Freedman B. Respectful service and reverent obedience. A Jewish view on making decisions for incompetent patients. *Hastings Cent Rep* 1996;26(4):31–37 and Rosner F. Jewish medical ethics. *J Clin Ethics* 1995;6:202–217.

80. For sources on Protestant Christian bioethics, see Bouma H III, Diekema D, Langerak E, et al. *Christian Faith, Health, and Medical Practice*. Grand Rapids, MI: William B. Eerdmans Publishing Co, 1989; Gustafson JM. *Ethics and Theology. Vol 2. Ethics from a Theocentric Perspective*. Chicago: University of Chicago Press, 1984; Hauerwas S. *A Community of Character: Toward a Constructive Christian Social Ethic*. South Bend, IN: University of Notre Dame Press, 1981; and Marty ME, Vaux KL, eds. *Health/Medicine and the Faith Traditions*. Philadelphia: Fortress Press, 1982.

81. Engelhardt HT Jr, Iltis AS. End-of-life: the traditional Christian view. *Lancet* 2006;366:1045–1049.

82. For sources on Catholic bioethics, see McCormick RA. *Health and Medicine in the Roman Catholic Tradition: Tradition in Transition*. New York: Crossroad, 1984; Pellegrino ED, Langan JP, Harvey JC. eds. *Catholic Prespectives on Medical Morals: Foundational Issues*. Boston: Kluwer Academic Publishers, 1989; Kelly MJ, ed. *Justice and Health Care*. St. Louis: Catholic Health Association of the US, 1985; and Griese ON. *Catholic Identity in Health Care: Principles and Practice*. Braintree, MA: Pope John Center, 1987. Christian scholars have written analyses of contemporary medical-ethical dilemmas from the perspective of Christian ethics. See, for example, Connors RB Jr, Smith ML. Religious insistence on medical treatment: Christian theology and re-imagination. *Hastings Cent Rep* 1996;26(4):23–30.

83. Markwell H. End-of-life: a Catholic view. *Lancet* 2006;366:1132–1135.

84. Markwell H. *Lancet* 2006:1135. I edited Markwell's summary. See also the complementary article addressing Catholic teaching on prolonging life: Panicola M. Catholic teaching on prolonging life: setting the record straight. *Hastings Cent Rep* 2001;31(6):14–25.

85. Sachedina A. End-of-life: the Islamic view. *Lancet* 2006;366:774–779.

86. This section has been abstracted from Hathrout H. Islamic basis for biomedical ethics. In Pellegrino E, Mazzarella P, Corsi P, eds. *Transcultural Dimensions in Medical Ethics.* Frederick, MD: University Publishing Group, 1992:57–72.

87. International Organization of Islamic Medicine. *Islamic Code of Medical Ethics-Kuwait Document.* Al Kuwait, Kuwait: International Organization of Islamic Medicine, 1981.

88. Sachedina A. *Lancet* 2006:775.

89. Firth S. End-of-life: a Hindu view. *Lancet* 2006;366:682–686. See also Flood G. *An Introduction to Hinduism.* Cambridge: Cambridge University Press, 1996.

90. Firth S. *Lancet* 2006:682–683.

91. Tucci G. Buddhism. In *Encyclopedia Britannica,* 15th ed. Chicago: University of Chicago, 1982:Macropedia, vol 3:374–403. See also Hughes JJ, Keown D. Buddhism and medical ethics: a bibliographic introduction. http://www.changesurfer.com/Bud/BudBioEth.html (Accessed June 12, 2007).

92. Keown D. End-of-life: the Buddhist view. *Lancet* 2006;336:952–955. See also Keown D. *Buddhism & Bioethics.* London: Palgrave, 2001.

Ethical Practice

2

The rules resulting from moral theory must be translated into practical concepts to be directly applicable at the bedside and in the clinic. This chapter introduces the concepts of ethical medical practice that form the moral foundation of the patient-physician relationship. These concepts are valid consent, competence, rationality, shared decision making, justified paternalism, and truth telling. Throughout this chapter, I use the erudite analyses of these concepts developed by Bernard Gert, Charles M. Culver, and K. Danner Clouser.[1] Understanding and using these concepts permit physicians to incorporate moral theory in their daily patient care.

VALID (INFORMED) CONSENT

Obtaining a patient's valid consent for any course of diagnosis or therapy forms the cornerstone of ethical medical practice. The requirement to obtain valid consent arises from the concepts of respect for patient self-determination and personal autonomy. The moral rule that prohibits one person from depriving another of freedom requires that physicians obtain patients' valid consent. Ordinarily, no one, including a clinician, has the right to touch a person's body without first obtaining that person's freely given consent. We acknowledge respect for autonomy by obtaining valid consent before we treat patients. The older and more commonly used term "informed consent" is inadequate in ethical practice because it implies incorrectly that

merely providing information to the patient is sufficient to validate the consent process.[2] Nevertheless, because of its acceptance in medical and legal circles, "informed consent" enjoys widespread popularity. I use "informed consent" synonymously with "valid consent" but only with the understanding that the consent has been obtained validly as discussed below.

Informed consent developed as a legal doctrine before it was explicitly articulated as an ethical doctrine. In American law, the ruling in *Schloendorff v. Society of New York Hospital* (1914), discussed in chapter 1, clarified that the patient's voluntary consent was legally required for elective surgery. In *Canterbury v. Spence* (1972), a federal appeals court clarified that a surgeon's legal duty was not simply to obtain the patient's voluntary consent for elective surgery but added the stipulation that the consent had to be *informed* by the surgeon's disclosing the "material risks" of treatment. The consent became legally valid only once the patient was aware of the material risks of treatment. Material facts were defined as the body of information patients needed to make a medical decision.[3]

Some physicians and surgeons have misinterpreted their duty to obtain valid consent as simply a cumbersome legal requirement to secure a patient's signature on a consent form. They may resent spending the time necessary to accomplish this task and fail to appreciate the extent to which they need to educate patients in order to satisfy the ethical requirements of valid consent. Despite our generally heightened awareness of consent issues, several studies have shown that the majority of clinicians have not integrated ethically adequate consent behaviors into their daily medical practices.[4] While there are differences in the legal and ethical requirements for valid consent,[5] and there remain unfortunately widespread legal myths about informed consent,[6] it is the more stringent ethical requirements that I discuss in this section.

Consent has three essential elements that must be satisfied to become ethically valid: 1) physicians must convey adequate information to the patient; 2) the patient's consent must be obtained freely and without coercion by individuals or agencies; and 3) the patient must be competent to consent or refuse. Consents obtained without satisfying all three elements are invalid except in situations in which surrogate consents are provided for incompetent patients, in certain medical emergencies, and in those instances in which paternalism can be justified.[7]

The most common exception to the otherwise uniform ethical requirement for consent is in the true medical emergency where there may be neither the time nor the availability of a surrogate decision maker to obtain proper consent. It would be foolish and tragic for physicians not to provide appropriate lifesaving therapy while awaiting proper consent. In this circumstance, the concept of implied consent usually authorizes physicians to provide urgent treatment. Emergency treatment is provided with the understanding that the patient or surrogate would have provided consent if doing so had been feasible. But in all other clinical circumstances, the consent of the patient or surrogate first should be obtained.

The emergency treatment doctrine permits treatment without consent in emergencies if three conditions can be satisfied: (1) the treatment in question represents the usual and customary standard of care for the condition being treated; (2) it would be clearly harmful to the patient to delay treatment awaiting explicit consent; and (3) patients ordinarily would be expected to consent for the treatment in question if they had the capacity do so.[8] The emergency treatment doctrine

provides the ethical and legal basis for emergency treatment with implied consent, an activity that is routinely conducted in emergency rooms on a daily basis.

The American Academy of Neurology Ethics and Humanities Subcommittee considered the applicability of the emergency treatment doctrine to the question of whether neurologists could prescribe intravenous recombinant tissue plasminogen activator (IV rtPA) for the emergency management of stroke without the consent of the patient or surrogate. In a 1999 position paper, the Committee decided that the emergency treatment doctrine did not apply to IV rtPA treatment of stroke because its use entailed significant short-term risks (intracranial hemorrhage), many patients refused the therapy because of these risks in an assessment of its risk-benefit profile, and IV rtPA did not represent the unequivocal standard of care in such cases. They argued that, given current outcome and consent data, IV rtPA administration required prior patient or surrogate consent even in emergency situations.[9]

Although some neurologists disagreed with this controversial opinion, most American neurologists' practices support it and most American hospitals require consent for IV rtPA treatment. In one study that looked for evidence of informed consent in patients receiving IV rtPA for threatened stroke, Rosenbaum and colleagues found that patients or surrogates had provided consent in 84% of cases whereas 16% of cases had no consent at all.[10] Some physicians have advocated for permitting IV rtPA for urgent use without any consent in certain circumstances, and its unconsented urgent use is permitted by law in some countries.[11] In a recent review Stephanie White-Bateman and colleagues agreed that patient or surrogate consent is necessary and emphasized the importance of determining a patient's capacity to provide consent in the presence of aphasia or other neurological deficits. They urged neurologists to develop a validated and reliable instrument for capacity determination in patients with acute stroke.[12]

How much and what type of information is adequate for consent purposes? Some have remarked cynically that patients must be given a medical education to fully satisfy consent requirements, especially those dictated by malpractice courts. Clearly such a standard is unnecessary and absurd. Information is adequate for consent purposes when it includes what a reasonable person would need to know in order to make the medical decision in question. By this standard, adequate information includes: (1) the basic facts of available therapies that might be effective for a given condition; (2) the significant risks and benefits of the available types of treatments, including no treatment at all; and (3) the course of therapy recommended by the physician and the reasons for the recommendation. The "reasonable person" standard satisfies the requirement for "material" information dictated by *Canterbury v Spence*.[13]

In a provocative paper, Heather Gert proposed that the correct standard of information transmitted by physicians during consent discussions should be that precise quantity of information that will prevent the patient from being surprised by later events as a result of the test or treatment.[14] This standard leaves to the physician's discretion the determination of what information to communicate and is consistent with the reasonable person standard, because reasonable people do not want to be surprised.

What are significant risks and benefits of therapy? The physician's duty to communicate risks varies as a function of their frequency and magnitude. Mild risks like skin rash that occur frequently (>0.1) should be disclosed, but mild risks like gastric upset that occur infrequently (<0.01) need not be disclosed. However, severe risks, such as disability or death, should be discussed even when they are an infrequent consequence (<0.001). Patients require this information because they need to balance the stated risks against the stated benefits according to their own values and health-care goals in order to make a rational decision.[15]

During the information-transmittal process, the physician imparts both fact and opinion to the patient. Both facts and opinions are necessary but, in the presentation, the physician should attempt to keep them separate. The facts should be presented in a clear and unbiased manner, with the physician taking care not to subtly or unsubtly exaggerate risks or benefits to influence the patient's decision unjustifiably. Then, after the facts are presented, the clinician should express an opinion about which treatment option she recommends and why. It would be wrong for her merely to recite a menu of options without also making a treatment recommendation.[16] The patient should be permitted to keep the physician's opinion about the recommended treatment course separate from the facts about the treatment. In this way, the patient, who may rank the risks and benefits differently from the physician, is permitted to disagree with the physician's opinion while agreeing with the facts.

Coercion must be absent for the consent to be valid because consent must be as free and unconstrained as possible. Bernard Gert and colleagues have defined coercion as "the use of such powerful negative incentives (for example, threats of severe pain or significant deprivation of freedom) that it would be unreasonable to expect a patient to resist them."[17] Subtle forms of coercion exist in addition to obvious ones. A clinician who threatens to abandon a patient who does not follow his advice with statements such as "I refuse to take care of you unless you follow my orders!" obviously is coercing the patient. But there are more subtle varieties of coercion. A physician who purposely exaggerates the risk of the unrecommended form of treatment or minimizes the risk of the recommended treatment is deceiving the patient by failing to provide correct information, and thus he is practicing subtle coercion. Making an emphatic treatment recommendation by presenting a factual basis for the recommendation is perfectly acceptable and does not count as coercion unless the physician exaggerates, threatens, or uses other manipulative behavior to force a particular decision.

Clinicians should be aware of the effects of "framing" on the subsequent medical choices of their patients. If they frame a choice in a biased way, this action may be considered a form of subtle coercion. Framing refers to *how* a physician portrays the facts in explaining medical situations to patients. The physician may consciously or subconsciously present information in a biased way by using shades of emphasis, voice inflection, facial expression, or gesture, or may blatantly misrepresent facts. How the patient responds to the information presented is contingent on how the clinician frames it.[18]

A clinician's leading questions contrive to frame issues in a predictable manner. For example, Murphy and colleagues studied how elderly patients responded to the choices they were offered concerning cardiopulmonary resuscitation (CPR). When the question was framed as, "Would you want us to do everything possible to save your life if your heart stopped beating?" predictably most patients responded "yes." But when the researchers framed the question differently, explaining the mechanics of CPR and honestly communicating the dismal outcomes of such therapy for people in their age groups, most patients then declined to give consent.[19] In this study, framing effects alone led to the complete reversal of an important health-care decision in a group of patients. Because of the powerful influence of framing, clinicians have an ethical duty to frame consent discussions in the fairest, least biased, and most accurate manner possible to eliminate subtle coercion and to promote free choice. Patients' decisions ideally should be made on the basis of applying correct facts to their personal preferences.

A subtle form of framing results from how physicians present clinical evidence to patients. Ronald Epstein and colleagues recently studied how to communicate clinical evidence to maximally promote patient understanding. They found that using relative risk reduction is misleading and absolute risk reduction is preferred, the order of information presented can bias patients' decisions, and that many patients could not understand percentages or confidence intervals. They recommended strategies to accomplish five communication tasks: (1) understand the patient's and family member's experience and expectations; (2) build partnerships; (3) provide evidence; (4) present recommendations informed by clinical judgment and patient preferences; and (5) check for understanding and agreement.[20]

Physicians obtaining informed consent from patients with low literacy have a heightened responsibility to communicate effectively.[21]

In some cases, providing additional information can help patients make important clinical decisions. In another CPR study, the effect of patient education on CPR decisions was measured. Elderly residents of a retirement community were surveyed about their CPR preferences in the event that they suffered cardiopulmonary arrest. One group of residents was given a careful educational program in which the true outcomes of CPR in the elderly were explained. The other group received no education. Not surprisingly, a significantly larger percentage of the group involved in the educational program refused CPR.[22] This study demonstrated that adequate information is important, in addition to objective, non-coercive framing, as a necessary component of valid consent. Jonathan Baron recently argued that because patients must weigh the benefits and risks of each treatment option, consent is best modeled as a utilitarian decision analysis.[23]

Capacity to Make Treatment Decisions

The third condition necessary for valid consent is that the patient has the capacity to make medical treatment decisions. Gert and colleagues have used the term "competence" as an abbreviated way of stating that the patient has the capacity to make medical decisions. In this clinical, nonlegal usage, "competence" signifies that the patient possesses the mental capacity to understand the relevant medical information, to appreciate the medical situation and the possible consequences of treatment decisions, and to manipulate this information rationally to reach a decision.[24] Other scholars shun "competence" because of its legal connotation and prefer the more cumbersome "capacity to make medical decisions."

Bernard Lo identified the four components of clinical competence: (1) the patient appreciates that she has a choice; (2) the patient appreciates the medical situation and prognosis as well as the risks, benefits and consequences of available and recommended treatments,

(3) the patient's decision is stable over time and is not impulsive; and (4) the patient's decision is consistent with her personal values and health-care goals.[25]

Obviously, competence is not an all-or-none capacity, and a person's degree of competence may change over time, often over a very short time in hospitalized, seriously ill patients. Competence also is task specific; thus, a person may be competent to write a will but not to play the piano. I have examined hospitalized patients with dementia or delirium who were competent to name a surrogate decision maker for themselves but incompetent to understand medical facts sufficiently to validly consent to therapy. Depending on their ability to appreciate and process the information conveyed during the consent process, patients can be classified into one of three groups: competent, partially competent, and incompetent.

Fully competent patients can make rational judgments about medical decisions because they are able to understand and process all necessary information. Thus they are able to provide valid consent or refusal for therapy. Partially competent patients, such as those with mild delirium or dementia, may understand that the physician is requesting their consent for certain therapy, but they cannot fully comprehend the issues involved. They are capable of providing only simple consent[26] but not valid consent.[27] Surrogate decision makers must corroborate a simple consent to make it valid.

Patients rendered incompetent by coma, profound delirium, or dementia cannot understand even the most basic facts of their existence, such as that the clinician is requesting their consent. These patients are unable to provide even a simple consent. Under these circumstances, surrogate decision makers must be approached for all medical decisions.[28] There is evidence from a recent study that physicians managing elderly patients with delirium failed to adequately assess their cognitive status, failed to obtain their consent, and failed to use surrogate decision makers consistently.[29]

In each clinical encounter, the physician should assess the competence of a patient to make a medical decision during the consent process. Many clinicians have observed, perhaps cynically, (as I also have observed in numerous clinical ethics consultations) that the competence of a patient becomes an issue in practice only when the patient disagrees with the physician's treatment plan. If the patient concurs with the treatment plan, her cognitive capacities are not further scrutinized. The clinical determination of competence usually does not require formal testing but rather results from observations made during the clinical encounter. In cases in which competence is questioned, more formalized mental status testing is necessary. In the most difficult cases, psychiatric consultation may provide helpful advice.

Treatment of the patient with Alzheimer's disease is another common setting in which competency questions arise in neurological practice. Alzheimer's patients comprise a spectrum from the partially competent to the utterly incompetent. Patients in early stages often are competent to give consent for treatment and complete a valid advance directive for medical care.[30] Patients with moderate dementia can be tested reliably for their ability to make a clinical decision by using structured interviews[31] or neuropsychological tests.[32] The specific bedside determination of clinical competence in the Alzheimer patient has been the subject of several studies. Bedside instruments have been developed and validated specifically to assess competence in various clinical contexts for consent by the Alzheimer patient.[33]

Neurologists often must determine decision-making capacity in patients with aphasia. Aphasic patients comprise a spectrum of severity and variability in language comprehension and expression.[34] Many aphasic patients retain adequate cognitive capacity but are unable to express their preferences for treatment or provide valid consent because of language dysfunction.[35] Clinicians should enlist the services of a speech-language pathologist trained in aphasia assessment to help determine the patient's capacity to consent.[36]

Rationality and Irrationality

Unlike competency, which refers to the capacity to make a treatment decision, rationality refers to the characteristics of a treatment decision once a patient has made it. Thus, competent patients can make both rational and irrational decisions.[37] The clinician who responds to a patient's treatment decision must consider both the competency of the patient and the rationality of the decision. Physicians have an ethical duty to help their patients reach medical decisions through a rational decision-making process by providing necessary information, answering questions clearly, and addressing fears and concerns.

Gert and colleagues have stipulated that "to act irrationally is to act in a way that one knows (justifiably believes), or should know, will significantly increase the probability that oneself, or those one cares for, will suffer death, pain, disability, loss of freedom, or loss of pleasure; and one does not have an adequate reason for so acting." A reason is "a conscious, rational belief that one's action will help anyone, not merely oneself or those one cares about, avoid some of the harms or gain some good, namely, ability, freedom, or pleasure, and this belief is not seen to be inconsistent with one's other beliefs by almost everyone with similar knowledge and intelligence." Reasons may be adequate or inadequate. A reason is adequate only "if any significant group of otherwise rational people regard the harm avoided or benefit gained as at least as important as the harm suffered." Actions that are not irrational are rational.[38]

In general, when a patient follows a physician's recommendation, she is acting rationally. This assertion is based on the assumption that physicians very seldom make irrational treatment suggestions to patients. But a patient who refuses a physician's treatment recommendation is not necessarily acting irrationally. The patient's decision becomes irrational only if the reasons behind her decision are inadequate and, as a result, would cause her to suffer unjustified and unnecessary harms that she could have avoided easily.

For example, an otherwise healthy young woman with depression may be competent, but her decision to refuse simple treatment may be irrational. She may understand her medical situation with perfect clarity, including that her depression may likely reverse with treatment. Yet the magnitude of her mental anguish is so great that she refuses food and all medical treatment. Her refusal in this circumstance is seriously irrational; hence, her physician is not ethically required to respect it. In this case, her physician can overrule her refusal, as outlined later in this chapter in the section on paternalism.

The law generally does not permit physicians to overrule their competent patients' refusal of treatment merely on the basis of irrationality. In practice, when a patient's refusal seems seriously irrational, the physician usually labels her as incompetent, which thereby permits the physician to overrule the patient's treatment refusal. Although this practice confounds the distinct concepts of rationality and competence, it is a common solution that permits clinicians to overrule their patients' decisions to refuse treatment when the refusals are seriously irrational.

The rationality of a particular decision may vary as a function of other medical circumstances. It would be seriously irrational for a young, otherwise healthy patient to refuse intravenous antibiotics that can easily cure her bacterial pneumonia in favor of an exercise and macrobiotic diet regimen to treat the pneumonia. The patient would likely suffer the serious evils of death or disability without adequate justification because the harms of treatment are so slight by comparison. However, the same decision made by a person of any age with widespread metastatic carcinoma in a terminal stage would count as a rational decision because the harms that the patient likely will suffer with or without antibiotic treatment are similar.

Brock and Wartman outlined the forms of irrational decisions commonly made by patients. Some patients have an irrational and childish bias toward the present and near future. They may be churlishly and unreasonably unwilling to undergo even a slight amount of pain or discomfort in the present to prevent much worse suffering in the future. Other patients may categorically deny the possibility of complications of a specific treatment, using the rationalization, "Oh, I know that won't happen to me." Like small children, other patients have an irrational fear of pain or medical experiences in general, causing them to delay, avoid, or refuse much needed medical treatment.[39] Clinicians have a nonmaleficence-based ethical duty to help patients avoid irrational thinking in their decision making.

Refusal of medical therapy on religious grounds constitutes an interesting example of rational vs. irrational decision making. The well-known refusal of Jehovah's Witnesses to receive blood or blood products (including their own previously banked blood), and their resulting willingness to die of an otherwise treatable condition to maintain this religious conviction, has been respected in American medicine for over a generation. The religious injunction against receiving blood or blood products has a biblical rationale and is a fundamental tenet of their religious belief system. While dying of an easily treatable medical condition may strike some as an irrational act, it would not be considered irrational using the definition of Gert and colleagues, because this belief is consistent and coherent with the Jehovah's Witness patient's other beliefs. Similar conclusions can be reached with the decisions of Christian Scientists to refuse medical treatment. Respect for these treatment refusals does not necessarily apply to their minor children, however, and physicians have successfully secured court orders enforcing life-saving treatment for children of Jehovah's Witnesses and Christian Scientists.[40]

Responding to Patients' Treatment Decisions

Once a patient has made a treatment decision, the physician must respond to it. The physician's response should take into account both the competence of the patient and the rationality of the decision. When a competent patient provides valid consent to a physician's recommended treatment plan, the treatment is implemented because it is implicit (though not always true) that the physician's recommendation is rational. A competent patient's valid refusal should be similarly honored unless that refusal is seriously irrational. In a later section, I consider those rare instances of justified paternalism in which it may be morally defensible for a clinician to override a competent patient's

decision to refuse treatment and to proceed with treatment without consent. The rationality of a refusal of life-sustaining treatment may be difficult to determine, particularly in the patient with a psychiatric condition,[41] and should be handled on a case-by-case basis as discussed in chapter 8.

With a partially competent patient, the physician should seek simple consent from the patient and make the consent valid by corroborating with a surrogate decision maker. The physician responds to simple consents made valid by corroboration in exactly the same way as he responds to valid consents from competent patients. With the incompetent patient, the surrogate must corroborate all consents necessary. Once the consent is corroborated, the physician responds as he would to any valid consent.

Physicians should understand patients' cognitive and emotional reactions in the decision-making process. Not all ostensibly rational decision making operates by entirely rational processes. Redelmeier and colleagues have identified several psychological mechanisms patients may employ that influence their decisions in unsystematic and irrational ways. The effect of physician framing on patients' decisions was discussed earlier. Some patients lack the mathematical capacity to appreciate quantitative estimates of risk and prefer to dichotomize risks erroneously as "all or none" or "dangerous or safe." Most patients rank suffering a loss as a worse outcome than the failure to gain an equivalent quantity. Memories of emotional and traumatic past experiences affect the decision making of some people and account for their tendency to disproportionately weigh options that avoid those particular risks.[42] All patients have biases of risk estimation that lead to less than fully rational decisions.[43] Physicians have the ethical duty to try to understand the psychology their patients use in making decisions. They also have the responsibility to guide their patients to think rationally by identifying the sources of irrational thought processes and helping patients overcome them.

Surveys have shown that in practice it is quite common for patients to defer decisions entirely to their physicians, particularly as they grow older and sicker. They may utter such phrases as, "I'll do whatever you think is best, doctor."[44] There is nothing morally wrong with acceding to this attitude as long as it represents a patient's valid choice. Indeed, it shows that physician beneficence is implicit in the patient-physician relationship. Sherlock has pointed out that physicians have a special moral duty in caring for the sick to guide them to make correct decisions because their illness may interfere with their ability to think clearly.[45] Similarly, Loewy argued that physicians need to assume the beneficent role of leading the patient to the right decision.[46] Some scholars have called the physician's role "high-quality decision counseling."[47] Ubel explained how physicians' recommendations improved patients' decision making by gently leading them to make the right decisions for themselves.[48] There is evidence that hospitalized patients show evidence of childlike judgment with impairment in rational thinking that requires careful physician guidance.[49] But clinicians should take care not to assume the role of complete decision maker too readily, and thereby disenfranchise patients who wish not to defer their right of self-determination.

Paternalism

Paternalism has a long and hallowed tradition in medical practice evolving from the fiduciary duty of a physician to identify and act in the best interest of the patient. Because the clinician alone possesses specialized knowledge and experience in diagnosing and treating illness, only he can define the proper course of diagnosis and treatment.[50] Old-time physicians traditionally are portrayed as making wise and prudent choices for patients who followed those decisions unquestionably and respectfully.

The current connotation of paternalism is clearly negative, conjuring an image of a physician arrogantly and egotistically proceeding with a course of treatment without the least consideration for the patient's wishes. To further understand the explicit meaning of paternalism and to examine whether a physician's paternalistic behavior may ever be justified, we need an explicit definition of paternalism.

Of the numerous scholars who have attempted to define paternalism, Gert and colleagues have achieved the greatest precision. According to their definition, A is acting paternalistically toward S if and only if: (1) A believes that his action benefits S; (2) A recognizes (or should recognize) that his action toward S is a kind of action that needs moral justification; (3) A does not believe that his action has S's past, present, or immediately forthcoming consent; and 4) A regards S as believing he (S) can make his own decision on this matter.[51]

In neurological practice, an example of a paternalistic act that satisfies this definition is a physician's purposeful withholding of information concerning the risks posed by a carotid endarterectomy, which the neurologist has recommended that the patient undergo to prevent future carotid territory strokes. The physician's intent in withholding the information is to benefit the patient by protecting her from worrying unnecessarily about fearsome complications. The neurologist may rationalize that the patient clearly needs the operation, so why worry her further with information about the surgical risks? Withholding the risks involved in the procedure violates the moral rule, "Do not deceive" and therefore requires moral justification. The competent patient generally wants and needs to know and understand the risks of surgical procedures in order to provide valid consent. The deception is carried out without the patient's consent, which she is capable of giving.

Paternalistic acts of medical decision making (unlike the previous example) are morally acceptable only when they can be adequately justified. Moral theories differ in their criteria for the justification of paternalism. Utilitarians simply would examine the consequences of the act to determine its morality. Deontologists would hold that because paternalism breaks a moral rule without the affected party's consent, it never can be justified. Gert and colleagues conclude that common morality permits the occasional justification of paternalistic acts but only when they satisfy the strict criteria for justifying the violation of a moral rule, as discussed in chapter 1.[52]

In the circumstance of treating a patient who has refused treatment, Gert and colleagues provide four criteria for the justification of this paternalistic act: (1) the harms the treatment will probably avoid or ameliorate must be very great, for example, death or permanent disability; (2) the harms imposed by the treatment must be, by comparison, very much less; (3) the patient's desire not to be treated must be seriously irrational; (4) rational persons must advocate publicly that the physician should force treatment in cases having the same morally relevant characteristics described by the first three criteria.[53]

The following case is an example of justified paternalism. A previously healthy young woman develops acute appendicitis and appendiceal rupture. An experienced general surgeon in a hospital emergency room makes the diagnosis with a high degree of certainty. The patient refuses to consent to an emergency appendectomy, however, because she does not wish to have an abdominal scar that she regards as ugly. She truly wishes to recover but believes that antibiotics will be sufficient to cure her. The patient offers no religious objections or any reasons other than cosmetic concern for refusing consent. The surgeon's compassionate explanations and reasoning do not alter the patient's decision. Neither can family members convince the patient. The clinician knows that the patient will likely die or have serious complications if surgery is not performed quickly; therefore, he sedates the patient and performs an emergency appendectomy without her consent and despite her refusal.

I believe that paternalism in this case is justified. The evils of death or serious disability that surgical intervention alleviates are great and far exceed the evils of creating a small surgical scar and going against the patient's will by treating without her consent. Her decision is clearly irrational given her otherwise excellent health and potentially long healthy life span. Rational persons would always want their lives saved if they could retain good health at a relatively tiny expense.

Paternalistic treatment in the absence of consent represents a courageous act by the physician because it exposes the physician to criminal charges of battery. Battery in most jurisdictions conceivably encompasses the performance of refused surgery. Physicians who treat without consent must be prepared to defend their action as morally correct using the rigorous justification of paternalism.[54] There will be very few examples of truly justified paternalistic acts in clinical practice. If the paternalistic act cannot be justified rigorously, the physician should not perform it.

This case differs in an important way from the well-publicized Quackenbush case. Mr. Quackenbush was a chronically ill, elderly diabetic who refused to consent to amputations of his gangrenous legs, which his attending surgeons had urged upon him in order to save his life. Mr. Quackenbush explained that he was going to die soon anyway and that he would rather die whole than to live a short while longer without his legs. His surgeons tried to have him declared incompetent because they strongly disagreed with his decision, but a psychiatrist found that Quackenbush clearly understood his choices and their implications. A court ruled that Quackenbush's physicians could not override his decision because he was competent and his decision was rational. Despite the fact that Quackenbush's decision differed from the strong recommendation of his surgeons, the court held that it was rational given the quality and quantity of his remaining life.[55]

The adequacy of patients' reasons to refuse recommended surgery in the context of their diagnoses and prognoses highlights the difference between the Quackenbush and the appendectomy cases. In the appendectomy case, the patient declined life-saving surgery that could have assured her continued excellent health because she did not wish to have a scar. This is simply an inadequate reason for an otherwise healthy young person to risk almost certain death, making her thinking seriously irrational. Conversely, the decision of a chronically ill, elderly patient who will die in the near future and, therefore, refuses to part with his legs, preferring to "die whole," constitutes an adequate reason because many others would share his ranking of harms and values.

Thus, Quackenbush's refusal can be classified as rational.

Physicians have several duties when competent patients make choices that appear to be irrational. First, they should attempt to ascertain that a patient's decision is truly irrational and does not arise from a religious belief or value judgment different from theirs. Because the adequacy of the reasons for a choice distinguishes rational from irrational choices, physicians should carefully explore the reasons for a particular choice and help patients think rationally by explaining medical facts calmly and reassuringly. Physicians should explain to patients how their decision is irrational because their desired health-care goals cannot be accomplished if they persist in such thinking and refuse proper treatment. Physicians should enlist family members and friends in an attempt to persuade the patient that she is making a serious error. Only in those rare instances in which true paternalism can be rigorously justified are physicians morally permitted to override a patient's unequivocal treatment refusal.[56] Psychiatrists commonly are justified in and legally protected for paternalistic acts including involuntary hospitalization, treatment, and even overriding a patient's previously executed psychiatric advance directive for care.[57]

Shared Medical Decision Making

The replacement of the paternalistic model of medical decision making with the shared decision-making model is a defining characteristic of early 21st century American medicine. In the shared decision-making model the physician and patient comprise a collaborative decision-making dyad. The clinician contributes specialized knowledge, training, and experience which are prerequisites to making medical decisions. The patient contributes her own unique knowledge of her values and health-care goals through which to interpret and evaluate the extent to which the available treatment options can fulfill those goals.[58] The patient and physician collaboratively and jointly arrive at a mutually agreeable medical decision through an ongoing communication process that culminates in valid consent.[59]

Physicians' participation in medical shared decision making should not be restricted to offering a menu of treatment options. Physicians should make a treatment recommendation and explain the reasons for the treatment recommendation by citing valid outcome data and how the recommended treatment will help the patient achieve her health-care goals.[60] The patient remains free to accept or reject the recommendation.

Not all patients wish to actively participate in medical decision making. The doctrine of shared decision making is sufficiently elastic to accommodate patients' varying wishes and needs to participate in the decisions. Most experienced physicians have evolved techniques to work collaboratively with their patients to strike a reasonable balance between physician direction and patient choice.[61] Robert McNutt viewed shared decision making metaphorically as a moving vehicle in which the patient serves as pilot and the physician as navigator.[62] Lynn Peterson and I epitomized shared medical decision making as "the best blending of physician expertise and patient choice."[63]

Shared medical decision making is the most accurate contemporary conceptualization of the doctrine of valid consent. Several clinics and hospitals have founded centers for shared medical decision making to provide current and valid outcome data to patients and their physicians to assist the decision-making process and make it evidence-based.[64] Shared decision-making centers often employ decision aids—balanced, evidence-based videos or written literature providing information on treatment options—to help people make deliberative treatment choices.[65] In some clinical decisions, such as surgery to repair an acute hip fracture, patients simply agree with the physician's treatment plan. But in other clinical decisions, such as whether to undergo elective orthopedic surgery, there may be no unequivocally "best" treatment option. These elective surgery decisions are particularly benefited by the use of decision aids and formal shared decision-making consultations.[66] Studies on the outcomes, benefits, and harms of shared decision making are ongoing.[67] A recent legal treatise on informed consent in the United States showed how it has evolved from a physician-centered process of consent to a patient-centered process of shared medical decision making.[68]

Practical Considerations in Obtaining Consent

Consent is a process, not an event. It is a continuing bidirectional dialogue between a patient and a physician during which information is exchanged, questions are answered, recommendations are offered, and a mutually agreeable decision is jointly reached. The specific requirements of information exchange in the consent process vary with the circumstances. In general, the more risky the proposed tests or treatments, the greater the duty for the physician to provide detailed information and extended explanations, and the greater the desirability of formalizing the consent documentation.[69]

Consent for outpatient treatment, such as that required for beginning a patient with a newly diagnosed seizure disorder on anticonvulsant medications, may be accomplished simply. In discussing the diagnosis, the neurologist explains that most patients with seizure disorders can be controlled on anticonvulsant medications, that there are a number of possible medications available, and that the goal is to find an effective medication that causes few or no side effects and can be taken conveniently. The neurologist makes a recommendation based on the seizure type, the patient's age, and other factors, and briefly explains the actions, dosage, side effects, and necessary monitoring for the medication. The patient is given the opportunity to ask questions and then agrees by accepting and filling the prescription for the medication. Many neurologists document that the discussion about side effects and monitoring has taken place. Some writers call this informal and abbreviated shared decision-making agreement "simple consent."[70]

Consent for invasive testing, such as cerebral contrast angiography, or potentially risky therapies such as carotid endarterectomy and IV rtPA for threatened stroke requires a more extensive and formalized educational process. Given the seriousness of the known risks of these interventions, patients must understand that they are being asked to accept significant short-term health risks for the potential long-term health benefits. The consent process should attempt to quantify the risks, to the fullest extent that they are known. Neurologists should first study the risk-benefit ratio to ascertain that the local risks are acceptably low to permit benefit to the patient. For example, if the surgeon performing the carotid endarterectomy has a relatively high surgical mortality and morbidity rate, the patient may fare better solely with medical treatment or should be referred to another surgeon with an acceptable surgical record. In any event, patients deserve to know these statistics as part of their consent process.[71] Nevertheless, one study of the extent of patients' understanding following a consent discussion for carotid endarterectomy showed that most patients had false and unrealistic expectations of both the benefits and risks of the surgery.[72] Some physicians and institutions have created detailed patient information booklets and videos to more thoroughly and systematically communicate the important information patients need to understand before providing consent for procedures.[73]

The required documentation of the process of obtaining consent varies among institutions. Most hospitals require a written consent form signed by the patient and witnessed by a third party testifying that the patient has been adequately educated about the proposed procedure and has given her free consent for surgery or other invasive and potentially dangerous diagnostic and therapeutic procedures. Some but not all institutions require a signed consent for a lumbar puncture. Signed consent forms are not usually necessary for simple outpatient medication prescriptions. But the signed form is not itself the consent. The consent form is merely the evidence of consent that formalizes the preceding consent dialogue between the physician and patient.

Consent of Minors

Obtaining valid consent from minors is an issue that arises frequently in pediatric practice. From a strictly legal perspective, only persons of majority age can give informed consent.

Thus, parents and guardians of minors must be approached to provide consent for children under age 18 years[74] unless the minors have been granted a legal status of emancipation by dint of marriage, childbearing, military service, financial independence, or other factors. Most states also have enacted varying "mature minor" laws. These laws stipulate certain medical procedures and categories of medical care that can be consented to solely by minors. Parental consent or, in many cases, even notification, is not required.

Over the past generation, pediatricians and others have increasingly recognized the validity of including older children and teenagers in the medical consent process. Numerous studies have shown that children over the age of 12 usually have cognitive capacities sufficient to allow them to understand the necessary facts to have the capacity to consent for treatment.[75] In 1995, the American Academy of Pediatrics Committee on Bioethics published an influential position paper asserting the rights of older children and teenagers to actively participate in providing permission for their own medical decisions.[76] The American Academy of Pediatrics opinion was based on an empirical study showing that 14-year-olds had the same ability as adults to make health-care decisions.[77]

The American Academy of Pediatrics defined the concept of "assent" of minors and distinguished it from consent. They asserted that to the greatest extent feasible, decision making involving older children and adolescents should include the assent of the patient in addition to participation by the parents and physician. They held that a minor's assent for testing or treatment should include at least the following elements:

"(1) helping the patient achieve a developmentally appropriate awareness of the nature of his or her condition; (2) telling the patient what he or she can expect with tests and treatment(s); (3) making a clinical assessment of the patient's understanding of the situation and the factors influencing how he or she is responding (including whether there is appropriate pressure to accept testing or therapy); and (4) soliciting an expression of the patient's willingness to accept the proposed care. Regarding this final point,

we note that no one should solicit a patient's views without intending to weigh them seriously. In situations in which the patient will have to receive medical care despite his or her objection, the patient should be told that fact and should not be deceived."[78]

The Academy also defined the role of parents in the consent process as providing "permission." They chose this word purposely to emphasize that the parents should only corroborate the assent of the older child, and that their agreement alone did not constitute a valid consent, particularly if the treatment was refused by the child. Thus for adolescents and older children, the American Academy of Pediatrics held that "Informed Consent = Patient Assent + Parental Permission." The Academy document also contained suggestions about resolving conflicts between parents and children and provided examples of various consent discussions at different ages and in different clinical circumstances.

Some bioethicists responded that the Academy's "child liberation" philosophy unwisely afforded vulnerable young people too much latitude to make bad decisions. For example, Lainie Ross argued that permitting a child to prevail in situations in which the child and parents disagree may not be in the child's best interests. She argued that the child's autonomy may be furthered more by deferring to the parents. Parents often prudently look to the long-term good of the child and may be willing to permit painful treatment now for expected long-term benefit later. By contrast, children often give more weight to their short-term comfort issues without adequately considering their long-term perspective. Ross argued that the child's long-term autonomy often may be furthered best by sacrificing her short-term autonomy.[79] Rhonda Hartman recently proposed how the American Academy of Pediatrics assent concept could be introduced into state laws.[80]

To some extent, the success of childhood assent for medical care depends on the nature of the medical condition and the treatment physicians recommend. The previous discussion centered on life-threatening illnesses, such as cancer, with morbid treatments. In a study of children with diabetes, Priscilla Alderson and colleagues showed that children could become "partners" in their diabetes care. The children studied showed an adult-like capacity to make clinical decisions affecting them that exceeded the capacity predicted by their parents and other adults.[81]

TRUTH TELLING AND DECEPTION

It is nearly always morally correct for physicians to tell patients the truth rather than to lie to or deceive them. However, like most moral rules, the duty to tell the truth (veracity) may be abrogated in certain justified circumstances. There are four areas in which some clinicians believe that it may be morally correct to deceive patients, other parties, or agencies: (1) misrepresenting patient data to insurance companies to secure payment; (2) delaying or not telling patients their diagnosis in cases of hopeless illness; (3) not fully disclosing to patients the risks of proposed diagnostic tests or therapies; and (4) using placebos. Purposeful deception in each of these instances is an example of medical paternalism because it violates the moral rule not to deceive, and the affected party is presumed to want to know the information in question. With careful analysis of each area, however, I conclude that paternalism cannot be justified in most instances and that deception, even with beneficent motives, nearly always is wrong.

Misrepresentation to Third-Party Payers

The incidence of deception in medical practice is unknown, but surveys have shown various types of paternalistic deception to be quite common. Novack and colleagues found that the majority of physicians taking part in a questionnaire study were willing to engage in limited forms of deception if, by doing so, they satisfied what they believed to be higher moral ideals. They found that over two-thirds of the responding physicians were willing to purposely misrepresent the indication for a diagnostic test to secure insurance payment for a patient who could not afford the test. Over half of those surveyed were willing to mislead

a wife about her husband's diagnosis of gonorrhea in order to save their marriage. One-third said that they would provide incomplete or misleading information to a patient's family if a medical error caused the patient's death. A small percentage of physicians were willing to lie to a mother about her adolescent daughter's pregnancy. In each of these instances, the surveyed physicians explained that they placed a higher value on maintaining their patients' confidentiality and welfare than on veracity for its own sake.[82] But, of course, deception by physicians in cases of medical error is almost entirely self-serving.

Two studies reported that high proportions of physicians would purposely deceive third-party payers to secure insurance payment for medical services. Freeman and colleagues found that over half of surveyed physicians would provide misleading or false information to secure payment for coronary bypass surgery and arterial revascularization, about one-third would do so for mammography and emergency psychiatric referral, but only 2% would do so for cosmetic rhinoplasty.[83] Similarly, Wynia and associates found that 39% of physicians reported the use of at least one of the following tactics of manipulation of the truth in the past year: (1) exaggerating the severity of a patient's condition; (2) changing a patient's billing diagnosis; or (3) reporting signs or symptoms that the patient did not have.[84]

A more recent study showed a smaller number of physicians who were willing to misrepresent facts to insurers. In a survey of 1617 physicians, Werner and colleagues found that 11% were willing to deceive insurers by misrepresentation to avoid a seemingly arbitrary coverage restriction. When given the choice, 77% of physicians said they would appeal the restriction and 12% would accept the ruling.[85] Physicians indicated a greater willingness to deceive when the appeals process was longer, the likelihood of a successful appeal was lower, and the health consequences for the patient were more severe.[86] A comparison study of 700 prospective jurors using the same survey by the same investigators showed that 26% of prospective jurors (more than twice the physicians' rate) were willing to deceive.[87]

The motive that physicians report for misrepresenting facts to third-party payers is to help their patients by manipulating the reimbursement system to assure payment. Many physicians believe the reimbursement system to be capricious and unfair, and they justify their behavior as patient advocacy and following an ethic of fidelity to their patients. Physicians in this circumstance are morally squeezed between fidelity to their patients and their duty as responsible professionals to tell the truth to insurers. Their willingness to deceive reflects this moral tension.[88] Their willingness to deceive appears to be a symptom of a flawed system in which physicians are asked to implement financing policies that conflict with their primary ethical obligations to their patients.[89] Of course, cynics may detect an additional self-serving financial motive in their action.

While this type of deception to insurers is understandable, is it morally acceptable as a case of justified paternalism? I think not. A criterion for the justification of paternalism is to publicly advocate that everyone follow the behavior in question in morally similar situations. But clearly we cannot advocate that everyone break the rules in an *ad hoc* fashion because that will result in consequences that may harm all patients. Erratic or *ad hoc* following and breaking of rules is inherently unfair and likely will harm patients other than those of the physician. A better solution is to work politically with patient advocacy groups to change the third-party reimbursement system by eliminating unfair provisions, and by improving disclosure by forcing better publication of the exact reimbursement provisions. But as long as insurance coverage and reimbursement rules appear arbitrary, capricious, unreasonably restrictive, and harmful to patients, physicians likely will continue to "game the system."[90]

Diagnostic Deception

During former times when available therapies were unable to improve the outcome of many illnesses, a number of physicians delayed or avoided telling their patients grim diagnoses, defending their position with the doctrine of medical paternalism. Physicians then generally believed that disclosing grim and untreatable diseases created more net harm than benefit. In contemporary neurology, this practice is rare but in some regions of the world continues to be defended for certain chronic or terminal diseases, such as amyotrophic lateral sclerosis, multiple sclerosis, and Alzheimer's disease.[91]

Physicians who practice deception by not disclosing diagnoses to patients or their families usually offer one or more of the following justifications: (1) telling the patient immediately would extinguish all hope and produce harm; (2) the enormous psychological burden a patient would experience in knowing for certain that she had an incurable disease would, itself, produce a negative impact on the course of her illness; (3) because the physician never can be entirely certain of the diagnosis, it would be wrong to burden the patient with what might truly be an uncertainty; (4) because the patient does not really wish to know the bad news, it would be wrong to force it on her; and (5) the patient probably would not understand the explanation, so it is therefore unnecessary to provide one.[92]

Paternalistic deception cannot be justified in the majority of these cases using the test of Gert and colleagues previously described because delaying or withholding a patient's diagnosis creates unnecessary and unjustifiable harms. Without receiving a diagnosis, patients may "doctor shop," undergoing repeated, dangerous, painful, and expensive testing until ultimately a clinician tells them the truth. Patients may suffer needless fear and anxiety thinking that their diagnosis is even worse than the one they may actually have. Moreover, if a clinician does not divulge the truth, the bond of trust that forms the basis of the patient-physician relationship will be damaged when the patient eventually learns of the deception. As a result, the angry patient may mistrust any future pronouncements from a physician.[93]

Most importantly, by delaying or withholding a known diagnosis, the physician deprives the patient of the opportunity to plan for future life events, such as marriage, childbearing, education, or employment, all activities that knowing the prognosis may influence. Paternalism is not justified because, if people knew that paternalism was allowed, the harms produced by failing to disclose a diagnosis would clearly exceed those avoided by doing so. Surveys of patients with multiple sclerosis and amyotrophic lateral sclerosis uniformly have shown that patients want to be told the truth about their diagnosis once it has been made.[94]

Clinicians also have an ethical responsibility to inform patients about their prognoses. Patients who have a terminal disease should be told in order to allow them the opportunity to make appropriate plans for employment, treatment, and other issues important in their lives. Although the exact prognosis often cannot be stated with certainty, patients should be given the same general prognostic information that physicians have. Paul Helft calls his continuous prognostic forecasting communication with advanced cancer patients an "intimate collaboration."[95] Clinicians should communicate the truth in a compassionate but accurate manner, without employing misleading euphemisms.

The question of whether a legal duty exists to convey prognosis was considered in the *Arato* case. The California Supreme Court found for the family of Miklos Arato, a terminally ill patient with metastatic pancreatic cancer who later sued his physicians for failing to inform him of his dismal prognosis, who claimed that it thereby invalidating his consent for medical treatment. The family asserted that had Mr. Arato been aware that he was terminally ill, he would have refused to undergo a radical pancreatectomy. In the broad dimension of their ruling, the court opined that "a physician is under a legal duty to disclose to the patient all material information—that is, information that would be regarded as significant by a reasonable person in the patient's position when deciding to accept or reject a recommended medical procedure—needed to make an informed decision regarding a proposed treatment." In the narrow dimension, however, the court ruled that physicians did not have a legal duty to convey to the patient specific statistical data on life expectancy because doing so was not the standard of medical practice in 1980.[96]

The American Medical Association Council on Ethical and Judicial Affairs (CEJA) recently affirmed the stand that it was unethical for physicians to withhold information from patients that they needed to make a medical decision. They decried the former concept of "therapeutic privilege" upon which some physicians supported their paternalistic claim to justify withholding information. The CEJA wrote: "Withholding medical information for patients without their knowledge or consent is ethically unacceptable."[97] The CEJA pointed out that physicians could adjust the timing of disclosure to optimally balance the benefits and harms in the patient's interest. Commentators pointed out some of the complications of this policy that may arise in practice but they supported the principle.[98]

Cultural factors are relevant to physicians' practices of telling the truth to patients.[99] In a number of cultures, such as Russian, Japanese, Arabic, Pakistani, and Hispanic, it is common to withhold bad diagnostic news from patients, such as the diagnosis of cancer.[100] Interestingly, this practice was also common in mainstream American culture as recently as 50 years ago.[101] The effect of cultural practices on clinicians' honesty to patients about the diagnosis of cancer was studied by Mary Anderlik and colleagues.[102] They found that 73% of surveyed physicians reported at least one request from family members during the 12-month study period to withhold the diagnosis of cancer from patients of Arabic or Middle Eastern origin and 51% from families of patients of Hispanic origin. Family requests to withhold prognostic information were similarly frequent. Clinicians faced with this problem must balance the need for cultural respect and sensitivity with the legitimate rights of patients.[103] In my practice, I try to reach a compromise between the duty to respect cultural values and to tell the truth by asking the patient how much she wishes to know about her diagnosis and prognosis and then respecting that wish.

How to Tell the Truth

Patients generally want and need to be told the truth about their diagnoses and prognoses, but the truth should be told in the right way with gentleness, compassion, reassurance, and hope.[104] Patients need to be told about the level of certainty of their diagnoses. They should be given the option of seeking second opinions if they wish, without fear of offending their physicians. Physicians should assist them in securing a desired second opinion. No matter how sick his patients become, the clinician should tell them that she will not abandon them, that she will be available when needed, and that she will prescribe treatment to improve the course of the illness when possible and to relieve symptoms to the best of her ability. The physician should make a pact with her patients to do everything possible to prevent suffering, particularly in the final stages of an illness. Patients should be given the option of participating in clinical treatment research protocols and assisted in finding ones in which to enroll.

In the case of multiple sclerosis (MS), for example, the physician should compassionately explain to the affected patient that her pre-existing concept of the disease has been slanted toward the most extreme examples as a result of images presented during fundraising drives. The patient should know that many cases of MS are benign and compatible with a more or less normal life. The clinician can explain the many treatments that slow the course of the disease and improve the lives of patients. In striving to educate the patient to the greatest extent possible, the clinician should suggest that the patient read educational books available about MS and enroll in the local chapter of the M.S. Society (or another society dedicated to her disease). In this way, patients can be told the truth about their diagnoses and prognoses in a manner consistent with the highest ethical standards of medical practice.

Clinicians often have psychological difficulty in breaking bad news to patients. Part of the difficulty many physicians experience results from anticipatory anxiety about the conversation and part from ignorance of effective communication skills. Communication techniques have been developed that permit physicians to deliver bad news in an optimal manner. By learning and perfecting these techniques, physicians can minimize their own sense of isolation as well as their patient's, achieve a common perception of the problem, provide information tailored to the patient's needs, pay attention to the risk of suicide, respond to patients' immediate discomforts, and ensure an adequate follow-up plan.[105]

In the earlier case in which a patient suffered paternalistic deception because she was not told about the risks posed by carotid endarterectomy, the clinician should have accurately stated the risks of stroke with and without surgery. Instead, she purposely minimized and concealed those risks in order to protect the patient from undue worry because the patient required the procedure in any event. This example of paternalism cannot be justified because, if publicly known, the harms produced exceed those avoided; therefore, rational persons would not advocate deception in such cases. Patients cannot provide valid consent without understanding the risks and benefits of proposed therapies. Rather than minimizing the surgical risks, the physician should accurately state the risks with and without surgery and then explain to the patient why she believes that those risks are justified by the greater benefits of future stroke reduction with endarterectomy.

The Placebo

Prescribing placebos is a common form of deception in medical practice.[106] Shapiro has defined the placebo as "any therapeutic procedure which is objectively without specific activity for the condition being treated." He further defined a placebo effect as "the psychological, physiological, or psychophysiological effect of any medication or procedure given with therapeutic intent, which is independent of, or minimally related to, the pharmacologic effects of the medication or to the specific effects of the procedure, and which operates through a psychological mechanism.[107] In this section, I discuss the ethics of the therapeutic use of placebos. I discuss ethical issues concerning placebo controls in research in chapter 19.

A placebo (Latin for "I will please") exerts powerful effects on many disorders, and the placebo effect is the basis for the efficacy of many agents in the pharmacopoeia, particularly the analgesics.[108] Because of the power of the placebo effect, studies of a drug's pharmacological efficacy generally must demonstrate that the drug's effect is greater than that produced by a placebo.[109] Placebos are particularly effective when used to relieve pain. Physiologically, placebos have been shown to stimulate the release of endorphins, which bind to opiate receptors in the brain to relieve pain. Opiate antagonists, such as naloxone, can block the effects of a placebo.[110] Thus, the placebo's effect as an analgesic ironically might not fit Shapiro's definition because it operates by a physiological and not a purely psychological mechanism.

Utilizing the placebo effect in therapy is not in itself unethical (particularly when deception is not used), and probably accounts for the improvement that many patients experience with treatment of a variety of chronic diseases. Prescribing placebos becomes morally questionable only when outright purposeful deception is employed. The deception can undermine the honesty and trust that forms the basis of the patient-physician relationship and may lead to further deception and dishonesty.[111] Deceptive placebo use is an example of paternalism. The American Medical Association Council on Ethical and Judicial Affairs recently ruled that the therapeutic use of placebo is ethical if deception is not used.[112]

Under what conditions is placebo prescription an ethically acceptable medical practice? Several scholars have proposed criteria. Sissela Bok identified five criteria: (1) placebos should be used only after a careful diagnosis; (2) no active placebos should be employed, merely inert ones; (3) no outright lie should be told and questions should be answered honestly; (4) placebos should never be given to patients who have asked not to receive them; and (5) placebos should never be used when other treatment is clearly called for or when all possible alternatives have not been weighed.[113]

Jonsen, Siegler, and Winslade have produced their own criteria for which they believe placebo use to be ethically sound: (1) the condition to be treated should be known as one that has a high response rate to a placebo, mild mental depression or postoperative pain being examples; (2) the alternative to a placebo is either continued illness or use of a drug with known toxicity, monoamine oxidase inhibitors or morphine being examples of drugs producing toxic effects: (3) the patient wishes to be treated and cured, if possible and (4) the patient insists on a prescription.[114]

Most recently, Lichtenberg and colleagues provided the following guidelines for the justified use of placebos in clinical practice: (1) the intentions of the physician must be benevolent with the sole concern the patient's well-being, with no conflicting economic or emotional interests; (2) a placebo is given in the spirit of assuaging the patient's suffering, not simply to mollify or silence her; (3) when proven ineffective, the placebo should be withdrawn immediately; (4) placebos should not be prescribed in place of more effective medications but considered when no treatment exists or patients are refractory to ordinary treatment because of inefficacy or unacceptable side effects; (5) physicians should respond honestly when asked questions about the placebo and its effects; and (6) the placebo should not be discontinued if it helps the patient.[115]

The paternalism of placebo use can be justified only in those cases in which the benefit that patients receive from relief of distressing symptoms outweighs the harms to them from deception. Patients can be told that the medication prescribed can be expected to help relieve symptoms in some people. The placebo should be discontinued if it produces no beneficial effect. Physicians should respond honestly if asked what the pill contains. Further deception should not be practiced.

The therapeutic expectation of the patient, based on the strength of the patient-physician relationship, is the greatest benefit induced by the placebo. Essential to a patient's clinical improvement are the physician's reassurance and prediction of her recovery. Howard Brody has called the placebo "the lie that heals."

He pointed out that the placebo is merely the vehicle that permits the strength of the patient-physician relationship to heal the patient.[116] Moerman and Jonas similarly pointed out that the placebo effect is better conceptualized as the "meaning response" because its benefit is produced by the meaning the prescription carries to the patient's understanding of her illness.[117] In this context, a placebo effect connotes a desirable outcome whereas a "nocebo effect" connotes an undesirable outcome.[118]

Placebos can be used during neurodiagnostic procedures also. Martin Smith and colleagues recently discussed the ethical issues involved in using intravenous saline therapy to provoke a nonepileptic, psychogenic seizure. They explained that in an attempt to show the absence of seizure activity on EEG during a suspected psychogenic seizure, many epileptologists suggest to the patient that an intravenous medication will provoke a seizure.

They then administer intravenous saline during EEG recording, hoping to provoke such an event.[119] Smith and colleagues point out that a "positive" response to the saline infusion indicates only that the patient is suggestible and does not exclude true epilepsy as a diagnosis. They also point out the harms that can develop in the patient-physician relationship when the deception is discovered and, as a result, patients lose trust in physicians.[120] Others have raised similar ethical concerns.[121]

*A better method to elicit psychogenic nonepileptic seizures would be to obtain continuous EEG and video recording or routine EEGs using suggestion but without employing deceptive procedures. Indeed, S. R. Benbadis and colleagues recently showed that the same success rate of provoking nonepileptic seizures can be obtained merely by suggestion during routine EEG activation procedures and without using a placebo.[122]

NOTES

1. I use the analyses of valid consent, competence, rationality, paternalism, and truth telling developed by Bernard Gert, Charles M. Culver and K. Danner Clouser in this chapter. See Gert B, Culver CM, Clouser KD. *Bioethics: A Return to Fundamentals*, 2nd ed. New York: Oxford University Press, 2006:213–282. See also their earlier, shorter works: Culver CM, Gert B. Basic ethical concepts in neurologic practice. *Semin Neurol* 1984;4:1–8; Gert B, Culver CM. Moral theory in neurologic practice. *Semin Neurol* 1984;4:9–13; and Gert B, Nelson WA, Culver CM. Moral theory and neurology. *Neurol Clin* 1989;7:681–696.

2. Culver CM, Gert B. *Semin Neurol* 1984:1–8.

3. See the discussion of informed consent as a legal doctrine in Bereford HR. *Neurology and the Law: Private Litigation and Public Policy*. Philadelphia: F.A.Davis Co, 1998:36–41.

4. See Brody H. Transparency: informed consent in primary care. *Hastings Cent Rep* 1989;19(5):5–9; Lidz CW, Meisel A. Osterweis M, et al. Barriers to informed consent. *Ann Intern Med* 1983;99:539–543; Mazur DJ. Why the goals of informed consent are not realized: treatise for informed consent for the primary physician. *J Gen Intern Med* 1988;3:370–380; Sulmasy DP, Lehmann LS, Levine DM, Faden RR. Patients' perceptions of the quality of informed consent for common medical procedures. *J Clin Ethics* 1994;5:189–194; and Braddock CL III, Fihn SD, Levinson W, Jonsen AR, Pearlman RA. How doctors and patients discuss routine clinical decisions: informed decision making in the outpatient setting. *J Gen Intern Med* 1997;12:339–345. An annotated bibliography reviewing published studies on this topic is available: Sugarman J, McCrory DC, Powell D, et al. Empirical research on informed consent: an annotated bibliography. *Hastings Cent Rep* 1999;29(1 Suppl):S1–S42.

5. See Meisel A. A "dignitary tort" as a bridge between the idea of informed consent and the law of informed consent. *Law Med Health Care* 1988;16:210–218. For general references on consent issues, see Berg JW, Appelbaum PJ. *Informed Consent: Legal Theory and Clinical Practice*, 2nd ed. New York: Oxford University Press, 2001; Katz J. *The Silent World of Doctor and Patient*. Baltimore: Johns Hopkins University Press, 2002; Faden RR, Beauchamp TL, King NMP. *A History and Theory of Informed Consent*. New York: Oxford University Press, 1986; Miller LJ. Informed consent. Parts I-IV. *JAMA* 1980;244:2100–2103, 2347–2350, 2556–2558, 2661–2662; Rosoff AJ. *Informed Consent: A Guide for Health Care Providers*. Rockville, MD: Aspen, 1981;

Rozovsky FA. *Consent to Treatment: A Practical Guide.* 2nd ed. Boston: Little, Brown, 1990; and Applebaum PS, Grisso T. Assessing patients' capacities to consent to treatment. *N Engl J Med* 1988;319:1635–1638. For the particular legal issues in obtaining consent from minors, see Holder AR. Minors' rights to consent to medical care. *JAMA* 1987;257:3400–3402 and Holder AR. Disclosure and consent problems in pediatrics. *Law Med Health Care* 1988;16:219–228. For a history of consent issues in neurology, see Faden AI, Faden RR. Informed consent in medical practice with particular reference to neurology. *Arch Neurol* 1978;35:761–764.

6. Meisel A, Kuczewski M. Legal and ethical myths about informed consent. *Arch Intern Med* 1996;156:2521–2526.

7. Gert B, Culver CM, Clouser KD. *Bioethics: A Return to Fundamentals*, 2nd ed. 2006:213–236.

8. Rosoff AJ. *Informed Consent* 14–19.

9. American Academy of Neurology. Consent issues in the management of cerebrovascular diseases. A position paper of the American Academy of Neurology Ethics and Humanities Committee. *Neurology* 1999;53:9–11. Although now there is greater evidence of efficacy of IV rtPA for threatened stroke than in 1999 (see Hacke W, Donnan G, Fieschi C, et al. Association of outcome with early stroke treatment: pooled analysis of ATLANTIS, ECASS, and NINDS rt-PA stroke trials. *Lancet* 2004;363:768–774), the fundamental issue remains unchanged that a non-trivial percentage of patients and surrogates refuse consent for its administration. The American Academy of Emergency Medicine stated, "It is the position of the American Academy of Emergency Medicine that objective evidence regarding the efficacy, safety, and applicability of tPA for acute ischemic stroke is insufficient to warrant its classification as standard of care." See Goyal DG, Li J, Mann J, Schriger DL. Position statement of the American Academy of Emergency Medicine on the use of intravenous thrombolytic therapy in the treatment of stroke. http://www.aaem.org/positionstatements/thrombolytictherapy.php (Accessed June 14, 2007).

10. Rosenbaum JR, Bravata DM, Concato J, Brass LM, Kim N, Fried TR. Informed consent for thrombolytic therapy for patients with acute ischemic stroke treated in routine clinical practice. *Stroke* 2004;35:e353–355.

11. For discussions of unconsented emergency administration of IV rtPA, see Fleck LM, Hayes OW. Ethics and consent to treat issues in acute stroke therapy. *Emerg Med Clin North Am* 2002;20:703–715 and Ciccone A. Consent to thrombolysis in acute ischaemic stroke: from trial to practice. *Lancet Neurology* 2003;2:375–378.

12. White-Bateman SR, Schumacher HC, Sacco RL, Appelbaum PS. Consent for intravenous thrombolysis in acute stroke: review and future directions. *Arch Neurol* 2007;64:785–792.

13. The legal and ethical basis for the reasonable person standard is reviewed in Piper A Jr. Truce on the battlefield: a proposal for a different approach to medical informed consent. *J Law Med Ethics* 1994;22:301–317.

14. Gert HJ. Avoiding surprises: a model for informing patients. *Hastings Cent Rep* 2002;32(5):23–32.

15. Culver CM. Gert B. *Semin Neurol* 1984;4:1–4.

16. Mazur DJ, Hickam DH, Mazur MD, Mazur MD. The role of doctor's opinion in shared decision making: what does shared decision making really mean when considering invasive medical procedures? *Health Expectations* 2005;8:97–1102.

17. Culver CM. Gert B. *Semin Neurol* 1984;4:1–4; Gert B, Nelson WA, Culver CM. *Neurol Clin* 1989;7:690–693.

18. See Tversky A, Kahneman D. The framing of decisions and the psychology of choice. *Science* 1981;211:453–458 and Malenka DJ, Baron JA, Johansen S, et al. The framing effect of relative and absolute risk. *J Gen Intern Med* 1993;8:543–548.

19. Murphy DJ. Do-not-resuscitate orders: time for re-appraisal in long-term-care institutions. *JAMA* 1988;260:2098–2101. These findings were confirmed in a later study in which the percentage of elderly patients requesting CPR dropped from 41% to as low as 5% after the patients were informed of the probability they would survive CPR. Murphy DJ, Burrows D, Santilli S, et al. The influence of the probability of survival on patients' preferences regarding cardiopulmonary resuscitation. *N Engl J Med* 1994;330:545–549. Data on CPR outcomes in the context of medical futility are reviewed in chapter 10.

20. Epstein RM, Alper BS, Quill TE. Communicating evidence for participatory decision making. *JAMA* 2004;291:2359–2366.

21. Shalowitz DI, Wolf MS. Shared decision-making and the lower literate patient. *J Law Med Ethics* 2004;32:759–764.

22. Schonwetter RS, Walker RM, Kramer DR, et al. Resuscitation decision making in the elderly: the value of outcome data. *J Gen Intern Med* 1993;8:295–300. See also Blackhall LJ. Must we always use CPR? *N Engl J Med* 1987;317:1281–1285.

23. Baron J. A decision analysis of consent. *Am J Bioethics* 2006;6:46–52. See his longer argument defending this concept in Baron J. *Against Bioethics.* Cambridge, MA: MIT Press, 2006.

24. Legal usage of the terms "competency" and "incompetency" refers to the capacity of a person to make independent decisions, a capacity that can be conferred only through formal legal proceedings. However, whenever I use the word "competence," I refer only to the clinical, non-legal usage defined in the text. It is more convenient to say "competence" than "the capacity to make medical decisions."

25. Lo B. Assessing decision-making capacity. *Law Med Health Care* 1990;18:193–201.

26. Gert B, Culver CM, Clouser KD. *Bioethics: A Return to Fundamentals,* 1997:131–148.

27. Other scholars have used the term "simple consent," not as defined by Gert and colleagues, but to describe patient consent for low-risk interventions that require a minimum of information and counseling. See Whitney SN, McGuire AL, McCullough LB. A typology of shared decision making, informed consent, and simple consent. *Ann Intern Med* 2003;140:54–59.

28. Gert B, Culver CM, Clouser KD. *Bioethics: A Return to Fundamentals,* 1997:131–148; Culver CM, Gert B. *Semin Neurol* 1984;4:1–4; and Gert B, Nelson WA, Culver CM. *Neurol Clin* 1989;7:691–693.

29. Auerswald KB, Charpentier PA, Inouye SK. The informed consent process in older patients who developed delirium: a clinical epidemiologic study. *Am J Med* 1997;103:410–418.

30. Finucane TE, Beamer BA, Roca RP, et al. Establishing advance medical directives with demented patients: a pilot study. *J Clin Ethics* 1993;4:51–54; and Goold SD, Arnold RM, Siminoff LA. Discussions about limiting treatment in a geriatric clinic. *J Am Geriatr Soc* 1993;41:277–281. The use of advance directives in the demented patient is considered further in chapter 15.

31. Karlawish JHT, Casarett DJ, James BD, Xie SX, Kim SYH. The ability of persons with Alzheimer disease (AD) to make a decision about taking an AD treatment. *Neurology* 2005;64:1514–1519.

32. Gurrera RJ, Moye J, Karel MJ, Azar AR, Armesto JC. Cognitive performance predicts treatment decisional abilities in mild to moderate dementia. *Neurology* 2006;66:1367–1372.

33. Alexander MP. Clinical determination of mental competence: a theory and a retrospective study. *Arch Neurol* 1988;45:23–26; Freedman M, Stuss DT, Gordon M. Assessment of competency: the role of neurobehavioral deficits. *Ann Intern Med* 1991;115:203–208; Marson DC, Ingram KK, Cody HA, Harrell LE. Assessing the competency of patients with Alzheimer's disease under different legal standards: a prototype instrument. *Arch Neurol* 1995;52:949–954; and Marson DC, Chatterjee A, Ingram KK, Harrell LE. Toward a neurologic model of competency: cognitive predictors of capacity to consent in Alzheimer's disease using three different legal standards. *Neurology* 1996;46:666–672. Daniel Marson and colleagues also have applied the same instrument to test competency in patients with Parkinson's disease. See Dymek MP, Atchison P, Harrell L, Marson DC. Competency to consent to medical treatment in cognitively impaired patients with Parkinson's disease. *Neurology* 2001;56:17–24. The topic of consent in the demented patient is considered further in chapter 15.

34. Goodglass H. *Understanding Aphasia.* New York: Academic Press, 1993.

35. Au R, Albert ML, Obler LK. The relation of aphasia to dementia. *Aphasiology* 1988;2:161–173.

36. Braunack-Mayer A, Hersh D. An ethical voice in the silence of aphasia: judging understanding and consent in people with aphasia. *J Clin Ethics* 2001;12:388–396.

37. See Brock DW, Wartman, SA. When competent patients make irrational choices. *N Engl J Med* 1990;322:1595–1599 and Kerridge I, Lowe M, Mitchell K. Competent patients, incompetent decisions. *Ann Intern Med* 1995;123:878–881.

38. Gert B, Culver CM, Clouser KD. *Bioethics: A Return to Fundamentals.* 1997:26–31.

39. Brock DW, Wartman SA. *N Engl J Med* 1990;332:1597–1598. For advice on how to respond to irrational denial as a psychological defense, see Ness DE, Ende J. Denial in the medical interview: recognition and management. *JAMA* 1994;272:1777–1781. For a look at how clinicians' determinations of patients' decision-making capacity can be more difficult than they first appear, see Morreim EH. Impairments and impediments in patients' decision making: reframing the competence question. *J Clin Ethics* 1993;4:294–307.

40. See Ridley DT. Jehovah's Witnesses' refusal of blood: obedience to scripture and religious conscience. *J Med Ethics* 1999;25:469–472; Muramoto O. Bioethics of the refusal of blood by Jehovah's Witnesses: should

bioethical deliberation consider dissidents' views? *J Med Ethics* 1998;24:223–230; Letsoalo JL. Law, blood transfusion, and Jehovah's Witnesses. *Med Law* 1998;17:633–638; and Groudine SB. The child Jehovah's Witness patient: a legal and ethical dilemma. *Surgery* 1997;121:357–358.

41. See the thoughtful discussion of the complexities in such cases in: Pomerantz SD, de Nesnera A. Informed consent, competency, and the illusion of rationality. *Gen Hosp Psychiatry* 1991;13:138–142.

42. Redelmeier DA, Rozin P, Kahneman D. Understanding patients' decisions. Cognitive and emotional perspectives. *JAMA* 1993;270:72–76. See also Merz JF, Fischoff B. Informed consent does not mean rational consent: cognitive limitations on decision-making. *J Legal Med* 1990;11:321–350.

43. These biases are fully described in Bogardus ST, Holmboe E, Jekel JF. Perils, pitfalls, and possibilities in talking about medical risk. *JAMA* 1999;281:1037–1041. See also Mazur DJ, Hickam DH. Patients' interpretation of probability terms. *J Gen Intern Med* 1991;6:237–240.

44. Ende J, Kazis L, Ash A, et al. Measuring patients' desire for autonomy: decision making and information-seeking preferences among medical patients. *J Gen Intern Med* 1989;4:23–30 and Strull W, Lo B, Charles G. Do patients want to participate in medical decision making? *JAMA* 1984;252:2990–2994.

45. Sherlock R. Reasonable men and sick human beings. *Am J Med* 1986;80:2–4.

46. Loewy EH. In defense of paternalism. *Theor Med Bioethics* 2005;26:445–468. Some scholars argue that physicians can make certain medical decisions without their patients consent or knowledge. See Whitney SN, McCullough LB. Physicians' silent decisions: autonomy does not always come first. *Am J Bioethics* 2007; 7(7):33–38.

47. Woolf SH, Chan ECY, Harris R, et al. Promoting informed choice: transforming health care to dispense knowledge for decision making. *Ann Intern Med* 2005;143:293–300.

48. Ubel PA. What should I do, doc? Some psychologic benefits of physician recommendations. *Arch Intern Med* 2002;162:977–980.

49. Cassell EJ, Leon AC, Kaufman SG. Preliminary evidence of impaired thinking in sick patients. *Ann Intern Med* 2001;134:1120–1123.

50. Wulff HR. The inherent paternalism in clinical practice. *J Med Philosophy* 1995;20:299–311.

51. Gert B, Culver CM, Clouser KD. *Bioethics: A Return to Fundamentals*, 2nd ed. 2006:238–252.

52. In their current edition, Gert and colleagues argued that an analysis to justify paternalistic acts should address the 10 questions that must be answered when justifying the violation of a moral rule. See Gert B, Culver CM, Clouser KD. *Bioethics: A Return to Fundamentals*, 2nd ed 2006:252–278. The simplified and clinically more accessible justification criteria presented here were proposed in their previous edition: Gert B, Culver CM, Clouser KD. *Bioethics: A Return to Fundamentals*, 1997:26–31.

53. Culver CM, Gert B. *Semin Neurol* 1984;4:7–8.

54. In such circumstances, it is desirable also to urgently contact the hospital risk management service or general counsel for legal and administrative advice. It may be possible or desirable to secure a court order for treatment that immunizes the physician.

55. *In re Quackenbush* 156 NJ Super 282, 383 A2d 785 (1978).

56. For example, see Marzuk PM. The right kind of paternalism. *N Engl J Med* 1985;113:1474–1476 and Carnerie F. Crisis and informed consent: analysis of a law-medicine malocclusion. *Am J Law Med* 1986;12:55–97.

57. Swanson JW, McCrary SV, Swartz MS, Van Dorn RA. Overriding psychiatric advance directives: factors associated with psychiatrists' decisions to preempt patients' advance refusal of hospitalization and medication. *Law Hum Behav* 2007;31:77–90.

58. On the shared medical decision-making model, see King JS, Moulton BW. Rethinking informed consent: the case for shared medical decision-making. *Am J Law Med* 2006;32:429–501; President's Commission for the Study of Ethical Problems in Medicine and Biomedical and Behavioral Research. *Making Health Care Decisions: The Ethical and Legal Implications of Informed Consent in the Patient-Practitioner Relationship.* Washington, DC: US Government Printing Office, 1982; Veatch RM. *The Patient-Physician Relation: The Patient as Partner*, Part 2. Bloomington: Indiana University Press, 1991:2–6; and Brock DW. The ideal of shared decision making between physicians and patients. *Kennedy Inst Ethics J* 1991;1:28–47. For an explanation of how autonomy has eclipsed paternalism in contemporary medical ethics, see Veatch RM. *A Theory of Medical Ethics.* New York: Basic Books, 1981 and Veatch RM. Autonomy's temporary triumph. *Hastings Cent Rep* 1984;14(5):18–40.

59. Charles C, Gafni A, Whelan T. Shared decision making in the medical encounter: what does it mean? (Or it takes at least two to tango). *Soc Sci Med* 1997;44:681–692.

60. Mazur DJ, Hickam DH, Mazur MD, Mazur MD. The role of doctor's opinion in shared decision making: what does shared decision making really mean when considering invasive medical procedures? *Health Expectations* 2005;8:97–1102.

61. See Quill TE, Brody H. Physician recommendation and patient autonomy: finding a balance between physician power and patient choice. *Ann Intern Med* 1996;125:763–769.

62. McNutt RA. Shared medical decision making: problems, process, progress. *JAMA* 2004;292: 2516–2518.

63. Bernat JL, Peterson LM. Patient-centered informed consent in surgical practice. *Arch Surg* 2006;141:86–92.

64. For example, see the offerings at the Dartmouth-Hitchcock Medical Center's Center for Shared Decision Making. http://www.dhmc.org/webpage.cfm?site_id=2&org_id=108&gsec_id=0&sec_id=0&item_id=2486 (Accessed May 8, 2007).

65. Barry MJ. Health decision aids to facilitate shared decision making in office practice. *Ann Intern Med* 2002;136:127–135; Ottawa Health Research Institute. *Patient Decision Aids.* http://decisionaid.ohri.ca/cochsystem .html (Accessed May 8, 2007); O'Connor AM, Stacey D, Entwhistle V, et al. Decision aids for people facing health treatment or screening decisions. *Cochrane Systematic Reviews* 2004. http://decisionaid.ohri.ca/docs/ Cochrane_Summary.pdf (Accessed May 8, 2007); and Foundation for Informed Medical Decision Making. Decision support: shared decision making programs, 2006. http://www.fimdm.org/decision_sdms.php (Accessed May 8, 2007).

66. Weinstein JN, Clay K, Morgan TS. Informed patient choice: patient-centered valuing of surgical risks and benefits. *Health Affairs* 2007;26:726–730.

67. For example, see Mazur DJ, Hickam DH. Patients' preferences for risk disclosure and role in decision making for invasive medical procedures. *J Gen Intern Med* 1997;12:114–117 and Levinson W. Kao A, Kuby A, Thisted RA. Not all patients want to participate in decision making: a national study of public preferences. *J Gen Intern Med* 2005;20:531–535.

68. King JS, Moulton BW. Rethinking informed consent: the case for shared medical decision-making. *Am J Law Med* 2006;32:429–501.

69. I discuss these points further in Bernat JL, Peterson LM. Patient-centered informed consent in surgical practice. *Arch Surg* 2006;141:86–92. See also Dagi TF. Changing the paradigm for informed consent. *J Clin Ethics* 1994;5:246–250.

70. Whitney SN, McGuire AL, McCullough LB. A typology of shared decision making, informed consent, and simple consent. *Ann Intern Med* 2003;140:54–59.

71. American Academy of Neurology. Consent issues in the management of cerebrovascular diseases. A position paper of the American Academy of Neurology Ethics and Humanities Subcommittee. *Neurology* 1999; 53:9–11.

72. Lloyd A, Hayes P, Bell PR, Naylor PR. The role of risk and benefit perception in informed consent for surgery. *Med Decision Making* 2001;21:141–149.

73. Ross N. Improving surgical consent. *Lancet* 2004;364:812–813. Universal procedure consent forms can improve the frequency of obtaining informed consent for procedures in the ICU. See Davis N, Pohlman A, Gehlbach B, et al. Improving the process of informed consent in the critically ill. *JAMA* 2003; 289:1963–1968.

74. Eighteen years is the age of majority in most American jurisdictions.

75. I have summarized and reviewed these data elsewhere: Bernat JL. Informed consent in pediatric neurology. *Semin Pediatr Neurol* 2001 (in press).

76. American Academy of Pediatrics Committee on Bioethics. Informed consent, parental permission, and assent in pediatric practice. *Pediatrics* 1995;95:314–317.

77. Weithorn LA. *Competency to Render Informed Treatment Decisions: A Comparison for Certain Minors and Adults.* Pittsburgh, PA: University of Pittsburgh Press, 1980. The methodology of this study recently was criticized and its conclusions questioned. See Deatrick JA, Dickey SB, Wright R, et al. Correlates of children's competence to make healthcare decisions. *J Clin Ethics* 2003;14:152–163.

78. American Academy of Pediatrics Committee on Bioethics *Pediatrics* 1995:315–316.

79. Ross LF. Health care decision making by children. Is it in their best interest? *Hastings Cent Rep* 1997;27(6):41–45. Other bioethicists have reached the opposite conclusion. See Hyun I. When adolescents "mismanage" their chronic medical conditions: an ethical exploration. *Kennedy Inst Ethics J* 2000; 10:147–163.

80. Hartman RG. Coming of age: devising legislation for adolescent medical decision-making. *Am J Law Med* 2002;28:409–453.

81. Alderson P, Sutcliffe K, Curtis K. Children's competence to consent to medical treatment. *Hastings Cent Rep* 2006;36(6):25–34.

82. Novack DH, Detering BJ, Arnold R, et al. Physicians' attitudes toward using deception to resolve difficult ethical problems. *JAMA* 1989;261:2980–2985.

83. Freeman VG, Rathore SS, Weinfurt KP, Schulman KA, Sulmasy DP. Lying for patients: physician deception of third-party payers. *Arch Intern Med* 1999;159:2263–2270.

84. Wynia MK, Cummins DS, VanGeest JB, Wilson IB. Physician manipulation of reimbursement rules for patients: between a rock and a hard place. *JAMA* 2000;283:1858–1865. The incidence of medical residents using deception with each other and their supervisors was determined in Green MJ, Farber NJ, Ubel PA, et al. Lying to each other: when internal medicine residents use deception with their colleagues. *Arch Intern Med* 2000;160:2317–2323.

85. Werner RM, Alexander GC, Fagerlin A, Ubel PA. Lying to insurance companies: the desire to deceive among physicians and the public. *Am J Bioethics* 2004;4:53–59.

86. Werner RM, Alexander GC, Fagerlin A, Ubel PA. The "hassle factor": what motivates physicians to manipulate reimbursement rules? *Arch Intern Med* 2002;162:1134–1139.

87. Alexander GC, Werner RM, Fagerlin A, Ubel PA. Support for physician deception of insurance companies among a sample of Philadelphia residents. *Ann Intern Med* 2003;138:472–475.

88. Bloche MG. Fidelity and deceit at the bedside. *JAMA* 2000;283:1881–1884.

89. Bogardus ST, Geist DE, Bradley EH. Physicians' interactions with third-party payers: is deception necessary? *Arch Intern Med* 2004;164:1841–1844.

90. Morreim EH. Gaming the system: dodging the rules, ruling the dodgers. *Arch Intern Med* 1991;151:443–447.

91. See Elian M, Dean G. To tell or not to tell the diagnosis of multiple sclerosis. *Lancet* 1985:291:27–28; Sencer W. Suspicion of multiple sclerosis: to tell or not to tell? *Arch Neurol* 1988;45:441–442; and Drickamer MA, Lachs MS. Should patients with Alzheimer's disease be told their diagnosis? *N Engl J Med* 1992;326:947–951. For similar discussions of telling the truth to cancer patients, see Freedman B. Offering truth: one ethical approach to the uninformed cancer patients. *Arch Intern Med* 1993;153:572–576 and Thomsen OO, Wulff HR, Martin A, et al. What do gastroenterologists in Europe tell cancer patients? *Lancet* 1993;341:473–476.

92. These points are discussed in Gillon R. Telling the truth and medical ethics. *Lancet* 1985;291:1556–1557. See also Weir R. Truth telling in medicine. *Perspect Biol Med* 1980;195–212; and Bok S. *Lying: Moral Choice in Public and Private Life.* New York: Vintage Books, 1978. For a review of the physician's legal duty to disclose serious diagnoses, see Capron AM. Duty, truth, and whole human beings. *Hastings Cent Rep* 1993;23(4):14.

93. Mushlin AI, Mooney C, Grow V, et al. The value of diagnostic information to patients with suspected multiple sclerosis. *Arch Neurol* 1994;51:67–72 and O'Connor P, Detsky AS, Tansey C, et al. Effect of diagnostic testing for multiple sclerosis on patient health perceptions. *Arch Neurol* 1988;45:553–556.

94. Elian M, Dean G. *Lancet* 1985;291:27–28; Burnfield A. Doctor-patient dilemmas in multiple sclerosis. *J Med Ethics* 1984;10:21–26; and Beisecker AE, Cobb AK, Ziegler DK. Patients' perspectives of the role of care providers in amyotrophic lateral sclerosis. *Arch Neurol* 1988;45:553–556.

95. Helft PR. An intimate collaboration: prognostic communication with advanced cancer patients. *J Clin Ethics* 2006;17:110–121.

96. *Arato v Avedon*, 5 Cal 4th 1172, 23 Call Rptr 2d 131, 858 P 2d 598 (1993); *Arato v Avedon*, 13 Cal App 4th 1325, 11 Cal Rptr 2d 169 (1992). The medicolegal implications of this confusing ruling were discussed in Annas GJ. Informed consent, cancer, and truth in prognosis. *N Engl J Med* 1994;330:223–225.

97. Bostick NA, Sade R, McMahon JW, Benjamin R. Report of the American Medical Association Council on Ethical and Judicial Affairs: Withholding information from patients: rethinking the propriety of "therapeutic privilege." *J Clin Ethics* 2006;17:302–306.

98. Sirotin N, Lo B. The end of therapeutic privilege? *J Clin Ethics* 2006;17:312–316.

99. Bowman K. What are the limits of bioethics in a culturally pluralistic society? *J Law Med Ethics* 2004;32:664–669.

100. For examples of studies of cross-cultural issues in truth telling, see Pellegrino ED. Is truth telling a cultural artifact? *JAMA* 1992;268:1734–1735; Jecker N, Caresse J, Pearlman R. Caring for patients in

cross-cultural settings. *Hastings Cent Rep* 1995;25(1):6–14; and Macklin R. Ethical relativism in a multicultural society. *Kennedy Inst Ethics J* 1998;8:1–22. The Pakistani practices are described in Moazam F. Families, patients, and physicians in medical decisionmaking: a Pakistani perspective. *Hastings Cent Rep* 2000;30(6):28–37. Japanese practices are described in Akabayashi A, Slingsby BT. Informed consent revisited: Japan and the U.S. *Am J Bioethics* 2006;6:9–14.

101. Oken D. What to tell cancer patients: a study of medical attitudes. *JAMA* 1961;175:1120–1128.

102. Anderlik MR, Pentz RD, Hess KR. Revisiting the truth-telling debate: a study of disclosure practices at a major cancer center. *J Clin Ethics* 2000;11:251–259.

103. On the delicate balance of physicians' duties to respect patients' cultural values and to tell the truth, see Kuczewski M, McCruden PJ. Informed consent: does it take a village? The problem of culture and truth telling. *Camb Q Healthc Ethics* 2001;10:34–46; and Hyun I. Waiver of informed consent, cultural sensitivity, and the problem of unjust families and traditions. *Hastings Cent Rep* 2002;32(5):14–22.

104. See the discussions on these points in Howard R. Should the diagnosis of Alzheimer's disease always be disclosed? In Zeman A, Emanuel LL, eds. *Ethical Dilemmas in Neurology.* London: W. B. Saunders Co, 2000:54–60 and Wessely S. To tell or not to tell? The problem of medically unexplained symptoms. In Zeman A, Emanuel LL, eds. *Ethical Dilemmas in Neurology.* London: W. B. Saunders Co, 2000:41–53.

105. See Quill TE, Townsend P. Bad news: delivery, dialogue, and dilemmas. *Arch Intern Med* 1991;151:463–468; Fallowfield L. Giving sad or bad news. *Lancet* 1993;341:476–478; Buckman R. *How to Break Bad News: A Guide for Health Care Professionals.* Baltimore: Johns Hopkins University Press, 1992; and Buckman R, Korsch B, Baile W. *A Practical Guide to Communication Skills in Clinical Practice* on CD ROM. Medical Audio Visual Communications, Inc, 1998 (http://www.mavc.com). For talking to children with dread diseases, see Lipson M. What do you say to a child with AIDS? *Hastings Cent Rep* 1993; 23(2):6–12.

106. For general references on placebo use in clinical medicine, see Harrington A (ed). *The Placebo Effect: An Interdisciplinary Exploration.* Cambridge, MA: Harvard University Press, 1997; and Shapiro AK, Shapiro E. *The Powerful Placebo: From Ancient Priest to Modern Physician.* Baltimore: Johns Hopkins University Press, 1997.

107. Shapiro AK. The placebo effect in the history of medical treatment: implications for psychiatry. *Am J Psychiatry* 1964;116:298–304.

108. Chaput de Saintonge DM, Herxheimer A. Harnessing placebo effects in health care. *Lancet* 1994;344:995–998. However, a recent meta-analysis of 130 placebo-controlled trials found little for evidence for significant placebo effects in clinical medicine other than for the treatment of pain and other subjective outcomes. See Hróbjartsson A, Gøtzsche PC. Is the placebo powerless? An analysis of clinical trials comparing placebo with no treatment. *N Engl J Med* 2001;344:1594–1602.

109. Gøtzsche PC. Is there logic in the placebo? *Lancet* 1994;344:925–926.

110. See Levine JD, Gordon NC, Fields HL. The mechanism of placebo analgesia. *Lancet* 1978;2:654–657 and Grevert P, Albert LH, Goldstein A. Partial antagonism of placebo analgesia by naloxone. *Pain* 1983;16:129–143.

111. See Adler HM, Hammett VO. The doctor-patient relationship revisited: an analysis of the placebo effect. *Ann Intern Med* 1973;78:595–598; Silber TJ. Placebo therapy: the ethical dimension. *JAMA* 1979;242:245–246; and Simmons B. Problems in deceptive medical procedures: an ethical and legal analysis of the administration of placebos. *J Med Ethics* 1978;4:172–181.

112. American Medical Association Council on Ethical and Judicial Affairs. Placebo use in clinical practice. CEJA Report 1-A-06 (2006). http://www.ama-assn.org/ama1/pub/upload/mm/369/ceja_recs_2i06.pdf (Accessed June 13, 2007).

113. Bok S. The ethics of giving placebos. *Sci Am* 1974;231(5):17–23.

114. Jonsen AR, Siegler M, Winslade WJ. *Clinical Ethics,* 2nd ed. New York: Macmillan, 1986:69–72.

115. I edited and shortened the criteria. See Lichtenberg P, Heresco-Levy U, Nitzan U. The ethics of the placebo in clinical practice. *J Med Ethics* 2004;30:551–554.

116. Brody H. The lie that heals: the ethics of giving placebos. *Ann Intern Med* 1982;97: 112–118.

117. Moerman DE, Jonas WB. Deconstructing the placebo effect and finding the meaning response. *Ann Intern Med* 2002;136:471–476.

118. Hahn RA. The nocebo phenomenon: concept, evidence, and implications for public health. *Prev Med* 1997;26:607–611.

119. The prevalence of using placebo provocation of nonepileptic seizures was studied in Schachter SC, Brown F, Rowan AJ. Provocative testing for nonepileptic seizures: attitudes and practice in the United States among American Epilepsy Society members. *J Epilepsy* 1996;9:249–252.

120. Smith ML, Stagno SJ, Dolske M et al. Induction procedures for psychogenic seizures: ethical and clinical considerations. *J Clin Ethics* 1997;8:217–229. See also the accompanying editorial: Howe EG. Deceiving patients for their own good. *J Clin Ethics* 1997;8:211–216.

121. Devinsky O, Fisher R. Ethical use of placebos and provocative techniques in diagnosing nonepileptic seizures. *Neurology* 1996;47:866–870.

122. Benbadis SR, Johnson K, Anthony K, et al. Induction of psychogenic nonepileptic seizures without placebo. *Neurology* 2000;55:1904–1905.

Professional Ethics and Professionalism

3

Neurologists, like all physicians and all learned professionals, are bound by a set of ethical duties to those whom they serve professionally. Physicians' ethical duties are owed primarily to their patients and secondarily to others: the families of patients, their fellow physicians, and society. This set of ethical responsibilities has been a defining characteristic of the medical profession since its beginnings and is intrinsic to the purpose and goals of medical practice. Rules arising from these ethical duties have been codified into standards of medical professional conduct since the time of Hippocrates[1] (see Appendix 3-1). These rules and duties comprise the subject of professional ethics.

Professional ethical duties of physicians exist because medicine is a learned profession dedicated primarily to the welfare of those whom physicians serve. In recognizing the benefits its citizens accrue from the services of physicians, society has granted the medical profession a high level of prestige, autonomy, income potential, and professional authority. Ethical duties of medical professionals can be conceptualized as the set of responsibilities that physicians owe their patients and society in return for society's authorization of them to act as privileged fiduciaries for its citizens' medical well-being. Physicians' singular ethical responsibility is to act in the best medical interests of their patients and to practice according to the profession's highest standards.

Under most circumstances, physicians' professional duties to patients, families of patients, and society are mutually compatible. Ethical dilemmas arise in those instances in which ethical duties to one or more of these parties conflict. For example, what is a neurologist's duty to protect those known to be at risk when he discovers that his patient with uncontrolled epilepsy continues to drive an automobile despite his careful counsel that doing so is unsafe and illegal? Similarly, what is a physician's duty when his HIV-positive patient refuses to inform his wife of his diagnosis and continues to practice unprotected sexual intercourse with her? Does the physician's duty to protect a third party known to be at risk for harm justify compromising his responsibility to maintain patient confidentiality? These dilemmas can be resolved only if clinicians understand their professional duties and analyze the goods and harms accrued by each action.

PROFESSIONALISM

Clinicians can understand professional ethics more readily by first identifying the characteristics of a learned profession. The term "profession" is derived from the Latin *professio*, meaning a public oath of fealty, or turning over one's obedience and loyalty to another.[2] The essence of professionalism is maintaining primacy of the concern for the welfare of those whom the professional serves above his own proprietary and personal interests. Medicine, law, and the clergy were the original learned professions. In an essay decrying the contemporary deprofessionalization of medicine,

49

Reed and Evans enumerated the defining characteristics of a learned profession:

1. The profession possesses a circumscribed and socially valuable body of knowledge.

2. The members of the profession determine the profession's standards of knowledge and expertise.

3. The profession attracts high-quality students who undergo an extensive socialization process as they are absorbed into the profession.

4. The profession is given authority to license practitioners by the state, with licensing and admission boards made up largely of members of the profession.

5. There is an ostensible sense of community and mutuality of interests among members of a profession.

6. Social policy and legislation that relate to the profession are heavily influenced by members of the profession through such mechanisms as lobbying and expert testimony.

7. The profession has a code of ethics that governs practice, the tenets of which are more stringent than legal controls.

8. A service orientation supersedes the proprietary interests of the professionals.

9. A profession is a terminal occupation, that is, it is the practitioners' singular and lifelong occupational choice.

10. A profession is largely free of lay control, with its practitioners exercising a high degree of occupational autonomy.[3]

The ethical duties of physicians *qua* professionals arise from these characteristics. Despite the unfortunate trend in the United States toward medical commercialization, medicine is a learned profession, not a business. All codes of professional conduct clearly require physicians to place the welfare of their patients before their own financial interests whenever the two interests conflict. Thus, the practices of kickback payments, fee-splitting, and unregulated physician ownership of free-standing facilities to which their patients are referred but in which they have no professional responsibility are not only unethical professional arrangements, they are objectionable behaviors because they lead ultimately to the commercialization and deprofessionalization of medicine.

Recognizing the need to rededicate a commitment to instilling professionalism in practicing physicians in the 21st century, the principal American and European internal medicine societies drafted *Medical Professionalism in the New Millennium: A Physician Charter*, a document that explains the meaning of medical professionalism and emphasizes its critical importance.[4] The Charter pointed out that professionalism constituted the basis of medicine's contract with society. It asserted three fundamental principles that underlie the ethical practice of medicine: (1) the primacy of patient welfare; (2) the principle of patient autonomy; and (3) the principle of social justice. Ten professional responsibilities of physicians flowed directly from these principles: (1) commitment to professional competence; (2) commitment to honesty with patients; (3) commitment to patient confidentiality; (4) commitment to maintaining appropriate relations with patients; (5) commitment to improving quality of care; (6) commitment to improving access to care; (7) commitment to a just distribution of finite resources; (8) commitment to scientific knowledge; (9) commitment to maintaining trust by managing conflicts of interest; and (10) commitment to professional responsibilities.[5]

The *Charter* has been endorsed by over 90 medical societies and certifying boards in the United States and Europe.[6] A contemporaneous effort by the Royal College of Physicians Working Party on Medical Professionalism produced a similar document with the same intent.[7] Some scholars endorsing the *Charter* pointed out its unintended limitations that resulted from viewing professionalism only from the physician perspective without also considering the views of society, patients, and other health workers.[8] The limits placed by United States law on the practice of medicine as a learned profession have been detailed.[9] Educational curricula dedicated to teaching professionalism continue to be created by medical schools and professional societies.[10] The Accreditation Council on Graduate Medical Education identified professionalism as one of six key proficiencies that must be learned by all residents in specialty training programs to maintain accreditation.[11] The American Academy of Neurology enumerated the humanistic dimensions of professionalism that are desirable for practitioners of neurology.[12]

ETHICAL DUTIES TO PATIENTS

Professional medical ethics focuses principally on the set of duties physicians owe their patients. This set of ethical obligations encompasses all the physician's responsibilities related to the initiation, maintenance, and discontinuation of the patient-physician relationship.[13]

The Patient-Physician Relationship

The patient-physician relationship has been modeled three ways: (1) as a covenantal relationship in which physician beneficence to the patient is a cardinal feature; (2) as a fiduciary relationship in which the physician as professional has a duty to grant primacy to the patient's interests in clinical decision making; and (3) as a contractual relationship in which, physicians have implicitly (and sometimes explicitly) agreed obligations to their patients.[14] The physician's contractual obligation, based on the fact that both the physicians and patients have agreed to be parties to an unwritten, implied contract, requires the physician to practice competently and to respect the patient's confidentiality, autonomy, and welfare. The patient also has implied reciprocal duties of honesty in disclosing symptoms and relevant medical history and of fidelity in cooperating with the agreed-upon treatment plan.[15] Patients and physicians thereby become partners who share the a goal of improving and maintaining the patient's health.[16] The patient has an additional personal responsibility to maintain her own health by adopting a healthy lifestyle.[17] A critical component in the relationship is accountability. Ezekiel and Linda

Emanuel have thoughtfully analyzed the various elements of accountability in health care and have devised a stratified model that balances physicians' professional, political, and economic accountability to patients, employers, payers, professional associations, investors, and the government.[18]

Marc Rodwin defined the concept of the fiduciary. The fiduciary is "a person entrusted with power or property to be used for the benefit of another and legally held to the highest standard of conduct." Rodwin cited eight criteria of fiduciaries: (1) they advise and represent others and manage their affairs; (2) they have specialized knowledge or expertise; (3) their work requires judgment and discretion; (4) the party the fiduciary serves cannot monitor the fiduciary's performance; (5) the relationship is based on dependence, reliance, and trust; (6) fiduciaries must be scrupulously honest; (7) they must not divulge confidential client information; and (8) they may not promote their own interests or those of third parties.[19] A physician's fiduciary role imparts ethical duties to maintain the primacy of the patient's interests.

Within certain bounds, the physician is free to initiate and to discontinue the patient-physician relationship. The appropriately trained physician should not decline to provide medical care for a patient merely on the basis of the patient's age, race, nationality, religion, gender, or sexual orientation. Once the relationship has been initiated, the physician has an obligation to continue to provide needed medical care until one of the following outcomes has occurred: (1) the patient ends the relationship; (2) the physician directs the patient's care back to the referring physician or to another physician; or (3) the physician determines that no further medical care is necessary or desirable. If the physician chooses to end the relationship and the patient requires or desires further medical care, the ethical duty of fidelity obliges the physician to help assure the continuity of care by assisting the patient in obtaining care from another physician.[20]

A physician's decision not to care for a patient should not be based solely on the patient's disease (assuming the competence to treat) or on a falsely exaggerated perception of personal medical risk. Physicians entering the medical profession make a moral commitment to care for sick patients. This commitment entails willingness to assume some degree of risk to one's health. Throughout the history of medicine, physicians have risked contracting communicable diseases from their patients such as tuberculosis, hepatitis, and plague. Most recently, this issue has resurfaced concerning the care of patients with human immunodeficiency virus (HIV) infections. Because HIV infection is a communicable and often fatal disease that can be contracted from a patient under certain circumstances, the question of whether a physician has the duty to treat HIV patients has arisen.[21] This topic is considered further in chapter 18.

There is a clear consensus on the physician's ethical duty to treat HIV patients. Medical societies, including the American Medical Association, the American College of Physicians, the Infectious Diseases Society of America, and the American Academy of Neurology, as well as the Surgeon General of the United States, have stated this responsibility formally.[22] Physicians have an ethical duty to treat sick patients, even if doing so exposes them to risk, because of the implicit and explicit moral commitment they made when entering the medical profession. Rather than refusing to care for HIV patients, each physician should take appropriate "universal precautions" to minimize his own health risks in treating patients who may have communicable diseases.[23]

Physicians need to understand and respect the health-care values and preferences of their patients. Physicians can take a "values history" in which they ask specific questions to better understand patients' treatment wishes. The values history can be especially useful for surrogate decision makers when they attempt to apply their understanding of the patient's values to a particular clinical situation that may have been unanticipated by the patient.[24] Patients' values and treatment preferences may be quite different from those of physicians and patients' surrogate decision makers. One limitation of relying on an established values history is that patients' values may change with time and circumstance. Nevertheless, in their attempt to help patients reach the correct treatment decisions, physicians should try to understand and respect patients' personal values.[25]

One controversial question that arises occasionally surrounds a physician's duty to provide or refer a patient for medical services that are lawful but violate the physician's moral or religious beliefs. Most people believe that physicians should not be forced to perform medical procedures with which they have moral opposition. But at the same time most people believe that patients have a right for access to legal treatments.[26] Many hospital regulations provide a "conscience-clause" mechanism for physicians or other health professionals to opt out of providing services, such as abortion, about which they have moral qualms. Many, but not all, hospital regulations also provide a mechanism for referring the patient elsewhere for these services. Farr Curlin and colleagues recently polled physicians about their judgments of the balance of ethical rights and obligations in such cases.[27] They found that 63% of physicians believed it was ethically acceptable to explain their moral objections to patients, 86% believed they were obligated to present all options, and 71% believed they were obligated to refer the patient elsewhere for desired services. Physicians who were male, religious, and morally opposed to the requested treatment were less likely to feel these obligations.

Confidentiality. Physicians must respect the confidentiality and privacy of patients. Information conveyed to a physician in the course of treating a patient should not be discussed publicly without the patient's consent. Similarly, the patient's medical record is a confidential document that should not be shared with a third party without the patient's consent unless required by law. If the law requires sharing the confidential document, the patient should at least be notified. The patient deserves access to the information contained in the medical record.

Confidentiality of medical records is becoming increasingly difficult to maintain because of the large number of allied personnel in hospitals who now have access to the record. Further, the copious photocopying and external distribution of records necessary for third-party health-care reimbursement also make confidentiality harder to maintain because the protection of records no longer can be assured once they leave the institution.[28]

The electronic medical record, now commonplace in many offices and most hospitals, improves efficiency but introduces a new set of confidentiality concerns. Currently, a huge range of confidential records can be accessed from any computer simply by gaining access to the system. This ease of access had created the need for enhanced electronic privacy systems to be installed.[29] Electronic mail (e-mail) now provides physicians and patients with a rapid means of communication but also raises confidentiality concerns that require vigilance.[30] Similarly, the internet has been used to communicate confidential patient information for clinical and research purposes, a field called "e-medicine."[31] In all instances, physicians must exercise constant vigilance to protect patients' confidentiality and privacy, including following institutional guidelines to protect the privacy of records in electronic media. Institutions can create secure internet links for patient-physician communication. Patients should be warned that there are categorical limits to the degree of protection of their confidentiality that physicians and systems can guarantee.

In response to concerns about the increasing difficulty in maintaining the confidentiality and privacy of medical records, the United States Congress enacted legislation in 2003 under the Health Insurance Portability and Accountability Act (HIPAA) creating the "Privacy Rule."[32] The "HIPAA regulations" (as they are generally known) comprise a compendium of detailed rules governing every conceivable aspect of using paper and electronic medical records. Its most basic rule for maintaining confidentiality is testing the "need to know." Only those persons or agencies with the need to know are permitted access to patient medical information. Primary or consulting clinicians caring for a patient obviously satisfy the need to know rule. But

anyone else who requests or sees information without a demonstrable need to know may be violating the regulation.

The HIPAA rules are so detailed and complex that many institutions have created compliance officers to study and understand them, to train personnel about the rules, and to assure they are followed consistently and faithfully. Their complexity has led to widespread misunderstandings of the actual provision of the HIPAA regulations.[33] Because of the fear of possibly violating a regulation and incurring the mandated punishment, some medical and office personnel have interpreted HIPAA regulations in an unnecessarily rigid way. Most practicing physicians have witnessed unfortunate instances in which the incorrect or over-zealous application of the HIPAA regulations produced harm to the very patients they were intended to protect by unjustifiably restricting appropriate medical communication among physicians and medical office personnel or the patient's family members.

Despite their complexity, there are gaps in the rules themselves, so situations arise that require interpretation. These gaps also offer opportunities for misinterpretation that can perversely impede proper physician-to-physician communication and create harms to patients. In some cases, physicians or office personnel may consider disclosing information that could violate the regulations to facilitate proper patient care. Bernard Lo and colleagues offered the following series of ethical guidelines for physicians and others to justify such incidental disclosures of medical information: (1) the communication should be necessary and effective for good patient care; (2) the risks of breaching confidentiality are proportional to the likely benefits; (3) the alternative means of communication are impractical; and (4) the communication practice should be transparent.[34] These commonsense guidelines should be followed in questionable cases. In general, an ethically correct action will be legally defensible.

Secrets. Physicians may be told unsolicited "secrets" about patients from well-wishing families and friends, with the admonition,

"Don't tell him I told you this." Examples of such secrets include a patient's covert drinking of alcohol, taking of illicit drugs, or refusing to follow prescribed medical therapy. Despite the admonition, physicians are not ethically obligated to withhold such "secrets" from their patients. Physicians can respond by encouraging the third party to speak directly to the patient about the matter. They also can urge the third party to encourage the patient to speak about it to the physician. Otherwise, the physician should inform well-wishing friends that he has an ethical obligation to disclose the information he has received to the patient, although he does not necessarily have to say from whom this information came.[35]

Communication. Physicians have the ethical obligation to communicate effectively with patients. Although effective communication is particularly important for obtaining consent, it is a critical component of the patient-physician relationship. Timothy Quill has enumerated several barriers to physician-patient communication that the clinician should identify and mitigate by using effective communication skills. Such barriers include: (1) verbal-nonverbal mismatch, in which the words a patient uses to answer a question are opposed diametrically and negated by his gestures; (2) cognitive dissonance, in which the patient "protests too much" that an obviously emotional factor is irrelevant to his problem; (3) unexpected resistance, in which the physician consciously or subconsciously overreacts to the patient's complaint; and (4) treatment inefficacy, in which treatments expected to be effective are ineffective for no apparent reason. To address these barriers, physicians need to acquire the basic communication and psychotherapeutic skills of acknowledgment, exploration, empathy, and legitimation.[36]

There are subconscious factors in the mind of the physician that can impact on the success of the patient-physician relationship. Novack and colleagues showed how increasing personal awareness of physicians about these factors improved the effectiveness of patient care. They suggested that physicians should become more aware of their beliefs and attitudes, their

feelings and emotional responses, their approach to challenging clinical situations (such as mistakes), and the importance of self-care (such maintaining an optimal balance between their personal and professional lives).[37] Several scholars have explained how the patient-physician relationship could become more therapeutic if the goal of the partnership could be shifted toward a greater patient orientation, a doctrine known as "patient-centered medicine."[38]

Physicians have the ethical duty to communicate effectively with consultants to whom the patient has been referred. Referring physicians should provide adequate information to permit consultants to identify the problem in question accurately. In turn, consultants should be clear and punctual in communicating their opinions to the referring physician. Facilitating this dialogue is an ethical duty because it promotes good patient care.[39] Consultants should be wary of informal "curbside consultation" in which they may be asked their opinions without an adequate opportunity to fully review the details of the case or examine the patient. In curbside consultations, generally it is safer to dispense factual information than opinion because the opinion may turn on assumptions (such as the accuracy of alleged findings on neurological examination) that may be erroneous.[40]

Public communication is another area in which physicians have ethical duties. Physicians should be cautious about providing medical opinions and specific advice during teleconferences and lectures, especially when they have not examined the patient and may have no relationship with the patient. The American Academy of Neurology Ethics, Law & Humanities Committee published a practice advisory to neurologists summarizing their ethical responsibilities when they publicly promote pharmaceuticals or medical equipment to patients.[41]

Empathy. Physicians should respect patients as persons and treat them with respect, courtesy, honesty, conscientiousness, and empathy. The precise meaning of empathy, however, remains a subject of debate.[42] Outside of medical practice, empathy refers to a mode of understanding of another person's suffering that involves emotional sharing and an affective resonance with the other person's feelings.[43] Yet, from the time of Sir William Osler's famous 1912 essay *Æquanimitas* in which he argued that by remaining emotionally detached from patients suffering, physicians could "see into" and "study" their patient's "inner life,"[44] the medical definition of empathy has restricted it to a cognitive state and not an affective state.

Organized medicine has followed Osler's advice. For example, a working group of the Society for General Internal Medicine defined empathy as "the act of acknowledging the emotional state of another without experiencing that state oneself."[45] Thus they distinguished empathy as "detached concern" from sympathy, in which the sympathetic person joined in the affective experience of the other person's suffering. But experienced physicians know that only by being engaged emotionally (to some extent) in another person's suffering can they be truly empathetic.[46]

The resolution of the affective-cognitive tension in empathy is for physicians to reach a balance permitting a limited degree of emotion that generates true empathy but creating enough detachment to allow the physician to treat the patient objectively.[47] In a frequently cited article, Howard Spiro asked if empathy was an innate characteristic or if it could be taught.[48] Fortunately, both the affective and cognitive components of empathy are amenable to learning. First, physicians can learn techniques to identify, understand, and regulate their own emotional responses to patient suffering to protect themselves and their objectivity.[49] Second, physicians can learn communications skills to project their understanding of the patient's feelings, even if they feel nothing themselves.[50] Suchman and colleagues showed that the basic empathic communication skills are recognizing when emotions are present but not directly expressed, inviting exploration of these unexpressed feelings, and effectively acknowledging these feelings so the patient feels understood.[51]

The physician-patient relationship becomes therapeutic because the physician treats the patient with kindness, respect, compassion, empathy and caring. Francis Weld Peabody epitomized the essence of ethical medical care in 1927 when he famously wrote: "One of the essential qualities of the clinician is interest in humanity, for the secret of the care of the patient is in caring for the patient."[52] In *Love in the Ruins*, the American physician-novelist Walker Percy explained the linkage between empathy and a physician's self-knowledge, "If you listen carefully to your patients, they will tell you not only what is wrong with them, but also what is wrong with you."[53]

Impediments. A patient has the right to decline a physician's suggested treatment plan, but a physician has no correlative obligation to provide a specific form of treatment at a patient's request, particularly if she believes that the treatment is not indicated or can be harmful. Sick patients may make requests for unorthodox treatments that are unproved, expensive, and potentially dangerous. In this instance, the physician has the duty to investigate the scientific basis of the treatment and the evidence for its efficacy. If this investigation reveals that the treatment is of no value, she should discuss these findings with the patient and dissuade the patient from pursuing such treatment. Although a chronically ill or dying patient may reason, "What have I got to lose?" he has much to lose. The fact that he may be beyond help does not mean that he is beyond being hurt. Harms that can be sustained from undergoing unorthodox treatments include pain, expense, physical side effects, displacement of possibly effective therapies or participation in a scientific treatment protocol, and false hope.[54] Physicians are ethically bound not to prescribe treatments that have predictably harmful net effects. Refusal to provide requested treatment on the grounds of medical futility is discussed in chapter 10.

Physicians at times may find themselves caring for a "hateful patient." Hateful patients include those who are antagonistic, self-destructive, manipulative, excessively dependent, poorly compliant, excessively demanding, or generally difficult to communicate with and care for.[55] "Hateful" refers to an affective response of physicians evoked by caring for such patients. In most circumstances, physicians have the right to discontinue the patient-physician relationship if they feel unable to provide proper care for such patients. The American Medical Association outlined the criteria for a physician to refuse to care for a noncompliant patient: (1) the patient is responsible for the noncompliant behavior because patients should not be punished for behavior that is beyond their control; (2) the treatment in question should not be lifesaving so patients are not required to pay for bad behavior with their lives; and (3) treatment of the patient would involve a clear and significant compromise of the care of other patients.[56]

Clinicians who continue to care for such patients, however, may find it a challenging and fulfilling experience because many difficult patients previously have been unable to relate successfully to other physicians. Expectations of desired therapeutic results in these patients should be lowered, and the physician satisfied with a reduced therapeutic relationship, but able to take consolation in helping a person whom other physicians have rejected.

Personal Conduct and Misconduct

The physician has a duty to practice competently and to restrict his practice to within the scope of his training, experience, and ability. Most states that require continued medical education for physician relicensure base this requirement largely on the clinician's ethical duty to maintain a practice according to the prevailing standards. Patients should be referred to a consultant if the referring physician is not competent to provide the specialized care. Physicians should refer patients only to competent consulting physicians.

Patients are vulnerable because of illness, fear, and dependency when they request the services of physicians. Physicians occupy a position of power in the patient-physician relationship and have a duty to exercise that power responsibly and in the patient's interest. In their powerful position, physicians must never exploit or otherwise abuse patients physically, sexually, psychologically, or financially.

It is unethical for a physician to have a sexual or romantic relationship with a current patient, even with the patient's consent. The propriety of conducting a sexual or romantic relationship with a former patient is controversial. There would be little problem for an emergency physician dating a patient he had seen once professionally several years ago for a sore throat. But the American Psychiatric Association ruled that it is always unethical for a psychiatrist to have a romantic relationship with a former patient because of the exploitation potential resulting from the previous professional relationship. The American Medical Association Council on Ethical and Judicial Affairs (AMA CEJA) opined that romantic relationships with former patients become unethical whenever "the physician uses or exploits trust, knowledge, emotions, or influence derived from the previous relationship."[57] Additionally, the AMA CEJA advises physicians to "refrain from sexual or romantic interactions with key third parties . . . [such as] spouses, partners, parents, guardians, and proxies of their patients . . . when it is based on the use or exploitation of trust, knowledge, influence, or emotions derived from a professional relationship."[58]

Physicians are entitled to charge patients or their insurers reasonable professional fees for services rendered to them or on their behalf. Compensation should be restricted to services actually delivered or supervised. It is unethical for physicians to receive a fee for making a referral (fee-splitting) or to obtain a commission from anyone for an item or service ordered for a patient (kickback) because these situations place the financial gain of the physician ahead of the welfare of the patient. Physicians should not order tests or charge patients or their insurers for inappropriate or unnecessary care or for care that has not been performed.

Physicians also are responsible for maintaining their own personal health to permit them to provide optimal care to patients. Chronically unhealthy practices, such as alcohol or other drug abuse, acute conditions such as influenza and sleep deprivation, and the emotionally spent state of "burnout" (discussed later in this chapter) may impair their ability to provide their patients with proper care.

Conflicts of Interest

Conflicts of interest are inherent in the contemporary practice of medicine because of the complex relationships physicians have evolved with hospitals, universities, employers, insurers, health maintenance organizations (HMOs), managed care organizations, pharmaceutical companies, and medical equipment manufacturers, in addition to their traditional relationships with patients.[59] Michael Davis defines a conflict of interest as follows: "A person has a conflict of interest if: (a) he is in a relationship with another requiring him to exercise judgment in the other's service; and (b) he has an interest tending to interfere with the proper exercise of judgment in that relationship."[60] Conflicts of interest are a problem in medicine both because they demote the primacy of the patient's interests, thereby straining the patient-physician relationship,[61] and because their presence diminishes the overall confidence of patients and the public in the medical profession. I discuss the pervasive professional conflicts of interest in research in chapter 19.

Some scholars distinguish between conflicts of interest and conflicts of obligation by emphasizing the financial dimensions of the former and the duty-based obligations of the latter. I consider them together because they form a spectrum and they are analyzed and resolved similarly. Some scholars distinguish further between a real conflict, a potential conflict, and an apparent conflict. Although real conflicts generally are the most serious problem, apparent conflicts also are a problem because they diminish patients' confidence in physicians' judgments.

Dennis Thompson defines a financial conflict of interest as "a set of conditions in which professional judgment concerning a primary interest (such as a patient's welfare or the validity of research) tends to be unduly influenced by a secondary interest (such as financial gain)."[62] In practical terms, a conflict exists when the physician stands to profit personally from a medical decision and the profit motive consciously or subconsciously affects the objectivity of the decision. Surveyed patients are concerned about physicians' financial incentives, particularly when they involve incentives to decrease the availability of expensive testing and treatment.[63]

The ethical resolution of a conflict of interest is straightforward: the patient's interest is paramount, so physicians should attempt to resolve all such conflicts in the interests of patients. Their secondary (usually financial) interest should not be permitted to dominate or appear to dominate the primary interest of quality medical care. A general test of the ethical nature of a conflict is posed by this question: would the physician be willing to permit public knowledge of the financial relationship in question and to advocate it? Michael Camilleri and Denis Cortese recently provided useful guidelines for physicians and clinical investigators to manage individual and institutional conflicts of interest in clinical practice.[64]

Self-Referral. A common example of a conflict of interest in the practice of neurology is "self-referral," the referral of a patient to a freestanding neuro-imaging center, clinical neurophysiology laboratory, or rehabilitation center partially or fully owned by the neurologist but in which the neurologist has no professional responsibilities. Physician-owned ambulatory-surgery centers, diagnostic testing facilities, and specialty hospitals now are common in the United States and growing at annual rates of 6.1%, 10.4%, and 20.3% respectively.[65] A neurologist's decision about the necessity of a magnetic resonance scan for the patient with a headache or electromyoneurography for the patient with hand numbness may be influenced consciously or subconsciously by the fact that he stands to profit more from the performance or reading of these laboratory tests than from the office visit.[66]

Patients may derive advantages from self-referral, however, that may justify the practice in some cases. Often it is more convenient and less expensive for the patient to receive a test in an office than in a hospital. Because communication between physicians in self-referral situations often is more efficient, results are more quickly known. Some freestanding diagnostic and treatment facilities can provide state-of-the-art care less expensively than hospitals because of lower overhead resulting from treating only insured patients whose conditions have favorable reimbursement rates and the increased operational efficiency resulting from a single focus of care. Finally, facilities of the same high quality may not be available to patients outside the self-referral sphere.

Conflicts of interest from self-referral are seductive and quickly can evolve into commonplace practices. In self-referral fee-for-service settings, neurologists may develop too low a threshold for ordering discretionary but expensive laboratory testing such as electromyography, electroneurography, electroencephalography, magnetic resonance scans, and computed tomography scans. The majority of patients referred to such practices often undergo one or more of these tests. The neurologist may convince himself that conducting such a thorough laboratory evaluation is providing the best and most comprehensive medical care for a patient. Controlled studies comparing the incidence of radiological tests and radiation therapy ordered in self-referral settings compared with those ordered in non-self-referral, fee-for-service settings have shown that the frequency is greater in self-referral settings.[67]

Resolution of this conflict of interest has three requirements. First, neurologists should not refer patients to free-standing diagnostic or treatment facilities in which they have a financial investment but no direct patient care responsibilities unless there is no other choice in the community.[68] There are now Medicare and Medicaid legal sanctions regulating or prohibiting self-referrals.[69] Second, neurologists should closely adhere to the indications of clinical practice guidelines published by medical societies when ordering or performing any laboratory tests for which they stand to gain financially. Finally, neurologists should disclose all such financial arrangements to patients.[70]

The Pharmaceutical Industry. A second common conflict of interest involves the relationship of the physician to the pharmaceutical industry. The pharmaceutical industry currently provides financial support to the medical profession by: (1) defraying the cost of medical journals through advertisements and block grants; (2) sponsoring educational conferences through speakers' bureaus, grants to conference organizers, or direct cash payments to resident physicians to defray travel expenses to these conferences; (3) paying physicians with direct gifts and travel junkets to attend educational conferences; and (4) sponsoring clinical pharmacological research.[71]

Financial support from the pharmaceutical industry has grown to such as extent that currently they pay over 50% of the cost of continuing medical education (CME) in the United States. Influential leaders of American medicine have decried this situation because it blurs the distinction between impartial education and targeted marketing and have called for a separation of CME from pharmaceutical company control.[72] Of course, the money for all these pharmaceutical company-sponsored activities ultimately comes from sales to patients or insurers of the companies' pharmaceutical products.

Eric Campbell and colleagues recently provided survey data on the extent of relationships between physicians and the pharmaceutical and medical device manufacturing industry. They found that 94% of physicians reported some type of relationship with the pharmaceutical industry; most of these involved receiving free meals in the workplace (83%) or drug samples (78%). Over one-third (35%) reported receiving reimbursements for costs associated with professional meetings or continuing medical education. Over one-quarter (28%) reported receiving income for giving lectures, consulting, or enrolling patients in clinical trials. Cardiologists were more than twice as likely as family practitioners to receive payments but family practitioners met more frequently with sales representatives. They wondered if their data were skewed by underreporting because of social desirability bias.[73]

Physicians are heavily influenced by physician-peer "educational" lectures and presentations, and physician-authored published review articles that have been assisted or ghost written by pharmaceutical or industrial staff.[74]

Many physicians serve on speakers' bureaus of pharmaceutical companies and receive sizable compensation for lectures to peers. Pharmaceutical companies retain "influence leaders" from academia to lecture at community hospitals and local medical societies to educate practicing physicians. Many of these lectures are high-quality, objective, and unbiased, but some are tantamount to marketing, particularly when discussing the newest off-label uses of prescription drugs that pharmaceutical sales representative are banned by FDA regulations from discussing themselves.[75] The American Academy of Neurology Ethics, Law & Humanities Committee outlined the ethical obligations of neurologists who are retained by pharmaceutical companies as spokesmen or advocates to patients.[76]

Under this influence, physicians may make decisions about prescription drugs that are not necessarily in the best interests of their patients, producing an inherent conflict of interest. Accepting gifts, favors, and other rewards may unduly influence physicians because of the personal gain they accrue. Although most physicians would claim immunity to this influence ("They can't buy me"), the giving of gifts creates good will and induces a sense of reciprocal obligation, thereby producing the effect pharmaceutical manufacturers desire.[77] A survey of attending and resident physicians showed that a majority of both groups believe that their integrity could be compromised by receiving such gifts.[78]

Despite physicians' nearly ubiquitous claims of immunity to such influence, there are clear data showing powerful effects. A recent study showed a positive correlation between the tangible benefits that university hospital physicians received from a pharmaceutical company and the likelihood that the physicians would recommend the company's medication on the hospital formulary list. Tangible benefits included accepting money to attend or speak at conferences and performing pharmaceutical company-sponsored research. The study also revealed a correlation between the likelihood of the physician's adding a given pharmaceutical company's drug to the hospital formulary and the fact that a company's pharmaceutical

representative and this physician had previous personal contact.[79] A study of medical students' exposure to pharmaceutical marketing showed a powerful effect on their attitudes.[80] Another study showed that restricting resident exposure to pharmaceutical sales representatives influenced future attitudes and behaviors of physicians.[81] Clinical trial investigators supported by the pharmaceutical industry are more likely to prescribe products of the sponsoring firm.[82]

To minimize the conflict of interest between medicine and the pharmaceutical industry, the American College of Physicians has promulgated several rules: (1) physicians should not accept gifts if doing so might influence the objectivity of their clinical judgment; (2) institutional medical educational directors who accept financial support from the pharmaceutical industry should develop and enforce policies to maintain complete control of the content of their educational programs; (3) professional societies should develop and follow guidelines to minimize gifts and other amenities provided to their members at meetings; and (4) physicians who participate in drug trials supported by the pharmaceutical industry should conduct their research according to accepted scientific principles.[83] The American College of Physicians has more recently established even more restrictive guidelines for its members governing their interaction with the pharmaceutical and medical equipment manufacturing industries.[84] Most recently, a group sponsored by the Institute of Medicine and American Board of Internal Medicine Foundation proposed the most stringent guidelines which eliminate or greatly modify current practices including gifts, pharmaceutical samples, CME, funds for physician travel, speakers' bureaus, ghostwriting, and consulting and research contracts.[85] Some institutions, such as Stanford University Medical Center, have moved to strictly follow them.

The American Medical Association Council on Ethical and Judicial Affairs also has issued ethical guidelines for physicians who consider accepting gifts from pharmaceutical companies. Gifts that primarily serve the interests of patients are acceptable, but those that primarily serve the interests of physicians (cash, junkets, tickets to events, expensive meals) are unacceptable. Based on this premise, the guidelines dictate five rules: (1) gifts that primarily benefit patients, for example, textbooks, are acceptable; (2) gifts of substantial value that do not benefit patients, including trips to meetings, are unacceptable; (3) gifts of nominal value, for example, notepads and pens, that are related to a physician's work are acceptable; (4) gifts with "strings attached" are unacceptable; and 5) unrestricted subsidies for independently planned and controlled educational meetings are acceptable.[86]

The Pharmaceutical Research and Manufacturers of America (PhRMA) recently promulgated a code of conduct governing the interaction of pharmaceutical sales representatives and health-care professionals.[87] The PhRMA Code bans some of the more egregious former practices but continues to permit many of the practices considered by physician advisory groups to produce conflicts of interest.[88] Ironically, many of the conflicts of interest between medicine and the pharmaceutical industry in the United States will be settled in the future, not by physicians' voluntarily improving their ethical conduct, but through their compliance with mandatory governmental regulation under the threat of federal prosecution.[89] For example, Medicare has increased its scrutiny and regulation of gifts and other amenities provided by pharmaceutical companies to physicians, for which Medicare ultimately pays through the Medicare D program. There is evidence that many physicians are accepting gifts of substantial value from pharmaceutical companies in violation of both the AMA and the PhRMA Code guidelines.[90]

Several academic medical centers recently have established policies that regulate the relationship between professional personnel and representatives of pharmaceutical and medical device companies more strictly than those permitted by the AMA or PhRMA. Stanford, the University of Michigan, the University of Pennsylvania, Yale, and Dartmouth-Hitchcock medical centers, for example, do not permit sales representatives on site and ban all gifts to physicians, nurses, and others, including meals and tokens of even trivial value such as pens and note paper.

HMO and Managed Care. A third common conflict exists between a salaried physician and his employer, a staff-model health maintenance organization (HMO). Administrative pressure may be exerted on the HMO physician to save money by admitting fewer patients, ordering fewer tests, and prescribing fewer and less expensive medications. In some HMOs, physicians are given monetary bonuses at the end of the year if they have achieved certain money-saving targets for the institution. The financial incentives for the HMO physician are opposite to those for the fee-for-service physician. Yet the HMO physician's financial arrangement is equally unethical if, because of personal gain, he is unduly influenced by what should be objective decisions about proper medical care.[91]

Physicians participating in managed care contracts also may be subject to the conflict of making more money by spending less on patients. Until recently, some managed care contracts were configured with financial incentives to limit spending on "big-ticket" items such as hospital admissions, emergency room visits, specialty consultations, expensive tests (such as MRI), and expensive treatments. Salary holdovers or other forms of financial kickbacks or bonuses were provided on a *pro rata* basis for money saved beyond a prefigured limit. The American Medical Association and the American Academy of Neurology, among other organizations, vociferously protested the ethics of these arrangements, claiming that the blatant conflict they create damages the patient-physician relationship by producing a secondary interest for the physician that is more powerful than his interest in patient care.[92] Subsequently, many states enacted regulations banning the most egregious, patient-damaging practices of managed care, such as salary holdovers and gag clauses.[93] Currently, many managed care plans have evolved to providing incentives for quality care, and no longer simply cost-savings.[94] Nevertheless, a survey showed that neurologists remain extremely concerned about the negative impact of managed care conflicts on their relationships with patients and on the quality of their medical care.[95]

The physician who is an HMO employee or participates in a capitated managed care contract experiences the ethical problem of double agency, also known as divided loyalties.[96] With conflicting interests, to whom does the physician owe primary allegiance: his patient or his employer-payer? Despite the obvious pressures from above, the physician's fiduciary duty remains to his patient, thus the patient's interests should remain paramount in such situations. It is just as unethical for physicians to accept payments for not performing indicated tests as it is for them to accept payments for performing or self-referring for tests that are not indicated. Both situations represent clear conflicts of interest.

In an ethically acceptable HMO and managed care contract, the patient's welfare should come before that of the company. Physicians employed by institutions have ethical responsibilities to the institutional administration to ensure their patients' health-care needs are met. They should act as professional advocates to assure that their patients receive excellent care. Physicians participating in capitated managed care contracts should enter only those free of blatant conflicts that damage the patient-physician relationship. States need to regulate insurers to ban rules that harm patients, such as kickbacks, or that intimidate physicians, such as threats of "de-selection" if they spend too much.[97] Managed care configurations designed specifically to minimize conflicts of interest should be implemented.[98] When conflicts are unavoidable, they should be fully disclosed and understood by the patients.[99] Maintaining the primacy of patients' interests will become increasingly more difficult to accomplish in the future with global health-care budgets and more explicit rationing of health care.[100]

In 2004, the American College of Physicians, in conjunction with the Harvard Pilgrim Health Care Ethics Program, published a series of guidelines on ethics in managed care that was endorsed by 16 medical specialty societies and other groups. The guidelines emphasize truth telling, maintaining the primacy of the patient-physician relationship and the patient's interests, responsible stewardship of society's finite resources, fostering an ethical environment for health-care provision, promoting quality medical care, ensuring confidentiality, the importance of patient consent and information, and adequate disclosure of conflicts of interest by the health plan and physicians.[101] These guidelines comprise a model for securing an ethical foundation to managed care contracts.

Even when physicians faithfully make decisions in their patients' interests, at times it may be difficult to convince patients that decisions are being made for their own good and not for another reason, such as to save money for the health-care system. There is evidence that patients have greater trust for their physicians in fee-for-service environments than in capitated and managed care environments.[102] I have had the disquieting personal experience of having a patient question if the reason I chose not to order a brain MRI in the setting of migraine was to "save the hospital money." Maintaining patients' trust in an overall system of divided loyalties is difficult and requires skillful communication[103] and a redoubling of fidelity to patients' best interests.[104]

ETHICAL DUTIES TO PATIENTS' FAMILIES

Physicians also have ethical duties toward families of patients. The family is usually the sick person's primary caregiver and often has the responsibility to execute the physician's orders for medications and other therapies. For many elderly or chronically ill patients, care provided by family members permits the patient to remain at home and avoids institutionalization. Therefore, the family is an indispensable partner in the care of many neurological patients and is deserving of thoughtful consideration by the physician.[105] Nonmaleficence-based ethical duties of clinicians require that the family caregiver of the chronically ill patient be considered as a third party in the patient-physician relationship.[106]

Physicians should explain the nature of the patient's illness and the rationale for therapy to the family caregivers. Answering questions and providing explanations will improve family compliance with the prescribed medical regimen and thus contribute to improving the patient's health. Counseling family members reduces their anxiety, fear, and suffering about the patient's illness. Counseling also gives the physician an opportunity to understand the family's perspective and to derive greater insight into the patient as a person and his reaction to his illness. These insights provide the physician with a more comprehensive and realistic view of the patient's illness.

Some physicians resent the time required to explain medical issues to family members, or treat family members' entreaties as bothersome and unnecessary intrusions. Given the essential role of the family in the care of the patient, a better ethic for relating to them is one of attempting to accommodate the family's needs with those of the patient.[107]

Physicians need to take precautions, however, that their solicitousness toward the family does not create a situation in which "the family becomes the patient." Although the interests of the family and patient usually are compatible, there are times when they diverge. The difficulty with the family becoming the patient in these instances is that the family's potentially conflicting interests may take precedence over those of the patient.

In neurological practice, this situation occurs commonly in the management of the demented patient. Family members may overwhelm physicians with the stresses they endure in caring for the demented patient at home. The interests of the family may tend to predominate in the patient's care in such cases because family members can be more vocal and can more readily contact the physician, who relies on them as the sole source of data about the patient's illness and home functioning. The resolution of this dilemma is discussed in chapter 15.

ETHICAL DUTIES TO OTHER PHYSICIANS AND TO THE MEDICAL PROFESSION

Ethical duties owed to medical colleagues and the medical profession include the responsibilities to teach, to recognize and help rehabilitate impaired physicians, and to comport oneself properly when participating in professional liability activities and physician advertising.

Teaching

From the time of Hippocrates, the duty to teach other physicians the art, science, and ethics of medicine has been a part of the code of medical conduct. The title "doctor" is derived from the Latin *docere*, meaning "to teach." The ethical basis for teaching trainees and colleagues, writing scientific and scholarly articles, and performing research is that patients ultimately become the beneficiaries of improved health. Of course, the "doctor as teacher" also refers to the physician's important duty to teach patients, so that with their increased understanding they are better able to maintain proper health and follow the physician's prescribed therapies.

Impaired and Incompetent Physicians

Physicians have a nonmaleficence-based ethical duty to colleagues and to patients to help in the recognition and rehabilitation of impaired physicians. Practicing physicians may become impaired by alcoholism, drug abuse, depression, dementia, and other medical and psychiatric disorders. Impairment may be induced by "burnout," a common symptom of midlife professionals in whom overwork, stress, inability to achieve goals, and chronic fatigue leads to emotional blunting, apathy, poor work performance, alcoholism, and drug addiction.[108] Medical care that impaired physicians provide is more likely to be substandard than care rendered by unimpaired colleagues. The patients of impaired physicians remain in jeopardy until the physician can be removed from practice and, when possible, treated and rehabilitated.[109] Medical societies and hospitals now devote considerable attention to maintaining physician health. They try to prevent burnout and its consequences by helping physicians to assure a proper balance between their professional obligations and their personal time with families and friends.[110]

Physicians have a similar nonmaleficence-based ethical duty to identify, report, and remove incompetent colleagues from medical practice in accordance with state legal requirements.[111] To this end, physicians should cooperate with the activities of governmental boards of medical practice. Participation in approved peer-review activities should be encouraged because it helps weed out incompetent physicians and contributes to the overall betterment of patient care.[112]

Physicians also have nonmaleficence-based duties not to criticize the judgment, skill, knowledge, or training of a colleague without adequate justification. When criticism is justified, however, it is wrong for a physician to ignore the misconduct or incompetence of a colleague, thus jeopardizing the future safety of the colleague's patients.[113]

Medical Malpractice

The medical malpractice arena is one of the most contentious sources of collegial friction among physicians. To prove medical malpractice, the medical tort system requires that an expert physician testify that a duty existed to practice competently, that the clinician breached this duty by failing to practice according to prevailing medical standards, that the patient has suffered the harm of a compensable injury, and that the substandard treatment caused the injury (see further discussion in chapter 4). Physicians have an ethical responsibility to participate in the medical malpractice system by testifying to the best of their ability about prevailing standards of practice. On the defendant's side, physicians should try to assist a colleague unjustly sued. For the plaintiff, physicians should assist in righting the wrong a patient sustained as a result of the careless or incompetent actions of another physician.[114] Proper participation on either side of a medical malpractice suit requires that physicians have a clear concept of their ethical duties to their colleagues.

Unfortunately, there are flaws in the medical tort system. For example, the system has been accused of being unfair, cumbersome, expensive, and plaintiff-oriented. These problems are compounded by the participation of "hired-gun" physicians: expert witnesses for the plaintiff who will slant their testimony for a fee in order to suit the needs of the plaintiff's

lawyer. Some physicians have responded to these inequities simply by refusing to participate in the system. I believe that physicians have an ethical duty to participate, however, both to assist their colleagues and to serve all patients. Only if ordinary practicing physicians are willing to testify to the proper standards of medical care can hired-gun expert witnesses be marginalized and excluded from the malpractice arena.

Physicians who choose to testify as expert witnesses have several duties that were made explicit in a statement from the American Academy of Neurology in 2006.[115] They should testify only about those subjects for which they are qualified as experts by training and experience. In testifying for either the plaintiff or the defendant, they should agree to participate only if they feel the case on their side has merit. Before giving testimony, they should review all the relevant records and be familiar with the prevailing standards of medical practice. In providing testimony, physicians should render opinions that are honest and accurate scientifically and clinically, and evidence-based when possible.[116] They should understand the relevant standard of medical care, appreciate the wide range of acceptable medical practices in similar cases, and not egotistically insist that every patient be treated only as they would do. They should take care to preserve their impartiality and objectivity by guarding against monetary rewards or suggestions from attorneys who retained them. Payment for their services should be reasonable and reflect the time they spent in reviewing records, discussing the case with attorneys, and testifying. Under no circumstances should any payment be contingent on the outcome of the case. The privacy and confidentiality of all parties should be maintained at all times. Experts should be aware that their testimony generates a legal record for which they may held accountable by peer review, and that if substandard, may become the basis for disciplinary action.[117]

Advertising

Advertising and other public representations in which physicians participate are ethically acceptable practices if they are truthful and maintain the dignity of the profession. Advertising becomes unethical if it is untruthful, misleading, deceptive, or unsubstantiated.[118] Physicians have an ethical duty to their colleagues and patients to represent their training, ability, and areas of competence accurately.

ETHICAL DUTIES TO SOCIETY

The physician and the medical profession have ethical duties to society for two reasons: society is ultimately the population of potential patients to whom each physician owes ethical duties, and society has granted the medical profession a unique role with attendant professional prerogatives that demand reciprocal duties. A defining characteristic of late twentieth-century medicine was the growing awareness of the physician's ethical duty to society, particularly in those instances in which that duty conflicts with a duty to patients.[119]

The potential tension between the physician's duties to patients and his obligations to society differs qualitatively from that of the attorney to his client and to society. The attorney's professional duty is to represent the interests of his client to the best possible advantage. Both in civil and criminal law, attorneys regularly represent clients who they suspect may be in the wrong. Other than in a few clearly defined exceptions, the attorney does not judge the guilt or innocence of clients or the ultimate merit of their claims. The attorney does not feel any professional responsibility to the opposing party if, because of his cleverness in handling his client's case, his client prevails in a lawsuit in which, arguably, the client was in the wrong. Rather, such an outcome would constitute the mark of a good attorney. In our legal system, "the truth" in a lawsuit is defined by the outcome of an impartial judicial process.

By contrast, the responsibilities of health prevention and stewardship demand that the physician must be concerned about the impact on other patients of his actions performed with the intent of helping his own patient. Unlike an attorney, a physician cannot ethically restrict his concern to the welfare of his patient, irrespective of others. The ethical good that a patient accrues from the patient-physician encounter is of paramount importance, but it also must be balanced against the harm other patients may sustain as an inevitable byproduct of the encounter. I believe that if more harm to others ensues, the physician should not pursue his action even though it is clearly intended to help his patient. Indeed, the physician's ethical duty to society has itself become enshrined in law, as the following examples illustrate.

The Duty to Protect Third Parties Known To Be at Risk

The clearest example of the conflict of duties is the situation in which a physician's duty to respect the confidentiality and privacy of a patient conflicts with his duty to protect the safety of other persons. The most widely publicized case in which this conflict was portrayed was the tragic death of Tatania Tarasoff. Ms. Tarasoff was a college student who terminated a romantic relationship with a young man. This man confided his anger and intent to murder her to a college psychologist. Although the psychologist contacted the campus police, the police chose not to pursue the matter following a preliminary investigation. The psychologist, knowing that the investigation had been dropped, did not warn Ms. Tarasoff directly, concluding that his responsibility to her had been satisfied. He believed that it would violate rules of patient confidentiality if he contacted her without his patient's consent, and furthermore, he was not certain that her boyfriend was serious about his threat. The estranged boyfriend later murdered Ms. Tarasoff.

The California Supreme Court held the psychologist liable for not warning Ms. Tarasoff directly when he learned that she remained in peril after the police investigation. The court argued:

> The therapist owes a legal duty not only to his patient, but also to his patient's would-be victim and is subject in both respects to scrutiny by judge and jury . . . Some of the alternatives open to the therapist, such as

warning the victim, will not result in the drastic consequences of depriving the patient of his liberty. Weighing the uncertain and conjectural character of the alleged damage done to the patient by such a warning against the peril to the victim's life, we conclude that professional inaccuracy cannot negate the therapist's duty to protect the threatened victim.[120]

The decision of the court was based partially on the discussion of the limits of patient confidentiality published by the American Medical Association in the *Principles of Medical Ethics.* According to the American Medical Association, "A physician may not reveal the confidence entrusted to him in the course of medical attendance . . . unless he is required to do so by law or unless it becomes necessary in order to protect the welfare of the individual or the community."[121]

Physicians have a similar duty to protect the safety of the general public, even when a particular person at risk cannot be identified. The most common example of this ethical and legal duty in medical practice is the requirement to notify responsible public health officials in instances of certain communicable diseases. This duty supersedes the duty to maintain patient confidentiality because third parties are at risk of infection, which could be prevented by the actions of responsible public health officials. In addition, the harm produced by violating patient confidentiality in such cases generally is much less than the harm rendered to innocent third parties who become infected unknowingly, making the physician's duty to the third party paramount.

The President's Commission for the Study of Ethical Problems in Medicine and Biomedical and Behavioral Research stipulated five conditions that, if satisfied, permit physicians to override their ordinary ethical duty to maintain patient confidentiality to protect others: (1) reasonable efforts to elicit voluntary consent to disclosure have failed; (2) there is a high probability that harm would occur if the information is withheld; (3) there is a high probability that the disclosed information would avert that harm; (4) there is a high probability that the harm inflicted on the third party would be serious; and (5) appropriate precautions would be taken to ensure that the only

information conveyed is that necessary to avert the harm.[122] Nevertheless, one ethicist advocates the unpopular opposing position that a physician's duty to maintain patient confidentiality should supersede any third party protection considerations.[123]

Analyzed in this context, the ethical conflict concerning the HIV-positive patient, presented earlier in the chapter, becomes easier to resolve. Because the HIV-positive man refuses to notify his wife and continues to practice unprotected sexual intercourse with her, he is clearly endangering her in a manner similar to Tarasoff's ex-boyfriend. The physician's ethical duty is to urge the man to tell his wife of his HIV-positive condition and to practice only "safe sex" with her. If the physician is unable to confirm his patient's compliance with these instructions, he has the duty to report the instance to responsible public health officials. If state law in his particular jurisdiction will not permit the public health department to notify the patient's partner, the physician has an ethical duty to notify the wife directly, in much the same way as Ms. Tarasoff's ex-boyfriend's psychologist should have done.[124] These specific duties have been codified as principles of professional conduct by the American Medical Association, the American College of Physicians, the Infectious Diseases Society of America, and the American Academy of Neurology, among other organizations.[125]

A similar ethical conflict in the practice of neurology surrounds the duty to maintain patient confidentiality versus the duty to notify a state motor vehicle bureau of the potential danger an uncontrolled epileptic or other neurologically impaired automobile driver poses to the public. State law varies in regulating this important duty. Some states require notification in cases of epilepsy or other impairment; others forbid it without patient consent.[126]

In those states that forbid notification without consent, the physician has the ethical duty to urge the patient either to notify the motor vehicle bureau or to provide consent for the physician to do so. If the patient refuses to grant permission, the physician should appeal to the family to contact the motor vehicles bureau. Both should be warned that automobile insurance for collision or liability may be voided if a claim investigation reveals that the patient failed to properly disclose his seizure disorder. Failing each of these attempts, if the patient continues to drive, the physician should notify the motor vehicle bureau directly because of his ethical duty to protect the safety of the general public who are known to be at risk.

The Duty to Promote Public Health

Physicians have a professional responsibility to society to promote measures to improve the public health of all citizens. This duty requires them generally to support measures to reduce pollution and chemical and physical contamination of air, water, and land; to limit smoking in public places; to work toward improved safety in automobiles, public conveyances, homes, and workplaces; to encourage healthy habits in diet and exercise; and to work toward the reduction of poverty, malnutrition, and violence.[127] Physicians have a special duty to work toward improved access to medical care, particularly among the disenfranchised members of society because reduced access adds to patients' disease burden and suffering.[128] Each physician has the ethical duty to provide voluntary uncompensated (*pro bono*) medical care for patients unable to afford it.[129] The daunting public health ethical issues raised by planning for an inevitable future influenza pandemic—compulsory vaccination, quarantine, and forced rationing of drugs, hospital beds, and ventilators—have been the subject of much recent work.[130]

The Duty to Conserve Medical Resources

As stewards of the communal monetary resources for health care, physicians have a duty not to squander the money that our society has devoted to maintain the health of its citizens. When physicians order unnecessary tests, consultations, and hospitalizations, perform unnecessary medical and surgical procedures, and prescribe treatments they know to be ineffective, they squander precious medical resources that then cannot be applied to serving others, incurring what economists call an

"opportunity cost." The rendering of technically appropriate medical and health care is not only best for patients, it is also a duty that clinicians owe to populations. Contemporary clinicians should try to avoid practicing "overcare," the false belief that the quantity of medical care equals the quality of medical care.[131]

Howard Hiatt captured the shared finite resource dilemma most accurately in his discussion of the term "medical commons," which he adapted from a theme developed by Garrett Hardin. In a famous article in *Science*, Hardin pointed out that individuals act to maximize their personal gain when they take disproportionately from the "commons," that is, from the shared resources of citizens intended to benefit all.[132] Only altruism, personal conscience, public laws, and an individual's innate sense of justice and personal responsibility act to constrain his disproportionate use of the commons. The simple knowledge that the commons would be destroyed if everyone took disproportionate shares does not seem to influence an individual's perception about how to maximize his personal gain. Hiatt pointed out that physicians who act only in their patients' interest, without concern for the "medical commons," will similarly contribute to the depletion of that commons, ultimately harming all patients.[133] Thus, all physicians should avoid disproportionate use of the medical commons even though their goal is to help their own patients. In a follow-up article 32 years later, Christine Cassel and Troyen Brennan pointed out that physicians' professional responsibility to protect the medical commons has only increased as the cost of medical care has skyrocketed.[134]

There is a conflict between a physician's ethical duty to "do everything possible" to help a patient and his duty to conserve medical resources for society. Some have argued that physicians should not make unilateral rationing decisions or act as restrictive "gatekeepers" because this role conflicts with their role as primary patient advocates.[135] Yet, physicians have duties to society that may complement and may conflict with their duties to patients. They should critically examine tests and treatments they order to assess efficacy and utility because ordering these procedures represents expending finite health-care resources that are then not available for other patients. Only physicians have the professional knowledge of medicine and know the particular "local" details of the patient necessary to make such decisions in an optimal manner. They should not abdicate responsibility for such decisions by deferring them to health-care administrators or managed care agencies, because nonphysicians may make poorer decisions, and patients overall may be harmed to a greater extent.[136] Therefore, physicians have a professional ethical duty to "set limits" by not ordering tests and treatments of zero or very marginal utility[137] as well as to be the ones making bedside rationing decisions such as determining who should be admitted to "the last bed in the ICU."[138]

A survey on attitudes of members of the American Academy of Neurology about rationing found a high acceptance of the professional responsibility for rationing care. Of surveyed practicing neurologists, 75% believed that they made daily decisions that rationed health care, 60% felt a professional responsibility to consider the financial impact on other patients of individual treatment decisions, and only 25% believed that no restrictions should be placed on prescribing expensive therapies because of the potentially harmful effect on other patients.[139]

The Duty to Government Agencies

Because government agencies have an impact on patients' health and welfare, physicians should comply with requests from these agencies within the constraints of law and rules of confidentiality. Physicians should attempt to cooperate with reasonable requests from insurance, compensation, reimbursement, and other official health agencies.

THE DUTY TO DISCLOSE MEDICAL ERRORS

The physician's duty to disclose medical errors impacts patients, families, colleagues, and society. The magnitude of the problem of medical error reached American public attention in 1999 with the publication of the National Academy of Sciences Institute of Medicine (IOM) report *To Err is Human*. This report claimed that at least 44,000 Americans died every year of medical errors, a number greater than those dying from motor vehicle accidents, breast cancer, or AIDS.[140] The public and governmental reaction was swift and severe, with innumerable projects and federal directives undertaken to understand and lessen this epidemic. Interestingly, earlier scholarly studies of this longstanding problem did not galvanize public attention prior to the IOM report.[141]

In a follow-up report five years later, Lucian Leape and Donald Berwick concluded that the IOM report had made a huge impact on directing attention to the problem of medical error but that progress to fix the problem was too slow. The authors recommended that the Agency for Healthcare Research and Quality should establish explicit and ambitious goals to solve the problem by 2010.[142] George Annas offered the further suggestion that increasing litigation against hospitals would reduce errors and improve the quality of care.[143] The United States Congress passed the Patient Safety and Quality Improvement Act of 2005 that relies on existing state error reporting systems but provides protection to clinicians who report minor errors to patient safety organizations.[144] Neurologists have a professional opportunity and an ethical responsibility to engage in effort to enhance patient safety.[145]

Albert Wu and colleagues defined a medical mistake as "a commission or an omission with potentially negative consequences for the patient that would have been judged wrong by skilled and knowledgeable peers at the time it occurred, independent of whether there were any negative consequences."[146] Errors can be categorized as system errors or individual errors. Leape further categorizes cognitive errors into slips, rule-based errors, and knowledge-based errors.[147] Errors are not simply thoughtfully-considered misjudgments but reflect a clear failure. The ethical question is whether physicians always must disclose errors to patients and families once they have been discovered.

Most ethicists and clinicians who have studied this question advocate a strong policy of disclosure of errors based on the duty to tell the truth.[148] The patient-physician relationship is based on honesty and its foundation of trust could be damaged if physicians were deceptive. Moreover, patients have the right to know what happened to them and to seek financial compensation when appropriate. Disclosure also allows patients to avoid worry about the cause of symptoms resulting from mistakes and to seek timely treatment for them. It is certainly understandable that, as a matter of reflexive self-protection, many physicians are not eager to admit mistakes, particularly those that injured patients. Fred Rosner and colleagues pointed out, however, medical errors in and of themselves do not necessarily constitute improper, negligent, or unethical behavior or erode trust in physicians, but the failure to disclose them may.[149] The physician who harms a patient through an error has an obligation to account for the act through acknowledgment and apology.[150] A patient's forgiveness for a medical error is customary when a physician admits an honest error, but it should not be automatic.[151]

How to disclose errors has been the subject of much study. In some cases, an adverse outcome that was presumed to have been caused by an error may, on later root-cause analysis, be determined not to have been caused by the error.[152] Therefore, some risk managers advocate the position that physicians should not prematurely jump to the conclusion that the adverse outcome was the result of an error unless it is transparently so. When causation is unclear, physicians can tell the patient or family that an adverse event occurred but it will take a root-cause analysis to determine exactly what happened. Physicians can apologize to patients for a poor outcome of treatment without necessarily claiming an error was made.[153] This is the position of the American Medical Association Council on Ethical and Judicial Affairs that advised, "Physicians must offer professional and compassionate concern toward patients who have been harmed, regardless of whether the harm was caused by a health-care error. An expression of concern need not be an admission of responsibility. When patient harm has been caused by an error, physicians should offer a general explanation regarding the nature of the error and the measures being taken to prevent similar occurrences in the future."[154]

Thomas Gallagher and colleagues surveyed physicians, asking how they would disclose errors. They found that 56% of respondents mentioned the adverse event but did not mention the word "error" whereas 43% would say an error had occurred; 19% would not volunteer any information about the cause of the error, and 63% would not give specific information about preventing future errors. Surgeons were only one-third as likely as medical physicians to disclose an error.[155]

The legal dimensions of the disclosure problem are noteworthy. Some physicians and hospital risk managers have the impression that disclosure of error is tantamount to admitting guilt in a forthcoming malpractice action. They thus recommend nondisclosure, hoping that the patient and family will not discover the error. But newer thinking in risk management advocates providing full disclosure, the so-called extreme honesty position.[156] According to this philosophy, honesty is the best policy in the long run because many malpractice actions are generated by the anger felt by patients or their families. Their anger would be expected to be greater if they accidentally discovered later that the physician had been deceptive, and would be expected to be less if the policy provided that patients always were told the truth about errors. In fact, there is evidence from several institutions that have implemented an extreme honesty policy that their malpractice liability has decreased.[157] As of June 2007, 30 states had enacted "apology laws" (and similar federal legislation also has been introduced) that ban physician apologies from being introduced as evidence against them in malpractice actions arising from alleged medical errors.[158]

Two surveys showed that the large majority of physicians, residents, and medical students claim they would disclose any significant errors they made to patients and their families.[159] Interestingly, the same clinicians would be less likely to disclose the errors if they had been made by another physician. But in another study, resident physicians reported mistakes they had made to their attending physicians only half the time and to their patients less than one quarter of the time.[160] Most surveyed patients want their physicians to disclose even minor errors to them.[161] Many scholars have advocated creating a more open and protected forum to allow physicians to admit errors and to discuss the means of preventing future errors

without the draconian legal consequences that might motivate them to deceive patients.[162] Such a system would be similar to the voluntary, non-punitive systems in place in many industries, most notably the airline industry. Not surprisingly, the admission of a medical error causes great personal distress in physicians.[163] Largely because of its punitive nature, our current system of medical malpractice is an obvious barrier to admitting medical errors and reducing them in the future.[164]

Appendix 3-1

An analysis of the professional oaths (e.g., Hippocratic oath) that physicians take during medical school graduation has revealed that most do not address the importance of respecting a patient's autonomy and being truthful with patients.[165] To compensate for these shortcomings, Edmund Pellegrino and David Thomasma drafted a contemporary oath for physicians that updates the Hippocratic oath and epitomizes the ethical basis for professionalism in medicine that I advocate in this chapter.[166]

I promise to fulfill the obligations I voluntarily assume by my profession to heal, and to help those who are ill. My obligations rest in the special vulnerability of the sick and the trust they must ultimately place in me and my professional competence. I therefore bind myself to the good of the patient in its many dimensions as the first principle of my professional ethics. In recognition of this bond, I accept the following obligations from which only the patient or the patient's valid surrogates can release me:

1. To place the good of the patient at the center of my professional practice and, when the gravity of the situation demands, above my own self-interest.

2. To possess and maintain the competence in knowledge and skill I profess to have.

3. To recognize the limitations of my competence and to call upon my colleagues in all the health professions whenever my patient's needs require.

4. To respect the values and beliefs of my colleagues in the other health professions and to recognize their moral accountability as individuals.

5. To care for all who need my help with equal concern and dedication, independent of their ability to pay.

6. To act primarily in behalf of my patient's best interests, and not primarily to advance social, political, or fiscal policy, or my own interests.

7. To respect my patient's moral right to participate in the decisions that affect him or her, by explaining clearly, fairly, and in language understood by the patient the nature of his or her illness, together with the benefits and dangers of the treatment I propose to use.

8. To assist my patients to make choices that coincide with their own values or beliefs, without coercion, deception, or duplicity.

9. To hold in confidence what I hear, learn, and see as a necessary part of my care of the patient, except when there is a clear, serious, and immediate danger of harms to others.

10. Always to help, even if I cannot cure, and when death is inevitable, to assist my patient to die according to his or her own life plans.[167]

11. Never to participate in direct, active, conscious killing of a patient, even for reasons of mercy, or at the request of the state, or for any other reason.

12. To fulfill my obligation to society to participate in public policy decisions affecting the nation's health by providing leadership, as well as expert and objective testimony.

13. To practice what I preach, teach, and believe and, thus, to embody the foregoing principles in my professional life.

NOTES

1. A chronological list of some of the more notable codes of medical ethics includes the *Oath of Hippocrates* (6th century B.C.), Maimonides's *Daily Prayer of a Physician* (12th century), Thomas Percival's *Medical Ethics or A Code of Institutes and Precepts Adapted to the Professional Conduct of Physicians* (1803), the World Medical Association's *Declaration of Geneva* (1948) and *International Code of Medical Ethics* (1949), and the American Medical Association's *Principles of Medical Ethics* (1980). A complete reprinting of the texts of these and other codes of medical ethics, with English translations of the ancient texts, can be found in the appendix of the Codes and Statements Related to Medical Ethics. In Reich WT, ed. *Encyclopedia of Bioethics* Vol 2. New York: Free Press, 1978:1721–1815. For commentaries on these codes, see Sohl P, Bassford HA. Codes of medical ethics: traditional foundations and contemporary practice. *Soc Sci Med* 1986;22:1175–1179. Medical specialty societies have produced codes of professional ethics for medical practitioners within their specialties. For those of relevance to the practice of neurology, see The American Academy of Neurology Code of Professional Conduct. *Neurology* 1993;43:1257–1260; Snyder L, Leffler C. The American College of Physicians Ethics Manual, 5th ed. *Ann Intern Med* 2005;142:560–582; and World Federation of Neurosurgical Societies/European Association of Neurosurgical Societies. Good practice: a guide for neurosurgeons. *Crit Rev Neurosurg* 1999;9:127–131. The American Medical Association frequently updates and reprints their code. See American Medical Association Council on Ethical and Judicial Affairs. *Code of Medical Ethics. Current Opinions with Annotations*, 2006–2007 ed. Chicago: American Medical Association, 2006. For professional codes outside the medical profession, see Gorlin RA. *Codes of Professional Responsibility.* 2nd ed. Washington, DC: Bureau of National Affairs, 1990.
2. Pellegrino ED, Thomasma DC. *For the Patient's Good. The Restoration of Beneficence in Health Care.* New York: Oxford University Press, 1988:66.
3. Reed RR, Evans D. The deprofessionalization of medicine: causes, effects, and responses. *JAMA* 1987;258:3279–3282. See also Wynia MK, Latham SR, Kao AC, Berg J, Emanuel LL. Medical professionalism in society. *N Engl J Med* 1999;341:1612–1616.
4. ABIM Foundation, ACP Foundation, European Federation of Internal Medicine. *Medical Professionalism in the New Millennium: A Physician Charter.* Philadelphia: American College of Physicians, 2005.
5. ABIM Foundation, ACP-ASIM Foundation, European Federation of Internal Medicine. Medical Professionalism in the New Millennium: A Physician Charter. *Ann Intern Med* 2002;136:243–246.
6. Blank L, Kimball H, McDonald W, Merino J. Medical Professionalism in the New Millennium: A Physician Charter: 15 months later. *Ann Intern Med* 2003;138:839–841.
7. See the description of the Royal College of Physicians Working Party on Medical Professionalism project in Horton R. Medicine: the prosperity of virtue. *Lancet* 2005;1985–1987.
8. Reiser SJ, Banner RS. The charter on medical professionalism and the limits of medical power. *Ann Intern Med* 2003;138:844–846. *JAMA* 2007;298:670–673. See also Cohen JJ, Cruess S, Davidson C. Alliance between society and medicine: the public's stake in medical professionalism. *JAMA* 2007;298:670–673.
9. Rosenbaum S. The impact of United States law on medicine as a profession. *JAMA* 2003;289:1546–1556.
10. For descriptions of professionalism curricula in undergraduate and graduate medical education, see Stern DT, Papadakis M. The developing physician—becoming a professional. *N Engl J Med* 2006;355:1794–1799; Goldstein EA, Maestas RR, Fryer-Edwards K, et al. Professionalism in medical education: an institutional challenge. *Acad Med* 2006;81:871–876; Goold SD, Stern DT. Ethics and professionalism: what does a resident need to learn? *Am J Bioethics* 2006;6:9–17; Inui TS. *A Flag in the Wind: Educating for Professionalism in Medicine.* Washington, DC: Association of American Medical Colleges, 2003; and Stern DT (ed). *Measuring Medical Professionalism.* New York: Oxford University Press, 2006.

11. The core competencies are described in Delzell JE Jr, Rinqdahl EN, Kruse RL. The ACGME Core Competencies: a national survey of family practice residency directors. *Fam Pract* 2005;37: 576–580.

12. American Academy of Neurology Ethics, Law and Humanities Committee. Humanistic dimensions of professionalism in the practice of neurology. *Neurology* 2001;56:1261–1263.

13. Much of the following discussion is based on the standards of professional conduct elaborated in the American Academy of Neurology Code of Professional Conduct. *Neurology* 1993;43:1257–1260, which I co-drafted with Dr. H. Richard Beresford in 1992 and revised in 1998. It can be accessed at: http://www.aan.com/about/board/code_of_conduct.cfm. I have also drawn from the American College of Physicians Ethics Manual. 3rd ed. *Ann Intern Med* 1992;117:947–960. For additional commentary on the contemporary patient-physician relationship, see Almy TP. The healing bond. Doctor and patient in an era of scientific medicine. *Am J Gastroent* 1980;73:403–407; Emanuel EJ, Emanuel LL. Four models of the physician-patient relationship. *JAMA* 1992;267:2221–2226; and Siegler M. Falling off the pedestal: what is happening to the traditional doctor-patient relationship. *Mayo Clin Proc* 1993;68:461–467.

14. On the covenantal model of the patient-physician relationship, see Pellegrino ED, Thomasma DC. *For the Patient's Good. The Restoration of Beneficence in Health Care.* New York: Oxford University Press, 1988. On the contractual model of the patient-physician relationship, see Brody H. The physician/patient relationship. In Veatch RM, ed. *Medical Ethics.* Boston: Jones and Bartlett Publishers, 1989:65–91 and Veatch RM. Models of ethical medicine in a revolutionary age. In: Gorovitz S, Macklin R, Jameton AL, et al. (eds). *Moral Problems in Medicine.* 2nd ed. Englewood Cliffs, NJ: Prentice-Hall, 1983:78–82.

15. On the duties of patients in the patient-physician relationship, see American Medical Association Council on Ethical and Judicial Affairs. Patient responsibilities. In *Code of Medical Ethics. Current Opinions with Annotations,* 2006–2007 ed. Chicago: American Medical Association, 2006:320–321 and Meyer MJ. Patients' duties. *J Med Philosophy* 1992;17:541–555.

16. Quill TE. Partnerships in patient care: a contractual approach. *Ann Intern Med* 1983;98:228–234; and Suchman AL, Botelho RJ, Hinton-Walker P. *Partnerships in Healthcare: Transforming Relational Process.* Rochester, NY: University of Rochester, 1998.

17. This responsibility has been elevated to a duty by some health insurance programs. West Virginia Medicaid requires its beneficiaries to sign a written agreement that enumerates member responsibilities for their own health. See Steinbrook R. Imposing personal responsibility for health. *N Engl J Med* 2006;355:753–756; and Bishop G, Bradley AC. Personal responsibility and physician responsibility—West Virginia's Medicaid plan. *N Engl J Med* 2006;355:756–758.

18. For discussions of the professional duty of accountability, see Emanuel EJ, Emanuel LL. What is accountability in health care? *Ann Intern Med* 1996;124:229–239 and Emanuel LL. A professional response to demands for accountability: practical recommendations regarding ethical aspect of patient care. *Ann Intern Med* 1996;124:240–249.

19. Rodwin MA. Strains in the fiduciary metaphor: divided physician loyalties and obligations in a changing health care system. *Am J Law Med* 1995;21:241–257.

20. For professional guidelines from the American Medical Association on how physicians should unilaterally end the patient-physician relationship, see www.ama-assn.org/ama/pub/ category/4609.html.

21. On the duty to treat HIV patients, see Zuger A, Miles SH. Physicians, AIDS, and occupational risk: historic traditions and ethical obligations. *JAMA* 1987;258:1924–1928; Emanuel EJ. Do physicians have an obligation to treat patients with AIDS? *N Engl J Med* 1988; 318:1686–1690; Freedman B. Health professions, codes, and the right to refuse to treat HIV-infectious patients. *Hastings Cent Rep* 1988;18(suppl 2):20–25; Annas G. Legal risks and responsibilities of physicians in the AIDS epidemic. *Hastings Cent Rep* 1988;18 (suppl 2):26–32; Gramelspacher GP, Siegler M. Do physicians have a professional responsibility to care for patients with HIV disease? *Issues Law Med* 1988;4:383–393; Tegtmeier JW. Ethics and AIDS: a summary of the law and a critical analysis of the individual physician's ethical duty to treat. *Am J Law Med* 1990;16:249–265; and Daniels N. Duty to treat or right to refuse? *Hastings Cent Rep* 1991;21(2):36–46.

22. American Medical Association Council on Ethical and Judicial Affairs. Ethical issues involved in the growing AIDS crisis. *JAMA* 1988;259:1360–1361; American College of Physicians Health and Public Policy Committee. The acquired immunodeficiency syndrome (AIDS) and infection with human immunodeficiency virus (HIV). *Ann Intern Med* 1988;108:460–469; American College of Physicians and Infectious Diseases Society of America. Human immunodeficiency virus (HIV) infection. *Ann Intern Med* 1994;120:310–319; American Academy of Neurology Ethics and Humanities Subcommittee. The ethical role

of neurologists in the AIDS epidemic. *Neurology* 1992;42:1116–1117. See also the discussion of the duty to treat in Simberkoff M. Ethical aspects in the care of patients with AIDS. *Neurol Clin* 1989;7:871–882.

23. For a discussion of universal precautions and the recommended practices to reduce physicians' occupational exposure to HIV, see chapter 18.

24. Lambert P, Gibson JM, Nathanson P. The values history: an innovation in surrogate decision-making. *Law Med Health Care* 1990;18:202–212.

25. Tsevat J, Cook EF, Green ML, et al. Health values of the seriously ill. *Ann Intern Med* 1995;122:514–520 and Tsevat J, Dawson NV, Wu AW, et al. Health values of hospitalized patients 80 years or older. *JAMA* 1999;279:371–375.

26. Charo RA. The celestial fire of conscience—refusing to deliver medical care. *N Engl J Med* 2005;352:2471–2473 and White KA. Crisis of confidence: reconciling religious health care providers' beliefs and patients' rights. *Stanford Law Rev* 1999;51:1703–1749.

27. Curlin FA, Lawrence RE, Chin MH, Lantos JD. Religion, conscience, and controversial clinical practices. *N Engl J Med* 2007;356:593–600.

28. Siegler M. Confidentiality in medicine: a decrepit concept. *N Engl J Med* 1982; 307:1518–1521 and Welch CA. Sacred secrets—the privacy of medical records. *N Engl J Med* 2001;345:371–372.

29. On electronic medical record privacy, see Gostin L. Health law information and the protection of personal privacy: ethical and legal considerations. *Ann Intern Med* 1998;127:683–690; Hodge JG, Gostin LO, Jacobson PD. Legal issues concerning electronic health information: privacy, quality, and liability. *JAMA* 1999;282:1466–1471; and the symposium Electronic medical information: privacy, liability & quality issues. *Am J Law Med* 1999; 25:191–421.

30. Mandl KD, Kohane IS, Brandt AM. Electronic patient-physician communication: problems and promise. *Ann Intern Med* 1998;129:495–500 and Spielberg AR. On call and online: sociohistorical, legal, and ethical implications of e-mail for the patient-physician relationship. *JAMA* 1998;280:1353–1359.

31. See discussions in Rind DM, Kohane IS, Szolovits P, Safran C, Chueh HC, Barnett GO. Maintaining the confidentiality of medical records shared over the internet and world wide web. *Ann Intern Med* 1997;127:138–141 and Kassirer JP. Patients, physicians, and the internet. *Health Affairs* 2000;19:115–123. For a recent description of the development and successful use of a secure internet link permitting patients to communicate with physicians and staff members, see Stone JH. Communication between physicians and patients in the era of e-medicine. *N Engl J Med* 2007;356:2451–2454. Stone made the provocative but unsubstantiated claim that unsecured e-mail communication between physicians and patients violated the Health Insurance Portability and Accountability Act (HIPAA) regulations because the medical center could not guarantee confidentiality of the e-mail message once it left the medical center. By this overly broad interpretation, an ordinary letter with test results sent by a physician to a patient also could be construed as a HIPAA violation for the same reason.

32. The HIPAA regulations are explained in Kulynych J, Korn D. The new federal medical-privacy rule. *N Engl J Med* 2002; 347:1133–1134; and Annas GJ. HIPAA regulations—a new era of medical-record privacy? *N Engl J Med* 2003;348:1486–1490. For further information and the regulation details, see http://www.cms.hhs.gov/HIPAAGenInfo/ (Accessed June 13, 2007) or http://www.hhs.gov/ocr/hipaa/ (Accessed July 3, 2007).

33. Wilson JF. Health Insurance Portability and accountability Act Privacy Rule cause concerns among clinicians and researchers. *Ann Intern Med* 2006;145:313–316. See also Sobel R. The HIPAA paradox: the privacy rule that's not. *Hastings Cent Rep* 2007;37(4):40–50.

34. Lo B, Dornbrand L, Dubler NN. HIPAA and patient care: the role for professional judgment. *JAMA* 2005;293:1766–1771.

35. Burnum JF. Secrets about patients. *N Engl J Med* 1991;324:1130–1133. See also Bok S. The professional secret: the limits of confidentiality. *Hastings Cent Rep* 1983;13(1):24–26.

36. Quill TE. Recognizing and adjusting to barriers in doctor-patient communication. *Ann Intern Med* 1989;111:51–57. For further analyses of patient-physician communication, see Zinn WM. Doctors have feelings too. *JAMA* 1988;259:3296–3298; Suchman AL, Matthews DA. What makes the patient-doctor relationship therapeutic? Exploring the connexional dimension of medical care. *Ann Intern Med* 1988;108:125–130; Matthews DA, Suchman AL, Branch WT Jr. Making "connexions": enhancing the therapeutic potential of patient-clinician relationships. *Ann Intern Med* 1993;118:973–977; Delbanco TL. Enriching the doctor-patient relationship by inviting the patient's perspective. *Ann Intern Med* 1992;116:414–418; and the classic work Katz J. *The Silent World of Doctor and Patient.* Baltimore: Johns Hopkins University Press, 2002.

37. Novack DH, Suchman AL, Clark W, Epstein RM, Najberg E, Kaplan C. Calibrating the physician: personal awareness and effective patient care. *JAMA* 1997;278:502–509.

38. Laine C, Davidoff F. Patient-centered medicine: a professional evaluation. *JAMA* 1996;275:152–156 and Balint J, Shelton W. Regaining the initiative: forging a new model of the patient-physician relationship. *JAMA* 1996;275:887–891.

39. Emanuel LL, Richter J. The consultant and the patient-physician relationship: a trilateral deliberative model. *Arch Intern Med* 1994;154:1785–1790.

40. Golub RM. Curbside consultations and the viaduct effect. *JAMA* 1998;280:929–930; Kuo D, Gifford DR, Stein MD. Curbside consultation practices and attitudes among primary care physicians and medical subspecialists. *JAMA* 1998;280:905–909; Keating NL, Zaslavsky AM, Ayanian JZ. Physicians' experiences and beliefs regarding informal consultation. *JAMA* 1998;280:900–904.

41. American Academy of Neurology Ethics, Law and Humanities Committee. Practice advisory: participation of neurologists in direct-to-consumer advertising. *Neurology* 2001;56:995–996.

42. For a recent comprehensive discussion of empathy, see Hojat M. *Empathy in Patient Care: Antecedents, Development, Measurement, and Outcomes.* New York: Springer, 2007.

43. Halpern J. What is clinical empathy? *J Gen Intern Med* 2003;18:670–674.

44. Osler W. *Æquanimitas.* New York: Norton, 1963:29, as quoted in Halpern *J Gen Intern Med* 2003:670.

45. Markakis K, Frankel R, Beckman H, Suchman A. Teaching empathy: it can be done. Presented at the Annual Meeting of the Society for General Internal Medicine, San Francisco, April 29, 1999, as quoted in Halpern *J Gen Intern Med* 2003:670.

46. See the discussion of empathy and suffering in Cassell EJ. *The Nature of Suffering and the Goals of Medicine.* New York: Oxford University Press, 1991:72–74. Jodi Halpern examined the philosophical structure of empathy in Halpern J. *From Detached Concern to Empathy: Humanizing Medical Practice.* New York: Oxford University Press, 2001.

47. Larson EB, Yao X. Clinical empathy as emotional labor in the patient-physician relationship. *JAMA* 2005;293:1100–1106.

48. Spiro H. What is empathy and can it be taught? *Ann Intern Med* 1992;116:843–846.

49. Meier DE, Back AL, Morrison RS. The inner life of physicians and the care of the seriously ill. *JAMA* 2001;286:3007–3014.

50. The communication techniques to build empathy are described in Coulehan JL, Platt FW, Egener B, et al. "Let me see if I have this right . . . ": Words that help build empathy. *Ann Intern Med* 2001;135:221–227 and Quill TE, Arnold RM, Platt F. "I wish things were different": expressing wishes in response to loss, futility, and unrealistic hopes. *Ann Intern Med* 2001;135:551–555.

51. Suchman AL, Markakis K, Beckman HB, Frankel R. A model of empathic communication in the medical interview. *JAMA* 1997;277:678–682.

52. Peabody FW. The care of the patient. *JAMA* 1927;88:877–882.

53. Percy W. *Love in the Ruins.* New York: Farrar, Strauss, and Giroux, 1971.

54. Brett AS, McCullough LB. When patients request specific interventions: defining the limits of the physician's obligation. *N Engl J Med* 1986;315:1347–1351. See also Eisenberg DM, Kessler RC, Foster C, et al. Unconventional medicine in the United States: prevalence, costs, and patterns of use. *N Engl J Med* 1993;328:246–252.

55. Groves JE. Taking care of the hateful patient. *N Engl J Med* 1978;298:883–887. See also Gunderman R. Illness as failure: blaming patients. *Hastings Cent Rep* 2000;30(4):7–11 and Sledge WH, Feinstein AR. A clinimetric approach to the components of the patient-physician relationship. *JAMA* 1997;278:2043–2048. The unique plight of the disruptive chronic hemodialysis patient who has been banished from care in ambulatory dialysis centers was described in: Smetanka SL. Who will protect the "disruptive" dialysis patient? *Am J Law Med* 2006;32:53–91.

56. Orentlicher D. Denying treatment to the noncompliant patient. *JAMA* 1991;265:1579–1582.

57. American Medical Association Council on Ethical and Judicial Affairs. Sexual misconduct in the practice of medicine. *JAMA* 1991;266:2741–2745 and American Psychiatric Association. *The Principles of Medical Ethics With Annotations Especially Applicable to Psychiatry.* Washington, DC: American Psychiatric Association, 1989. For a review of court cases involving sexual activity between doctors and patients, see Johnson SH. Judicial review of disciplinary action for sexual misconduct in the practice of medicine. *JAMA* 1993;270:1596–1600. See also Dehlendorf CE, Wolfe SM. Physicians disciplined for sex-related offenses. *JAMA* 1998;279:1883–1888 and Morrison J, Wickersham P. Physicians disciplined by a state medical board. *JAMA* 1998;279:1889–1893.

58. American Medical Association Council on Ethical and Judicial Affairs. Sexual or romantic relations between physicians and key third parties. In *Code of Medical Ethics. Current Opinions with Annotations*, 2006–2007 ed. Chicago: American Medical Association, 2006:258–259.

59. Bernat JL, Goldstein ML, Ringel SP. Conflicts of interest in neurology. *Neurology* 1998;50:327–331.

60. Davis M. Conflicts of interest revisited. *Business and Professional Ethics Journal* 1993;12(4):21–41.

61. John Lantos traced the 50-year history of strains on the patient-physician relationship imposed by American health insurance and managed care. Lantos J. The doctor-patient relationship in the post-managed care era. *Am J Bioethics* 2006;6:29–32. For a personal impassioned essay on the same subject as it applies to the practice of neurology, see McQuillen MP. Values in conflict: neurology before and after the advent of managed care. *Semin Neurol* 1997;17:281–285.

62. Thompson DF. Understanding financial conflicts of interest. *N Engl J Med* 1993;329:573–576.

63. Pereira AG, Pearson SD. Patient attitudes toward physician financial incentives. *Arch Intern Med* 2001;161:13132–1317.

64. Camilleri M, Cortese DA. Managing conflict of interest in clinical practice. *Mayo Clin Proc* 2007;82:607–614.

65. Iglehart JK. The emergence of physician-owned specialty hospitals. *N Engl J Med* 2005;352:78–84.

66. Armour BS, Pitts MM, MacLean R, et al. The effect of explicit financial incentives on physician behavior. *Arch Intern Med* 2001;161:1261–1266. For a thoughtful analysis of the ethics and consequences of different physician reimbursement models, see Lantos J. RVUs blues: how should docs get paid? *Hastings Cent Rep* 2003;33(3):37–45.

67. Hilman BJ, Joseph CA, Mabry MR, et al. Frequency and costs of diagnostic imaging in office practice: a comparison of self-referring and radiologist-referring physicians. *N Engl J Med* 1990;323:1604–1608; Mitchell JM, Sunshine JH. Consequences of physicians' ownership of health care facilities—joint ventures in radiation therapy. *N Engl J Med* 1992;327:1497–1501; and Swedlow A, Johnson G, Smithline N, Milstein A. Increased costs and rates of use in the California worker's compensation system as a result of self-referral by physicians. *N Engl J Med* 1992;327:1502–1506.

68. American Medical Association Council on Ethical and Judicial Affairs. Conflicts of interest. Physician ownership of medical facilities. *JAMA* 1992;267:2366–2369. See also Relman A. "Self-referral"—What's at stake? *N Engl J Med* 1992;327:1522–1524; Morreim EH. Conflicts of interest: profits and problems in physician referrals. *JAMA* 1989:262:390–394; McDowell TN Jr. Physician self-referral arrangements: legitimate business or unethical "entrepreneurialism." *Am J Law Med* 1989;15:61–109; and Scott E, Mitchell JM. New evidence of the prevalence and scope of physician joint ventures. *JAMA* 1992;268:80–84.

69. Crane TS. The problem of physician self-referral under the Medicare and Medicaid anti-kickback statute. *JAMA* 1992;268:85–91. See also American College of Physicians. Understanding the fraud and abuse laws: guidance for internists. *Ann Intern Med* 1998;128:678–684.

70. Miller TE, Sage WM. Disclosing physician financial incentives. *JAMA* 1999;281:1424–1430.

71. Blumenthal D. Doctors and drug companies. *N Engl J Med* 2004;351:1885–1890. For more extended discussions, see Santoro MA, Gorrie TM. *Ethics and the Pharmaceutical Industry*. New York: Cambridge University Press, 2005; and Graham Dukes MN. *The Law and Ethics of the Pharmaceutical Industry*. Amsterdam: Elsevier, 2006.

72. Relman AS. Separating continuing medical education from pharmaceutical marketing. *JAMA* 2001;285:2009–2014; and Elliott C. Pharma goes to the laundry: public relations and the business of medical education. *Hastings Cent Rep* 2004;34(5):18–23. For an impassioned argument from a prominent medical editor that the financial incentives pharmaceutical companies provide to physicians are tarnishing the soul of medicine, see Angell M. *The Truth about Drug Companies: How They Deceive Us and What To Do About It*. New York: Random House, 2004.

73. Campbell EG, Gruen RL, Mountford J, Miller LG, Cleary PD, Blumenthal D. A national survey of physician-industry relationships. *N Engl J Med* 2007;356:1742–1750.

74. Choudhry NK, Stelfox HT, Detsky AS. Relationships between authors of clinical practice guidelines and the pharmaceutical industry. *JAMA* 2002;287:612–617.

75. For an account of how a pharmaceutical firm employed opinion leaders to increase physicians' prescriptions for (and impressively boost sales of) a product for off-label uses, see Steinman MA, Bero LA, Chren MM, Landefeld CS. Narrative review: the promotion of gabapentin: an analysis of internal industry documents. *Ann Intern Med* 2006;145:284–293.

76. American Academy of Neurology Ethics, Law and Humanities Committee. Practice advisory: participation of neurologists in direct-to-consumer advertising. *Neurology* 2001;56:995–996.

77. Chren MM, Landefeld S, Murray TH. Doctors, drug companies, and gifts. *JAMA* 1989;262:3448–3451. For a review of the extent of the financial relationship between the medical and pharmaceutical professions, see Noble RC. Physicians and the pharmaceutical industry: an alliance with unhealthy aspects. *Perspect Biol Med* 1993;36:376–394.

78. McKinney WP, Schiedermayer DL, Lurie N, Simpson DE, Goodman JL, Rich EC. Attitudes of internal medicine faculty and residents toward professional interaction with pharmaceutical sales representatives. *JAMA* 1990;264:1693–1697.

79. Chren MM, Landefeld CS. Physicians' behavior and their interactions with drug companies. A controlled study of physicians who requested additions to a hospital drug formulary. *JAMA* 1994;271:684–689.

80. Sierles FS, Brodkey AC, Cleary LM, et al. Medical students' exposure to and attitudes about drug company interactions. *JAMA* 2005;294:1034–1042.

81. McCormick BB, Tomlinson G, Brill-Edwards P, Detsky AS. Effect of restricting contact between pharmaceutical company representatives and internal medicine residents on posttraining attitudes and behavior. *JAMA* 2001;286:1994–1999.

82. Psaty BM, Rennie D. Clinical trial investigators and their prescribing patterns: another dimension to the relationship between physician investigators and the pharmaceutical industry. *JAMA* 2006;295:2787–2790.

83. American College of Physicians. Physicians and the pharmaceutical industry. *Ann Intern Med* 1990; 112:624–626.

84. Coyle SL. Physician-industry relations. Part 1: individual physicians. *Ann Intern Med* 2002;136:396–402 and Coyle SL. Physician-industry relations. Part 2: organizational issues. *Ann Intern Med* 2002;136:403–406.

85. Brennan TA, Rothman DA, Blank L, et al. Health industry practices that create conflicts of interest: a policy proposal for academic medical centers. *JAMA* 2006;295:429–433.

86. American Medical Association Council on Ethical and Judicial Affairs. Gifts to physicians from industry. In American Medical Association Council on Ethical and Judicial Affairs. *Code of Medical Ethics. Current Opinions with Annotations*, 2006–2007 ed. Chicago: American Medical Association, 2006:212–214, 216–224. For a catalogue of national and international guidelines on accepting gifts from pharmaceutical firms and industry, see Noble RC. *Perspect Biol Med* 1993;36:376–394.

87. Pharmaceutical Research and Manufacturers of America. *PhRMA Code on Interactions with Healthcare Professionals*. Washington, DC: Pharmaceutical Research and Manufacturers of America, 2004.

88. Some of the reasons that the PhRMA Code is insufficient to mitigate serious conflicts of interest are enumerated in Brennan TA, Rothman DA, Blank L, et al. Health industry practices that create conflicts of interest: a policy proposal for academic medical centers. *JAMA* 2006;295:429–433.

89. Studdert DM, Mello MM, Brennan TA. Financial conflicts of interest in physicians' relationships with the pharmaceutical industry—self-regulation in the shadow of federal prosecution. *N Engl J Med* 2004; 351:1891–1900.

90. Ross JS, Lackner JE, Lurie P, Gross CP, Wolfe S, Krumholz HK. Pharmaceutical company payments to physicians: early experiences with disclosure laws in Vermont and Minnesota. *JAMA* 2007;297:1216–1223.

91. See Hillman AL. Health maintenance organizations, financial incentives, and physicians' judgments. *Ann Intern Med* 1990;112:891–893; Hillman AL. Financial incentives for physicians in HMOs: is there a conflict of interest? *N Engl J Med* 1987;317:1743–1748; and Egdahl RH, Taft CH. Financial incentives to physicians. *N Engl J Med* 1986;315:59–61. For conflicts arising in third-party health care payment, see Perry CB. Conflicts of interest and the physician's duty to inform. *Am J Med* 1994;96:375–380.

92. American Medical Association Council on Ethical and Judicial Affairs. Ethical issues in managed care. *JAMA* 1995;273:330–335 and American Academy of Neurology Ethics and Humanities Subcommittee. Managed care and neurologists: ethical considerations. *Neurology* 1997;49:321–322.

93. See Hellinger FJ. The expanding scope of state legislation. *JAMA* 1996;276:1065–1070; Miller TE. Managed care regulation: in the laboratory of the states. *JAMA* 1997;278:1102–1109; and Brody H, Bonham VL Jr. Gag rules and trade secrets in managed care contracts: ethical and legal concerns. *Arch Intern Med* 1997;157:2037–2043. For a review of the liability of managed care organizations, see Mariner WK. The Supreme Court's limitation of managed-care liability. *N Engl J Med* 2004;351:1347–1352.

94. Dudley RA, Luft HS. Managed care in transition. *N Engl J Med* 2001;344:1087–1092.

95. Bernat JL, Ringel SP, Vickrey BG, Keran C. Attitudes of US neurologists concerning the ethical dimensions of managed care. *Neurology* 1997;49:4–13.

96. Toulmin S. Divided loyalties and ambiguous relationships. *Soc Sci Med* 1986;23;783–787.

97. Liner RS. Physician deselection: the dynamics of a new threat to the physician-patient relationship. *Am J Law Med* 1997;23:511–537.

98. See Pearson SD, Sabin JE, Emanuel EJ. Ethical guidelines for physician compensation based on capitation. *N Engl J Med* 1998;339:689–693 and Hall MA, Berenson RA. Ethical practice in managed care: a dose of realism. *Ann Intern Med* 1998;128:395–402.

99. Gunderson M. Eliminating conflicts of interest in managed care organizations through disclosure and consent. *J Law Med Ethics* 1997;25:192–198.

100. Sullivan WM. What is left of professionalism after managed care? *Hastings Cent Rep* 1999;29(2):7–13.

101. Povar GJ, Blumen H, Daniel J, et al. Ethics in practice: managed care and the changing health care environment. Medicine as a Profession Managed Care Ethics Working Group Statement. *Ann Intern Med* 2004;141:131–136.

102. Kao AC, Green DC, Zaslavsky AM, Koplan JP, Cleary PD. The relationship between method of physician payment and patient trust. *JAMA* 1998;280:1708–1714.

103. Levinson W, Gorawara-Bhat R, Dueck R, et al. Resolving disagreements in the patient-physician relationship: tools for improving communication in managed care. *JAMA* 1999;282:1477–1483.

104. For essays explaining how conflicted physicians can maintain patients' trust, see Shortell SM, Waters TM, Clarke KWB, Budetti PP. Physicians as double agents: maintaining trust in an era of multiple accountabilities. *JAMA* 1998;280:1102–1108; Bloche MG. Clinical loyalties and the social purposes of medicine. *JAMA* 1999;281:268–274; and Pearson SD. Caring and cost: the challenge for physician advocacy *Ann Intern Med* 2000;133:148–153.

105. Carter JH, Nutt JG. Family caregiving: a neglected and hidden part of health care delivery. *Neurology* 1998;51:1245–1246.

106. See American Medical Association Council on Scientific Affairs. Physicians and family caregivers: a model for partnership. *JAMA* 1993;269:1262–1264; Nelson JL. Taking families seriously. *Hastings Cent Rep* 1992;22(4):6–12; Blustein J. The family in medical decision making. *Hastings Cent Rep* 1993;23(3):6–13; and Hardwig J. What about the family? *Hastings Cent Rep* 1990;20(2):5–10.

107. Levine C, Zuckerman C. The trouble with families: toward an ethic of accommodation. *Ann Intern Med* 1999;130:148–152 and Levine C, Zuckerman C. Hands on/hands off: why health care professionals depend on families but keep them at arm's length. *J Law Med Ethics* 2000;28:5–18.

108. Spickard A, Gabbe SG, Christensen JF. Mid-career burnout in generalist and specialist physicians. *JAMA* 2002;288:1447–1450. Burnout can begin during medical school and residency training. See Shanafelt TD, Bradley KA, Wipf JE, Back AL. Burnout and self-reported patient care in an internal medicine residency program. *Ann Intern Med* 2002;136:358–367; Thomas NK. Resident burnout. *JAMA* 2004;292:2880–2889; and Dyrbye LN, Thomas MR, Shahafelt TD. Medical student distress: causes, consequences, and proposed solutions. *Mayo Clin Proc* 2005;80:1613–1622.

109. Shore JH. The Oregon experience with impaired physicians on probation: an eight-year follow-up. *JAMA* 1987;257:2931–2934; Talbott GD, Gallegos KV, Wilson PO, et al. The Medical Association of Georgia's impaired physicians program. Review of the first 1,000 physicians: analysis of specialty. *JAMA* 1987;257: 2927–2930; Herrington RE, Benzer DG, Jacobs GR, et al. Treating substance-use disorders among physicians. *JAMA* 1982;247:2253–2257; and Walzer RS. Impaired physicians: an overview and update on the legal issues. *J Legal Med* 1990;11:131–198.

110. On how physicians can maintain their health in a stressful workplace, see Shanafelt TD, Sloan JA, Habermann TM. The well-being of physicians. *Am J Med* 2003;114:513–519; Mechanic D. Physician discontent: challenges and opportunities. *JAMA* 2003;290:941–946; and Zuger A. Dissatisfaction with medical practice. *N Engl J Med* 2004;350:69–75.

111. American Medical Association Council on Ethical and Judicial Affairs. Reporting impaired, incompetent, or unethical colleagues. In *Code of Medical Ethics. Current Opinions with Annotations*, 2006–2007 ed. Chicago: American Medical Association, 2006:274–275.

112. See Leape L, Fromson JA. Problem doctors: is there a system-level solution? *Ann Intern Med* 2006;144:107–115; and Curran WJ. Medical peer review of physician competence and performance: legal immunity and the anti-trust laws. *N Engl J Med* 1987;316:597–598.

113. See Morreim EH. Am I my brother's warden? Responding to the unethical or incompetent colleague. *Hastings Cent Rep* 1993;23(3):19–27.

114. For a general review of the duties of physician expert witnesses, see Beresford HR. *Neurology and the Law: Private Litigation and Public Policy*. Philadelphia: FA Davis Co, 1998:111–130; Kunin CM. The expert witness in medical malpractice litigation. *Ann Intern Med* 1984;100:139–143; and Herz DA. Neurosurgical liability: the expert witness. *J Neurosurg* 1992;76:334–335. For how physicians participate in the medical tort

system, see Beresford HR. *Neurology and the Law*, 1998:13–60; and Jacobson PD. Medical malpractice and the tort system. *JAMA* 1989;262:3320–3327. For the actual impact of malpractice suits against neurologists, see Bernat JL. Council on Medical Specialty Societies Professional Liability Report: Neurologists in medical malpractice: suggestions for future action. *Neurology* 1985;35:28A, 93–95; Safran A. Expert witness testimony in neurology: Massachusetts experience 1980–1990. *Neurol Chron* 1992;2(7):1–6; and Glick TH. Malpractice claims: outcome evidence to guide neurologic education? *Neurology* 2001;56:1099–1100.

115. Williams MA, Mackin GA, Beresford HR, et al. American Academy of Neurology qualifications and guidelines for the physician expert witness. *Neurology* 2006;66:13–14. The American Medical Association has similar guidelines. See American Medical Association Council on Ethical and Judicial Affairs. Medical testimony. In *Code of Medical Ethics. Current Opinions with Annotations*, 2006–2007 ed. Chicago: American Medical Association, 2006: 286–287.

116. Hurwitz B. How does evidence based guidance influence determinations of medical negligence? *BMJ* 2004;329:1024–1028.

117. For discussions on how medical societies should and do enforce standards of expert testimony, see Freeman JM, Nelson KB. Expert medical testimony: responsibilities of medical societies. *Neurology* 2004;63:1557–1558; Sagsveen MG. American Academy of Neurology policy on expert medical testimony. *Neurology* 2004;63:1555–1556; and Milunsky A. Lies, damned lies, and medical experts: the abrogation of responsibility by specialty organizations and a call for action. *J Child Neurol* 2003;18:413–419.

118. Irvine DH. The advertising of doctor's services. *J Med Ethics* 1991;17:35–40.

119. I explored this theme further in Bernat JL. Ethical and legal duties of the contemporary physician. *The Pharos* 1989;5(2):29–32. See also Havard JDJ. The responsibility of the doctor. *Br Med J* 1989;299:503–508.

120. *Tarasoff v Regents of the University of California*, Cal Supreme Ct (17 Cal 3rd 425, July 1, 1976). This case was cited and discussed in Beauchamp TL, Childress JF. *Principles of Biomedical Ethics*. 2nd ed. New York: Oxford University Press, 1982:282. See also the discussion in Veatch RM. *A Theory of Medical Ethics*. New York: Basic Books,1981:108–140.

121. American Medical Association. *Principles of Medical Ethics of the American Medical Association*. Chicago: American Medical Association, 1957. This quote is cited in Beauchamp TL, Childress JF. *Principles of Biomedical Ethics*, 1982:283. The use of the *Tarasoff* precedent in analyzing the duty to protect sexual partners of HIV-seropositive patients has been discussed further in Dickens BM. Legal limits of AIDS confidentiality. *JAMA* 1988;259:3449–3451 and Reamer FG. AIDS: The relevance of ethics. In, Reamer FG, ed. *AIDS & Ethics*. New York: Columbia University Press, 1991:8–10. For an opposing viewpoint, claiming that *Tarasoff* is not applicable to the duty to warn in HIV, see Ainslie DC. Questioning bioethics: AIDS, sexual ethics, and the duty to warn. *Hastings Cent Rep* 1999;29(5):26–35.

122. President's Commission for the Study of Ethical Problems in Medicine and Biomedical and Behavioral Research. *Screening and Counseling for Genetic Conditions: The Ethical, Social, and Legal Implications of Genetic Screening, Counseling, and Education Programs*. Washington, DC: US Government Printing Office, 1983:44.

123. Kipnis K. A defense of unqualified medical confidentiality. *Am J. Bioethics* 2006;6:7–18.

124. State laws vary on the legal duty to notify partners at risk of contracting AIDS. Notifying partners is a legal requirement in some jurisdictions. Many jurisdictions indemnify physicians who warn sexual partners of HIV-positive patients. See Bayer R. Public health policy and the AIDS epidemic: an end to HIV exceptionalism. *N Engl J Med* 1991;324:1500–1504; Brennan TA. AIDS and the limits of confidentiality: the physician's duty to warn contacts of seropositive individuals. *J Gen Intern Med* 1989;4:242–246; and O'Brien RC. The legal dilemma of partner notification during the HIV epidemic. *J Clin Ethics* 1993;4:245–252. For a more general treatment of the problem of breaking confidentiality to benefit other patients, see Veatch RM. *A Theory of Medical Ethics*, 1981:141–176. See also the further discussion of this subject in chapter 17.

125. American Medical Association Council on Ethical and Judicial Affairs. *JAMA* 1988;259:1360–1361; American College of Physicians Ethics Manual. 3rd ed. *Ann Intern Med* 1992;117:947–960: American College of Physicians and Infectious Diseases Society of America. *Ann Intern Med* 1994;120:310–319; and The American Academy of Neurology Code of Professional Conduct. *Neurology* 1993;43:1257–1260.

126. For specific information on state law as it pertains to the epileptic driver, see Krumholz A, Fisher RS, Lesser RP, et al. Driving and epilepsy: a review and reappraisal. *JAMA* 1991;265:622–626 and Berg AT, Engel J Jr. Restricted driving for people with epilepsy. *Neurology* 1999;52:1306–1307. For general information about physicians' legal liability for the epileptic driver, see Beresford HR. Legal implications of epilepsy. *Epilepsia* 1988;29(suppl 2):S114-S121 and Hughes JT, Devinsky O. Legal aspects of epilepsy. *Neurol Clin* 1994; 12:203–223.

127. Paraphrasing Rudolph Virchow, Michael Marmot argued that "physicians . . . need to be the natural attorneys of the disadvantaged." Marmot M. Harveian Oration: Health in an unequal world. *Lancet* 2006;368:2081–1094.

128. For a study showing that reduced access to medical care led to inadequate risk factor modification and recurrent cardiovascular events, see Levine DA, Kiefe CI, Houston TK, Allison JJ, McCarthy EP, Ayanian JZ. Younger stroke survivors have reduced access to physician care and medications: National Health Interview Survey from years 1998–2002. *Arch Neurol* 2007;64:37–42. For additional evidence of the harmful effect on health resulting from reduced access to medical care, see Fontanarisa PB, Rennie D, DeAngelis CD. Access to care as a component of health system reform. *JAMA* 2007;297:1128–130.

129. See American Medical Association Council on Ethical and Judicial Affairs. Caring for the poor. *JAMA* 1993;269:2533–2537 and American College of Physicians. Access to health care. *Ann Intern Med* 1990; 112:641–661.

130. Lo B, Katz MH. Clinical decision making during public health emergencies: ethical considerations. *Ann Intern Med* 2005;143:493–498; Salmon DA, Teret SP, Macintyre CR, Salisbury D, Burgess MA, Halsey NA. Compulsory vaccination and conscientious or philosophical exemptions: past, present, and future. *Lancet* 2006;367:436–442; Hick JL, O'Laughlin DT. Concept of operations for triage of mechanical ventilation in an epidemic. *Acad Emerg Med* 2006;13:223–229; and Gostin LO. Medical countermeasures for pandemic influenza: ethics and the law. *JAMA* 2006;295:554–556. See also two recent symposia: Symposium: Public Health Law and Ethics. *J Law Med Ethics* 2002;30:136–304; and The Proceedings of the Public's Health and the Law in the 21st Century: Fourth Annual Partnership Conference. *J Law Med Ethics* 2005;33:3–118.

131. Friedman E. Doctors and rationing: the end of the honor system. *Primary Care* 1986; 13:349–364.

132. Hardin G. The tragedy of the commons. *Science* 1968;162:1243–1248.

133. Hiatt HH. Protecting the medical commons: who is responsible? *N Engl J Med* 1975;293:235–241.

134. Cassel CK, Brennan TE. Managing medical resources: return to the commons? *JAMA* 2007;297: 2518–2521.

135. Sulmasy DP. Physicians, cost control, and ethics. *Ann Intern Med* 1992;116:920–926. For a similar opinion citing physicians' intrinsic conflicts of "double agency" in their attempt to conserve societal resources, see Angell M. The doctor as double agent. *Kennedy Inst Ethics J* 1993;3:279–286. The essential role of any system of medical ethics to address costs was emphasized in Lamm RD. Redrawing the ethics map. *Hastings Cent Rep* 1999;29(2):28–29. That ethics should be basis of any rationing plan was emphasized in: Pellegrino ED. Is rationing ever ethically justified? *Pharos* 2002;65(3):18–19.

136. Baily MA. Managed care organizations and the rationing problem. *Hastings Cent Rep* 2003;33(1):34–42.

137. The ethical duty of physicians to set limits is discussed in Callahan D. *Setting Limits: Medical Goals in an Aging Society*. New York: Simon & Schuster, 1987; Welch HG, Bernat JL, Mogielnicki RP. Who's in charge here? Maximizing patient benefit and professional authority by physician limit setting. *J Gen Intern Med* 1994;9:450–454; Murphy DJ, Povar GJ, Pawlson LG. Setting limits in clinical medicine. *Arch Intern Med* 1994;154:505–512; and Ubel PA, Arnold RM. The unbearable rightness of bedside rationing: physician duties in a climate of cost containment. *Arch Intern Med* 1995;155:1837–1842.

138. Truog RD, Brock DW, Cook DJ, et al. Rationing in the intensive care unit. *Crit Care Med* 2006; 34:958–963.

139. Holloway RG, Ringel SP, Bernat JL, Keran CM, Lawyer BL. US neurologists: attitudes on rationing. *Neurology* 2000;55:1492–1497.

140. Kohn LT, Corrigan JM, Donaldson MS, eds. *To Err is Human. Building a Safer Health System*. Washington, DC: National Academy Press, 1999. Some scholars claimed that the number of deaths estimated in this report was exaggerated. See McDonald CJ, Weiner M, Hui SL. Deaths due to medical errors are exaggerated in Institute of Medicine report. *JAMA* 2000;284:93–95 and the rebuttal by Leape LL. Institute of Medicine medical error figures are not exaggerated. *JAMA* 2000;284:95–97.

141. See, for example, Bogner MS, ed. *Human Error in Medicine*. Hillsdale, NJ: Erlbaum Associates, 1994.

142. Leape LL, Berwick DM. Five years after *To Err is Human*: What have we learned? *JAMA* 2005;293: 2384–2390.

143. Annas GJ. The patient's right to safety—improving the quality of care through litigation against hospitals. *N Engl J Med* 2006;354:2063–2066.

144. The provisions and limitations of the act are discussed in Fassett WE. Patient Safety and Quality Improvement Act of 2005. *Ann Pharmacother* 2006;40:917–924.

145. Glick TH, Rizzo M, Stern BJ, Feinberg DM. Neurologists for patient safety: where we stand, time to deliver. *Neurology* 2006;67:2119–2123. For a report on how commonly errors are made and adverse events

occur on hospitalized stroke patients, see Holloway RG, Tuttle D, Baird T, Skelton WK. The safety of hospital stroke care. *Neurology* 2007;68:550–555.

146. Wu AW, Cavanaugh TA, McPhee SJ, Lo B, Micco GP. To tell the truth: ethical and practical issues in disclosing medical mistakes to patients. *J Gen Intern Med* 1977;12:770–775.

147. Leape LL. Error in medicine. *JAMA* 1994;272:1851–1857.

148. In addition to those works already cited, see Smith ML, Forster HP. Morally managing medical mistakes. *Camb Q Healthc Ethics* 2000;5:38–53; Finkelstein D, Wu AW, Holtzman NA, Smith MK. When a physician harms a patient by a medical error: ethical, legal, and risk-management considerations. *J Clin Ethics* 1997;8:330–335; Baylis F. Errors in medicine: nurturing truthfulness. *J Clin Ethics* 1997;8:336–340; Zoloth L, Rubin SB (eds). *Margin of Error: The Ethics of Mistakes in the Practice of Medicine.* Hagerstown, MD: University Publishing, 2000; Vincent C. Understanding and responding to adverse events. *N Engl J Med* 2003;348: 1051–1056; and Sharpe VA. Promoting patient safety: an ethical basis for policy deliberation. *Hastings Cent Rep* 2003;33(5Suppl):S1–S19.

149. Rosner F, Berger JT, Kark P, Potash J, Bennett AJ. Disclosure and prevention of medical errors. *Arch Intern Med* 2000;160:2089–2092.

150. Gallagher TH, Levinson W. Disclosing harmful medical errors to patients: a time for professional action. *Arch Intern Med* 2005;165:1819–1824.

151. Berlinger N. Avoiding cheap grace: medical harm, patient safety, and the culture(s) of forgiveness. *Hastings Cent Rep* 2003;33(6):28–36.

152. Chassin MR, Becher EC. The wrong patient. *Ann Intern Med* 2002;136:826–833.

153. Lazare A. Apology in medical practice: an emerging clinical skill. *JAMA* 2006;296:1401–1404.

154. American Medical Association Council on Ethical and Judicial Affairs. Ethical responsibility to study and prevent error and harm. In *Code of Medical Ethics. Current Opinions with Annotations*, 2006–2007 ed. Chicago: American Medical Association, 2006:242–243.

155. Gallagher TH, Garbutt JM, Waterman AD, et al. Choosing words carefully: how physicians would disclose harmful medical errors to patients. *Arch Intern Med* 2006;166:1585–1593. There is little difference between surveyed physicians in Canada and the United States, suggesting that the liability crisis in the USA is responsible for failure to disclose. See Gallagher TH, Waterman AD, Garbutt JM, et al. US and Canadian physicians' attitudes and experiences regarding disclosing errors to patients. *Arch Intern Med* 2006;166:1605–1611. Thomas Gallagher and colleagues recently reviewed the subject of medical error disclosure. See Gallahger TH, Studdert D, Levinson W. Disclosing harmful errors to patients. *N Engl J Med* 2007;356:2713–2719.

156. Kraman SS, Hamm G. Risk management: extreme honesty may be the best policy. *Ann Intern Med* 1999;131:963–967 and Wu AW. Handling hospital errors: is disclosure the best defense? *Ann Intern Med* 1999;131:970–972.

157. Personal communication with Dr. Thomas H. Gallagher, October 4, 2006.

158. Tabler NG Jr. Should physicians apologize for medical errors? *Health Lawyer* 2007;19(3):23–26.

159. Sweet MP, Bernat JL. A study of the ethical duty of physicians to disclose errors. *J Clin Ethics* 1997;8:341–348; and Gallagher TH, Levinson W. Disclosing harmful medical errors to patients: a time for professional action. *Arch Intern Med* 2005;165:1819–1824.

160. Wu AW, Folkman S, McPhee SJ, Lo B. Do house officers learn from their mistakes? *JAMA* 1991; 265:2089–2094.

161. Witman AB, Park DM, Hardin SB. How do patients want physicians to handle mistakes? A survey of internal medicine patients in an academic setting. *Arch Intern Med* 1996;156:2565–2569; Gallagher TH, Waterman AD, Ebers AG, Fraser VJ, Levinson W. Patients' and physicians' attitudes regarding the disclosure of medical errors. *JAMA* 2003;289:1001–1007; and Mazor KM, Simon SR, Yood RA, et al. Health plan members' views about disclosure of medical errors. *Ann Intern Med* 2004;140:409–418.

162. Volpp KGM, Grande D. Residents' suggestions for reducing errors in teaching hospitals. *N Engl J Med* 2003;348:851–855.

163. West CP, Huschka MM, Novotny PJ, et al. Association of perceived medical errors with resident distress and empathy: a prospective longitudinal study. *JAMA* 2006;296:1071–1078.

164. Gostin L. A public health approach to reducing error: medical malpractice as a barrier. *JAMA* 2000;283:1742–1743.

165. Dickstein E, Erlen J, Erlen JA. Ethical principles contained in currently proposed medical oaths. *Acad Med* 1991;10:622–624. See also Orr RD, Pang N, Pellegrino ED, Siegler M. Use of the Hippocratic Oath: a review of twentieth century practices and a content analysis of oaths administered in medical schools in the US

and Canada in 1993. *J Clin Ethics* 1993;8:377–388. On the historical aspects of the Hippocratic Oath, see Markel H. "I swear by Apollo"—on taking the Hippocratic Oath. *N Engl J Med* 2003;350:2026–2029. On the relevance of the Hippocratic Oath to contemporary medical ethics, see Miles SH. *The Hippocratic Oath and the Ethics of Medicine.* New York: Oxford University Press, 2003.

166. From Pellegrino ED, Thomasma DC. *For the Patient's Good. The Restoration of Beneficence in Health Care.* New York: Oxford University Press, 1988:205–206. (© Oxford University Press, reprinted with permission.)

167. The context makes clear that the statement "assist my patient to die" refers to providing optimum palliative care and to discontinuing unwanted medical therapies, but it does not refer to physician-assisted suicide or active euthanasia.

Clinical Ethics and the Law

4

The ideal standards of medical conduct are dictated by medical ethics. A parallel and frequently overlapping standard of medical conduct is that regulated by the law. Generally speaking, the law dictates standards of physicians' professional conduct that are minimally acceptable to society. By contrast, medical ethics sets aspirational standards of professional conduct that an ideal physician should practice. In short, the law says what physicians *must* do whereas medical ethics says what physicians *should* do.

Medical ethics and the law have similar intents because both establish rules governing professional conduct. Although ethics is an ancient discipline, much of medical ethical analysis is of more recent vintage and has appropriated concepts first developed in law. For example, the legal doctrine of informed consent was developed before an analogous doctrine evolved in medical ethics. Similarly, the legal rules surrounding the obligations of fiduciaries, the avoidance of professional conflicts of interest, and the protection of rights of self-determination were well-developed legal doctrines before they became medical ethical doctrines. Thus, the content of medical ethics and law overlaps substantially.

The interaction between contemporary medical ethics and law is complex and symbiotic. Judiciaries and legislatures try to achieve ends similar in some ways to those of physicians during ethical deliberations. The legal system works to enact just laws and interpret them to respect and protect persons and society as a whole, whereas the medical profession tries to identify the medically and morally correct action to benefit and protect each patient. Indeed, in many judicial decisions on clinical issues, ethical reasoning has been utilized as the foundation of legal arguments.[1] In many areas, the proscriptions and aspirations of the law are as demanding as those of medical ethics.

Just as clinicians need not be moral philosophers to make ethically sound decisions, neither do they require formal legal training to make appropriate clinical decisions. But having a working knowledge of the basic theory and operation of the law is useful because it permits clinicians to place proper emphasis on the role of law and legal process in their medical practices. There are relatively few times when legal considerations are paramount in making clinical decisions. This chapter explores the relationship of ethics and law, and highlights the relatively minor constraints that the law exerts on medical practice in contrast to the fundamental demands that medical ethics exerts on medical practice. I discuss specific legal rulings pertaining to individual neurological disorders in the remaining chapters.

There are three general medico-legal references with which neurologists should be familiar. Neurologists seeking an in-depth discussion of the legal issues in neurological practice should consult the authoritative monograph by neurologist and law professor H. Richard Beresford.[2] Neurologists interested in important American judicial precedent-setting cases relevant to medical ethics should consult the accessible monograph by Jerry Menikoff,[3] and those interested in the application of American law to critically ill and dying patients should consult the indispensable, encyclopedic reference work by Alan Meisel and Kathy Cerminara.[4]

THE LAW

Legal scholars find it difficult to precisely define "the law"; it is easier to describe its purpose and function. Operationally, the law refers to the set of general and specific rules governing the conduct of individuals in their interactions with each other and with society.[5] The law creates a system to adjudicate conflicts, solve problems, and adapt to change. It governs and protects individuals in their relations with each other, the state, institutions, and organizations. The law imposes penalties on those found guilty of breaking its civil and criminal rules. Finally, it comprises a superstructure that organizes society both by codifying the minimum standards of personal, professional, and institutional conduct and by permitting the orderly redress of a broad range of wrongs.[6]

The vast corpus of law can be classified into overlapping descriptive categories. Statutory law refers to the body of legislation enacted within a jurisdiction, including civil and criminal statutes. Common law refers to a process of judicial decision making, used most extensively in the United States, Canada, and England, in which judgments are rendered after a careful study of individual cases. Case law judgments result in the gradual evolution and articulation of general legal principles and the establishment of judicial precedents that influence subsequent decisions. Criminal law is statutory law enacted to prohibit the most severe acts of antisocial behavior, to punish perpetrators, and thereby to protect society by discouraging others from committing these acts. Civil law—statutory law enacted to protect personal interests—permits an injured party to receive compensation from a wrongdoer who harmed the party through intent or negligence. Administrative law consists of a body of regulations propounded by

agencies to clarify the interpretation of relevant statutes. The term *the law* can refer to any or all of these categories.[7]

Several categories of law are relevant to medical practice. The law governing medical malpractice is an example of tort law, itself a branch of civil law. The law regulating decisions to withhold or withdraw life-sustaining treatment is an example of common law, in which judicial precedents including high state court decisions and rulings of the U.S. Supreme Court have established certain principles and rights. Statutory law is exemplified by state laws governing the determination of death and the use of advance directives. Criminal law encompasses the determination of homicide, which may become relevant to medical practice if physicians act directly to take a patient's life, even for compassionate motives or with the patient's consent, as discussed in chapter 9. The "Baby Doe" regulations, insuring mandatory treatment of some severely-ill newborns, are an example of administrative laws and are discussed in chapter 13.

CONFLICTS BETWEEN CLINICAL ETHICS AND THE LAW

In an ideal world, medical ethics and the law would never conflict. Laws would be drafted carefully and completely to incorporate and epitomize ethical behaviors that would ultimately benefit individuals, institutions, and society. Each law would reflect and codify the morally correct behavior of an individual or institution in every foreseeable situation. In such a world, all case law emanating from judiciaries and all statutory law enacted by legislatures would be based on ethical arguments about what is right and just, and would clearly and comprehensively codify normative ethical behaviors.

In practice, however, the law considers factors in addition to those of ethics. Case law may be biased by the judge's innate concept of justice, influenced by personal philosophical or political views, as discussed in chapter 1. The law evolves in a process of repeated statutory amendments and case law precedents in a continual attempt to codify the requirements of ethical behavior as well as the rights and responsibilities of individuals and society. In the medical context, this activity is most apparent in the series of famously adjudicated cases of the right to refuse life-sustaining treatment encompassing *Quinlan* to *Cruzan* (discussed in chapter 8) in which many of the legal questions were framed in ethical and constitutional terms. Despite these accomplishments, law lags behind the requirements of ethics, ostensibly attempting to follow and capture these requirements.

In the real world, medical ethics and the law may conflict in those instances in which a law has been written inadequately to recapitulate ideal ethical conduct. Laws intended to protect individuals or institutions may be drafted clumsily or may generate unanticipated and seemingly perverse consequences. If their negative consequences ultimately become paramount, these laws will need to be amended or repealed because they have become dysfunctional, harming the very individuals and institutions they were enacted to protect, or harming others unjustly.

Most statutory laws are drafted in general language with the anticipation that they will be clarified later by judicial deliberation during the litigation of individual cases. Case law, produced by a series of judicial decisions, is an evolving, iterative process in which precedents are cited and analyzed. Through this process, the theory and meaning of the law are scrutinized to distill its essence and intent, leading to its gradual perfection.

Society empowers judges with authority to suspend certain laws and grant exceptions to them in justified cases. This power is based on society's acceptance that the language of a law may not always be sufficiently clear and comprehensive to dispense proper justice. Although all citizens, including physicians, have an ordinary communal duty to follow the law, public interest is served best when exceptions to laws can be granted in those instances in which they are justified ethically.

Occasionally, physicians encounter situations in which their perceived ethical duty to patients conflicts with the law. If physicians, in their usual practice of following the law, find that doing so in a particular instance clearly produces more harm than good to a patient or others, if possible, they should contact a hospital attorney and seek a court order legally authorizing them to make an exception to the law. If such an order cannot be obtained with sufficient timeliness to permit physicians to protect the interest of those for whom they are responsible, generally they should act in accordance with the ethically correct decision, even if doing so conflicts with the law. In these unusual cases, seeking advice from the hospital attorney is essential.

In those rare instances in which following the law violates the requirements of medical ethics and a person is directly and avoidably harmed as a result, as a general rule, physicians are best advised to adhere to the obligations imposed by medical ethics. But because knowingly violating a law in such a circumstance could constitute civil disobedience, physicians who do so must be prepared to justify that such an action was courageously following the ethically correct behavior in response to an imperfect law. Physicians then should work within the political system to revise laws that systematically conflict with the mandates of ethics. In such potential conflicts of ethics and law, the best maxim for physicians to follow is: "Good ethics makes good law."

THE UNEASY RELATIONSHIP BETWEEN LAW AND MEDICINE

In contemporary American society, law and medicine have evolved an uneasy relationship. Marshall Kapp and Bernard Lo identified four reasons for the breakdown of their formerly collegial relationship.[8] First, a general challenge to authority figures is a defining characteristic of contemporary American life. Physicians' assertions no longer go unconditionally unchallenged, especially by other professionals such as attorneys. Second, the political movement asserting personal rights has expanded from the civil rights arena into the rights of patients. Because of public pressure, legislators have enacted statutes and administrative regulations to further protect patients' rights. Similarly, judicial interpretations of individual cases have highlighted the legal rights of patients, often against those of physicians. Third, the rise of consumerism has changed the distribution of power in the patient-physician relationship, making it more of an equal partnership by emphasizing patient autonomy over medical paternalism. Fourth, public financing of medical care through Medicare and Medicaid has thrust the legal system into the role of auditing the quality of medical care physicians provide, thus protecting the public investment.[9]

There are additional pragmatic reasons why physicians may be wary of lawyers and the law. First, and most importantly, contemporary American physicians nearly unanimously believe that the medical malpractice establishment systematically victimizes physicians, unjustly rewards lawyers, encourages lawsuits (because of the contingency fee structure), fails to provide efficient compensation for deserving patients, and generally falls short in dispensing proper justice.[10] Nearly all clinicians have been involved in a malpractice suit or know another who has. They are only too familiar with the details of how lawyers subject defendant physicians to years of harassment, intimidation, and unfair and insulting allegations.[11] The practice of most liability insurance companies to settle unmeritorious malpractice suits that they consider a "nuisance," rather than to pursue more expensive courtroom litigation, compounds the physicians' sense of injustice. The high prevalence of malpractice suits in some communities has instigated an unfortunate change in physicians' attitudes. Some physicians have come to fear prospective patients as potential plaintiffs and to loathe interactions with lawyers.

A second reason that provokes physicians to avoid legal interactions is the intimidating power of the law and lawyers. A patient or family's verbal or veiled threat to pursue legal action often is sufficient to win whatever demand either makes on the physician. Many physicians understandably lack the courage to endure a legal battle that they could avoid simply by capitulating to the demand. However, a poor medical decision may be made as a result of this capitulation, causing harm. Physicians would be better served to courageously stand by their medical judgments when these comprise the medically and ethically right course of action, but this decision is understandably difficult.

Third, because many physicians do not understand the law, they fear it and are suspicious of lawyers. For example, many physicians (and some lawyers) share the fallacious notion that anything not specifically permitted by law is therefore prohibited.[12] These physicians become unnecessarily and undesirably preoccupied with legalistic process to the detriment of good patient care. Before they make certain medical decisions, particularly those to cease or reduce life-sustaining medical treatment, some clinicians erroneously believe that they require legal permission.[13] Patients and their families may be harmed by this legalistic attitude because it inappropriately and unnecessarily insinuates a legal process into medical decision making with its consequent delays and misguided diffusion of authority.

There is a cultural reason for the American preoccupation with legal process. In his classic work *Democracy in America* (1835), Alexis de Tocqueville observed a quintessential American propensity to transform moral dilemmas into legal problems. He pointed out that Americans turn not to moral philosophy, religion, or cultural norms for insight and guidance on the right course of action, but to the courts.[14]

Van McCrary and Jeffrey Swanson examined the prevalence of legal defensiveness among physicians and its causes and effects. They found that 25% of surveyed Texas physicians who treat critically ill and terminally ill patients adopted a position of extreme legal defensiveness about clinical decision making, and found an inverse relationship between physicians' knowledge of relevant laws and their degree of legal defensiveness.[15] Their posture of legal defensiveness created conflicts between the physician and the critically ill or terminally ill patient and family resulting in an adversarial relationship that was counter-therapeutic.[16] The same investigators showed that, with increasing experience, physicians lessened their legal defensiveness to the betterment of patient care.[17] They also showed how highly publicized state judicial decisions influenced physicians' legal defensiveness, such as that seen in New York following the *O'Connor* decision, discussed further in chapter 15.[18]

Fourth, physicians may receive unsound legal advice from hospital attorneys and risk managers. Hospital attorneys and risk managers have the responsibility to protect their institution, which at times may lead them to provide unnecessarily conservative advice. In cases in which physicians wish to withdraw life-sustaining treatment, they may advise continuation of life-sustaining treatment, ostensibly to protect the hospital or medical staff against perceived potential liability. Hospital attorneys also may recommend that the safest legal course for a physician planning to terminate life-sustaining treatment in a certain case is first to secure a court order.

A hospital attorney should voice her opinions to the administration about the potential legal consequences of particular options. Administrators then should choose the option that appears most prudent. Because some administrators and managers are markedly averse to risk, they may prefer options that maximize the protection of the institution and the physicians. Although such options may be legally sound insofar as the institution's narrow interests are concerned, they may not be in the patient's or family's best interests. And most importantly, these options may not necessarily represent good medical care.[19] There are convincing arguments that maintaining an attitude of strong patient advocacy represents the best legal advice an attorney can provide her hospital.[20]

The most poignant example of the devastating effect of overly conservative legal advice from a hospital attorney occurred in the Linares case. Sammy Linares was six months old when he aspirated a deflated balloon at a birthday party. He suffered cardiopulmonary arrest and hypoxic-ischemic brain damage sufficient to result in a persistent vegetative state (PVS). Thereafter, he was totally dependent on a ventilator and had failed many attempts at ventilator weaning. Sammy's attending physician explained to his parents that there was no hope for his recovery: he would never regain consciousness or be able to be weaned from the ventilator. But because of advice from the hospital's legal counsel, the physician further explained that he was not permitted to follow the wishes of the parents to terminate the use of the ventilator unless they first obtained a court order. Inexplicably, despite the parents' obvious financial and educational limitations, no one in the hospital attempted to assist them in seeking such an order.

Mr. Linares visited Sammy frequently and, at one point, he was restrained by the nursing staff when tried to disconnect Sammy from the ventilator. After Sammy had been in PVS for nine months, his father, apparently motivated by compassion and desperation, entered the intensive care unit and held the nursing staff at gunpoint while he personally disconnected the ventilator. Mr. Linares held his son in his arms for an hour until he was certain that Sammy had died. At various times during the ordeal he said, "I'm not here to hurt anyone . . . I did it because I love my son and my wife. I only wanted him to be at rest." Mr. Linares then surrendered to the police. He received a suspended sentence on a misdemeanor weapons charge, but a grand jury, apparently moved by his compassionate motive, refused to hand down an indictment for attempted criminal homicide.[21]

The physicians in the Linares case were led to believe that they had no choice than to continue ventilatory therapy that neither they nor the family wanted, and that represented inappropriate care given his prognosis and the parents' treatment preferences. Although the hospital attorneys may have given the physicians and administrators proper legal advice based on their interpretation of Illinois law, clearly the wrong decision had been made. It appears that Sammy's physicians felt bound to follow advice of legal counsel and believed the law prevented them from giving appropriate medical treatment. These physicians' broader interest was in protecting the welfare of Sammy Linares, whereas the hospital attorneys' interests lay in protecting the institution and its staff physicians. Because their fear of violating the law was judged to be of prime importance, Sammy's physicians did not or could not make the ethically correct decision.

Overly conservative legal advice may have a more pernicious and enduring effect on physicians' thinking than the direct effects of legal advice in a particular case. Physicians may develop a false belief that formal legal proceedings represent the best or only resolution of a patient's complex medical-ethical problem. Not only is this belief incorrect, but it encourages the physician, consciously or subconsciously, to misconstrue a patient's ethical conflict as a legal one.[22] Physicians should retain responsibility for their patients' medical care and should not willingly transfer it to, or unnecessarily allow it to be usurped by, a lawyer or court of law.[23]

Fifth, physicians are understandably intimidated by criminal law, particularly the increasing and disturbing tendency for cases of extreme medical negligence to be subjected to criminal prosecution. One area where practicing clinicians may encounter the criminal justice system is when law enforcement officials wish to interview hospitalized patients who may have experienced, witnessed, or perpetrated a crime. Physicians may be unsure how to balance patient confidentiality with the requirements of law, particularly given the fact that state and federal regulations and professional guidelines governing this activity are minimal. Paul Jones and colleagues developed five guidelines for physicians: (1) respect for patient autonomy permits the competent patient to decide whether to speak with the police; (2) police interviews should not interfere with medical care unless competent patients accept the risk of harm; (3) patient privacy should be respected by strict adherence to HIPAA regulations as discussed in chapter 3; (4) clinicians should maintain professional boundaries by clarifying that they have no role in the criminal justice operation; and (5) hospitals should proactively form committees to develop guidelines governing the interaction of medical and other personnel with the law enforcement system.[24]

Finally, physicians should not ask the law to grant them unconditional immunity from liability for their medical decisions. Although no physician wishes to be a party to civil or criminal litigation, her best protection is to practice medicine according to the highest ethical standards. Requesting absolute immunity from legal liability before making a potentially controversial

decision (such as termination of life-sustaining treatment) is unnecessary, time-consuming, and inefficient. In the end, the request may backfire, as occurred in the tragic case of the anencephalic Baby K discussed in chapter 10.

Insisting upon unconditional immunity represents poor medical practice for other reasons. It incorrectly displaces the focus of decision-making responsibility to the court, where it does not belong. This decision rightfully belongs to the principals involved: the physician, the patient, surrogate decision maker, family, and health-care facility. Requests for unconditional immunity foster poor patient care because of delays and deferral of responsibility. Finally, requests for immunity are of questionable morality because they place the self-interest of the physician (in trying to guarantee her absolute protection) above the interest of the patient.[25]

Attorneys also have grounds to distrust physicians. Many attorneys regard the negative attitudes that physicians harbor against the medical malpractice system to be largely their own fault because physicians have failed to properly police their profession to weed out incompetent colleagues and improve patient safety. Attorneys further view physicians' attempts to pursue tort reform and other institutionalized means of providing immunity from liability simply as the machinations of a special interest group to protect itself. They believe that a robust malpractice system remains the best public protection against physicians' carelessness and incompetence.

Despite these differences and conflicts, physicians and lawyers share much common ground. They share a set of core social and ethical values, interests, and experiences that define both physicians and attorneys as professionals, particularly their fiduciary duties to their patients/clients.[26] Further, they share respect for individual patient/client autonomy, a commitment to reason and the rule of law, and the use of professional judgment and experience as grounds for decision making.[27] They should use these shared values to lessen antagonism, build better professional relationships, and work together to solve mutual problems such as: (1) the optimum way to conserve medical resources while accommodating individual patient autonomy and social concepts of fairness; and (2) the design of an improved patient safety system that maintains appropriate accountability but permits a confidential reporting system.[28] One example of their past cooperation was during the development of the Patients' Bill of Rights.[29]

In an ideal world, physicians and lawyers would have mutual respect and work together toward a common goal—the betterment of health and the protection of personal and institutional rights. For their part, physicians should concentrate on identifying and following the medically and ethically correct course of action in patient management and try not be unnecessarily preoccupied with legalistic concerns.

STANDARDS OF SURROGATE DECISION MAKING

The doctrine of valid consent, described in chapter 2, requires physicians to obtain a competent patient's free and informed consent before embarking on diagnostic testing or treatment. Respect for patients' rights of self-determination and the duty to promote patients' medical welfare predicate this ethical and legal responsibility of clinicians. Competent patients are partners with their physicians in a shared decision-making process in which the physician contributes her specialized knowledge, skills, and experience and the patient contributes her unique values and preferences for health care.[30] The right of competent patients to give or refuse consent extends to instances in which they are profoundly paralyzed and have difficulty with communication, as discussed in chapter 14.

When a patient is incompetent, a surrogate decision maker must be identified from whom the physician obtains valid consent for tests or treatment. In the ideal circumstance, the patient previously will have named a legally authorized surrogate in a durable power of attorney or a document appointing a health-care agent. In the absence of a legally authorized surrogate, an informal surrogate must

be chosen. In the selection of a surrogate decision maker, physicians should consider the urgency of the situation and the existence of suitable candidates, such as family members or guardians. When an emergency situation arises, the physician in charge must make a rapid decision that she believes to be in the patient's best interest. But in a non-emergency situation, the nuclear family generally serves as the appropriate surrogate decision maker. There are several reasons to justify this practice: (1) family members usually have the greatest concern about the patient's welfare; (2) family members are most knowledgeable about the patient's health-care values and goals; (3) family members form a social unit that should be recognized as a unitary decision maker; and (4) there is a common law basis for respecting the wishes of family members in the absence of a prior formal surrogate appointment.[31] Physicians can respect the wishes of the family as a surrogate assuming the family speaks with one mind and is not divided. The problem of handling the divided family is considered in chapter 2.

Surrogate decision makers cannot properly execute their important role in making health-care decisions for incompetent patients without understanding the standards that guide their decision making. Three general decision-making standards are recognized in ethics and the law: the standards of expressed wishes, substituted judgment, and best interests. Different jurisdictions have cited these standards in rulings with varying degrees of emphasis. I discuss these three standards in descending order of their ethical power, a hierarchy based upon their ability to recapitulate the decision that would have been made by the patient and thus respecting the patient's autonomy.[32]

Expressed Wishes

Surrogate decision makers first should try to follow wishes expressed previously by patients when they were competent that pertain to the current clinical situation. For example, if the patient had expressly stated that she did not wish to receive cardiopulmonary resuscitation in the event of expected cardiopulmonary arrest, the surrogate should insist that the physician write a Do-Not-Resuscitate order. Patients' written advance directives (such as living wills or proxy appointment written directives, discussed later) are an important place to search for their expressed wishes.

Following the standard of expressed wishes most closely respects a patient's autonomy by permitting her to continue to consent for or refuse specific medical treatment despite the fact that she now is incompetent. The practical problem with this standard is that most patients cannot possibly have anticipated and discussed their preferences in the numerous specific clinical states that later may occur. Even written wishes expressed in a living will (see below) usually are too vague and ambiguous to be of use except in the most general way. Thus, though it is powerful ethically, this standard often cannot be applied in practice.

Substituted Judgment

When a surrogate does not know the patient's expressed wishes, she should attempt to reproduce the decision the patient would have made by applying the patient's values and preferences to the situation in question.[33] This process of making a judgment by "walking in the patient's shoes" is known as the standard of substituted judgment. Success in executing true substituted judgment requires the proxy to have a clear concept of the patient's healthcare preferences, goals, and values as well as the courage to apply and uphold them despite her own potential misgivings. Preferences of the patient may be evident from written directives, conversations the proxy had with the patient, or deductions the proxy can make based on the way in which the patient has lived her life.[34]

Substituted judgment is an ideal that does not succeed fully in clinical practice. Its practical limitations were illustrated convincingly in a study of spouses' predictions of patients' choices for undergoing cardiopulmonary resuscitation (CPR). Each spouse surveyed was asked to predict whether or not the patient would choose to undergo CPR if the patient's heart stopped beating. Several scenarios in

which this event could occur were depicted. Spouses were assumed to be the ideal surrogate to employ a standard of substituted judgment because of their intimate knowledge of the patient. However, spouses chose incorrectly in over one-third of the cases, usually stating that the patients would wish CPR when in fact they would not. Physicians also erred by a similar percentage in their predictions of patients' wishes. Tellingly, when the physicians erred, they usually predicted that the patients would refuse CPR when in fact they would consent.[35]

These same errors in substituted judgment have been replicated in several subsequent similar studies, showing only a modest level of accuracy when spouses, children, and other surrogates attempt to replicate patients' treatment decisions. David Shalowitz and colleagues performed a meta-analysis on 16 studies of surrogate decision making using a substituted judgment standard for end-of-life decision making. They found 151 hypothetical scenarios involving 2,595 surrogate-patient pairs, with a collective analysis of 19,526 patient-surrogate paired responses. Overall, surrogates predicted patients' treatment preferences with 68% accuracy. Surrogates' treatment preference accuracy was improved neither by patient designation of surrogates nor by prior discussion of patients' treatment preferences.[36]

In one study, chosen surrogate decision makers scored no better than volunteers picked randomly to answer a questionnaire listing clinical scenarios about the treatment choices that patients preferred.[37] Most of the substituted judgment errors in these studies were committed because surrogates misunderstood patients' true wishes and had failed to discuss them in advance. One study in England showed that patients' relatives could not exercise a substituted judgment because they did not know the patients' CPR wishes. Their decisions presumed what the patients wanted and accorded with those of the physicians.[38] Some legal scholars have expressed doubt that the doctrine of substituted judgment, originally created to settle property disputes, ever can be applied usefully to medical decision making.[39]

Suggestions to improve the accuracy of substituted judgments have included requiring the use of a decision-making syllogism in which the patient's values are stated explicitly as a premise,[40] encouraging the use of concurrent written explicit directives, and most importantly, emphasizing the need for patients while healthy to engage their chosen surrogates in detailed conversations about their health-care values and treatment choices in anticipation of possible future incompetence. Jeffrey Berger recently emphasized that surrogates' substituted judgments also should take into account what most patients really care about, namely the effect of the clinical decision on those whom the patient loves.[41]

Best Interest

In instances in which a surrogate decision maker lacks reliable evidence of the patient's values and preferences, substituted judgments cannot be made. Here, the surrogate must rely on more objective grounds to decide which treatment course is best for the patient. Examples of such objective grounds include the degree of the patient's suffering with or without treatment, the likelihood of her recovery, and the impact on the family. This decision-making process, known as the best interest standard, asks how a reasonable person would balance the anticipated burdens borne as a result of a proposed treatment course against the benefits accrued from it. If the burdens exceed the benefits, a reasonable person using a utilitarian analysis would conclude that is in the patient's best interest not to proceed with treatment.[42]

Best interest judgments are made routinely in infants and young children whose stated health-care preferences do not exist, by state-appointed surrogates who do not know the patients they represent, and by any surrogate who does not know the patient's values and preferences. The best interest standard is less powerful ethically than the substituted judgment standard because the latter permits physicians to respect the patient's personal autonomy and self-determination despite her present incompetence. No such goals are possible with a best interest standard. From a best

interest decision-making process, a third party can only make a reasoned judgment of what she thinks is best for the patient without applying the patient's personal ranking of health-care goals and values.

The best interest standard has been justifiably criticized because it requires a judgment about the patient's quality of life which, although it attempts to be objective, remains inherently subjective.[43] Survey studies have shown that physicians systematically underestimate the quality of their elderly patients' lives and the important meaning to them of even a limited quality of life. Thus, physicians or surrogates could make treatment decisions based on an erroneous concept of a patient's best interest.[44] The personal preferences of spouses and physicians also influence their perceptions of patients' preferences.[45] Decisions of physicians and surrogates reached by a best interest process may be seriously flawed, therefore, because they may differ systematically from the decisions the patients would have made for themselves.

Attempts have been made to enhance the objectification of best interest determinations, to make them less ad hoc, and to make them depend less on the surrogate's attitude about the patient's quality of life. For example, James Drane and John Coulehan devised a biopsychosocial model of best interest decision making designed to incorporate and properly weigh all relevant factors in the surrogate's decision.[46] This attempt to systematize the best interest standard will help reduce some of its inherent subjectivity but does not compensate for its ultimate reliance on a judgment about the patient's quality of life.

Both best interest determinations and substituted judgments are imperfect decision-making processes. In executing their difficult task, surrogates first should try to employ the expressed wishes standard. When the patient's expressed wishes are unknown, they should decide by substituted judgment to the best of their ability. With no knowledge whatsoever of the patient's values, they should employ a best interest process but should attempt to objectify assessing the burdens and benefits of treatment and to exercise caution and prudence when rendering quality of life determinations for elderly or disabled patients. Hospitals should draft policies stipulating the procedures for decision making using the best interest standard when patients lack a surrogate decision maker and advance directives.[47]

ADVANCE DIRECTIVES FOR MEDICAL CARE

The advance directive is the most powerful extension of the competent patient's right of self-determination. The physician who respects a patient's advance directive fulfills her ethical duty to respect the autonomy of a person. Theoretically, an advance directive is superior to a substituted judgment or best interest determination because, as an expressed wish, it does not attempt to reproduce a patient's decision, it *is* the decision.[48] Physicians have an ethical duty to attempt to follow relevant advance directives to the fullest extent possible and a legal duty to follow those that are legally authorized.

Advance directives are of two principal types: (1) written instructional statements of a patient's wishes for treatment in different anticipated clinical situations; and (2) written appointments designating surrogate decision makers whose authority is activated when a patient becomes incompetent. Often, the appointment is accompanied by written instructions. There are advantages and disadvantages of each type of advance directive.[49] Both have been incorporated into statutory law in the majority of states in the United States and in several other countries.[50]

Advance directives are a tool to help execute the broader concept of advance care planning. Advance care planning encompasses patients' prudent anticipation of future medical events and their clear communication to their family and physicians of how they wish to be treated if these events should occur.[51] Advance care planning includes patients' understanding of their diagnosis, the burdens of treatment, the possible outcomes and their likelihood, and their treatment preferences based on their health-care values and goals.[52] Patients should communicate clearly with their physicians and close family members to insure that both groups understand their wishes for future treatment and are willing to uphold them.[53] Many nursing homes and other chronic care facilities require the completion of an advance care plan to determine in advance what level of treatment to provide in anticipated situations. Unfortunate instances of unwanted and unnecessary aggressive treatment may result from the absence of such advance care plans.[54] Advance directives have value when they help in correctly formulating care plans.

Living Wills

The written instructional directive popularly known as the "living will" and called the "terminal care document" in some jurisdictions states the patient's preferences for future treatment in certain anticipated circumstances. Commonly, living wills contain language such as "If I am ever terminally ill without reasonable hope for recovery, I wish to be permitted to die naturally without receiving life-sustaining treatments." Although the impetus for executing living wills usually is to limit or terminate life-sustaining treatment in the event of terminal illness, they are not categorically restricted to termination of treatment and may be designed to indicate a wish for maximum medical treatment.[55] As a rule, living wills become activated only in the setting of terminal illness. Most but not all states have statutes permitting living will directives.

Most written directives are brief general statements but others are more expansive, with details of particular clinical scenarios and instructions, for example, about whether artificial hydration and nutrition are considered therapies to be withheld. Instructional directives on state-authorized forms are legal documents that require the signature of patient and witnesses. The precise language of written directives and the regulations regarding their execution and implementation, such as the definition of terminal illness, vary from state to state. Some states, such as Ohio, have chosen to legislate lengthy and onerous conditions before a patient can exercise the directive.[56] In all jurisdictions, the living will directive becomes activated only in the presence of a terminal illness that must first be certified by a physician.

One advantage of the written directive is that it provides a clear and convincing account of a patient's treatment preference at the time the directive was executed. The directive's formality and signatures attest to the fact that the patient had given serious and thoughtful consideration to the statements contained within it. Courts usually view such written directives as more reliable evidence of the carefully considered wishes of the patient than statements made in casual conversations.[57]

Limitations of Written Directives

Written advance directives have several disadvantages. The language in which the majority of them are drafted is vague and ambiguous.[58] For example, does a persistent vegetative state count as a "terminal illness"? Is artificial hydration and nutrition considered a "life-sustaining medical treatment" that can be discontinued? The answers to these and other potential ambiguities remain unclear in the majority of written directives. Despite the fact that the patient may think she is clearly stating her wishes, he physician and proxy later may have the unenviable task of attempting to interpret the meaning of these vague statements and apply them to a particular clinical situation.[59]

Some scholars have addressed the inherent ambiguity of written directives by designing highly detailed written documents that attempt to clarify all ambiguous terms. These directives also portray several specific paradigmatic clinical scenarios complete with prognosis and level of disability, and specify the precise form of treatment and life-sustaining interventions that the patient wishes in each case.[60] Some directives are many pages in length and filled with technical details and checklists.

The difficulty with such sophisticated directives is that they can be used successfully only by the minority of highly educated patients. Although the directives may be streamlined to present the material graphically, as in a checklist, they contain technical information that most non-physicians find difficult to comprehend. I saw an elderly patient who attempted to complete such a directive with the result that it contained internally contradictory statements about her wishes. In a subsequent discussion, her daughter explained that her mother simply misunderstood the technical jargon. Further, even obsessively detailed written directives cannot anticipate every possible clinical situation; thus, ambiguity of interpretation remains an unresolved problem in many cases.[61]

Another problem with written instructional directives is that patients' values and health-care goals may change over time, especially with aging and advancing disease. A young person in vigorous health may wish to die rather than to live in a disabled state. Older people, however, may be more willing to derive pleasure from limited states of activity. Should a directive written at age 30 stating that the patient would prefer to die rather than to live with a particular degree of disability maintain its force 40 years later when the patient may be quite satisfied to live at a diminished functional level?[62] Also, patients who become ill may change their minds about the desirability of treatment and negate even recent directives they made when they were healthy.[63] Indeed, there is little evidence that decisions patients make when healthy accurately predict the choices they make when their death is imminent.[64]

Periodic updates of written instructional directives can help keep an advance directive contemporaneously accurate, but the essential problem remains. In chapter 15, we return to this problem in its most difficult version: what is a clinician's ethical and legal duty toward the demented patient who appears happy and wants to continue living although she had previously executed a written directive stating that she wanted to be permitted to die by withholding artificial or oral hydration and nutrition if she were ever in a demented state?[65]

The degree of stability of directives over short periods of time has been the subject of several studies. In one study, researchers presented clinical vignettes containing specific treatment choices to outpatients and other volunteers. In three interviews, conducted over a two-year period, the subjects demonstrated a high rate of consistency in their treatment choices. The stability of their choices increased over time in those patients who had the opportunity to discuss them with their physician.[66] However, in another study of the stability of treatment preferences over approximately a year, 80% of patients changed at least one of twelve choices.[67] In an interesting recent study, not only did treatment preferences change over a two-year follow up interval, but the patients were generally unaware that they had changed.[68]

One study showed a surprisingly poor correlation between the statements made by patients on legally executed written directives and their subsequent responses to survey questions about their health-care preferences.[69] In another study, 55% of the outpatients participating were unable to identify the correct definition of a term commonly used in the living will.[70] A study of patients completing the Maryland advance directive form showed a disturbing level of internal inconsistency between responses on the form and responses to more specific scenarios presented to the patients.[71] Such data raise vexing questions about the extent to which patients truly understand the meaning and implications of their signed written statements and cast doubt on their significance as the clear and convincing statement of patients' wishes.

Written directives are inadequate advance care plans by themselves. Written directives are most useful and valid in the short term when they stimulate a discussion between patients and physicians about the details of selected treatments and the meaning of specific treatment choices.[72] Several prominent clinical ethicists have declared the living will a failure as a solitary advance directive.[73] Experienced physicians, particularly in ICU settings, find written directives are difficult to apply to patient care.[74] One study showed written directives rarely were of value in decisions for chronically ill outpatients.[75] The President's Council on Bioethics forcefully concluded "Advance instruction directives (or living wills), though valuable to some degree and in some circumstances, are a limited and flawed instrument for addressing most of the decisions caregivers must make for those entrusted to their care." The Council urged surrogate appointments as the best advance directive mechanism.[76]

Patients should discuss their treatment wishes with their physician, family, and surrogate.[77] In the setting of an established physician-patient relationship, a living will executed with careful instruction and explanation from a patient's physician about the terms and implications used in the document can help the patient to ensure that her health-care preferences will be respected if she should become incompetent and terminally ill. Although there is evidence that the mere presence of an advance directive does not stimulate a discussion with the physician,[78] educational interventions with physicians can improve patient-physician communication to make the directives more useful.[79] There is evidence that patients who have had discussions with their physicians about advance directives are more satisfied with their care.[80] One recent study showed that patients who had completed a living will were more likely to die at home or a nursing home than in a hospital.[81]

Despite the authority granted to written advance directives, it is ethically justifiable to overrule them in certain instances. The most common case is when a surrogate decision maker overrules a patient's previous written directive because an unexpected deterioration in the patient's health has rendered it no longer applicable. For example, a patient may have executed a written directive requesting cardiopulmonary resuscitation and other rescue treatments when he was in robust health. But during a hospitalization for routine surgery, he suffered two strokes rendering him paralyzed, globally aphasic, and requiring permanent institutionalization for nursing care. His health-care agent has the discretion to overrule his previous request for CPR because his agent knows that now the patient would not wish to undergo it because it no longer can restore his robust health.[82]

Health-Care Surrogate Appointments

Shortly after the living will became popular, another advance directive mechanism was introduced, the health-care surrogate appointment. The surrogate appointment permits a patient, while competent, to authorize another person to make her health-care decisions in the event that later she becomes incompetent. Such a legally authorized surrogate is known variously in different states as durable power of attorney for health care, health-care agent, health-care proxy, or health-care surrogate. As in living will legislation, states have authorized the printing of legal forms for durable power of attorney for health care for the patient to complete and the patient and surrogate to sign, with co-signatures of witnesses.

All states have provisions for naming durable powers of attorney for financial matters. The "durable" modifier refers to the fact that such appointments are not nullified by the patient's subsequent incompetence. The health-care surrogate is a modification of the durable power of attorney wherein the surrogate's authority is restricted specifically to health-care decisions. Lawful surrogates generally have the same authority as the patient had before she became incompetent. The health-care surrogate must be approached to obtain valid consent before the patient can receive non-emergency diagnosis or treatment exactly as a competent patient would be. Some states restrict the authority of the agent to refuse artificial hydration and nutrition unless the patient had expressly refused it in the written portion of the directive. The state-by-state specific legal provisions for surrogates have been tabulated.[83]

States permit competent adults to name their chosen surrogate but the surrogate must consent to play this role and in some states sign the form. Most commonly, patients choose a spouse, sibling, or mature child. Most states will not permit the patient to choose her physician to serve as a surrogate, but some scholars have argued that the patient's longstanding physician with clear knowledge of the patient's wishes would be ideal to serve in that role.[84] One study showed that 10% to 15% of patients prefer a non-family member to serve as surrogate, particularly in the setting of family strife or perceived conflicts of interest.[85]

Appointing a health-care surrogate has several advantages over creating written instructional directives. Most importantly, it permits greater flexibility because the surrogate can use her discretion to interpret the general wishes of the patient in the context of a specific clinical situation. In a living will, the patient must anticipate all possible clinical contingencies and stipulate in advance what treatment she would like to receive in each case. By contrast, the health-care surrogate can make a novel but intelligent judgment, applying the known values and wishes of the patient to a unique and previously unanticipated situation.[86] Also, activation of the durable power of attorney for health-care does not require terminal illness but rather only that the patient lacks the capacity to make health-care decisions. For these reasons and from my clinical experience as an ethics consultant, I conclude that the surrogate appointment is superior to the living will as an advance directive, particularly because surrogate appointment documents also provide patients the opportunity to leave specific written instructions. Clinicians should encourage their patients to complete a surrogate appointment.[87]

The health-care surrogate and the patient's physician have a unique relationship that has some of the features of the patient-physician relationship.[88] Physicians need to advise surrogates and provide them information and counsel to help them to successfully fulfill their difficult, lonely, and anxiety-ridden role. Surrogates struggle to faithfully represent their understanding of the patient's wishes but may be pressured from family or friends for a different course of action. The surrogate-physician relationship should be collaborative because both surrogate and physician share the goal of improving the patient's health and following the patient's directives.

Surrogate decision making has limitations. The frequent errors that occur in practice when a surrogate attempts to make a substituted judgment decision were discussed previously. Conflicts of interest can occur when the surrogate's decision is made more in her own interest than in the patient's interest.[89] Equally disturbing are the reports of cases in which the surrogate has chosen a course of treatment or non-treatment that is diametrically opposite the one which the physician understood the patient to want when the patient was competent.[90] This mismatch of patient's and surrogate's wishes produces a serious and ongoing conflict over defining appropriate treatment that, in my experience, frequently results in asking for an ethics committee to try to resolve it.

A study of patients completing the California Durable Power of Attorney directive and controls who were not offered advance directives revealed the provocative finding that there was no difference in health outcomes, medical treatments, or charges that both groups received.[91] However, in a more recent study, patients completing advance directives were found to incur lower costs of hospitalization for their terminal illness, presumably by avoiding costly life-sustaining treatment.[92] These data need to be monitored in the future to evaluate the impact of advance directives on the clinical care of patients.

Legality and Public Acceptance

Currently, all 50 states and the District of Columbia have statutory provisions for health-care agent appointments, living wills, or both.[93] The American Medical Association and the American Academy of Neurology, among other medical societies, support the use of legal advance directives.[94] A majority of surveyed physicians supported more widespread use of advance directives.[95] Surveyed hospital inpatients and outpatients indicate that most want a greater opportunity to complete advance directives.[96] Yet, the large majority of patients have not completed a living will or health-care surrogate appointment.

There are several impediments to patients executing advance directives. First is the obvious psychological barrier raised when patients consider death or disability. Most people would prefer to avoid thinking about and planning for such emotionally upsetting subjects. Second is the lack of knowledge about the availability and meaning of advance directives. In one study, less than 40% of the patients with a Do-Not-Resuscitate order knew the definition of a living will.[97] Third, adverse patient demographic factors, particularly educational level and socioeconomic status, have been shown to impede the execution of advance directives.[98] Fourth, prior to 1990, most hospitals did not routinely inquire about the existence of advance directives or offer

assistance to patients who wished to complete them.[99] Finally, even among hospitalized patients who had completed advance directives, the existence of the advance directive frequently went unrecognized or was not honored during the hospital admission.[100]

One study identified five barriers that made physicians reluctant to discuss advance directives with patients: physicians showed (1) lack of understanding of the purpose of advance directives; (2) erroneous beliefs about the appropriateness of advance directives; (3) lack of knowledge of how to execute an advance directive; (4) concern about time constraints for the discussion; and (5) lack of comfort in the discussion.[101] While most studies have shown that outpatients generally wish to discuss directives with their physicians,[102] the SUPPORT study provocatively found that a majority of critically ill inpatients without advance directives preferred not to do so.[103] Another study showed a greater willingness of physicians to discuss advance directives if they perceived that the patient's prognosis was less favorable, such as in the setting of HIV.[104] One study assessing how physicians communicate with patients showed that even physicians who discussed advance directives did not ask patients about their values or their attitudes toward prognostic uncertainty.[105] Improvement in physicians' communication skills may help reduce this barrier.

The Patient Self-Determination Act of 1990

The Patient Self-Determination Act (PSDA) of 1990 was enacted to encourage more hospitalized patients to complete advance directives.[106] It was drafted in the wake of the publicity surrounding the U.S. Supreme Court *Cruzan* decision and the awareness that Nancy Cruzan, like most citizens, had not completed a living will or health-care surrogate appointment. Had Ms. Cruzan completed an advance directive prior to entering a persistent vegetative state, the answer to the vexing question of whether to permit her parents' wish to discontinue her artificial hydration and nutrition (discussed in chapter 12) would have been clear. The PSDA was predicated on the assumption that better medical decision making and improved patient care would result if more patients completed advance directives.

The PSDA applies to all hospitals, skilled nursing facilities, hospices, home health agencies, personal care agencies, and health maintenance organizations that receive revenues from Medicare or Medicaid. The act requires that each institution have in place a mechanism to determine whether patients being admitted have an advance directive. If they do not, the institution must provide them with written information upon their admission stating the patient's legal rights to refuse life-prolonging therapy and to complete a lawful advance directive. This information must also include the relevant portion of the hospital's policy on this issue.[107]

Several concerns have been raised about the impact of the PSDA on patient care. Ideally, the execution of an advance directive would represent the culmination and formalization of an ongoing dialogue between a patient and a physician about the patient's wishes for future medical treatment. However, the PSDA requires only that advance directive information be presented to patients without stipulating how they can be educated to fully understand its meaning and intent. In some institutions, this teaching obligation may be assigned to a clerk or employee who has neither a relationship with the patient nor any knowledge of her. With such an arrangement, the potential exists for patients to misunderstand the information presented and to execute misleading, inaccurate, or incomplete directives. Because a discussion with a physician is not mandated by the PSDA, an educational effort directed at institutional employees is necessary to prevent the act from producing potential harm.[108]

Some critics have expressed fears that the PSDA could be used as a cost-containment strategy. By employing such a strategy, institutions could subtly or explicitly encourage patients to agree to have their lives shortened in order to reduce costly terminal hospital and nursing home admissions.[109] Studies of the impact of advance directives on the costs of medical care, however, are conflicting, with some finding no difference in costs of hospitalization for those who had completed advance directives compared to those who had not, and others finding cost savings from advance directives.[110]

The wide sweep of the PSDA has been criticized because it requires that *all* patients admitted to health-care facilities undergo education toward completing an advance directive. For some groups, this timing is undesirable. For example, it is probably unwise to encourage elderly patients admitted to psychiatric facilities with depression to complete advance directives. They may make decisions that do not represent their true wishes because of temporary irrationality resulting from their illness.[111]

The practical impact of the PSDA was studied in two medical school teaching hospitals. The advance directive practices of a group of patients made before the passage of the PSDA were compared with those of a matched group made after the Act became law. After the passage of the PSDA, there was a small but significant increase in the number of patients who had discussed general end-of-life issues with their surrogates but no increase in the number of patients who had held detailed discussions about specific therapeutic interventions. There was no increase in the proportion of patients who discussed advance care planning with their physicians, except among the subgroup of patients in poorer health. Overall, while there was a significant increase in patients who had carried out verbal advance directive planning, there was not a significant increase in the use of formal written directives. Thus, the PSDA apparently has stimulated more general discussions with families and surrogates about advance care planning but has resulted in no greater completion of specific written advance directives.[112] Additional studies of a similar nature should be conducted to follow the future impact of the PSDA.

HEALTH-CARE SURROGATE ACTS

An alternative to relying on patients to complete advance directives is to legislate a mechanism creating a default mode for medical decision making in the absence of prior advance directives. Because fewer than 25% of American citizens complete an ordinary will, it is unrealistic to believe that many more will complete an advance directive, no matter how great the incentives or the mandates from such laws as the PSDA. Several states have drafted health-care surrogacy acts that take effect in the absence of advance directives and in the context of specific illnesses by which the patient is rendered incompetent. These acts automatically designate legally authorized surrogate decision makers from a priority list beginning with close family members, the very people most patients would have voluntarily authorized to be their surrogate if they had made prior efforts to do so.[113]

Health-care surrogacy acts were created as a default mode to facilitate medical decision making for ill, incompetent patients in the absence of advance directives. Some states restrict the authority to certain circumstances. For example, in New York, the law covers only Do-Not-Resuscitate orders. Other states limit the applicable legal authority to only certain classes of patients, such as to adults (in Florida). Still other states limit the authority to stipulated diagnoses. In Oregon, only patients who are both comatose and terminally ill fall under this act.[114] In some states, the breadth of authority of default surrogates is less than of Durable Powers of Attorney for Health Care appointed by patients.

Under the Illinois Health Care Surrogate Act, for example, surrogates are named if advance directives are absent and if patients have one of three qualifying conditions: (1) a terminal disease; (2) permanent unconsciousness; or (3) an incurable or irreversible disorder that will ultimately cause death even with life-sustaining treatment. Relatives are chosen first as surrogates; but, if a relative is not available, a close friend is selected. Physicians are given the dual roles of determining if patients have a qualifying condition and of counseling surrogate decision makers.[115]

Patients retain the right to execute advance directives in which they stipulate how they wish to be treated. For example, if they fear that legally appointed default surrogates may discontinue treatment before they wish it to

be stopped, they can execute advance directives to insist that treatment be continued. All prior directives executed by the patient take precedence over surrogacy laws because the latter become activated only in the absence of prior advance directives.

Some state legislatures have opposed drafting surrogacy laws, largely because of the fear that the legally authorized surrogate automatically named may not necessarily be the same person the patient would have chosen. In my experience, this mismatch is particularly prevalent among gay and lesbian patients who have become dissociated from their families. Many such patients may wish to have their partner serve as surrogate and not a family member, as would be automatically provided by the law.[116] Of course, the ideal solution here is preventive: the patient can name his or her partner as durable power of attorney for health care, a move that would preclude the implementation of the surrogacy law action.

I believe that both advance directives and health-care surrogacy laws are desirable. If executed properly, advance directives can permit the patient's precise wishes to be followed, whereas health-care surrogacy laws can function as a default means to facilitate decision making in the absence of advance directives. Both are complementary mechanisms, and ideally each protects the patient's interests by assuring that only desired treatments are conducted. Implementing both mechanisms helps assure that health-care decisions for incompetent patients can be made by those who can best make them.

Linda and Ezekiel Emanuel have proposed an alternative to the imperfect written and proxy appointment models of decision making.[117] In their communitarian approach, communities of patients would jointly decide on health-care goals and preferences that would apply to all persons within the community, including incompetent patients without advance care directives. The most basic unit of community in the Emanuel system is the health-care organization. Patients could choose health-care organizations that reflect their personal health-care preferences. Members of health-care communities would agree to abide by rules on which they mutually decided. The decisions of how to spend finite health-care dollars within each health-care community would be chosen democratically. The Emanuels argued that a communitarian system more closely satisfies the ethical goals of justice and respect for autonomy than does our present system.

MEDICAL MALPRACTICE

Medical malpractice is the most visible and highly feared legal constraint on neurological practice. In legal theory, medical malpractice usually is not categorized as a breach of contract between physician and patient. Rather, it is classified within a branch of civil law known as the law of torts. The word "tort" is derived from the Latin *tortus*, meaning twisted or crooked (tortuous), and is defined as a non-criminal wrongful act other than a breach of contract.

A claim of medical malpractice can be sustained in a legal proceeding only when it fulfills four criteria: (1) the physician has a duty to provide the patient with medical care that meets a certain defined standard; (2) the professional conduct of the physician falls below that standard of medical care; (3) the patient has sustained a compensable injury; and (4) there is a causal relationship between the physician's substandard medical care and the compensable injury sustained by the patient.[118]

Legal obligations physicians owe to patients include the duty to possess necessary training and knowledge and the duty to exercise reasonable skill and care.[119] Analyses of malpractice claims data reveal that neurologists have a 30% to 40% risk of being sued for malpractice at some time during their career, that fewer than 5% of these suits proceed to trial, and that neurologists prevail in about 80% of cases.[120] Neurologists are sued most frequently for three allegations: (1) failure to diagnose; (2) production of adverse drug reactions; and (3) failure to provide proper treatment.[121] If a clinician can be shown to have fulfilled the four criteria in the preceding paragraph, she may be found negligent. In a recent in-depth study of 42 neurology malpractice claims,

"authentic, preventable harm" had occurred in 24 cases. Of the harm cases, 46% occurred in outpatient care. Most cases resulted from poor communication with patients and other clinicians, lack of follow-through on tests and treatments, failure to diagnose, and complications of imaging procedures.[122]

To pursue a claim against the physician, the plaintiff's attorney retains an expert witness to testify that the defendant physician did not meet the prevailing standards of medical care in her practice[123] and that the failure to practice properly caused the plaintiff's alleged injuries. The defendant physician's attorney, in turn, retains an expert witness to testify that she did not practice below the legal standard of care, that the injury sustained by the patient was not causally related to the defendant's practice, or that the patient suffered no compensable injury. Because the legal standard of care is defined by practicing physicians, both expert witnesses usually are clinicians practicing within or closely allied to the specialty of the defendant physician.

There is widespread belief among physicians that there is a malpractice crisis in the United States with rampant lawsuits filed by avaricious attorneys for any poor outcome of care, record payouts, rising insurance premiums, and lowered availability of insurance coverage.[124] As one means of responding to the crisis, physicians' professional organizations have lobbied intensely for malpractice law (tort) reform, with model policies intended to mitigate many of the exacerbating factors, such as excessive attorney contingency fees, and permitting arbitration and other means of screening unmeritorious cases and settling meritorious cases out of court.[125] Despite the counterclaims by attorneys that the crisis is the fault of careless physicians and greedy insurance companies, there are clear data showing the inefficiency and exorbitant overhead costs of malpractice litigation.[126]

Current Ethical Issues

Three ethical issues currently dominate the subject of medical malpractice. The first encompasses the ethical duty of retained expert witnesses to render opinions that are impartial, honest, and representative of accepted medical practice. (See chapter 3.) Unfortunately, some physicians serving as expert witnesses do not attempt to remain impartial and use the court as a forum for proffering their tendentious or unproved hypotheses rather than providing evidence-based testimony.[127] More disturbingly, a small subclass of professional expert witnesses derives a living from malpractice testimony. Among these professional experts are "hired guns" who are notorious for their willingness to slant their opinions to fulfill the needs of the plaintiff's attorney.

The most effective solution to the problem of the unqualified, charlatan, eccentric, or professional expert witness is for medical societies to formulate and enforce guidelines governing the professional conduct of expert witnesses. Medical societies can aggressively enforce disciplinary policies to assure that their self-imposed guidelines are followed. Enforcement should be conducted by medical specialty society peers and can include punitive actions, such as censure or expulsion from the society when unprofessional conduct has been clearly proved.[128] Practicing physicians should be encouraged to participate as experts in meritorious malpractice cases to give courts accurate descriptions of the prevailing standards of medical practice. Many of the guidelines require that physicians testifying as experts maintain active medical practices with only a small proportion of their professional time devoted to legal work. The American Academy of Neurology has recently published guidelines for expert witness testimony[129] as discussed in chapter 3.

A second ethical issue of malpractice is physicians' practice of "defensive medicine" in response to the fear they may be charged with failure to diagnose.[130] Defensive medicine is an ethical problem because it leads to unnecessary testing that squanders resources and can physically harm patients from complications of testing.[131] The effect of defensive medicine was studied in a recent survey of 595 neurologists in the United States.[132] When given six case scenarios, all of which involved uncertainty, neurologists cited malpractice concerns as an

important justification for ordering tests that otherwise they would not have ordered. The neurologists also markedly overestimated their risk of incurring a malpractice suit based on available claims data. Excessive testing has the effect of transferring test utility from the patient (for medical care) to the physician (for self-protection), and increasing the costs while diminishing the quality of care.[133]

The third ethical dilemma of medical malpractice surrounds the potential professional liability of a physician who, for reasons of mandatory cost constraints, orders fewer tests or treatments. If a patient claims injury as a result of the physician's alleged failure to diagnose or treat, does the physician's duty to contain medical costs alter the usual standards of physicians' duties in medical malpractice determination?

Consider the case of a neurologist employed by a health maintenance organization (HMO) or under contract with a managed care organization (MCO) that dictates that she must practice under guidelines explicitly restricting the number of computed tomography (CT) or magnetic resonance (MR) scans she can order. She examined a young woman for newly developed throbbing unilateral headaches. The patient's neurological examination was normal, and the physician diagnosed common migraine. The neurologist judged that the probability that this patient had a structural brain lesion causing the headaches was too low to justify "spending" one of her limited CT scans. She explained to her patient that a CT scan was not indicated in this case. The patient continued to complain of headaches and came under the care of another neurologist six months later. The second neurologist ordered a CT scan that revealed a large meningioma. Following its excision, the patient complained of memory loss. She sued her original neurologist for failing to diagnose her meningioma and for injuries she sustained from its removal. The plaintiff's expert neurologist witness testified that nowadays all patients suffering with new headaches should undergo neuroimaging with a CT or MR brain scan. The defendant neurologist explained that her professional prerogative to order CT scans was constrained and that, according to her practice pattern, the patient should not have had a scan because the chance that it would have been positive was too small. In finding for the plaintiff, the judge ruled that the cost constraint factor was irrelevant in defining the proper standard of medical care the defendant physician should have given the patient.

There is a lively debate among legal scholars about the relevancy of cost constraints to malpractice defense.[134] Haavi Morreim represents one camp that has argued that physicians' duties to constrain costs are on a "collision course" with malpractice law and that it is physicians who will be injured in the collision. Current malpractice standards reflect only duties that physicians owe to their individual patients. They do not acknowledge the validity of a physician's decision that may potentially hurt an individual patient but arguably is the right decision because of its overall impact on others. Morreim argues that the only way to prevent the collision is to restructure the standards of malpractice law to take into account cost containment as well as other duties physicians have to society.[135]

Mark Hall represents the opposing view. He argued that the law has the capacity to accommodate varying standards of medical care that reflect practice patterns across a spectrum of several different economic arrangements. He pointed out that it is physicians, after all, who define the standards of medical care. He willingly acknowledged that cost containment is a relevant factor in medical decision making, and pointed out that once cost containment considerations become institutionalized in medical practices, they too will represent a standard of care. Thus, future physicians who take these constraints into account will practice according to these standards of care. Because the legal system can accommodate these varying practice patterns, no radical change in the law is needed.[136]

One possible solution to the potential collision between malpractice liability and cost constraint obligations is the development of medical practice parameters that incorporate justifiable cost constraint considerations.[137] Practice parameters ("practice guidelines") are developed by expert physicians and endorsed by medical societies to delineate the evidence-based standards of medical care for particular clinical problems.[138] Because the guidelines represent best quality practice, physicians are expected to follow them unless the specific circumstances of caring for an individual patient create an adequate justification for varying from them.[139] Given the reality of cost constraint requirements for future patient care, cost factors can be incorporated into accepted practice parameters. Once in effect, these practice parameters could serve as a potent justification for using cost constraints as a malpractice defense. In this case, the defendant physician's attorney could have used the powerful defense that the American Academy of Neurology published a practice parameter stating that neuroimaging in the young patient with a normal neurological examination and a diagnosable migraine was unnecessary.[140]

Viewing clinical practice guidelines as best quality care illustrates their potential for creating legal liability. In malpractice proceedings, some lawyers have argued that a physician's failure to follow accepted practice guidelines is *prima facie* evidence of practicing below the standard of care. Varying from the dictates of clinical practice guidelines is not necessarily practicing beneath the standard of care when physicians can adequately explain and justify why they did so. While it is the nature of such guidelines to permit justified exceptions, they confer the responsibility on clinicians to account for the variation.

Some scholars have argued that following clinical practice guidelines may be unethical when they limit treatment options available to patients.[141] But here I emphasize the important distinction between medical society quality practice guidelines and managed care organization (MCO) proprietary guidelines. Following medical society clinical practice guidelines is not unethical when they represent high quality care. But the requirement to follow MCO proprietary guidelines designed only to save money is unethical when they harm patients.[142] Further complicating the discussion is the fact that proprietary guidelines may be misleadingly and self-servingly called quality measures when they are simply cost-control measures.[143] Barbara Redman has shown how medical ethical principles must be integrated into proprietary practice guidelines to make them ethical.[144]

The use of a written contractual agreement offers a possible solution to these conflicts. Patients could bargain with physicians, health maintenance organizations, or insurers and negotiate a contract stipulating the standard of care they prefer. In exchange for lowering the standard of care applicable in a medical malpractice action, patients could receive a reduction in health insurance premiums. For example, a patient could agree to limit the potential malpractice recovery she would receive only to instances of "gross negligence" or "willful misconduct" resulting from the medical care given by her physician. Patients could be given the choice to save money on premiums by waiving their rights to recover damages from physicians' actions that did not fall to these severe depths.[145]

Another potential solution is to rely on the doctrine of "enterprise liability." This increasingly accepted legal doctrine provides that if the HMO or MCO physician has followed the HMO or MCO network guidelines and rules, she is immunized from personal professional liability from a malpractice suit filed on the grounds of the failure to order tests or treatments not allowed in the guidelines. Enterprise liability holds that because the HMO or MCO established and enforced the rules, only it can be held directly liable in such an action.[146]

The federal Employee Retirement Income Security Act (ERISA) immunizes MCOs from liability for decisions with harmful consequences made by its physicians to save costs.[147] In a noteworthy decision, the U.S. Supreme Court ruled that an MCO did not breach its fiduciary duty to its subscribers under ERISA, even though the case featured clear and direct financial incentives to the physician for cutting costs.[148] The Supreme Court ruled that not only is rationing to contain costs routine in the United States but it is also a matter of national policy.[149] However, in a Fifth Circuit Court of Appeals case, the court ruled that lawsuits against MCOs for negligence or malpractice in state courts are not exempted by ERISA.[150] A future decision by the U.S. Supreme Court on this question would definitively answer this ambiguous interplay between state and federal law.

NOTES

1. For an analysis of the problems resulting from laws using the language of bioethics, see Schneider CE. Bioethics in the language of the law. *Hastings Cent Rep* 1994;24(4):16–22.

2. Beresford HR. *Neurology and the Law: Private Litigation and Public Policy*. Philadelphia: F A Davis Co, 1998.

3. Menikoff J. *Law and Bioethics: An Introduction*. Washington, DC: Georgetown University Press, 2001.

4. Meisel A, Cerminara KL. *The Right to Die: The Law of End-of-Life Decisionmaking*, 3rd ed. Aspen Publishers, Inc, 2004.

5. Waltz JR, Inbau FE. *Medical Jurisprudence*. New York: Macmillan, 1971:4. In his famous dictionary, Dr. Samuel Johnson quipped that "the law is the last result of human wisdom acting on human experience."

6. Beresford HR. *Legal Aspects of Neurologic Practice*. Philadelphia: FA Davis Co, 1975:5.

7. Beresford HR. *Legal Aspects of Neurologic Practice*. 1975:3–5.

8. Kapp MB, Lo B. Legal perceptions and medical decision making. *Milbank Q* 1986;64(suppl 2):163–202.

9. On the conflicts between law and ethics, see Stone AA. Law's influence on medicine and medical ethics. *N Engl J Med* 1985;312;309–312; Kapp MB. Medicine and law: a symbiotic relationship? *Am J Med* 1985;78:903–907; and Dickens BM. Patients' interests and clients' wishes: physicians and lawyers in discord. *Law Med Health Care* 1987;15(3):110–117. For two volumes of thoughtful essays addressing the impact of

law on contemporary medicine and medical ethics, see Annas GJ. *Standard of Care: The Law of American Bioethics.* New York: Oxford University Press, 1993; and Annas GJ. *Judging Medicine.* Clifton, NJ: Humana Press, 1988.

10. For example, in a survey of child neurologists, 70% believed the malpractice system was unfair and 90% believed it should be reformed. Ethics and Practice Committees of the Child Neurology Society. Child neurologist as expert witness: a report of the Ethics and Practice Committees of the Child Neurology Society. *J Child Neurol* 1998;13:398–401.

11. For a discussion of the negative psychological reactions of physicians to malpractice suits, see Weiler PC. *Medical Malpractice on Trial.* Cambridge, MA: Harvard University Press, 1991:6–7; Charles SC, Wilbert JR, Kennedy EC. Physicians' self-reports of reactions to malpractice litigation. *Am J Psychiatry* 1984;141:563–565; and Charles SC, Wilbert JR, Franke KJ. Sued and nonsued physicians' self-reported reactions to malpractice litigation. *Am J Psychiatry* 1985;142:437–440.

12. See the debunking of this and other legal myths in Meisel A. Legal myths about terminating life support. *Arch Intern Med* 1991;151:1497–1502.

13. For example, in a survey conducted by the American Academy of Neurology, 40% of neurologists wrongly believed that they needed to consult legal counsel before withdrawing a patient's life-sustaining therapy. See Carver AC, Vickrey BG, Bernat JL, Keran C, Ringel SP, Foley KM. End of life care: a survey of U.S. neurologists' attitudes, behavior, and knowledge. *Neurology* 1999;53:284–293.

14. de Tocqueville A. *Democracy in America.* Chicago: University of Chicago Press, 2000. I relied on a summary in Paris JJ, Ferranti J, Reardon F. From the Johns Hopkins baby to Baby Miller: what have we learned from four decades of reflection on neonatal cases? *J Clin Ethics* 2001;12:207–214.

15. McCrary SV, Swanson JS, Perkins HS, Winslade WJ. Treatment decisions for terminally ill patients: physicians' legal defensiveness and knowledge of medical law. *Law Med Healthcare* 1992;20:364–376.

16. Swanson JS, McCrary SV. Medical futility decisions and physicians' legal defensiveness: the impact of anticipated conflict on thresholds for end-of-life treatment. *Soc Sci Med* 1996;42:125–132.

17. McCrary SV, Swanson JW, Coulehan J, Faber-Langendoen K, Olick RS, Belling C. Physicians' legal defensiveness in end-of-life treatment decisions: comparing attitudes and knowledge in states with different laws. *J Clin Ethics* 2006;17:15–26.

18. McCrary SV, et al. *J Clin Ethics* 2006:22–24.

19. For a discussion and illustration of the poor advice physicians sometimes receive from hospital risk managers, see Macklin R. *Enemies of Patients.* New York: Oxford University Press, 1993:15–16, 52–76; and Kapp MB. Are risk management and health care ethics compatible? *Perspect Healthcare Risk Manage* 1991;11(4):1–5.

20. Herb A. The hospital-based attorney as patient advocate. *Hastings Cent Rep* 1995;25(2):13–19.

21. For details of the Linares case and commentary about its significance, see the symposium Gostin L, ed. Family privacy and persistent vegetative state. *Law Med Health Care* 1989;17:295–346. The quotations of Mr. Linares are from Lantos JD, Miles SH, Cassel CK. The Linares affair. *Law Med Health Care* 1989;17:309. One tangible benefit of the Linares tragedy was that the state of Illinois thereafter impaneled a task force on life-sustaining treatment that drafted a statute that became the Illinois Health Care Surrogate Act of 1991.

22. Kapp MB, Lo B. *Milbank Q* 1986;64(suppl 2):179–180.

23. See a judge's explicit warning to physicians in *In re Nemser,* 273 NYS 2d 624, 629 (Sup Ct NY County, 1966) as discussed in Capron AM. The burden of decision. *Hastings Cent Rep* 1990;20(3):36–41. In his ruling, the judge in *Nemser* decried: "the current practice of members of the medical profession and their associated hospitals of shifting the burden of their responsibilities to the courts, to determine, in effect, whether doctors should proceed with certain medical procedures . . . [and the] . . . ultra-legalistic maze we have created to the extent that society and the individual have become enmeshed and paralyzed by its unrealistic entanglements!" In a similar vein, Dr. Franz J. Ingelfinger warned in a *New England Journal of Medicine* editorial that if physicians continued to rely on the courts "to resolve essentially medical matters" that the medical profession's unfortunate "dependence on the lawyer in reaching essentially medical decisions will continue." Ingelfinger FJ. Legal hegemony in medicine. *N Engl J Med* 1975;293:825–826. For a further discussion of how the advice of risk management lawyers hired by hospitals can contribute to poor patient care, see Macklin R. *Enemies of Patients,* 1993:52–76.

24. Jones PM, Appelbaum PS, Siegel DM. Law enforcement interviews of hospital patients: a conundrum for clinicians. *JAMA* 2006;295:822–825.

25. Annas G. Reconciling *Quinlan* and *Saikewicz*: Decision making for the terminally ill incompetent. *Am J Law Med* 1979;4:389–391.

26. Jacobson PD, Bloche MG. Improving relations between attorneys and physicians. *JAMA* 2005;294: 2083–2085.

27. Hadorn DC. Emerging parallels in the American health care and legal-judicial systems. *Am J Law Med* 1992;18:73–96.

28. Budetti PP. Tort reform and the patient safety movement: seeking common ground. *JAMA* 2000;293:2660–2662.

29. Reece S. The circuitous journey to the Patients' Bill of Rights: winners and losers. *Albany Law Rev* 2000–2001;65:17–95.

30. For a comprehensive legal analysis of how shared decision-making has evolved from informed consent, see King JS, Moulton BW. Rethinking informed consent: the case for shared medical decision-making. *Am J Law Med* 2006;32:429–501. Earlier works include Brock DW. The ideal of shared decision making between physicians and patients. *Kennedy Inst Ethics J* 1991;1:28–47; and Veatch RM. *The Patient-Physician Relation: The Patient as Partner*. Part 2. Bloomington: Indiana University Press, 1991:2–6.

31. President's Commission for the Study of Ethical Problems in Medicine and Biomedical and Behavioral Research. *Making Health Care Decisions: The Ethical and Legal Implications of Informed Consent in the Patient-Practitioner Relationship*. Washington, DC: US Government Printing Office, 1982:181–183. For a discussion of the covenant theory of the family as a unitary decision maker, see Doukas DJ. Autonomy and beneficence in the family: describing the family covenant. *J Clin Ethics* 1991;2:145–148.

32. Bernat JL. Plan ahead: how neurologists can enhance patient-centered medicine. *Neurology* 2001;56:144–145.

33. American Medical Association Council on Ethical and Judicial Affairs. Surrogate decision making. In, *Code of Medical Ethics. Current Opinions with Annotations*, 2006–2007 ed. Chicago: American Medical Association, 2006:232–233. http://www.ama-assn.org/ama1/pub/upload/mm/369/ceja_4a01.pdf (Accessed June 15, 2007).

34. President's Commission for the Study of Ethical Problems in Medicine and Biomedical and Behavioral Research. *Making Health Care Decisions*, 1982:177–179; and Buchanan AE, Brock DW. *Deciding For Others: The Ethics of Surrogate Decision Making*. Cambridge: Cambridge University Press, 1989:112–116.

35. Uhlmann RF, Pearlman RA, Cain KC. Physicians' and spouses' predictions of elderly patients' resuscitation preferences. *J Gerontol* 1988;43:M115–M121.

36. Shalowitz DI, Garrett-Mayer E, Wendler D. The accuracy of surrogate decision makers: a systematic review. *Arch Intern Med* 2006;166:493–497.

37. Suhl J, Simons P, Reedy T, et al. Myth of substituted judgment: surrogate decision making regarding life support is unreliable. *Arch Intern Med* 1994;154:90–96.

38. Sayers GM, Beckett N, Waters H, Turner C. Surrogates' decisions regarding CPR, and the fallacy of substituted judgment. *J Clin Ethics* 2004;15:334–345.

39. Harmon L. Falling off the vine: legal fictions and the doctrine of substituted judgment. *Yale Law J* 1990;100:1–71.

40. Baergon R. Revising the substituted judgment standard. *J Clin Ethics* 1995;6:30–38.

41. Berger JT. Patients' interest in their family members' well-being: an overlooked, fundamental consideration within substituted judgments. *J Clin Ethics* 2005;16:3–10.

42. President's Commission for the Study of Ethical Problems in Medicine and Biomedical and Behavioral Research. *Making Health Care Decisions*, 1982:179–180; and Buchanan AE, Brock DW. *Deciding for Others: The Ethics of Surrogate Decision Making*, 1989:122–133. For a general discussion of the interests of patients, see Wikler D. Patient interests: clinical implications of philosophical distinctions. *J Am Geriatr Soc* 1988,36: 951–958.

43. Pearlman RA, Jonsen A. The use of quality of life considerations in medical decision-making. *J Am Geriatr Soc* 1985;33:344–352.

44. Uhlmann RF, Pearlman RA. Perceived quality of life and preferences for life-sustaining treatment in older adults. *Arch Intern Med* 1991;151:495–497.

45. Schneiderman LJ, Kaplan RM, Pearlman RA, et al. Do physicians' own preferences for life-sustaining treatment influence their perceptions of patients' preferences? *J Clin Ethics* 1993;4:28–33 and Pearlman RA, Uhlmann RF, Jecker NS. Spousal understanding of patient quality of life: implications for surrogate decisions. *J Clin Ethics* 1992;3:114–121.

46. Drane JF, Coulehan JL. The best-interest standard: surrogate decision making and quality of life. *J Clin Ethics* 1995;6:20–29.

47. For an example of such a hospital policy, see Hyun I, Griggins C, Weiss M, Robbins D, Robichaud A, Daly B. When patients do not have a proxy: a procedure for medical decision making when there is no one to speak for the patient. *J Clin Ethics* 2006;17:323–330.

48. For a conceptual defense of the desirability of advance directives, see Buchanan A, Brock DW. Deciding for others. *Milbank Q* 1986;64(suppl 2):17–94; Buchanan AE, Brock DW. *Deciding for Others: The Ethics of Surrogate Decision Making,* 1989:87–109; and Conard AF. Elder choice. *Am J Law Med* 1993;19:233–283.

49. For general background on advance directives, see Schneiderman LJ, Arras JD. Counseling patients to counsel physicians on future care in the event of patient incompetence. *Ann Intern Med* 1985;102:693–698; Emanuel L. Advance directives: what have we learned so far? *J Clin Ethics* 1993;4:8–16; Annas GJ. The health care proxy and the living will. *N Engl J Med* 1991;324:1210–1213; and Orentlicher D. Advance medical directives. *JAMA* 990;263:2365–2367.

50. Gillick MR. Advance care planning. *N Engl J Med* 2004;350:7–8. For a state-by-state list of advance directive legislation, see Health Care Power of Attorney and Combined Advance Directive Legislation, September 1, 2004 http://www.abanet.org/aging/legislativeupdates/docs/ HCPA-CHT04.doc (Accessed June 15, 2007).

51. Gillick MR. A broader role for advance medical planning. *Ann Intern Med* 1995;123:621–624; Miles SH, Koepp R, Weber EP. Advance end-of-life treatment planning: a research review. *Arch Intern Med* 1996;156:1062–1068.

52. Fried TR, Bradley EH, Towle VR, Allore H. Understanding the treatment preferences of seriously ill patients. *N Engl J Med* 2002;346:1061–1066.

53. Tulsky J. Beyond advance directives: importance of communication skills at the end of life. *JAMA* 2005;294:359–365.

54. Lynn J, Goldstein NE. Advance care planning for fatal chronic illness: avoiding commonplace errors and unwanted suffering. *Ann Intern Med* 2003;138:812–818. David Goldblatt reported two neurological cases to illustrate that the physician, patient, and surrogate must work together in advance of need, to make advance directives most effective. See Goldblatt D. Who's listening? Advance directives are not always directive. *The Neurologist* 2001;7:180–185.

55. Kapp MB. Response to the living will furor: directives for maximum care. *Am J Med* 1982;72:855–859. For example, the South Carolina living will form contains this language: DIRECTIVE FOR MAXIMUM TREATMENT. I want my life to be prolonged to the greatest extent possible within the standards of accepted medical practice, without regard to my condition, the chances I have for recovery, or the cost of the procedures. *S.C. Code Ann* § 62-5-504 (Law. Co-op, Supp, 1995).

56. Minogue B, Reagan JE. Can complex legislation solve our end-of-life problems? *Camb Q Healthc Ethics* 1994;3:115–124.

57. This point was emphasized by the *Cruzan* and the *O'Connor* courts. See the discussion of how these cases encouraged the use of written directives in Rouse F. Advance directives: where are we heading after Cruzan? *Law Med Health Care* 1990;18:353–359. The criteria for a patient's capacity to complete an advance directive is described in Silberfeld M, Nash C, Singer PA. Capacity to complete an advance directive. *J Am Geriatr Soc* 1993:41:1141–1143.

58. Thompson T, Barbour R, Schwartz L. Adherence to advance directives in critical care decision making: vignette study. *BMJ* 2003;327:1011–1014.

59. See Eisendrath SJ, Jonsen AR. The living will: help or hindrance? *JAMA* 1983; 249:2054–2058 and Sehgal A, Galbraith A, Chesney M, et al. How strictly do dialysis patients want their advance directives followed? *JAMA* 1992;267:59–63.

60. Emanuel LL, Emanuel EJ. The medical directive: a new comprehensive advance care document. *JAMA* 1989;261:3288–3293 and Cantor NL. My annotated living will. *Law Med Health Care* 1990;18:114–122.

61. Brett AS. Limitations of listing specific medical interventions in advance directives. *JAMA* 1991;266: 825–828.

62. Robertson JA. Second thoughts on living wills. *Hastings Cent Rep* 1991;21(6):6–9.

63. Lee MA, Smith DM, Fenn DS, Ganzini L. Do patients' treatment decisions match advance statements of their preferences? *J Clin Ethics* 1998;9:258–262.

64. Meier DE, Morrison RS. Autonomy reconsidered. *N Engl J Med* 2002;346:1087–1089.

65. Dworkin R. Autonomy and the demented self. *Milbank Q* 1986;64:4–16.

66. Emanuel LL, Emanuel EJ, Stoeckle JD, et al. Advance directives: stability of patients' treatment choices. *Arch Intern Med* 1994;154:209–217 and Danis M, Garrett J, Harris R, et al. Stability of choices about life-sustaining treatments. *Ann Intern Med* 1994;120:507–573.

67. Kohut N, Sam M, O'Rourke K, MacFadden DK, Salit I, Singer PA. Stability of treatment preferences: although most preferences do not change, most people change some of their preferences. *J Clin Ethics* 1997;8:124–135.

68. Gready RM, Ditto PH, Danks JH, Coppola KM, Lockhart LK, Smucker WD. Actual and perceived stability of preferences for life-sustaining treatment. *J Clin Ethics* 2000;11:334–346.

69. Schneiderman LJ, Pearlman RA, Kaplan RM, et al. Relationship of general advance directive instructions to specific life-sustaining treatment preferences in patients with serious illness. *Arch Intern Med* 1992;152:2114–2122.

70. Joos SK, Reuler JB, Powell JL, et al. Outpatients' attitudes and understanding regarding living wills. *J Gen Intern Med* 1993;8:259–263.

71. Hoffman DE, Zimmerman SI, Tompkins CJ. The dangers of directives or the false security of forms. *J Law Med Ethics* 1996;24:5–17.

72. Lo B, Steinbrook R. Resuscitating advance directives. *Arch Intern Med* 2004;164:1501–1506.

73. Fagerlin A, Schneider CE. Enough: the failure of the living will. *Hastings Center Rep* 2004;34(2):30–42; and Lynn J. Why I don't have a living will. *Law Med Health Care* 1991;19:101–104. Harry Perkins recently criticized all advance directives as fundamentally flawed because they presuppose more control over future care than is realistic. He suggested that advance care planning instead focus on emotionally preparing patients and families for future crises. Perkins HS. Controlling death: the false promise of advance directives. *Ann Intern Med* 2007;147:51–57.

74. Prendergast TJ. Advance care planning: pitfalls, progress, promise. *Crit Care Med* 2001;29 (suppl):N34–N39.

75. Dexter PR, Wolinsky FD, Gramelspacher GP, Eckert GJ, Tierney WM. Opportunities for advance directives to influence medical care. *J Clin Ethics* 2003;14:173–188.

76. President's Council on Bioethics. *Taking Care: Ethical Caregiving in our Aging Society.* September 2005. http://www.bioethics.gov/reports/taking_care/chapter5.html (Accessed June 15, 2007).

77. Bernat JL. Plan ahead: how neurologists can enhance patient-centered medicine. *Neurology* 2001; 56:144–145.

78. Virmani J, Schneiderman LJ, Kaplan RM. Relationship of advance directives to physician-patient communication. *Arch Intern Med* 1994;154:909–913.

79. Hanson LC, Tulsky JA, Danis M. Can clinical interventions change care at the end of life? *Ann Intern Med* 1997;126:381–388.

80. Tierney WM, Dexter PR, Gramelspacher GP, Perkins AJ, Zhou X-H, Wolinsky FD. The effect of discussions about advance directives on patients' satisfaction with primary care. *J Gen Intern Med* 2001; 16:32–40.

81. Degenholz HB, Rhee Y, Arnold RM. Brief communication: the relationship between having a living will and dying in place. *Ann Intern Med* 2004;141:113–117.

82. Lynn Peterson and I discussed the special circumstances in which health care agents are justified in overruling patients' previously written directives in Bernat JL, Peterson LM. Patient-centered informed consent in surgical practice. *Arch Surg* 2006;141:86–92.

83. The American Bar Association maintains a list of advance directive legislation state-by-state. See Health Care Power of Attorney and Combined Advance Directive Legislation, September 1, 2004. http://www.abanet.org/aging/legislativeupdates/docs/HCPA-CHT04.doc (Accessed June 15, 2007). For a commentary on model statute design, see Sabatino CP. The legal and functional status of the medical proxy: suggestions for statutory reform. *J Law Med Ethics* 1999;27:52–68.

84. Rai A, Siegler M, Lantos J. The physician as health care proxy. *Hastings Cent Rep* 1999;29(5):14–19.

85. Emanuel EJ, Weinberg, DS, Gonin R, et al. How well is the Patient Self-Determination Act working? An early assessment. *Am J Med* 1993;95:619–628.

86. For an impassioned argument why an experienced bioethicist rejects the living will in favor of the health care surrogate appointment, see Lynn J. Why I don't have a living will. *Law Med Health Care* 1991;19:101–104.

87. Goldblatt D. A messy, necessary end: health care proxies need our support. *Neurology* 2001;56: 148–152.

88. Post LF, Blustein J, Dubler NN. Introduction: the doctor-proxy relationship: an untapped resource. *J Law Med Ethics* 1999;27:5–12. See also the symposium on this topic in *J Law Med Ethics* 1999;27:5–86.

89. Hardwig J. The problem of proxies with interests of their own: toward a better theory of proxy decisions. *J Clin Ethics* 1993;4:20–27.

90. McClung JA. Time and language in bioethics: when patient and proxy appear to disagree. *J Clin Ethics* 1995;6:39–43; Schneiderman LJ, Teetzel H, Kalmanson AG. Who decides who decides? When disagreement occurs between the physician and the patient's appointed proxy about the patient's decision making capacity. *Arch Intern Med* 1995;155:793–796; Spike J, Greenlaw J. Ethics consultation: refusal of beneficial treatment by a surrogate decision maker. *J Law Med Ethics* 1995;23:202–204; Gillick MR, Fried T. The limits of proxy decision making: undertreatment. *Camb Q Healthc Ethics* 1995;4:172–177; Terry PB, Vettese M, Song J, et al. End-of-life decision making: when patients and surrogates disagree. *J Clin Ethics* 1999;10:286–293; and Alpers A, Lo B. Avoiding family feuds: responding to surrogate demands for life-sustaining interventions. *J Law Med Ethics* 1999;17:74–80.

91. Schneiderman LJ, Kronick R, Kaplan RM, et al. Effects of advance directives on medical treatments and costs. *Ann Intern Med* 1992;117:599–606.

92. Weeks WB, Kofoed LL, Wallace AE, Welch HG. Advance directives and the cost of terminal hospitalization. *Arch Intern Med* 1994;154:2077–2083. However, these authors use of the term "advance directives" includes patients' oral responses to physicians' questions during their final hospitalizations.

93. See Emanuel LL, Barry MJ, Stoeckle JD, et al. Advance directives for medical care—a case for greater use. *N Engl J Med* 1991;324:889–895.

94. Orentlicher D. *JAMA* 1990;263:2365–2367 and American Academy of Neurology. *Resolution on Legislation Regarding Durable Power of Attorney for Health Care.* Minneapolis: American Academy of Neurology, 1989.

95. Davidson KW, Hackler C, Caradine DR, et al. Physicians' attitudes on advance directives. *JAMA* 1989;262:2415–2419.

96. Emanuel LL, Barry MJ, Stoeckle JD, et al. Advance directives for medical care—a case for greater use. *N Engl J Med* 1991;324:889–895.

97. Stolman CJ, Gregory JJ, Dunn D, et al. Evaluation of patient, physician, nurse, and family attitudes toward do not resuscitate orders. *Arch Intern Med* 1990;150:653–658.

98. Sugarman J, Weinberger M, Samsa G. Factors associated with veterans' decisions about living wills. *Arch Intern Med* 1992;152:343–347.

99. McCrary SV, Botkin JR. Hospital policy on advance directives: do institutions ask patients about living wills? *JAMA* 1989;262:2411–2414.

100. Danis M, Southerland LI, Garrett JM, et al. A prospective study of advance directives for life-sustaining care. *N Engl J Med* 1991;324:882–888; and SUPPORT principal investigators. A controlled trial to improve care for seriously hospitalized patients. The Study to Understand Prognosis and Preferences for Outcomes and Risks of Treatment. *JAMA* 1995;274:1591–1598.

101. Morrison RS, Morrison EW, Glickman DF. Physician reluctance to discuss advance directives. An empiric investigation of potential barriers. *Arch Intern Med* 1994;154:2311–2318. Some of the practical barriers preventing neurologists from encouraging and assisting their patients to complete advance directives were discussed in Goldblatt D. A messy, necessary end: health care proxies need our support. *Neurology* 2001;56:148–152.

102. Reilly BM, Magnussen CR, Ross J, Ash J, Papa L, Wagner M. Can we talk? Inpatient discussions about advance directives in a community hospital. Attending physicians' attitudes, their inpatients' wishes, and reported experience. *Arch Intern Med* 1994;154:2299–2308.

103. Hofmann JC, Wenger NS, Davis RB, et al. Patient preferences for communication with physicians about end-of-life decisions. *Ann Intern Med* 1997;127:1–12. The SUPPORT study is described in detail in chapter 8.

104. Sugarman J, Kass NE, Faden RR, Goodman SN. Catalysts for conversations about advance directives: the influence of physician and patient characteristics. *J Law Med Ethics* 1994;22:29–35.

105. Tulsky JA, Fischer GS, Rose MR, Arnold RM. Opening the black box: how do physicians communicate about advance directives? *Ann Intern Med* 1998;129:441–449.

106. For details of the provisions of the PSDA, see La Puma J, Orentlicher D, Moss RJ. Advance directives on admission: clinical implications and analysis of the Patient Self-Determination Act of 1990. *JAMA* 1991;266:402–405; Greco PJ, Schulman KA, Lavizzo-Mourey R, et al. The Patient Self-Determination Act and

the future of advance directives. *Ann Intern Med* 1991;115:639–643; and White ML, Fletcher JC. The Patient Self-Determination Act: on balance, more help than hindrance. *JAMA* 1991;266:410–412.

107. Wolf SM, Boyle P, Callahan D, et al. Sources of concern about the Patient Self-Determination Act. *N Engl J Med* 1991;325:1666–1671. See also the symposium on the Patient Self-Determination Act in *Camb Q Healthc Ethics.* 1992;1:97–126. For a study of how states vary in their implementation of the PSDA, see Teno JM, Sabatino C, Parisier L, et al. The impact of the Patient Self-Determination Act's requirement that states describe law concerning patients' rights. *J Law Med Ethics* 1993;21:102–108.

108. Wolf SM, Boyle P, Callahan D, et al. *N Engl J Med* 1991:1666–1671.

109. McIntyre KM. Implementation of advance directives. For physicians, a legal dilemma becomes an ethical imperative. *Arch Intern Med* 1992;152:925–929.

110. Schneiderman LJ, Kronick R, Kaplan RM, et al. *Ann Intern Med* 1992:599–606 and Weeks WB, Kofoed LL, Wallace AE, Welch HG. *Arch Intern Med* 1994:2077–2083.

111. Ganzini L, Lee MA, Heintz RT, et al. Is the Patient Self-Determination Act appropriate for elderly persons hospitalized for depression? *J Clin Ethics* 1993;4:46–50.

112. Emanuel EJ, Weinberg, DS, Gonin R, et al. How well is the Patient Self-Determination Act working? An early assessment. *Am J Med* 1993;95:619–628.

113. Menikoff JA, Sachs GA, Siegler M. Beyond advance directives—health care surrogate laws. *N Engl J Med* 1992;327:1165–1169. See also Portman RM. Surrogate decision-making legislation: the next frontier in life-sustaining treatment policy. *J Health Hosp Law* 1991;24:311–319.

114. Menikoff JA, Sachs GA, Siegler M. *N Engl J Med* 1992:1166.

115. Menikoff JA, Sachs GA, Siegler M. *N Engl J Med* 1992:1166–1167.

116. See Steinbrook R, Lo B, Moulton J, Saika G, Hollander H, Volberding PA. Preferences of homosexual men with AIDS for life-sustaining treatment. *N Engl J Med* 1986;314:457–460.

117. Emanuel LL, Emanuel EJ. Decisions at the end of life: guided by communities of patients. *Hastings Cent Rep* 1993;23(5):6–14. The communitarian model of medical ethics is further described in Emanuel EJ. *The Ends of Human Life: Medical Ethics in a Liberal Polity.* Cambridge, MA: Harvard University Press, 1991.

118. Waltz JR, Inbau FE. *Medical Jurisprudence,* 1971:40–41 and Beresford HR. *Neurology and the Law,* 1998:29–45. For a more comprehensive reference works on medical malpractice, see Danzon PM. *Medical Malpractice: Theory, Evidence, and Public Policy.* Cambridge, MA: Harvard University Press, 1985; and Sage WM, Kersh R, eds. *Medical Malpractice and the U.S. Health Care System.* New York: Cambridge University Press, 2006.

119. Waltz JR, Inbau FE. *Medical Jurisprudence,* 1971:44–48.

120. Beresford HR. *Neurology and the Law,* 1998:3–5.

121. Beresford HR. *Legal Aspects of Neurologic Practice,* 1975:68–85. See also Bernat JL. Council on Medical Specialties Societies Professional Liability Report: neurologists in medical malpractice, suggestions for future action. *Neurology* 1985;35: 28A, 93–95 and Glick TH. Malpractice claims: outcome evidence to guide neurologic education? *Neurology* 2001;56:1099–1100. Michael Weintraub recently discussed neurologists' malpractice liability for either prescribing or not prescribing intravenous tissue plasminogen activator (t-PA) in patients with threatened stroke. See Weintraub MI. Thrombolysis (tissue plasminogen activator) in stroke: a medicolegal quagmire. *Stroke* 2006;37:1917–1922.

122. Glick TH, Cranberg LD, Hanscom RB, Sato L. Neurologic patient safety: an in-depth analysis of malpractice claims. *Neurology* 2005;65:1284–1286.

123. States differ in whether they permit determining the standard of care based on prevailing local or national practices. See Lewis MH, Gohagan JK, Merenstein DJ. The locality rule and the physician's dilemma: local medical practices vs. the national standard of care. *JAMA* 2007;297:2633–2636.

124. Studdert DM, Mello MM, Brennan TA. Medical malpractice. *N Engl J Med* 2004;350:283–292.

125. Kachalia A, Choudhry NK, Studdert DM. Physician responses to the malpractice crisis: from defense to offense. *J Law Med Ethics* 2005;33:416–428.

126. Studdert DM, Mello MM, Gawande AA, et al. Claims, errors, and compensation payments in medical malpractice litigation. *N Engl J Med* 2006;354:2024–2033.

127. Hurwitz B. How does evidence based guidance influence determinations of medical negligence? *BMJ* 2004;329:1024–1028.

128. For example, see The American Academy of Neurology Code of Professional Conduct and The American Academy of Neurology Disciplinary Action Policy. In *American Academy of Neurology 2006–2007*

Membership Directory and Resource Guide. St. Paul, MN: American Academy of Neurology, 2006:387–394. http://www.aan.com/globals/axon/assets/2500.pdf (Accessed June 15, 2007).

129. Williams MA, Mackin GA, Beresford HR, et al. American Academy of Neurology qualifications and guidelines for the physician expert witness. *Neurology* 2006;66:13–14.

130. Studdert DM, Mello MM, Sage WM, et al. Defensive medicine among high-risk specialist physicians in a volatile malpractice environment. *JAMA* 2005;293:2609–2617.

131. The increasing prevalence of the practice of defensive medicine was measured in Kessler DP, Summerton N, Graham JR. Effects of the medical liability system in Australia, the UK, and the USA. *Lancet* 2006;368:240–246.

132. Birbeck GL, Gifford DR, Song J, Belin TR, Mittman BS, Vickrey BG. Do malpractice concerns, payment mechanisms, and attitudes influence test-ordering decisions? *Neurology* 2004;62:119–121.

133. DeKay M, Asch D. Is the defensive use of diagnostic tests good for patients, or bad? *Med Decision Making* 1998;18:19–28.

134. Morreim EH. Cost constraints as a malpractice defense. *Hastings Cent Rep* 1988;18(2):5–10; Hall MA. The malpractice standard under health care cost containment. *Law Med Health Care* 1989;17:347–355; Morreim EH. Stratified scarcity: redefining the standard of care. *Law Med Health Care* 1989;17:356–357; and Hirshfeld EB. Economic considerations in treatment decisions and the standard of care in medical malpractice litigation. *JAMA* 1990;264:2004–2012.

135. Morreim EH. *Hastings Cent Rep* 1988;18(2):5–10; Morreim EH. *Law Med Health Care* 1989; 17:347–355; and Morreim EH. Cost containment and the standard of medical care. *Calif Law Rev* 1987; 75:1719–1763.

136. Hall MA. The malpractice standard under health care cost containment. *Law Med Health Care* 1989;17:347–355.

137. On the development and use of practice guidelines, see Hirshfeld EB. Practice parameters and the malpractice liability of physicians. *JAMA* 1990;263:1556–1562; Hirshfeld EB. Should ethical and legal standards for physicians be changed to accommodate new models for rationing health care? *U Penn Law Rev* 1992;140:1809–1846; Rosenberg J, Greenberg MK. Practice parameters: strategies for survival into the nineties. *Neurology* 1992;42:1110–1115; Bierig JR, Hirshfeld EB, Kelly JT, et al. Practice parameters: malpractice liability considerations for physicians. In: Wecht CH, ed. *Legal Medicine* 1991. Salem, NH: Butterworth Legal Publishers, 1991:207–225; Havighurst CC. Practice guidelines as legal standards governing physician liability. *Law and Contemporary Problems.* 1991;54:87–117; and Woolf SH. Practice guidelines: a new reality in medicine. III. Impact on patient care. *Arch Intern Med* 1993;153: 2646–2655.

138. Franklin GM, Zahn CA. AAN clinical practice guidelines: above the fray. *Neurology* 2002; 59:975–976.

139. A common reason to justify varying from clinical practice guidelines is in caring for the patient with multiple conditions, where the presence of a comorbidity may make a guideline inapplicable. See Tinetti ME, Bogardus T Jr, Agostini JV. Potential pitfalls of disease-specific guidelines for patients with multiple conditions. *N Engl J Med* 2004;351:2870–2874.

140. Quality Standards Subcommittee, American Academy of Neurology. Practice parameter: the utility of neuroimaging in the evaluation of headache in patients with a normal neurological examination (summary statement). Report of the Quality Standards Subcommittee of the American Academy of Neurology. *Neurology* 1994;44:1353–1354.

141. Halpern J. Can the development of practice guidelines safeguard patient values? *J Law Med Ethics* 1995;23:75–81.

142. Berger JT, Rosner F. The ethics of practice guidelines. *Arch Intern Med* 1996;156:2051–2056.

143. Bernat JL. Quality of neurological care: balancing cost control with ethics. *Arch Neurol* 1997;54:1341–1345.

144. Redman BK. Ethical issues in the development and use of guidelines for clinical practice. *J Clin Ethics* 1996;7:251–256.

145. Havighurst CC. Private reform of tort-law dogma. *Law and Contemporary Problems* 1986;49:134–183. I am grateful to Dr. H. Richard Beresford for explaining these options.

146. Havighurst CC. Vicarious liability: relocating responsibility for the quality of medical care. *Am J Law Med* 2000;26:7–29.

147. Mariner WK. Liability for managed care decisions: the Employee Retirement Income Security Act (ERISA) and the uneven playing field. *Am J Public Health* 1996;86:863–869.

148. 120 S. Ct. 2143 (2000). The implications of this case are discussed in Mariner WK. What recourse?— Liability for managed care decisions and the Employee Retirement Income Security Act. *N Engl J Med* 2000;343:592–596 and Gostin LO. Managed care, conflicts of interest, and quality. *Hastings Cent Rep* 2000;30(5):27–28.

149. Bloche MG, Jacobson PD. The Supreme Court and bedside rationing. *JAMA* 2000;284:2776–2779.

150. *New York State Conference of Blue Cross and Blue Shield Plans v. Travelers Ins. Co.*, 514 US 645, 654 (1995).

The Hospital Ethics Committee and the Ethics Consultant

5

Hospital ethics committees have evolved over the past several decades to provide an interdisciplinary forum for the discussion of ethical problems arising in inpatient care. These committees also help educate hospital staff members about clinical-ethical issues and advise hospital administrators about the design and implementation of policies on clinical subjects with ethical dimensions. The ultimate intent of these committees is to improve the quality of patient care by resolving conflicts, clarifying treatment plans, and optimizing hospital policies. Because nearly identical ethics committees have evolved in chronic care and rehabilitation facilities, I use the more inclusive term institutional ethics committee (IEC) to refer to them. In this chapter, I review the role and success of the contemporary institutional ethics committee and contrast it with the roles of the institutional review board and the infant care review committee. I then review empirical data on the benefits and harms of having clinical ethics consultants perform ethics consultations. I end with a short consideration of the emerging field of organizational ethics.

EVOLUTION OF THE INSTITUTIONAL ETHICS COMMITTEE

The contemporary institutional ethics committee is not a direct-line descendant of any single progenitor but rather evolved over the last several decades in the context of several concurrent traditions.[1] With the development of chronic hemodialysis in the 1960s, multidisciplinary hospital committees were impaneled to select which patients should receive it.[2] In 1971, the preamble of the *Medico-Moral Guide* of the Canadian Catholic bishops recommended the establishment of "medical-moral committees" in all Catholic hospitals and other health facilities. These committees were charged with educating hospital personnel about medical-moral problems. They served as a forum to interpret Roman Catholic religious doctrines in the context of patient care, to write hospital policies that reflected Catholic teachings, and to communicate these policies to the hospital staff. Medical-moral committees were multidisciplinary in composition, with representatives from all hospital services relevant to inpatient care.[3]

In a law review article in 1975, Karen Teel suggested that all hospitals should form similar but secular multidisciplinary ethics committees to help advise physicians about clinical-ethical issues arising in their care of patients.[4] The following year, the *Quinlan* court in New Jersey formally adopted this suggestion in its influential ruling. The *Quinlan* court enlarged Teel's proposed scope of the committee's role to include confirming the prognosis of critically ill patients, assisting physicians and families in the resolution of ethical dilemmas involving hospitalized patients, and acting generally as would a court of law to protect patients' rights and interests.[5] Subsequently, and with relatively few exceptions, other high courts have asserted

109

that a properly functioning hospital ethics committee could replace much of the need for routine judicial review of controversial cases.[6]

In the mid-1970s, several hospitals impaneled "prognosis committees" when it became recognized that establishing the prognosis of severely ill patients was a prerequisite to ethical decision making about their care. The most well known and longest functioning prognosis committee was the Optimum Care Committee of the Massachusetts General Hospital.[7] Attending physicians consulted this committee for assistance with ethically troubling cases. Its mission was to clarify prognosis, facilitate communication, re-establish treatment objectives, and maximize the support of physicians authorized to make difficult treatment decisions. Some prognosis committees subsequently evolved into IECs, while others, such as in New Jersey under the influence of *Quinlan*, have remained oriented to establishing the prognosis of critically ill patients.

The 1982 and 1983 reports of the President's Commission for the Study of Ethical Problems in Medicine and Biomedical and Behavioral Research further consolidated the role and value of IECs. The Commission not only opined that IECs were justified, it also suggested that their more widespread implementation could lessen the need of referring clinical-ethical dilemmas involving hospitalized patients to courts for judicial review.[8] The Commission argued that a properly functioning IEC, like a court of law, could provide standardized procedures and multidisciplinary impartial oversight of decisions that would protect patients' rights and interests.

Subsequently, a number of professional societies, including the American Medical Association, the American Hospital Association, the American Academy of Pediatrics, the American Academy of Neurology, and the New York State Task Force on Life and the Law endorsed the formation of IECs in hospitals.[9] In 1987, Maryland became the first state to require that all hospitals establish patient care advisory committees, whose role was essentially identical to those of the IEC.[10] A 1992 New Jersey law for hospital licensing required the presence of an ethics or prognosis committee.[11] The Maryland Health-Care Decisions Act required that conflicts or disagreements among family members of similar authority over decisions to terminate life-sustaining treatment of patients must be referred to the hospital's IEC.[12]

Since 1991, the standards of the Joint Commission on Accreditation of Healthcare Organizations (JCAHO) have made the presence of an IEC or similar body essentially mandatory in American hospitals and nursing homes. The JCAHO standards require that all health-care facilities have in place a "mechanism" to ensure "rights of patients and organizational ethics." These rights and ethical standards include formulating advance directives, determining when to withhold resuscitative services and withdraw life-sustaining treatment, deciding what care and treatment are appropriate at the end of life, providing informed consent, and resolving conflicts in treatment decisions.[13] Although the JCAHO does not mandate how this mechanism must be accomplished, most hospitals have chosen to fulfill it by impaneling IECs.

Ethics committees proliferated during the 1980s. A 1983 survey performed for the President's Commission to determine the prevalence of IECs found that they were functioning in only 4.3% of the hospitals with greater than 200 beds and in no hospitals with fewer than 200 beds.[14] A 1987 survey showed that 60% of American hospitals had IECs.[15] Community surveys in the early 1990s estimated the number of hospitals with IECs to be in the 65% to 85% range,[16] although one large survey in 1992 by the American Hospital Association found IECs in only 51% of the nearly 6,000 surveyed hospitals.[17] A 1992 survey of hospitals in the U.S. Department of Veterans Affairs disclosed that about 90% had IECs.[18] The most recent and comprehensive survey sampled 600 hospitals in the United States. Ethics consultation services operated in 81% of all hospitals and in 100% of hospitals with more than 400 beds.[19]

A common pattern for the ontogeny of an IEC is for interested hospital staff members to form a clinical ethics study group. After a few years of self-study, the group assumes the responsibility for educating other hospital staff members on clinical-ethical issues. The hospital administration may then authorize the group as an official IEC and request that the newly formed IEC review hospital policies on clinical-ethical issues and make recommended improvements. In its most productive stage, the IEC reviews clinical-ethical dilemmas of hospitalized patients on request. Expert members of the group can provide requested on-site clinical ethics consultations.

Many mature IECs have experienced a "midlife crisis" in which their previous functions and directions have been questioned and their future role debated. Some midlife committees lost the clear direction they previously followed and found themselves performing fewer clinical consultations than they did in earlier stages of development.[20] The departure of energetic founding members is one explanation. Secondly, once hospital staff members have become educated and more sophisticated about clinical ethics practices, demand diminishes for the simpler consultations. Lastly, many non-IEC hospital staff members, particularly nurses and social workers, have become more knowledgeable about clinical ethics as a result of the Patient Self-Determination Act (PSDA) of 1990 and the rise of the clinical ethics movement. The mature stage and ultimate fate of the IEC remain to be determined.

STRUCTURE OF THE INSTITUTIONAL ETHICS COMMITTEE

The essential feature of the IEC is its multidisciplinary composition, as originally suggested by the *Quinlan* court.[21] In theory, a multidisciplinary committee cannot easily be dominated by the parochial interests of a single physician, another professional, or a service. A functioning multidisciplinary process permits the committee to represent the broad interests of the hospitalized patient properly, as each professional member and represented service contributes a unique perspective to help define the totality of the patient's interests. A balanced, multidisciplinary IEC also has the greatest chance of achieving a functioning democratic process.

Ethics committees are multidisciplinary in two dimensions: professional training and hospital service. Most committees are composed of at least a physician, nurse, chaplain, social worker, patient advocate, administrator, and lawyer. It is useful to have professional members representing hospital services in which ethical problems commonly arise, including intensive care, emergency room, operating room, psychiatry, neurology, pediatrics, quality assurance, and risk management. Most committees restrict the participation of the hospital counsel to an advisory role, recognizing the potential conflict between the lawyer's duty to protect the institution and medical staff and the committee's interest in protecting the patient.[22] It is desirable for the IEC to have access to the services of a professional with training in clinical ethics or moral philosophy. One study found that the moral reasoning of philosophers and theologians serving as medical ethicists was more sophisticated than the moral reasoning of physicians[23] but others have found that the moral reasoning of an ordinary IEC member is no better than that of an average person.[24] Many committees also contain non-staff lay members who represent the community and its values.[25] Active participation of the lay member helps diminish the tendency for the committee to orient its interests in favor of the hospital.

Within the institutional bureaucracy, the IEC may be placed under the medical staff or under the hospital administration, depending on the purpose of the committee. Committees functioning under the direction of the medical staff may be less threatening to physicians and hence more easily accepted by the medical staff. Such committees may more easily fulfill a consultation role. Further, their case consultations and minutes may be shielded to a greater extent by peer review protection statutes. As a result, however, such committees tend to be dominated by physicians and may lack true multidisciplinary composition and functioning. Committees functioning under the hospital administration are less likely to be dominated by physicians, but they run the risk that the hospital's interests may be considered over those of patients in those rare situations in which the two interests conflict. Another choice is for the committee to bypass hospital administration and report directly to the hospital Board of Trustees.[26]

The optimal size of the IEC varies with the function and size of the institution. Small hospitals or nursing homes may have IECs with 6 to 12 members; larger institutions may have up to 25 members. It is desirable for the members to function as a team under the leadership of a chairperson skilled at maintaining order, focus, and egalitarianism. Small and rural hospital IECs have unique characteristics and practical problems resulting from their small size and isolation.[27] The prevalence, activities, and types of case consultations of IECs within nursing homes have been surveyed.[28]

Most IECs have closed meetings to maximize patient confidentiality and foster the development of a close working relationship of members. When specific clinical cases are discussed, patients and their families ideally should have access to the committee, but many committees do not offer this service. Most committees record minutes. Advantages of recording the minutes include enhanced member and IEC accountability, the creation of a useful teaching resource, and a reduction of the opportunity for subsequent misunderstanding. However, the issue of IEC members' legal liability can be affected both positively and negatively if minutes are recorded.[29] In our hospital, IEC minutes containing clinical consultation reports and summaries of discussion are considered quality improvement documents and thereby shielded from legal discovery under the state peer review protection statute.

FUNCTIONS OF THE INSTITUTIONAL ETHICS COMMITTEE

Surveys have shown that most IECs execute three principal functions: education, policy review and development, and clinical consultation and case review.[30] Many mature committees, like that which I chair, have appointed three working subcommittees, each staffed and dedicated to fulfilling one of these three functions. Some committees that report to the facility's administration have been assigned clinical ethics quality assurance as a fourth role.

Education

Nearly all IECs fulfill a twofold educational role: teaching IEC members and other hospital staff members about clinical-ethical subjects. Most committees begin as self-study groups. Many new committee members read the American Hospital Association's ethics committee handbook or other handbooks designed to educate IEC members.[31] Members then identify journal articles and books about key clinical-ethics subjects for their fellow IEC members to read and study. After several years of self-study, IEC members may organize educational conferences featuring outside expert speakers to assist in educating the remainder of the hospital staff.[32] The hospital administration relies on successfully functioning committees to maintain an ongoing clinical-ethical educational program for the entire hospital staff. For example, in our hospital's ethics committee, liaison members are recruited from each hospital department to assist departmental ethics teaching. The educational role is expanded in many committees to teaching patients and their families in the context of a clinical-ethical consultation.

Policy Review

Most IECs fulfill institutional policy review and drafting functions. Hospital administrators may work with members of the IEC or permit the IEC alone to draft policies with ethical dimensions. Such institutional policies include Do-Not-Resuscitate (DNR) orders, withholding and withdrawing medical treatment, brain death determination, organ procurement, informed consent, advance directives, medical futility, and decision making in children and incompetent patients. Many of these policies are required by governing agencies and laws. For example, the JCAHO requires that hospitals maintain policies on certain clinical-ethical issues, such as DNR orders. The PSDA of 1990 requires all hospitals receiving Medicare or Medicaid revenues to maintain policies that require requesting and educating patients about advance directives and their right to accept or refuse medical treatment.[33] A useful compendium of existing selected policies on clinical-ethical subjects from leading hospitals is available for IEC members to guide them in the development of new policies.[34]

Clinical Consultations

Clinical consultations provided by the IEC are its most important and controversial role. Conclusions or recommendations offered by members in clinical matters are only advisory. While their advice can be powerfully influential, IECs are not authorized to make treatment decisions.[35] The attending physician of record has the ultimate responsibility for the patient's medical care. In the Department of Veterans Affairs and in many other hospitals, IECs call themselves "ethics advisory committees" to stress this limited clinical authority. In many IECs, the members serve as an expert panel to discuss clinical-ethical dilemmas arising in patient care. In the course of the panel hearing, the ethical dimensions of the case are outlined, the process of decision making is inspected, and the merits and harms of various treatment options are debated. Many committees have reported that clinicians participating in the discussions have gained a clearer idea of ethically acceptable treatment options as they make their subsequent decision.[36]

The experience of the Optimum Care Committee of the Massachusetts General Hospital exemplifies how much influence an IEC can wield. The committee reported 20 cases in which it recommended that the attending physician overturn the family's decision to request cardiopulmonary resuscitation (CPR) for patients who were critically ill. The committee cited data indicating that CPR in each case would be futile. As a result, in each case the attending physician wrote a DNR order in opposition to the family's request.[37] I am unaware of another example in which an IEC has assumed this influential clinical responsibility.

Many IECs have evolved a practice in which all requests for clinical consultations are directed to the chairperson, who then decides the best way to respond to the request. The chairperson can consider a range of possible responses to address the question raised in the most appropriate way. For example, when the request is simply for factual information, a short verbal consultation may be given without convening the committee. In cases in which controversy about an ethical issue appears to result from poor communication, the chairperson can make a limited and discreet inquiry and render informal advice to assist the parties in improving their communication, or the chairperson can schedule a conference of all principals to discuss their differences of opinion. Some ethics committees facing large numbers of consultation requests perform proactive screening using a printed form.[38]

When the chairperson finds that the issue is one of a patient's prognosis, she can respond by assembling specialist physicians and others to specifically address this issue. She may perform an ethics consultation herself or employ other ethics consultants on the committee. The chairperson also may impanel the consultation subcommittee or the entire committee and arrange a family meeting, including relevant practitioners, nurses, the patient, and family members. The ability of the chairperson to use her discretion and choose the appropriate mode of IEC response increases its clinical value.

There is a wide spectrum of rules that different IECs employ regarding who is empowered to trigger a clinical consultation, how the IEC responds to the request, who is permitted to attend a family meeting on the issue, and when a formal note will be made in the medical record. It is preferable to permit anyone of moral or legal standing in the patient's care to request a consultation: physicians, nurses,[39] other members of the health-care team, the patient, or patient's family members. A seasoned chairperson can decide the most useful and appropriate way to respond to each request. A medical record note summarizing the reason for the involvement of the IEC, the major points raised in the discussion, and options or recommendations usually is desirable in a formal consultation unless the responsible physician does not want it.

Most IECs use the consensus model of deliberation. In the consensus model, the case is discussed in its entirety with inputs from all participating and relevant parties, including the committee members, the patient, and the patient's physicians, nurses, and family members. All participants are given the opportunity to speak and explain their positions. The chair maintains order, assures democratic process, and attempts to achieve consensus once the ethical issue has been clarified and the full range of issues, opinions, and feelings have been expressed. In the consensus model, the chair employs the process of clinical pragmatism, discussed in chapter 6.[40] The process, efficacy, and outcomes of ethics consultations are considered later in the chapter in the discussion of ethics consultants.

In one survey, chairs of IECs reported that they were consulted most frequently about end-of-life issues. They felt most unsuccessful in dealing with administrative ethical issues. They believed that problems including the cost of medical care, managed care, and rationing were important ethical issues that fell within the purview of their committee. They felt they succeeded to a greater extent in educating non-physician hospital professionals about clinical ethics than physicians. They were uncertain how effective they had been is settling disputes and what value others attributed to their activities.[41] In another survey the most common ethical dilemmas leading to ethics consultations were end-of-life issues including futility and withdrawal of life-sustaining treatment in 74%, patient autonomy and surrogacy issues in 57%, and conflicts between principals involved in the patient's care in 39%.[42]

In a recent report of 255 clinical ethics consultations performed during 1995–2005 at the Mayo Clinic, Keith Swetz and colleagues found that: 40% of consultations involved intensive care unit patients; 40% of the patients died during the hospitalization; and that the most common underlying diseases were malignancy, neurological disease, and cardiovascular disease. Most consultations involved more than one ethical issue. The most common themes were the adequacy of patient decision-making capacity (82%), staff member disagreement with the care plan (76%), end-of-life and quality-of-life issues (60%), goals of care/medical futility (54%), and withholding/withdrawing medical treatment (52%).[43] These cases are similar to those we have seen over the past decade by the Dartmouth-Hitchcock Medical Center Bioethics Committee.

Other Roles

Hospital administrators have assigned some IECs a quality assurance role of performing mandatory audits on all cases with clinical-ethical dimensions. For example, some committees have been assigned the role of reviewing all cases with DNR orders to ascertain compliance with hospital policy in regard to mandatory physician signatures and progress notes. Others have been asked to systematically review orders that limit or terminate medical treatment to make sure that they comply with hospital policies of informed consent.[44] Committee members should carefully consider the auditing function before agreeing to perform it. Case audit is a quality assurance function and, by being mandatory, is contrary to the voluntariness of the committee's usual clinical functions. Although the clinical consultation role is voluntary and non-binding, a mandatory auditing role may result in corrective or disciplinary action. Physicians who are aware that committees must also perform audits may be reluctant to engage them in case consultations.

A few IECs have become politically active in advising state legislators as they draft laws that involve bioethical issues. For example, our IEC assisted New Hampshire legislators in the drafting of the state advance directives law in the early 1990s, and during its 2006 revision.[45] The IEC at George Washington University Hospital reported on its experience helping legislators amend the Health-Care Decisions Act in the District of Columbia.[46] These extracurricular activities are justified because IEC members understand the workings of relevant health laws in practice and can provide critical advice to legislators on the likely clinical consequences of their implementation.

PITFALLS AND LIMITATIONS OF INSTITUTIONAL ETHICS COMMITTEES

The potential benefit of having an IEC perform clinical consultations is that the education of the requesting physician and staff about the scope of ethically acceptable treatment alternatives may help safeguard the interests of the patient and lead to improved patient care. The potential risk of IEC clinical involvement is that the physician may abdicate decision-making responsibility to a distant committee that lacks accountability, and create a circumstance that may result in poorer patient care.[47] The ultimate balance of these two opposing effects will determine the justification of the continued involvement of ethics committees in clinical consultations.[48]

To prevent an unaccountable IEC from usurping a physician's decision-making responsibility, the precise role of the IEC must be restricted specifically to exclude the primary responsibility for making decisions concerning a patient's care. Committees should be conducted solely as advisory groups to help educate medical and hospital staff members and thereby increase the breadth of available treatment options for the patient. By reviewing the decision-making details of cases, committees also can function in an oversight capacity to assure that patients' rights are protected.

Committee proceedings should not produce independent patient care decisions. At all times, the responsibility for making decisions concerning patient care must rest with the attending physician of record. If the IEC chooses to make a treatment recommendation, the attending physician should treat the advice like that of any other consultant. She can choose to follow it or ignore it, depending on her judgment of what is best for the patient.[49]

The major value of the IEC is in its process and not necessarily in its product.[50] In many instances, the committee's chief benefit will have been accomplished simply because the principals in a difficult case were afforded the opportunity to sit down together, jointly hear the patient's diagnosis, prognosis, treatment options, and treatment preferences, and discuss the ethical and care issues calmly and rationally. Facilitating this discussion is an important role of the IEC because the patient's interests are further protected by the development of consensus resulting from improved staff communication.

Committees require accurate clinical information to debate ethical issues properly. One limitation of some IECs is their near total reliance on secondhand information presented by physicians, nurses, social workers, and others. Secondhand information may be inaccurate, vague, and misleading. Committees should secure primary information sources by interviewing the principals directly and reviewing the medical record and other documents to obtain correct and current information before analyzing and debating the ethical issues. Clinical ethics consultants (discussed later) optimally fill this role.

Committees should attempt to minimize the interpersonal problems inherent in any committee activity. A common pitfall is "groupthink," the tendency of well meaning but conflict-averse committee members to reach a consensus before important areas of disagreement have been identified and honestly resolved. Groupthink can produce an overwhelming desire to achieve consensus and thereby act to prematurely terminate discussion of alternative viewpoints and conflicting data. Groupthink can hurt the patient if it causes the IEC to fail to consider certain potentially beneficial options carefully.[51]

The IEC usually cannot recapitulate the complete impartiality of judicial review. The professionals serving on the committee often are colleagues or friends of physicians and others bringing cases before the committee. These pre-existing relationships may color the objectivity of committee members and affect the outcome of the discussion. Moreover, physician colleagues often think alike, as a consequence of training. Committee members should try to remain impartial and focus on maintaining the patient's rights and best interests.

Another interpersonal problem is the tendency for unassertive committee members to be influenced unduly by strong and persuasive members. Department chairpersons and other influential and strong-willed members may carry their aura of authority with them into the committee meeting. They may intimidate more junior members, stifle dissenting opinion, and diminish democratic process. Lawyers can dominate the committee by overemphasizing concern for liability and other legal issues, misdirecting the committee's emphasis away from the patient's welfare to a preoccupation with legal considerations or hospital interests. Robert Weir has cautioned appropriately that IECs should remain "ethical advisors" and not become "legal watchdogs."[52]

If IECs are to succeed in a clinical consultative role, patients and families must be guaranteed proper access to them. Committees should not be restricted for use solely by physicians. Patients and families should be allowed to trigger consultations and discuss their concerns with the committee. Similarly, IEC proceedings should be available to all parties involved in the case.[53]

MEDICOLEGAL ASPECTS OF INSTITUTIONAL ETHICS COMMITTEES

Many people believe and several courts have ruled that properly functioning ethics committees can serve as local and more accessible substitutes for formal judicial review. The success rates of committees vary in this capacity. Even in those IECs best fulfilling their duty to recapitulate impartial judicial review, there remain three unresolved medicolegal questions. First, in which instances should IECs urge the referral of a case to court for formal judicial review? Second, in their rulings, how do courts consider the findings and conclusions of an IEC? Third, what is the professional liability of an IEC member faithfully discharging her responsibilities as a member of the hospital staff?

Ethics committees can supplant formal judicial review in many but not all cases. Committees should recommend that clinicians refer cases for judicial review in four general circumstances. First is the incompetent patient with no legally authorized surrogate about whom there is an irreconcilable conflict between family decision makers regarding the kind and level of proposed treatment. A judge can appoint a legally authorized surrogate from the family or a guardian *ad litem*, thereby protecting the patient and secondarily protecting the physician and institution from having disgruntled family members take legal action. Second are those rare instances where there is an intractable conflict between what is in the best interest of the patient and what is in the best interest of the institution. Third, when there is objective evidence that, because of conflicts of interest, the surrogate decision maker is not deciding in the patient's best interests, the court should be asked to appoint a new surrogate. Fourth, when there is neither a surrogate decision maker nor an advance directive to guide the physician, and hospital policy and state law fail to provide an alternative remedy, a

formal guardian *ad litem* should be appointed by the court.[54]

Courts have varied on how they weigh the findings and conclusions of IECs. The *Quinlan* court believed that the IEC could be an effective substitute for judicial review. However, in the more recent case of *In re L.H.R.*, the highest court in Georgia ignored the recommendation of the IEC. At issue was whether a child in a persistent vegetative state with no hope of recovery could be removed from the ventilator. Such a treatment plan was agreed to by the parents, physicians, guardian *ad litem*, and IEC. The *L.H.R.* court ruled that IECs were unnecessary in such cases and their recommendations irrelevant.[55] One justification the court cited for ignoring the findings of the IEC was the committee's lack of procedural rigor, in comparison with formal judicial process.

In two other jurisdictions, IEC findings and recommendations have been cited and used as evidence. In *In re Torres*, the findings of three IECs were relied on in the court's finding that a comatose man could be removed from a ventilator. More than one IEC reviewed the case because the patient had become comatose while in one hospital but was transferred to other hospitals. The *Torres* court ruled that IECs "are uniquely suited to provide guidance to physicians, families, and guardians when ethical dilemmas arise." In two Massachusetts Supreme Judicial Court cases, *Saikewicz* and *Spring*, the courts rejected the idea that ethics committees were an adequate substitute for judicial review but permitted the consideration of ethics committee views as valid findings during judicial review.[56]

Susan Wolf pointed out that courts should seriously consider the proceedings of an IEC only if the committee has followed a properly executed due process in handling the ethics consultation. Without developing such a theory of process, members of IECs would lack accountability and responsibility for their actions and conclusions, and insufficient patient care could result. The committee's theory of process should be patient-centered and complement the substantive, patient-centered ethical principles and values the IEC embraces.[57]

The professional liability of an IEC member is small but real. Institutional employees serving as IEC members usually are indemnified by their institution for professional liability arising from their service. Lay members from the community probably should ascertain their indemnification as well. There is reason to believe that professional liability for IEC members is minimal because the committee serves only in an advisory capacity and the members strive to represent the best interests of the patient from each of their professional perspectives. Nevertheless, ethics committee members are held to standards of professional competence and behavior and potentially can be liable for negligence.[58]

Some scholars have advocated providing IEC members with immunity from civil and criminal liability. Such immunity would be granted on the basis that IEC members are acting in good faith within the established rules of the hospital. Further, like hospital peer review committees, IECs may feel that their members require immunity in order to function properly. If blanket immunity is given, however, the accountability of IEC members risks being diminished. I am in agreement with those who believe that blanket immunity should not be granted to IEC members because each member should maintain proper accountability for her actions and conclusions.[59]

I am aware of only a single case of a patient who sued an IEC. Elizabeth Bouvia, a young woman with severely debilitating cerebral palsy who was totally and permanently dependent on others for her daily care, refused further oral, enteral, and parenteral hydration and nutrition when hospitalized. She stated that she wished to die in order to escape a life of unmitigated misery. Her physician overruled her refusal of treatment and ordered her to be forcibly fed. In 1986, Ms. Bouvia sued her physician and hospital to reverse this action. She also sued the hospital ethics committee for concurring with her physician's treatment plan but the suit was dropped in 1990.[60]

THE INFANT CARE REVIEW COMMITTEE

Albert Jonsen and colleagues initially proposed that an infant care review committee (ICRC) or infant bioethics committee should function as a mechanism to improve medical decision making when ethical issues arise in the care of severely ill neonates. The ICRC subsequently was endorsed by the American Academy of Pediatrics and the President's Commission for the Study of Ethical Problems in Medicine and Biomedical and Behavioral Research. Now ICRCs are mandated by legislation accompanying the "Baby Doe" regulations and by the Joint Commission on Accreditation of Healthcare Organizations.[61] The ICRC has a role and function almost identical to that of the IEC, except that the oversight role of the ICRC is restricted to the optimum care of the hospitalized infant.

Some scholars have emphasized the distinction between the ICRC mandated by the "Baby Doe" regulations and the infant bioethics committee recommended by both the President's Commission and the American Academy of Pediatrics. The former must convene within 24 hours of a disagreement between the infant's family and the physician concerning termination of life-sustaining therapy. Some scholars feel that the ICRC, unlike the infant bioethics committee, is not primarily concerned about the ethics of the situation.[62] However, because most institutions have only one committee serving both functions, this distinction usually is irrelevant in practice. Therefore, I refer to both committees as ICRCs.

Four unique characteristics of the critically ill hospitalized infant distinguish the role of the ICRC from that of the IEC in overseeing ethical issues in a comparably ill hospitalized adult: (1) infants are "never competent" human beings, therefore a standard of substituted judgment in making decisions is impossible and only a best interest standard can be used; (2) prognoses of severely ill infants usually are less definite than those of comparably ill adults; (3) decisions to terminate treatment of severely ill infants have inescapable political overtones that have been linked to politically sensitive public controversies, e.g, abortion; and (4) federal regulations mandate certain types of medical treatment for disabled infants.[63]

Institutions have taken varied approaches to staffing ICRCs. In some institutions the ICRC is a subcommittee of the IEC. In others the ICRC includes all IEC members and a few neonatologists who are not members of the IEC. The IEC and the ICRC are identical in some hospitals, with certain meetings of the

IEC dedicated periodically to ICRC case review. Some larger institutions empanel two entirely separate committees. A 1990 survey showed that 52% of American hospitals had functioning ICRCs.[64] The remainder are community hospitals and other health-care facilities without neonatology services.

The American Academy of Pediatrics believes that the ICRC should have the same educational, clinical, and policy drafting functions as a standard IEC with one important difference. The ICRC's consultative function should include mandatory review of all infant patients (except those who are imminently dying) for whom the parents and attending physicians propose to terminate life-sustaining treatment.[65]

In one survey, neonatologists were asked about the value of the ICRC in their daily practices. Most respondents said that they did not need ICRCs because they had received training in clinical ethics and felt comfortable in making clinical decisions concerning critically ill neonates in conjunction with the parents and other professionals through discussions at multidisciplinary infant care conferences. Further, those surveyed indicated that the Baby Doe regulations had made no significant impact on their decision-making practices, even on those critically ill neonates whose cases raised ethical questions.[66]

In two thoughtful critiques, George Annas and Robert Weir pointed out that the ultimate success of ICRCs depends not on mere assertions of their theoretical value, but rather on their clinical accuracy, efficiency, and social acceptability. ICRCs will improve current decision-making practices in critical care neonatology only if they can help guarantee the interests of infants over those of the institution and other parties.[67] A successful multidisciplinary infant care conference probably can accomplish much the same oversight role as the ICRC.

THE INSTITUTIONAL REVIEW BOARD

Contemporaneous with the growth of IECs, institutional review boards (IRBs) evolved to protect the safety, health, and welfare of humans serving as research subjects.[68] The IRB was developed in response to public concern about the ethical conduct of researchers following such well publicized research scandals as the Tuskegee syphilis study. Over the past two decades, the IRB has become institutionalized as the trusted protector of human research subjects.[69] Some confusion between the IRB and IEC may result from the European practice of referring to IECs as "clinical ethics committees" and IRBs as "research ethics committees."

Federal regulations mandate a systematic review by the IRB whenever research is conducted on human subjects. Research is defined in the federal statute as an activity carried out with the intent to develop "generalizable knowledge."[70] All medical schools, hospitals, research institutes, and other institutions that conduct research on human subjects must impanel IRBs. These boards convene periodically to review and approve or disapprove all research protocols involving human subjects.

The IRB mandate to protect human research subjects derives from the federal "common rule" that requires investigators to observe strict rules of informed consent and safety and carry out scientifically sound protocols.[71] Overall, the IRB must certify that: (1) the rights and welfare of research subjects are protected; (2) the risk to the research subject is outweighed by the sum of the potential benefits to the subject and future subjects; and (3) the informed consent of the subject is obtained.[72]

IRB activities are governed by the Department of Health and Human Services Office of Human Research Protection (OHPR), which in 2000 replaced the less visible NIH Office for Protection from Research Risks. The OHPR is charged with educational, quality improvement, and investigational duties to supervise IRB oversight. The FDA has established an analogous Office for Good Clinical Practice to coordinate its protection of research subjects receiving investigational drugs and devices. IRBs thus operate under federal and local rules.

The IRB and the IEC share concerns regarding the ethical behavior of professionals, but it is essential to understand their different missions. The IRB regulates ethical issues in research whereas the IEC serves as a forum to discuss ethical issues in patient care. The IRB review of research is mandatory whereas the IEC clinical review is solely advisory. The IRB operates according to federal guidelines whereas the IEC is entirely controlled locally. The IRB holds open meetings but those of the ethics committee are closed. Approval by the IRB is a necessary step before investigators can begin any research protocol using human subjects.[73] Operation of the IRB in approving clinical research protocols is considered further in chapter 19.

Ezekiel Emanuel and colleagues recently analyzed the problems commonly experienced by IRBs and proposed means to improve their functioning.[74] They identified structural problems including inconsistent regulations and guidelines, a lack of a mechanism for resolving ethical issues, a lack of guidance on resolving institutional conflicts of interest, unnecessary repetition in reviewing cooperative clinical trials, inadequate funding, and haphazard education. They identified procedural problems including a cumbersome review process, IRB members' lack of expertise, unhelpful adverse event reporting, and a preoccupation with informed consent documents. They proposed six reforms to address the problems: (1) accreditation of IRBs and institutional protections; (2) credentialing of IRB personnel; (3) centralized IRBs to systematize policies; (4) legislative proposals to fix the problems of funding, personnel training, and conflicts of interest; (5) OHRP initiatives to simplify processes and establish a quality improvement program; and (6) compliance with the recommendations of the Institute of Medicine's study *Responsible Research* to apply federal protection to all research, improve the process of informed consent, improve safety monitoring systems, develop outcome measures, and provide a no-fault compensation system for research injuries.[75] Michelle Mello and colleagues catalogued the lawsuits against IRBs and investigators, commenting that these suits may stimulate improved oversight and reform.[76]

THE CLINICAL ETHICS CONSULTANT

Most experienced ethics committees have learned that their clinical consultation role can be executed more successfully by trained ethics consultants than by the entire committee. Mature committees have formed clinical ethics consultation services headed by ethics consultants. Clinical ethics consultants are professionals with training and experience in clinical ethics whose assistance is sought at the bedside to help resolve ethical dilemmas arising in patient care.[77]

Ethics consultants have several advantages over ethics committees in performing clinical ethics consultations. First, the consultant can respond to urgent requests in a more timely manner than can a committee. Second, the consultant can more easily gain direct access to primary patient data through chart reviews and interviews. Third, the consultant can be expected to possess more expertise in clinical ethics than other committee members. Fourth, the ethics consultation can be used to educate house staff in clinical ethics. Finally, an organized ethics consultation service can more easily keep systematic data available to conduct reviews and to perform empirical research.[78]

Four models of ethics consultation have been used successfully in different institutions. In the "pure committee" model, the committee as a whole responds to the consultation request. In the "committee member as consultant" model, one member of the IEC is selected to serve as the ethics consultant in each case. In the *ex post facto* committee review model, the ethics consultant performs the consultation and later presents the case to the whole committee at a regularly scheduled meeting. In the "pure consultation" model, only the ethics consultant is involved and no presentation is made to an IEC.[79] I have found the consultant and *ex post facto* committee review model to work most successfully in practice.

In a consensus statement, John Fletcher and Mark Siegler summarized the goals of clinical ethics consultations: (1) to maximize benefit and minimize harm to patients, families, healthcare professionals, and institutions by fostering a fair decision-making process that honors the wishes of patients and their surrogates and respects cultural values; (2) to facilitate the resolution of conflicts respectfully with consideration of the interests, rights, and responsibilities of those involved; (3) to inform institutional policy development, quality improvement, and resource utilization by understanding ethical problems and by promoting ethical standards; and (4) to educate individuals in clinical ethics to assist them in resolving ethical problems.[80] An additional goal is to reduce moral distress among all parties.[81]

The effective clinical ethics consultant serves as patient advocate, professional colleague, case manager, negotiator, mediator, and educator. Clinical ethics consultants therefore should possess the following skills: (1) ability to identify and analyze moral problems in patient care; (2) ability to use good clinical judgment; (3) ability to communicate effectively with the health-care team, family, and patient; (4) ability to negotiate and mediate; (5) ability to teach; and (6) ability to facilitate conflict resolution.[82]

The American Society for Bioethics and Humanities (ASBH) published a report of a national task force that studied hospital ethics consultations and recommended core competencies for clinical ethics consultants and standards for their consultations.[83] The ASBH task force classified the core competencies for ethics consultants into the following three categories and subcategories: (1) *core skills*: ethical assessment skills, process skills, and interpersonal skills; (2) *core knowledge*: knowledge of moral reasoning and ethical theory, common bioethical issues and concepts, health-care systems, clinical context, the local health-care institution and its policies, beliefs and perspectives of patient and staff, codes of ethics and professional conduct, and relevant health law; and (3) *character*: personal virtues of tolerance, patience, compassion, honesty, courage, prudence, humility, and integrity.[84]

How many currently practicing ethics consultants fulfill the ASBH competency requirements? One study of the competency of ethics consultants in Maryland in 2000 concluded that approximately two-thirds lacked the competencies recommended by the ASBH task force.[85] Although the need for further training and standardization is obvious, the ASBH task force recommended against certifying ethics consultants for several reasons: (1) the fear of further displacing the physician as the primary decision maker; (2) the fear of undermining disciplinary diversity; (3) the fear of institutionalizing one particular view of morality;

(4) the difficulty of devising reliable tests to show competency; and (5) the need to develop a new bureaucracy to oversee this field.[86]

Hospital ethics consultants come from a variety of disciplines including medicine, nursing, law, philosophy, theology, and social work. The ASBH report was silent on the issue of the minimal professional background or credentials for ethics consultants other than their need to possess the core competencies listed above. I believe it is essential that clinical ethics consultants have a background in clinical medicine sufficient to clearly understand the clinical context in which ethical problems arise. Clinical decisions may be made as a result of the ethics consultation, so the consultants need to adequately understand the medical facts.[87] Clinical understanding also improves the credibility of the ethics consultation service to the medical and nursing staff. Those services in which ethics consultants have been reported to achieve the greatest success have included the primary participation of practicing physicians. Many hospitals combine physician ethics consultants with those from other disciplines.

Of the various approaches the consultant can take, there is now a consensus that the ethics facilitation approach is the most successful.[88] The consultant begins by gathering relevant data through a careful review of the patient's medical record and relevant documents such as advance directives. She then interviews the patient and other principals involved in the case, including physicians, nurses, and family members. The consultant then formulates and analyzes the clinical-ethical problem by clarifying the ethical concepts in question and related matters, such as legal and policy issues. She helps identify the range of morally acceptable options and works collaboratively with the principals to mediate, negotiate, and implement a solution to the problem.[89]

A growing number of ethics consultations are being requested for assistance in conflict resolution. Robert Orr and Dennis deLeon explained how the ethics consultant can function as an implicit or explicit third party negotiator, mediator, or arbitrator to help resolve conflicts.[90] In negotiation, the third party enters the conflict at the invitation of one of the warring parties and serves as a partisan to advance that party's position. In mediation, the third party is invited by both sides, is neutral, [91] and works to facilitate a process to resolve the conflict. In arbitration, a neutral third party is invited by both sides, as in mediation, but then is empowered by both parties with the authority to decide which side should prevail.[92] One study of the process of ethics consultation showed the frequent use of techniques of mediation and negotiation.[93] Some hospitals have created mediation-medical advisory panels to resolve disputes arising in end-of-life care.[94] Mediation techniques can be taught and used successfully by many hospital professionals to defuse conflicts over the use of life-sustaining treatments,[95] a problem that is particularly common in intensive care units.[96]

Relationships between the clinical ethics consultant and the IEC vary. In most services, the consultant is the chair or co-chair of the IEC. In only a few institutions do the IEC and ethics consultants function entirely separate from one another. Ideally, the consultant later presents her completed findings to the whole committee for advice and consent. The formal case presentation and discussion educate the less experienced IEC members and provide valuable critical feedback for the consultant. Interested clinicians who are committee members can accompany consultants for training purposes.[97]

There is a limited literature assessing the outcomes of ethics consultants and IEC case consultation successes or failures. An impediment to performing these studies has been the lack of standardized criteria outlining successful outcomes.[98] A conference in 1995 developed methodological standards for future studies,[99] including defining desirable outcome measures [100] and recommending appropriate evaluation tools.[101] Nevertheless, there are numerous obstacles to objectively assessing outcomes of ethics consultations that make the effort complex.[102]

A large recent survey assessed the practice of ethical consultation in American hospitals. The median number of consultations in each hospital performed annually was three. Most professionals performing ethics consultations were physicians (34%), nurses (31%), social

workers (11%), and chaplains (10%). Only 41% of these consultants had received formal, supervised training in ethics consultation. Formal recommendations were always offered by 65% of consultants, never by 6%, and sometimes by the rest. Nearly all committees (95%) permitted any relevant professional to order an ethics consultation. Only 54% of consultants or committees always interviewed the patient; the remainder did so infrequently or not at all. Consultants documented the consultations in the medical record in 72% of cases and the remainder kept records in internal files. Only 28% of ethics committees or consultants regularly collected and evaluated the consultations they had performed over a time interval.[103]

Several studies have examined the impact of ethics consultations on patient care. In one study of 44 ethics consultations, 14 were found to have identified previously unrecognized ethical issues and 18 changed patient management considerably. The most frequently overlooked issue concerned inappropriate family decision making for incompetent patients. The most frequent changes in management involved the writing of DNR orders.[104]

In another study, 71% of 51 consultation requests were found to be "very important" in clarifying ethical issues, improving patient management, or educating concerned parties in medical ethics. Clinicians requested assistance with issues of withholding or withdrawing medical therapy in 49% of the cases, with issues of resuscitation in 37%, and with issues of legality in 31%.[105]

In a third study, more than 90% of the surveyed respondents found the consultation helpful in clarifying ethical issues, educating the team, increasing confidence in clinical decisions, and assisting patient management. In only 36% of the cases, however, did significant changes in patient management result from the consultant's suggestions.[106]

A fourth study examined a community hospital ethics consultation service and compared the findings with similar services in a university hospital. Consultations in the community hospital were requested for issues related to terminating life sustaining treatment in 74% of the cases, resolving disagreements in 46%, and assessing patient competence in 30% of the cases. Those requesting the consultation rated the advice as helpful or very helpful in 86% of the cases. These community hospital data were similar to data from a university hospital that the same group of researchers had previously collected and analyzed.[107]

The only randomized clinical trial studying the effects of ethics consultation on limiting nonbeneficial life-sustaining treatments in the intensive care unit found that ethics consultations were useful in resolving conflicts with families over life-sustaining treatments. The ethics consultation intervention led to a mean reduction in hospitalization duration of about three days, a reduction in ICU stays of 1.5 days, and a reduction of 1.7 days of ventilator treatment among patients who died in the hospital. A subsequent satisfaction survey showed that 87% of physicians, nurses, and patients/surrogates reported that the ethics consultation was helpful in addressing the treatment conflict.[108] In an accompanying editorial, Bernard Lo pointed out that the study raised four questions: (1) How can institutions increase the frequency of ethics consultations to resolve treatment disputes in intensive care units? (2) What components of the ethics consultation are associated with desirable outcomes? (3) How can the goals of ethics consultations be broadened to address palliative care? (4) How can ethics consultations enhance the quality of medical education?[109]

Lawrence Schneiderman and colleagues recently reported a series of cases culled from their randomized controlled trial of ethics consultations,[110] in which surrogates, physicians, or nurses later expressed dissatisfaction with the ethics consultation.[111] Of those surveyed after an ethics consultation, 3% of physicians, 4% of nurses, and 13% of surrogates were dissatisfied. Subsequent interviews of these persons yielded a miscellany of sources of their dissatisfaction. Some surrogates disagreed with the treatment plan, thought mistakes were being covered up, or felt badgered by physicians to discontinue life-sustaining therapy. Physicians were unhappy because they disagreed with the treatment plan or found the process of consultation unhelpful. Nurses were dissatisfied usually because they disagreed with

the treatment recommendations. But more than 80% of surrogates and more than 90% of physicians and nurses gave favorable reviews of the consultation.

One survey examined why physicians chose not to order ethics consultations. The reasons cited by physician respondents were: (1) the physician should remain the primary decision maker and not defer medical decisions to an unaccountable committee; (2) ethical deliberation does not provide helpful answers to tough clinical problems; (3) medical ethics is not a useful field of study; and (4) the committee will give binding advice on cases brought to it.[112] While some of these beliefs could be changed by improvements in physician education, some show the respondents' fear of nonclinicians inadvertently harming clinical care. This finding underscores the necessity of maintaining physicians as primary members of any ethics consultation service. In another study of internists hesitation to use ethics consultations, 29% felt they were too time consuming, 15% stated that they made the situation worse, 11% said the consultants were unqualified, 9% said the consultations were unhelpful, and 9% claimed that the solutions offered were inconsistent with good medical practice.[113]

One emerging reason why some clinicians request ethics consultation is to try to resolve economic dilemmas in patient care, a finding analogous to the finding that some psychiatric consultations were masked requests for ethical discussion.[114] In one report, covert economic dilemmas included trying to minimize the "unnecessary" expense of chronic care, dealing with non-altruistic motives (wishing to save money) of a family member who made a surrogate decision against surgical treatment, and addressing the obligation of insurers to pay for costly organ transplantation.[115]

Another reason for requesting ethics consultations is a concern over the legal ramifications of medical decision making. Questions about the law often are intertwined with questions about clinical ethics. Most articles and textbooks on clinical ethics also discuss relevant laws and legal decisions.[116] Indeed, one active ethics consultation service found that 30% of its requested ethics consultations involved medicolegal issues.[117]

One study in 1991 examined the consistency of ethics consultants' opinions and found a disturbing lack of substantive agreement among different ethics consultants reviewing the same cases. Experienced ethics committee members and ethics consultants were asked to give their advice on seven paradigmatic cases of patients in a persistent vegetative state (PVS). Agreement was found only in the "easy" case in which the patient's advance directive and the family both requested discontinuation of life sustaining treatment for the patient.[118] The investigators repeated the study in 2003, after the publication of guidelines on the care of patients in PVS (discussed in chapter 12) and found the identical results.[119] These findings suggest that there may be less consensus and standardization in ethics consultants' recommendations than is commonly believed. If these findings are representative of ethics consultants' recommendations in general, the ethics consultants should understand that their ability to foster a process to help promote a harmonious resolution of interpersonal conflicts may be at least as useful as their substantive and procedural recommendations.

One study in 2000 examined the effect of ethics consultations on health-care costs. Although the intent of ethics consultations is not to lower costs, the investigators found that 20 of the 29 consultations performed during the study period lowered hospital costs by approximately $300,000. By clarifying concepts of surrogate decision making, medical futility, and patients' rights, the consultations led directly to reduced costs as a result of fewer hospital days, avoided resuscitations, and avoided surgical and diagnostic procedures. By comparison, the direct costs of the ethics consultation service during the study period were approximately $12,000.[120]

Ethics consultants should try to practice "preventive ethics" because ethical conflicts in progress are more difficult to solve than they are to prevent. Preventive ethics refers to the application of the principles and practical strategies of preventive medicine to clinical ethics.[121] Because many ethical problems evolve over time without a sudden onset, there may be a "window of opportunity" in which timely intervention prevents the ethical problem from developing. After this time has passed, it may no longer be possible to obtain the necessary information to resolve the problem. For example, discussing advance directives with a patient in detail before the patient becomes cognitively incapacitated prevents the need to speculate later about what the patient's wishes would have been. Some hospital ethics consultation services conduct regular rounds in intensive care units for preventive purposes.

There are two emerging and unresolved professional ethics issues concerning ethics consultants. The medicolegal issue is whether clinical ethicists and bioethicists should be permitted to testify as expert witnesses in court.[122] Some courts have permitted their testimony once their *bona fides* have been established. But given the absence of ethicist certification, this activity immediately raises the question of whether their education and training justifies their role as experts, and there remains no established standard for their testimony.[123]

A second issue in the growing tendency for ethics consultants to be hired by private corporations to analyze and ethically justify their research programs.[124] One highly visible example that provoked bioethics controversy involved the private Ethics Advisory Board retained by Advanced Cell Technology, which provided ethical approval for the company's research on cloned human embryos. Responding to critics, the Board justified its decision on scientific and ethical grounds.[125] At least one bioethicist has suggested that the conflicts of interest produced by industry funding of bioethics programs and consultants should cause journal editors to limit or ban the publication of their articles.[126] Some ethics scholars also see an intrinsic conflict of interest in performing ethics consultations. This concern can be mitigated if consultants refuse to act as agents and maintain their focus on doing the right thing.[127]

THE "NEUROETHICIST"

Neurologists and neurosurgeons with training in clinical ethics can serve a unique function on IECs and as ethics consultants, a role that

Ronald Cranford called the "neuroethicist."[128] Many issues provoking clinical ethics consultations in the general hospital surround the prognosis of patients who are severely brain damaged or paralyzed, including patients with brain death, those in coma after cardiac arrest or in a persistent vegetative state, and those suffering from dementia, stroke, and locked-in syndrome. Neurologists and neurosurgeons can combine their specialized knowledge of and experience with these states with their knowledge of clinical ethics to provide a unique combination of clinical-ethical advice.[129]

Neuroethicists can help correct misconceptions and incorrect definitions of clinical states that may confound ethical discussions. For example, even experienced intensive care unit physicians and nurses remain confused about the definition of brain death and the criteria used to establish it.[130] Similarly, whether patients are in a persistent vegetative state or other states of impaired consciousness may become a critical factor in the decision to terminate life-sustaining treatment. These basic clinical determinations often are erroneous and poorly understood.[131] The neuroethicist can help to clarify the exact diagnosis and prognosis of the critically ill patient to lay the foundation for a coherent discussion of their ethical dilemmas.

ORGANIZATIONAL ETHICS

The concept of organizational ethics is based on the premise that not only should clinicians behave ethically in their practices but health-care organizations also should behave ethically in their operations, services, and activities. All business and operational decisions of health-care organizations that affect patients ultimately are based on values. The values professed and practiced by organizations through their regulations and operations comprise the subject of organizational ethics.[132]

In 1992, the American Hospital Association (AHA) created the first national standards with the publication of *Ethical Conduct for Health Care Institutions*[133] but the JCAHO brought this concept to widespread American public attention in 1994 through its required standards. The AHA advised hospitals to conduct themselves through their corporate decisions in an ethical manner that emphasizes community orientation and justifies public trust. The JCAHO currently recommends that hospitals develop a program of "integrated" ethics in health care encompassing clinical ethics, organizational ethics, and community ethics.[134] The American Hospital Association has initiated a nationwide project to encourage member hospitals to develop local organizational ethics plans.

The numerous attempts to define organizational ethics were reviewed and analyzed by Robert Potter. Potter has synthesized these attempts into his preferred definition: "organizational ethics is the discernment of values for guiding managerial decisions that affect patient care." He explains that clinical ethics involves the discernment of values for guiding clinical decisions that affect patient care, while organizational ethics involves the discernment of values that guide managerial decisions that affect patient care.[135] Some institutions have broadened this definition to encompass managerial decisions that affect employees and the professional staff.

Catherine Myser and colleagues illustrated the difference between clinical ethical issues and organizational ethical issues. Examples of clinical ethical issues include withholding and withdrawing treatment, the doctrines of best interest and substituted judgment, and physician-assisted suicide. Examples of organizational issues include issues of business and research ethics resulting from partnerships with for-profit organizations, policy issues related to capitated managed care contracts, and reproductive care issues resulting from the merger of a secular institution with a Roman Catholic institution.[136] Confidentiality is both a clinical ethical issue and an organizational ethical issue because it can be protected or violated by both clinicians and organizations.[137] Similarly, the duty to disclose errors in patient care has both clinical and organizational ethical dimensions.[138] Quality improvement programs span organizational and clinical ethics.[139] There are a few differences but also many similarities between clinical ethical analysis and organizational ethical analysis.[140]

Susan Goold pointed out the important analogy between patients' trust in health-care institutions and their trust in physicians which forms the core of the patient-physician relationship.[141]

Institutions have taken varying approaches to implementing programs of organizational ethics. Some institutions have charged the IEC with the additional role of organizational ethics. Other institutions have impaneled separate organizational ethics committees to oversee this role. Some institutions hold meetings of high level administrators to discuss and analyze strategic decisions affecting patients in ethical terms. Others hold conferences in which past decisions are studied by ethical analysis. Some institutions have established a code of ethical practice that they publish and try to uphold in their day-to-day corporate decisions.[142]

The latest trend is to combine organizational and clinical ethics (and, according to some models, research ethics) into a program called "integrated ethics."[143] Integrated ethics programs recognize that ethical cases often are symptoms of underlying and more generalized ethical issues that can respond to proactive, systems level interventions. They create functional linkages between ethics program leaders and administrative leadership that mitigate the "silo" problem in which clinical ethics consultation is isolated from institutional ethical practices.[144] Programs of integrated ethics elucidate ethical conflicts, establish ethical principles for handling them, educate people about ethical practices, evaluate the ethical practices to permit continuous quality improvement, and enhance effective institutional execution of ethical practices.[145]

Appendix 5-1: Standards for Bioethical Consultation

The following policy standards for bioethics consultation were formulated by John Fletcher and serve to summarize many of the major points of this chapter:[146]

1. Ethics consultations must be offered in the framework of an institutional policy that defines the ethics committee's task to provide ethics consultation on request under certain conditions.

2. There should be an "open" policy as to who can request consultation, with a process to explore the context of the request and the degree to which other efforts to address the problem have reached an impasse.

3. Policy must prohibit intimidation or punishment of anyone requesting ethics consultation.

4. The patient's attending physician should be notified (if he or she is not the requestor), and the chair of the ethics committee, who has authority to mediate and continue the consultation process over an attending physician's refusal, should be involved.

5. The patient or the incapacitated patient's surrogate should be notified (if he or she is not the requestor) and given an opportunity to consent to the consultation.

6. If the consultation is refused by the patient or surrogate, it may not continue, and consultants may not access the patient's chart or room, as would be the case if consent were given.

7. Patients or surrogates who refuse consultation must be reported to the chair of the committee who has the authority to provide resources for the clinical staff to discuss the type of ethical problem(s) involved without using the patient's chart and without identifying the patient.

8. If health-care providers have data indicating that the consequences of continued refusal of consultation and/or ensuing conflict are harming the patient or violating professional standards of care, the chair of the committee may convene a small ad hoc group of ethic committee members and other consultants to attempt to resolve the conflict. Notification of the meeting and an

opportunity to attend must be given to the patient or surrogate.

9. All recommendations of ethics consultants or the ethics committee are advisory only; final responsibility for decisions and outcomes of cases rest with the primary decision makers, as defined by state law and/or required by the dynamics of the case.

10. All ethics consultations that proceed with patient or surrogate consent should be recorded in the progress notes of the patient chart.

11. All ethics consultations and *ad hoc* group meetings on controversial cases must be reported to the full committee in writing (with precautions as to confidentiality) on a regular basis.

12. The committee should provide oversight and evaluation of ethics consultation activities, give training toconsultants, develop a selection process for choosing consultants, and nominate them for membership on the clinical staff for privileges and terms as consultants.

13. The clinical staff of the institution has the final responsibility of appointing, and setting terms of, ethics consultants.

14. Patients should not be charged for ethics consultation, but the institution should support the costs of training and administration of the ethics committee's programs, including ethics consultation.

NOTES

1. The early history of institutional ethics committees (IEC) has been documented in Rosner F. Hospital medical ethics committees: a review of their development. *JAMA* 1985;253:1693–1697. For other historical perspectives, see Cranford RE, Jackson DL. Neurologists and the hospital ethics committee. *Semin Neurol* 1984;4:15–21 and Fleetwood JE, Arnold RM, Baron RJ. Giving answers or raising questions? The problematic role of institutional ethics committees. *J Med Ethics* 1989;15:137–142.
2. These committees (nicknamed "God squads") captured public fascination when the journalist Shana Alexander reported on their life and death decision-making power in an article in Life Magazine. See Alexander S. They decide who lives, who dies. *Life* 1962;53(Nov 9):102–125. Their interesting history was told in Jonsen AR. The God Squad and the origins of transplantation ethics and policy. *J Law Med Ethics* 2007;35:238–240.
3. See Kosnik AR. Developing a health facility medical-moral committee. *Hosp Prog* 1974;55:40–44.
4. Teel K. The physician's dilemma: a doctor's view: what the law should be. *Baylor Law Rev* 1975;27:6–9.
5. *In re Quinlan*, 70 NJ 10, 355 A 2d 647 (1976). See chapters 8 and 12 for further discussions of the medicolegal impact of the *Quinlan* ruling.
6. These rulings are thoroughly reviewed in Meisel A, Cerminara KL. *The Right to Die: The Law of End-of-Life Decisionmaking*, 3rd ed. Gaithersburg, MD: Aspen Publishers, 2004.
7. Optimum care for hopelessly ill patients: a report of the Clinical Care Committee of the Massachusetts General Hospital. *N Engl J Med* 1976;295:362–364.
8. President's Commission for the Study of Ethical Problems in Medicine and Biomedical and Behavioral Research. *Deciding to Forego Life-Sustaining Treatment: Ethical, Medical, and Legal Issues in Treatment Decisions*. Washington, DC: US Government Printing Office, 1983:160–165 and President's Commission for the Study of Ethical Problems in Medicine and Biomedical and Behavioral Research. *Making Health Care Decisions: The Ethical and Legal Implications of Informed Consent in the Patient-Practitioner Relationship*. Washington, DC: US Government Printing Office, 1982:187–188.
9. American Medical Association Judicial Council. Guidelines for ethics committees in health care institutions. *JAMA* 1985;253:2698–2699; New York State Task Force on Life and the Law. *Do Not Resuscitate Orders*. New York: New York State Task Force on Life and the Law, 1986; and American Academy of Pediatrics Committee on Bioethics. Institutional ethics committees. *Pediatrics* 2001;107:205–209. For citations of endorsements from other societies, see Cranford RE, Van Allen EJ. The implications and applications of institutional ethics committees. *Bull Am Coll Surg* 1985:70(6):19–24.
10. Hollinger PC. Hospital ethics committees required by law in Maryland. *Hastings Cent Rep* 1989;19(1):23–24. This legislation definitely increased the number of hospitals in Maryland with ethics

committees. However, many of the newly formed committees were inactive because, although the law mandated the committee's existence, it did not require its successful function. See Hoffmann DE. Does legislating hospital ethics committees make a difference? A study of hospital ethics committees in Maryland, the District of Columbia, and Virginia. *Law Med Health Care* 1991;19:105–119.

11. New Jersey Administrative Code Title 8 § 486–5.1 (March 16, 1992).

12. Maryland Health General Code Annotated, § 5–606(b).

13. Joint Commission on Accreditation of Healthcare Organizations. *Accreditation Manual for Hospitals.* Chicago: Joint Commission on Accreditation of Healthcare Organizations, 2006.

14. Youngner SJ, Jackson DL, Coulton C, et al. A national survey of hospital ethics committees. In, President's Commission for the Study of Ethical Problems in Medicine and Biomedical and Behavioral Research. *Deciding to Forego Life-Sustaining Treatment: Ethical, Medical, and Legal Issues in Treatment Decisions.* Washington, DC: US Government Printing Office, 1983:443–457.

15. These data were quoted in Fleetwood JE, Arnold RM, Baron RJ. *J Med Ethics* 1989:137.

16. Ross JW, Glaser JW, Rasinski-Gregory D, et al. *Health Care Ethics Committees: The Next Generation.* Chicago: American Hospital Publishing Corporation, 1993:ix.

17. These data were quoted in Fletcher JC, Hoffman DE. Ethics committees: time to experiment with standards. *Ann Intern Med* 1994;120:335–338.

18. Lomax KJ, Fraser JE. A survey of ethics advisory committees in V.A. medical centers. V.A. National Center for Clinical Ethics, White River Junction, VT, 1992 (unpublished data).

19. Fox E, Myers S, Pearlman RA. Ethics consultation in United States hospitals: a national survey. *Am J Bioethics* 2007;7(2):13–25.

20. Several reasons for the midlife crisis of ethics committees are discussed in Blake DC. The hospital ethics committee: health care's moral conscience or white elephant? *Hastings Cent Rep* 1992;22(1):6–11.

21. One judge in *Quinlan* wrote: "In the real world and in relationship to the momentous decision contemplated, the value of additional views and diverse knowledge is apparent." *In re Quinlan,* 355 A2d 647, 669 (NJ 1976).

22. Lance Lightfoot discussed his conflicted role as an in-house hospital attorney serving on his hospital's ethics committee in Lightfoot L. The ethical health lawyer. Incompetent decisionmakers and withdrawal of life-sustaining treatment: a case study. *J Law Med Ethics* 2005;33:851–856.

23. Self DJ, Skeel JD, Jecker NS. A comparison of the moral reasoning of physicians and clinical medical ethicists. *Acad Med* 1993;68:852–855.

24. Dobrin A. Moral reasoning of members of hospital ethics committees: a pilot study. *J Clin Ethics* 2003;14:270–275.

25. There is a large literature describing the structure and functioning of ethics committees. See, in particular, Ross JW, Glaser JW, Rasinski-Gregory D, et al. *Health Care Ethics Committees: The Next Generation,* 1993; Cranford RE, Jackson DL. *Semin Neurol* 1984;4:15–21; Cranford RE, Doudera AE Jr. *Institutional Ethics Committees and Health Care Decision Making.* Ann Arbor, MI: Health Administration Press, 1984; Fleetwood JE, Arnold RM, Baron RJ. *J Med Ethics* 1989:137–142; and Meisel A, Cerminara KL. *The Right to Die: The Law of End-of-Life Decisionmaking,* 3rd ed. Gaithersburg, MD: Aspen Publishers, 2004.

26. For a discussion of the administrative issues in the design and working of an IEC, see Fost N, Cranford RE. Hospital ethics committees: administrative aspects. *JAMA* 1985;263:2687–2692.

27. See Niemira DA. Grassroots grappling: ethics committees at rural hospitals. *Ann Intern Med* 1988; 109:981–983; Niemira DA, Orr RD, Culver CM. Ethics committees in small hospitals. *J Rural Health* 1989; 5:19–32; Cook AF, Hoas H, Guttmannova K. Bioethics activities in rural hospitals. *Cambr Q Healthc Ethics* 2000;9:230–238; and Nelson W, Lushkov G, Pomerantz A, Weeks WB. Rural health care ethics: is there a literature? *Am J Bioethics* 2006;6:44–50.

28. Brown B, Miles SH, Aroskar M. The prevalence and design of nursing home ethics committees. *J Am Geriatr Soc* 1987;35:1028–1033 and Glasser G, Zweibel N, Cassel C. The ethics committee in the nursing home: results of a national survey. *J Am Geriatr Soc* 1988;36:150–156.

29. Fost N, Cranford RE. Hospital ethics committees: administrative aspects. *JAMA* 1985;263:2687–2692.

30. McGee G, Spanogle JP, Caplan AL, Penny D, Asch DA. Successes and failures of hospital ethics committees: a national survey of ethics committee chairs. *Camb Q Healthc Ethics* 2002;11:87–93; and Wilson RF, Neff-Smith M, Phillips D, et al. Hospital ethics committees: are they evaluating their performance? *HEC Forum* 1993;5:1–34.

31. Ross JW, Glaser JW, Rasinski-Gregory D, et al. *Health Ethics Committees: The Next Generation*, 1993. For a recently published handbook, see Post LF, Blustein J, Dubler NN. *Handbook for Health Care Ethics Committees.* Baltimore: John Hopkins, 2007.

32. Interestingly, there is little evidence of a significant effect of ethics education on the moral reasoning, moral competency, or moral development of medical professionals. See Bardon A. Ethics education and value prioritization among members of U.S. hospital ethics committees. *Kennedy Inst Ethics J* 2004;14:395–406.

33. The PDSA is discussed further in chapter 4.

34. Monagle JF, Thomasma DC. *Medical Ethics: Policies, Protocols, Guidelines & Programs.* Gaithersburg, MD: Aspen Publishers, 2006 (annually updated).

35. American Medical Association Council on Ethical and Judicial Affairs. Ethics consultations. In *Code of Medical Ethics. Current Opinions with Annotations*, 2006–2007 ed. Chicago: American Medical Association, 2006:295–296.

36. Berchelmann K, Blechner B. Searching for effectiveness: the functioning of Connecticut clinical ethics committees. *J Clin Ethics* 2002;13:131–145; and Forde R, Vandvik IH. Clinical ethics, information, and communication: review of 31 cases from a clinical ethics committee. *J Med Ethics* 2005;31:73–77.

37. Brennan TA. Incompetent patients with limited care in the absence of family consent: a study of socioeconomic and clinical variables. *Ann Intern Med* 1988;109:819–825. For a more general report on the Optimum Care Committee's operation in decisions to terminate medical treatment, see Brennan TA. Ethics committees and the decision to limit care: the experience at the Massachusetts General Hospital. *JAMA* 1998;260:803–807. One of the Committee's decisions to overturn a family's refusal of a DNR order led to the highly publicized lawsuit against the Massachusetts General Hospital by the family of Catherine Gilgunn. A jury verdict was handed down in favor of the defendant hospital and physicians. This case is discussed further in chapter 10.

38. Morgenstern L. Proactive bioethics screening: a prelude to bioethics consultation. *J Clin Ethics* 2005;16:151–155.

39. For an extended study on the reasons nurses order ethics consultations and the barriers they encounter, see Gordon EJ, Hamric AB. The courage to stand up: the cultural politics of nurses' access to ethics consultation. *J Clin Ethics* 2006;17:231–254.

40. Fins JJ, Bachetta MD, Miller FG. Clinical pragmatism: a method of moral problem solving. *Kennedy Inst Ethics J* 1997;7:129–145 and Martin PA. Bioethics and the whole: pluralism, consensus, and the transmutation of bioethical methods into gold. *J Law Med Ethics* 1999;27:316–327.

41. McGee G, Spanogle JP, Caplan AL, Penny D, Asch DA. Successes and failures of hospital ethics committees: a national survey of ethics committee chairs. *Camb Q Healthc Ethics* 2002;11:87–93.

42. DuVal G, Sartorius L, Clarridge B, Gensler G, Danis M. What triggers requests for ethics consultations? *J Med Ethics* 2001;27(Suppl 1):i24–i29.

43. Swetz KM, Crowley ME, Hook CC, Mueller PS. Report of 255 clinical ethics consultations and review of the literature. *Mayo Clin Proc* 2007;82:686–691.

44. See Ross JW, Glaser JW, Rasinski-Gregory D, et al. *Health Care Ethics Committees: The Next Generation*, 1993: 154–156.

45. New Hampshire RSA 137-J (2006).

46. Mishkin DB, Povar G. The District of Columbia amends its Health-Care Decisions Act: bioethics committees in the arena of public policy. *J Clin Ethics* 2005;16:292–298.

47. Emphasizing the lack of accountability of ethics committees, a New York judge warned: "Deferring the decision to an 'ethics committee' merely shifts the burden of decision to another unqualified tribunal, further removing it from the family or guardian where it rightfully belongs." *In re Storar*, 434 NYS 2d 46, 47 (App Div 1980).

48. Seigler M. Ethics committees: decision by bureaucracy. *Hastings Cent Rep* 1986;16(3):22–24 and Seigler M, Singer PA. Clinical ethics consultation: Godsend or "God" squad? *Am J Med* 1998;85:759–760. For a discussion of the accountability of IECs, see Fry-Revere S. Some suggestions for holding bioethics committees and consultants accountable. *Camb Q Healthc Ethics* 1993;2:449–455. For an analysis of the success of ethics committees at protecting the interests of patients, see Hoffmann DE. Evaluating ethics committees: a view from the outside. *Millbank Q* 1993;71:677–701.

49. Restricting the authority of IECs to an advisory role is carefully stipulated by the American Hospital Association in its guidelines. See American Hospital Association. Guidelines: Hospital committees on biomedical ethics. In Ross JW, ed. *Handbook for Hospital Ethics Committees.* Chicago: American Hospital Publishing Co, 1986:57, 110–111.

50. Fleetwood J, Unger SS. Institutional ethics committees and the shield of immunity. *Ann Intern Med* 1994;120:320–325.

51. Lo B. Behind closed doors: promises and pitfalls of ethics committees. *N Engl J Med* 1987;317:46–50. For further reflections on the fallacies of committee-made decisions, see Moreno JD. Ethics by committee: the moral authority of consensus. *J Med Philosophy* 1988;14:411–432 and Moreno JD. What means this consensus? Ethics committees and philosophical tradition. *J Clin Ethics* 1990;1:38–43.

52. Weir RF. Pediatric ethics committees: ethical advisors or legal watchdogs? *Law Med Health Care* 1987;15:99–108.

53. See Agich GJ. Youngner SJ. For experts only? Access to hospital ethics committees. *Hastings Cent Rep* 1991;21(5):17–25 and Lo B. *N Engl J Med* 1987:46–50.

54. The indications for seeking formal judicial review are discussed further in chapter 8.

55. *In re L.H.R.*, 253 GA 439, 321 SE 2d 716. This case is discussed in Wolf SM. Ethics committees in the courts. *Hastings Cent Rep* 1986;16(3):12–15.

56. *In re Torres*, 357 NW 2d 232 (Minn 1984); *Superintendent of Belchertown v Saikewicz*, 373 Mass 728, 370 NE 2d 417; and *In re Spring*, 380 Mass 629, 405 NE 2d 115. See discussion of these cases in Wolf SM. *Hastings Cent Rep* 1986;16(3):12–15 and in chapter 15.

57. Wolf SM. Ethics committees and due process: nesting rights in a community of caring. *Maryland Law Rev* 1991;50:798–858 and Wolf SM. Toward a theory of process. *Law Med Health Care* 1992;20:278–290.

58. The liability issue is authoritatively reviewed in Meisel A, Cerminara KL. *The Right to Die: The Law of End-of-Life Decisionmaking*, 3rd ed. Gaithersburg, MD: Aspen Publishers, 2004. The theoretical legal basis for liability of ethics consultants based on negligence is discussed in Duval G. Liability of ethics consultants: a case analysis. *Camb Q Healthc Ethics* 1997;6:269–281.

59. See Fleetwood J, Unger SS. *Ann Intern Med* 1994:320–325; Fletcher JC, Hoffman DE. *Ann Intern Med* 1994:335; and Cohen M, Schwartz R, Hartz J, et al. Everything you always wanted to ask a lawyer about ethics committees. *Camb Q Healthc Ethics* 1992;1:33–39.

60. *Bouvia v Superior Court*, 225 Cal Rptr 297, 300, 1986. The poignant case of Elizabeth Bouvia is discussed further in Steinbrook R, Lo B. The case of Elizabeth Bouvia: starvation, suicide, or problem patient? *Arch Intern Med* 1986;146:161–164 and in chapter 14. For general references on the civil and criminal liability of hospital ethics committee members, see Cranford RE, Hester FA, Ashley BZ. Institutional ethics committees: issues of confidentiality and immunity. *Law Med Health Care* 1985;13:52–60; and Ross JW, Glaser JW, Rasinski-Gregory D, et al. *Health Care Ethics Committees: The Next Generation*, 1993:133–143.

61. Jonsen AR, Phibbs RJ, Tooley WH, et al. Critical issues in newborn intensive care: a conference report and policy proposal. *Pediatrics* 1975;55:756–768; American Academy of Pediatrics Infant Bioethics Task Force and Consultants. Guidelines for infant bioethics committees. *Pediatrics* 1984;74:306–310; President's Commission for the Study of Ethical Problems in Medicine and Biomedical and Behavioral Research. *Deciding to Forego Life-Sustaining Treatment: Medical, Ethical, and Legal Issues in Treatment Decisions*, 1983.

62. Caplan A, Cohen CB. Imperiled newborns. *Hastings Cent Rep* 1987;17(6):5–32.

63. The Baby Doe regulations are discussed further in chapter 13.

64. Fleming GV, Hud SS, LeBailey SA, et al. Infant care review committees. The response to federal guidelines. *Am J Dis Child* 1990;144:778–881.

65. American Academy of Pediatrics Infant Bioethics Task Force and Consultants. *Pediatrics* 1984;74:309. But more recently, the American Academy of Pediatrics opined that freestanding ICRCs should be dissolved and the function of ICRCs folded into the general IEC. See American Academy of Pediatrics Committee on Bioethics. Institutional ethics committees. *Pediatrics* 2001;107:205–209. However, several institutions have had longstanding successfully functioning ICRCs. See Fleischman AR. An infant bioethical review committee in an urban medical center. *Hastings Cent Rep* 1986;16(3):16–18 and Kleigman RM, Mahowald MB, Youngner SJ. In our best interests: experience and workings of an ethics review committee. *J Pediatrics* 1986;108:178–187.

66. Carter BS. Neonatologists and bioethics after Baby Doe. *J Perinatol* 1993;13:144–150. See the extended discussion of the Baby Doe regulations in chapter 13.

67. Annas GJ. Ethics committees in neonatal care: substantive protection or procedural diversion? *Am J Publ Health* 1984;74:843–845 and Weir RF. *Law Med Health Care* 1987:99–108.

68. May WW. The composition and function of ethical committees. *J Med Ethics* 1975;1:23–29. For general references on the composition and functioning of the IRB, see Levine R.J. *Ethics and the Regulation of Clinical Research*. 2nd ed. New Haven: Yale University Press, 1988:321–363 and Robertson JA. Ten ways to improve IRBs. *Hastings Cent Rep* 1979;9(1):29–33.

69. For a comprehensive and succinct summary of how IRBs currently function to protect human subjects, see Wagner RM. Ethical review of research involving human subjects: when and why is IRB review necessary? *Muscle Nerve* 2003;28:27–39. For a more detailed account directed at educating new IRB members, see Mazur DJ. *Evaluating the Science and Ethics of Research on Humans. A Guide for IRB Members.* Baltimore: Johns Hopkins University Press, 2007.

70. 45 *Code of Federal Regulations* § 46.102(e) (rev March 8, 1983). For the complete regulations concerning IRBs and the protection of human research subjects published by the Department of Health and Human Services, see President's Commission for the Study of Ethical Problems in Medicine and Biomedical and Behavioral Research. *Protecting Human Subjects: The Adequacy and Uniformity of Federal Rules and their Implementation.* Washington, DC: US Government Printing Office, 1981:87–108.

71. Steinbrook R. Improving protection for research subjects. *N Engl J Med* 2002;346:1425–1430.

72. National Institutes of Health Office of Extramural Research and Office of Protection from Research Risks. *Protecting Human Research Subjects: Institutional Review Board Guidebook.* Washington, DC: US Government Printing Office, 1993 and Dr. David Kimmel, personal communication, November 1, 1993.

73. Lind SE. The institutional review board: an evolving ethics committee. *J Clin Ethics* 1992;3:278–282.

74. Emanuel EJ, Wood A, Fleischman A, et al. Oversight of human participants research: identifying problems to evaluate reform proposals. *Ann Intern Med* 2004;141:282–291.

75. Institute of Medicine. *Responsible Research: A Systems Approach to Protecting Research Participants.* Washington, DC: National Academies Press, 2002.

76. Mello MM, Studdert DM, Brennan TA. The rise of litigation in human subjects research. *Ann Intern Med* 2003;139:40–45.

77. The history and early development of clinical ethics consultation services have been outlined in La Puma J, Schiedermayer DL. Ethics consultation: skills, roles, and training. *Ann Intern Med* 1991;114:155–160. For general references on ethics consultants, see Purtillo R. Ethics consultation in the hospital. *N Engl J Med* 1984;311:983–986; Fletcher JC, Quist N. Jonsen AR, eds. *Ethics Consultation in Health Care.* Ann Arbor, MI: Health Administration Press, 1989; La Puma J, Toulmin SE. Ethics committees and ethics consultants. *Arch Intern Med* 1989;149:1109–1112; La Puma J, Schiedermayer D. *Ethics Consultation: A Practical Guide.* Boston: Jones and Bartlett, 1994; and Baylis FE (ed). *The Health Care Ethics Consultant.* Totawa, NJ: Humana Press, 1994.

78. Singer PA, Pellegrino ED, Siegler M. Ethics committees and consultants. *J Clin Ethics* 1990;1:263–267.

79. Singer PA, Pellegrino ED, Siegler M. *J Clin Ethics* 1990:265–266.

80. Fletcher JC, Siegler M. What are the goals of ethics consultation? A consensus statement. *J Clin Ethics* 1996;7:122–126.

81. Craig JM, May T. Evaluating the outcomes of ethics consultation. *J Clin Ethics* 2006;17:168–180.

82. La Puma J, Schiedermayer DL. *Ann Intern Med* 1991:156–157.

83. American Society for Bioethics and Humanities. *Core Competencies for Health Care Ethics Consultation.* Glenview, IL: American Society for Bioethics and Humanities, 1998. See the summary of this report in Aulisio MP, Arnold RM, Youngner SJ. Health care ethics consultation: nature, goals, and competencies. *Ann Intern Med* 2000;133:59–69. See the several thoughtful commentaries on this report published in the *Journal of Clinical Ethics* 1999;10:3–56.

84. American Society for Bioethics and Humanities. *Core Competencies for Health Care Ethics Consultation.* 1998:11–23.

85. Hoffman D, Tarzian A, O'Neil A. Are ethics committee members competent to consult? *J Law Med Ethics* 2000;28:30–40.

86. American Society for Bioethics and Humanities. *Core Competencies for Health Care Ethics Consultation.* 1998:31–32.

87. For an argument defending why primary clinical ethics consultants should be physicians, see Braddock CH 3rd, Tonelli MR. Too much ethics, not enough medicine: clarifying the role of clinical expertise for the clinical ethics consultant. *J Clin Ethics* 2001;12:24–30.

88. Aulisio MP, Arnold RM, Youngner SJ. *Ann Intern Med* 2000;59–61.

89. La Puma J, Schiedermayer DL. Must the ethics consultant see the patient? *J Clin Ethics* 1990;1:56–59. For an account of the consensus model of resolving ethical dilemmas, see Kuczewski M. Two models of ethical consensus, or what good is a bunch of bioethicists? *Camb Q Healthc Ethics* 2002;11:27–36.

90. Orr RD, deLeon D. The role of the clinical ethicist in conflict resolution. *J Clin Ethics* 2000;11:21–30. See also West MB, Gibson JM. Facilitating medical ethics case review: what ethics committees can learn from mediation and facilitation techniques. *Camb Q Healthc Ethics* 1992;1:63–74.

91. On the limits of mediator neutrality, see Gibson K. Mediation in the medical field: is neutral intervention possible? *Hasting Cent Rep* 1999;29(5):6–13.

92. Orr RD, deLeon D. *J Clin Ethics* 2000:21–22.

93. Jurchak M. Report of a study to examine the process of ethics case consultation. *J Clin Ethics* 2000; 11:49–55.

94. Buchanan SF, Desrochers JM, Henry DB, Thomassen G, Barrett PH Jr. A mediation-medical advisory panel model for resolving disputes about end-of-life care. *J Clin Ethics* 2002;13:188–202.

95. Back AL, Arnold RM. Dealing with conflict in caring for the seriously ill: "it was just out of the question." *JAMA* 2005;293:1374–1381.

96. Breen CM, Abernethy AP, Abbott KH, Tulsky JA. Conflict associated with decisions to limit life-sustaining treatment in intensive care units. *J Gen Intern Med* 2001;16:283–289. The concept of medical futility that often is cited in such decisions is discussed in chapter 10.

97. For a comparison of the relative merits of three models of ethics consultation, see Cohen CB. Avoiding "Cloudcuckooland" in ethics committee case review: matching models to issues and concerns. *Law Med Health Care* 1992;20:294–299.

98. See, for example, Schierton LS. Measuring hospital ethics committee success. *Camb Q Healthc Ethics* 1993;2:495–504. See also Fletcher JC. Standards for evaluation of ethics consultation. In Fletcher JC, Quist N, Jonsen AR, eds. *Ethics Consultation in Health Care*. Ann Arbor, MI: Health Administration Press, 1989:173–184.

99. Tulsky JA, Fox E. Evaluating ethics consultation: framing the questions. *J Clin Ethics* 1996;7:109–115 and Fox E. Concepts in evaluation applied to ethics evaluation research. *J Clin Ethics* 1996;7:116–121.

100. Fox E, Arnold RM. Evaluating outcomes in ethics consultation research. *J Clin Ethics* 1996;7:127–138.

101. Tulsky JA, Stocking CB. Obstacles and opportunities in the design of ethics consultation evaluation. *J Clin Ethics* 1996;7:139–145 and Fox E, Tulsky JA. Evaluation research and the future of ethics consultation. *J Clin Ethics* 1996;7:146–149.

102. Craig JM, May T. Evaluating the outcomes of ethics consultation. *J Clin Ethics* 2006;17:168–180.

103. Fox E, Myers S, Pearlman RA. Ethics consultation in United States hospitals: a national survey. *Am J Bioethics* 2007;7(2):13–25.

104. Perkins HS, Saathoff BS. Impact of medical ethics consultations on physicians: an exploratory study. *Am J Med* 1988;85:761–763.

105. La Puma J, Stocking CB, Silverstein MD, et al. An ethics consultation service in a teaching hospital: utilization and evaluation. *JAMA* 1988;260:808–811.

106. Orr RD, Moon E. Effectiveness of an ethics consultation service. *J Fam Pract* 1993; 36:49–53.

107. La Puma J, Stocking CB, Darling CM, et al. Community hospital ethics consultant: evaluation and comparison with a university hospital service. *Am J Med* 1992;92:346–351.

108. Schneiderman LJ, Gilmer T, Teetzel HD, et al. Effect of ethics consultations on nonbeneficial life-sustaining treatments in the intensive care setting: a randomized controlled trial. *JAMA* 2003;290:1166–1172. The issue of medical futility usually invoked in a dispute over the value of "unbeneficial treatment" is discussed in chapter 10.

109. Lo B. Answers and questions about ethics consultations. *JAMA* 2003;290:1208–1210.

110. Schneiderman LJ, Gilmer T, Teetzel HD, et al. Effect of ethics consultations on nonbeneficial life-sustaining treatments in the intensive care setting: a randomized controlled trial. *JAMA* 2003;290: 1166–1172.

111. Schneiderman LJ, Gilmer T, Teetzel HD, Dugan DO, Goodman-Crews P, Cohn F. Dissatisfaction with ethics consultations: the Anna Karenina principle. *Camb Q Healthc Ethics* 2006;15:101–106. They called their findings the "Anna Karenina principle" because the miscellany of reasons for dissatisfaction with ethics consultations was reminiscent of the famous first line in Tolstoy's novel: "Happy families are all alike; every unhappy family is unhappy in its own way."

112. Davies L, Hudson LD. Why don't physicians use ethics consultation? *J Clin Ethics* 1999;10:116–125.

113. DuVal G, Clarridge B, Gensler G, Danis M. A national survey of U.S. internists' experiences with ethical dilemmas and ethics consultation. *J Gen Intern Med* 2004;19:251–258.

114. Perl M, Shelp EE. Psychiatric consultation masking moral dilemmas in medicine. *N Engl J Med* 1982;307:618–621.

115. Schiedermayer DL, La Puma J. Ethics consultations masking economic dilemmas in patient care. *Arch Intern Med* 1989;149:1303–1305.

116. Spielman B. Invoking the law in ethics consultation. *Camb Q Healthc Ethics* 1993;2:457–467.

117. La Puma J, Stocking CB, Silverstein MD, et al. *JAMA* 1988:808–811.

118. Fox E, Stocking C. Ethics consultants' recommendations for life-prolonging treatment of patients in a persistent vegetative state. *JAMA* 1993;270:2578–2582.

119. Fox E, Daskal FC, Stocking C. Ethics consultants' recommendations for life-prolonging treatment of patients in persistent vegetative state: a follow-up study. *J Clin Ethics* 2007;18:64–71.

120. Heilscser BJ, Meltzer D, Siegler M. The effect of clinical ethics consultation on healthcare costs. *J Clin Ethics* 2000;11:31–38.

121. Forrow L, Arnold RM, Parker LS. Preventive ethics: expanding the horizons of clinical ethics. *J Clin Ethics* 1993;287–294 and Cohn F, Goodman-Crews P, Rudman W, Schneiderman LJ, Waldman E. Proactive ethics consultation in the ICU: a comparison of value perceived by healthcare professionals and recipients. *J Clin Ethics* 2007;18:140–147.

122. Imwinkelried EJ. Expert testimony by ethicists: what should be the norm? *J Law Med Ethics* 2005;33:198–221.

123. Scofield G. Motion(less) *in limine. J Law Med Ethics* 2005;33:821–833.

124. Brody B, Dubler N, Blustein J, et al. Bioethics consultation in the private sector. *Hastings Cent Rep* 2002;32(3):14–20.

125. Green RM, DeVries KO, Bernstein J, et al. Overseeing research on therapeutic cloning: a private ethics board responds to its critics. *Hastings Cent Rep* 2002;32(3):27–33.

126. Elliott C. Should journals publish industry-funded bioethics articles? *Lancet* 2006;366:422–424. For a balanced analysis of the conflicts of interest problem among paid bioethicists, see Sontag DN. What is wrong with "ethics for sale"? An analysis of the many issues that complicate the debate about conflicts of interest in bioethics. *J Law Med Ethics* 2007;35:175–186.

127. Meyers C. Clinical ethics consulting and conflict of interest: structurally intertwined. *Hastings Cent Rep* 2007;37(2):32–40.

128. Cranford RE. The neurologist as ethics consultant and as a member of the institutional ethics committee: the neuroethicist. *Neurol Clin* 1989;7:697–713.

129. I have discussed the role of the neurologist as ethics consultant further in Bernat JL. Ethical considerations in the locked-in syndrome. In Culver CM, ed. *Ethics at the Bedside.* Hanover, NH: University Press of New England, 1990:87–98.

130. Youngner SJ, Landefeld S, Coulton CJ, et al. "Brain death" and organ retrieval. A cross-sectional survey of knowledge and concepts among health professionals. *JAMA* 1989;261:2205–2210.

131. The extent of incorrect clinical determinations of persistent vegetative state was described in Multi-Society Task Force on PVS. Medical aspects of the persistent vegetative state. Part I. *N Engl J Med* 1994;330:1499–1508.

132. For a current review of organizational ethics, with a particular application to urgent care issues, see Suter RE. Organizational ethics. *Emerg Med Clin North Am* 2006;24:579–603.

133. American Hospital Association. *Management Advisory: Ethical Conduct for Health Care Institutions.* Chicago: American Hospital Association, 1992.

134. Joint Commission on Accreditation of Healthcare Organizations. *Ethical Issues and Patient Rights across the Continuum of Care.* Oakbrook, IL: Joint Commission on Accreditation of Healthcare Organizations, 1998.

135. Potter RL. On our way to integrated bioethics: clinical/organizational/communal. *J Clin Ethics* 1999;10:171–177.

136. Myser C, Donehower P, Frank C. Making the most of disequilibrium: bridging the gap between clinical and organizational ethics in a newly merged healthcare organization. *J Clin Ethics* 1999;10:194–201.

137. Hall R. Confidentiality as an organizational ethics issue. *J Clin Ethics* 1999;10:230–236.

138. Johnson KM, Roebuck-Colgan K. Organizational ethics and sentinel events: doing the right thing when the worst thing happens. *J Clin Ethics* 1999;10:237–241. The ethical duty to disclose medical errors is discussed in chapter 4.

139. Fox E, Tulsky JA. Recommendations for the ethical conduct of quality improvement. *J Clin Ethics* 2005;16:61–71 and Mills AE, Rorty MV, Werhane PH. Clinical ethics and the managerial revolution in American healthcare. *J Clin Ethics* 2006;17:181–190. A recent consensus conference identified the ethical issues in quality improvement and suggested recommendations for action. See Lynn J, Baily MA, Bottrell M, et al. The ethics of using quality improvement methods in health care. *Ann Intern Med* 2007;146:666–673.

140. Hirsch NJ. All in the family—siblings but not twins: the relationship of clinical and organizational ethics analysis. *J Clin Ethics* 1999;10:210–215.

141. Goold SD. Trust and the ethics of health care institutions. *Hastings Cent Rep* 2001;31(6):26–33.

142. Bishop LJ, Cherry MN, Darragh M. Organizational ethics and health care: expanding bioethics to the institutional arena. *Kennedy Inst Ethics J* 1999;9:189–208.

143. See Seeley CR, Goldberger SL. Integrated ethics: a synecdoche in healthcare. *J Clin Ethics* 1999; 10:202–209.

144. Foglia MB, Pearlman RA. Integrating clinical and organizational ethics. A systems perspective can provide an antidote to the "silo" problem in clinical ethics consultation. *Health Prog* 2006;87(2):31–35.

145. I am indebted to Prof. Paul J. Reitemeier, a leader in developing the integrated ethics program for the Department of Veterans Affairs hospital system, for explaining the elements of integrated ethics.

146. Fletcher JC. Commentary: constructiveness where it counts. *Camb Q Healthc Ethics* 1993;2:426–434. (© Cambridge University Press, reprinted with permission).

Resolving Ethical Dilemmas

6

Clinical-ethical dilemmas can be defined as clinical problems in which all feasible solutions require breaking a moral rule. Whether to continue painful aggressive treatment of an incompetent, gravely ill patient in order to preserve his life or to provide only palliative treatment and allow him to die in order to prevent his suffering is a common example of a clinical-ethical dilemma. Both solutions can be defended on moral grounds but both decisions also break moral rules. The dilemma can be resolved first if one decides whether, when, why, and how it is justified to break a moral rule, usually by appealing to a higher moral duty through a process of rigorous analysis. Second, non-moral clinical facts must be ascertained and clarified, including the patient's prognosis, outcomes and degrees of suffering with various treatment courses, and the patient's or surrogate's preference for aggressive or palliative treatment in this circumstance.

Not all ethical problems encountered in clinical practice rise to the level of dilemmas. Ethical issues can complicate clinical decisions, for example, when clinicians sense that a patient's valid consent to treatment is not being respected properly, when clinicians feel it is justified to make minor decisions for patients without their knowledge, when clinicians are uncertain what to do when incompetent patients have not made explicit their wishes for life-sustaining treatment, and when patients make poor clinical decisions and clinicians are uncertain whether to respect and follow them. Resolving medical-ethical

problems and dilemmas requires gathering and processing correct medical and social facts as well as applying sound ethical reasoning.[1] Experienced clinical ethicists frequently cite the maxim: "Good ethics begins with good facts."

Clinicians and philosophers have offered systematic approaches to resolving medical-ethical problems and dilemmas that require consideration of both moral and clinical issues. These approaches differ in their degree of rigor and practicality. They comprise a spectrum from the purely analytical to the purely practical. The moral philosopher Bernard Gert's method is the most rigorous method of justifying the morality of an act that violates a moral rule but requires additional information to apply usefully in a clinical context. Principlism offers an accessible and popular guide to ponder ethical issues but provides no means for reconciliation in situations in which the principles conflict (such as the common tension between duties to promote autonomy and practice beneficence). The principle of double effect is analytical but can be applied to only one type of medical-ethical predicament, though admittedly a common and important one. Casuistry is an iterative system of ethical analysis that relies less on principle than on precedent.

The methods for resolving ethical problems offered by ethicists Mark Siegler, Bernard Lo, John Fletcher, and the American College of Physicians are generally less rigorous but more practical. They require physicians to thoughtfully and systematically consider the medical and social factors most relevant to the decision. Clinical pragmatism relies on fusing a scientific approach to studying problems with an interpersonal process of mediation in settling disputes. Whichever approach a clinician finds most useful and adopts, it should be practiced systematically for the same reason a clinician systematically performs the elements of a physical examination. In this chapter, I present outlines of the more prominent of these approaches for clinicians to consider adopting in their practices. I end with several comments about the limits of clinical ethics expertise and the extent to which expert ethical opinion is objective or is based on a subjective political interpretation of ethical concepts.

The first step in any approach is to recognize that an ethical problem exists. Every clinician can measure her degree of discomfort with a clinical problem. When the discomfort results from trying to decide if a situation is morally (as opposed to medically) right or wrong, an ethical problem may be present. Some scholars have coined the term "moral distress" to refer to a situation in which physicians or nurses intuitively sense an ethical problem by analyzing their feelings of moral discomfort in response to the problem.[2] The identification, analysis, and resolution of moral distress has been most thoughtfully studied by scholars in nursing ethics.[3] Moral distress can be generated by: (1) clinical situations such as perceiving that a patient is receiving inappropriate life-sustaining treatment or is being treated without having provided adequate informed consent; (2) internal factors, such as when disempowered nurses or house officers feel powerless to change the wrong direction of a patient's medical care; or (3) external factors such as those generated by an institutional culture that is harmful to patients, lack of administrative support, or compromised care resulting from pressures to reduce costs.[4]

ETHICAL PROBLEMS ARE COMMON IN NEUROLOGICAL PRACTICE

Neurologists encounter ethical problems frequently in their practice. Perhaps the most common issue arising in outpatient practice is the extent to which a patient's informed consent conforms to modern concepts of shared decision making and patient-centered medicine, as discussed in chapter 2. The balance of free patient choice and paternalistic physician guidance to make the "right" choice is delicate and requires physicians to possess virtues such as compassion and respect and to have excellent communication skills. The ideal location of the balance point varies among patients: some patients wish to maintain free rein to choose their own treatment; others request and follow their physician's advice. The wise physician intuitively understands each patient and adjusts her approach accordingly. But how should a wise physician act when a patient makes a clearly bad decision?

Ethical issues of nearly equal frequency arise from a physician's decision to perform testing while trying to make a challenging diagnosis. Some physicians rely heavily on their experience to reach diagnoses and believe that ordering many tests to exclude rare disorders is wasteful and unnecessary. Other physicians believe it is their professional responsibility to prove the diagnosis beyond reasonable doubt, a belief that may be enhanced consciously or subconsciously by financial considerations (for example, income from self-referral for electrodiagnostic testing), and by the practice of defensive medicine to prevent lawsuits. The ethical question is the extent to which physicians' duties to conserve and not squander society's finite resources should impact on clinical decisions about patients under their care, as discussed in chapter 3.

Ethical issues arise commonly in the care of patients who are at the end of life. Advance planning for end-of-life care is essential in patients with ALS and other fatal neuromuscular diseases. The clinician must know and uphold each patient's choice with regard to a feeding gastrostomy tube, ventilator, and other life-sustaining treatments (chapter 14). Advance care planning for patients with Alzheimer's disease includes encouraging them to execute advance directives early in their illness that will govern future decisions about feeding tubes and other treatments in order to ensure that their wishes are followed (chapter 15). Ethical issues in palliative care of dying patients include the debates about the propriety of palliative sedation or physician-assisted suicide (chapter 9). Whether to provide continued intensive treatment for hopelessly, critically ill and dying patients in intensive care units raises the ethical, legal, and societal question of whether physicians are justified in asserting medical futility as grounds for refusing to order further life-sustaining treatment (chapter 10). The vexing decision of parents and neonatologists of to continue or stop life-sustaining treatment of a profoundly brain-damaged infant contains numerous ethical considerations (chapter 13).

The satisfactory resolution of these and other medical-ethical problems requires a systematic approach combining moral analysis and ascertaining the relevant clinical facts. Philosophers and clinicians have recommended procedural approaches to resolving these problems, allowing clinicians to consider the relative merits of both formal and practical analyses. I next offer examples of some of the most useful ones.

FORMAL APPROACHES

Formal approaches to resolving ethical dilemmas use analytical tools devised to dissect and rigorously study the question at hand. They use methods of analytic philosophy to identify and classify the nature of the problem, and they provide a rigorous means to decide whether the violation of a moral rule is justified. Usually, they need to be linked to relevant medical and social facts and a process to settle a dispute that takes into account patient and surrogate preferences. They are a prerequisite for resolving clinical-ethical dilemmas but are insufficient alone.

Gert's Method

Bernard Gert's analytical method to justify the violation of a moral rule (presented in chapter 1) is the most formal and rigorous technique to analyze and justify the morality of an act. It complements the more procedural

approaches I later consider. Gert poses ten questions that must be sequentially answered for one to justify the violation of a moral rule.[5] I will illustrate the value of using Gert's analysis to examine the morality of providing palliative sedation to a patient dying of ALS who has refused further ventilator treatment, but who may die more quickly with the sedation than without it. Is such an act, which could be construed to violate the moral rule: "Do not kill," morally acceptable?

1. *What moral rules are being violated?* The moral rule arguably being violated is: "Do not kill." Some commentators (including me) claim that a physician's act to discontinue a ventilator that has been refused by an ALS patient is not killing but allowing her to die because the disease is fatal in the absence of life-sustaining therapy that the patient has a right to refuse.[6] But for the purposes of applying Gert's method to rigorously justify a moral rule violation, we will accept that the act could be construed as a type of killing.

2. *What harms are being avoided, prevented, or caused?* The harm avoided is unnecessary suffering while dying that can be prevented by timely and appropriate palliative medical treatment.

3. *What are the relevant desires and beliefs of the person toward whom the rule is being violated?* The patient should be asked if he will consent to palliative sedation. Most patients prefer not to suffer from air hunger or other preventable sources of suffering while dying, and readily agree to or demand proper palliative treatment.

4. *Is the relationship between the person violating the rule and the person toward whom the rule is being violated such that the former has a duty to violate moral rules with regard to the latter independent of the latter person's consent?* Physicians should always seek consent for therapy when possible. It is usually possible in patients with ALS because, although they may have some cognitive impairment, it is usually not sufficient to render them incompetent.

5. *What goods (including kind, degree, proba-bility, duration, and distribution) are being promoted by the violation?* The goods are freedom from pain and suffering. Indeed, the moral rule: "Do not cause pain" is being followed by (arguably) violating the moral rule: "Do not kill."

6. *Is the rule being violated toward a person in order to prevent her from violating a moral rule when the violation would be unjustified or weakly justified?* No.

7. *Is the rule being violated toward a person because he has violated a moral rule unjustifi-ably or with weak justification?* No.

8. *Are there any alternative actions or policies that would be preferable?* No. Palliative treat-ment is customary and, as a matter of excellent end-of-life care, should be required during removal of ventilation in ALS patients and in any other patients capable of suffering.

9. *Is the violation being done intentionally or only knowingly?* The violation is being done knowingly. The intent is not to kill the patient but to permit the patient to die comfortably. The goal is palliation.

10. *Is the situation an emergency such that no per-son is likely to plan to be in that kind of situa-tion?* No, ventilator discontinuation usually is performed after a process of informed consent or refusal that yields a treatment plan to discontinue the ventilator.

Analyzing the violation of the moral rule: "Do not kill" in this way justifies the act of pro-viding palliative sedation during ventilator removal is the ALS patient, even though the act could be construed as violating the moral rule: "Do not kill."

Double Effect

The principle of double effect is an analytical technique to justify the morality of a single act that produces two morally opposite effects, one beneficial and one harmful, the former intended and the latter foreseen but unintended. The principle was devised by the-ologians to justify the morality of an act that

otherwise could be considered immoral because it caused harm in a predictable way. Over the past two generations medical ethi-cists have adopted and applied the principle to difficult cases in clinical medicine to ana-lyze the morality of clinical decisions that have double effects. Advocates of the princi-ple have provided five criteria all of which must be present to justify the morality of sin-gle acts that produce double effects:

1. The act must not be intrinsically wrong.

2. The intended effect must be the good effect, even though the bad effect may be foreseen.

3. The bad effect must not be a means to the end of creating the good effect.

4. The act is undertaken for a proportion-ately serious reason.

5. The good resulting from the act must exceed the evil produced by the bad effect.[7]

Clinical examples of the principle of dou-ble effect are common. Consider the case in which a physician prescribes a palliative dose of morphine to relieve a dying patient's pain and shortness of breath, but the patient dies sooner than he would have without the mor-phine because of respiratory depression. (The acceleration of death in this setting has been grossly overestimated and, in fact, occurs only rarely in clinical practice.[8]) The intent of the physician was to relieve the patient's pain and shortness of breath and the choice of drug and the dosage administered were appropri-ate for palliative purposes. The acceleration of death was a foreseen but unavoidable and unintended consequence. The physician, therefore, has performed an act with a double effect: one intended and the other foreseen but unintended. Is the prevention or pallia-tion of pain and air hunger morally justifiable despite the simultaneous occurrence of accel-eration of the moment of death?

The physician's act in our example is moral because it satisfies the five conditions for the principle of double effect: (1) giving mor-phine in the dosage administered to relive suffering is not intrinsically wrong; in fact it is an accepted element of excellent palliative care; (2) relieving suffering was the desired effect even though a small risk of death was foreseen; (3) death was not the means for providing the desired effect because the morphine relieved suffering independent of accelerating death; (4) prevention of suffering during dying is important and is a clear goal of palliative medicine; and (5) prevention of suffering in a dying patient exceeds the evil of possibly dying slightly sooner.

Once the principle of double effect has established that the act is morally acceptable, the consent of the patient or surrogate also is necessary. The patient or surrogate should be adequately informed that a palliative dosage of morphine is indicated but possibly may accelerate the moment of death. If she has consented to receiving a palliative dosage of morphine with this knowledge and if the criteria for double effect have been satisfied, the act is morally justified.

Principlism

The four well-known "principles of biomedical ethics" advocated by Tom Beauchamp and James Childress were discussed in chapter 1. The Georgetown "principles" of autonomy, nonmaleficence, beneficence, and justice are cited widely in bioethics analysis. Danner Clouser, Bernard Gert, and Charles Culver correctly pointed out their shortcomings as ethical principles[9] but they remain useful as easily-recalled and understood concepts for clinicians to sequentially consider in the analysis of clinical-ethical problems. Their lack of rigor and the absence of means to resolve situations in which they conflict limit their usefulness as a moral system as discussed in chapter 1.

Casuistry

Casuistry is a time-honored method of case-by-case ethical analysis with roots in antiquity, common law, and early Christian theology. It was used by Roman Stoics, Chinese Confucians, Jewish Talmudists, Muslim Qur'anic commentators, medieval European scholastics, and most recently and prominently, Roman Catholic Jesuits. Casuistry attempts to resolve moral dilemmas by applying general moral or religious rules embodied in precedent-setting cases to novel situations that seem to elude ethical resolution because they pose conflicting duties. Casuists argue by analogy: they explore the aptness of precedents for settling new questions.

Casuistry relies on developing a consensus on index cases on which everyone can agree. They end their analysis by developing the so-called "rebuttable conclusion": a penultimate stopping point that might or might not withstand another round of critical scrutiny. Involved parties are expected to review the reasoning that yielded this conclusion and to accept it or reject it as decisive in the new situation. Casuistry was a dominant mode of ethical analysis over centuries of scholarship and is used currently in the development of case law. Casuistry has experienced a revival of popularity in contemporary clinical ethics.[10]

Casuistic analysis is most prevalent today in judicially written case law. In their interpretation of statutory, administrative, and constitutional law, judges cite and apply relevant legal precedents. Each new ruling adds a new layer to the growing corpus of existing case law. The current judge's fresh insights and connections to previous decisions further clarifies the meaning of the law and helps to distill the essential concept on which the law was based and extends its reach to novel cases.

PRACTICAL APPROACHES

Clinical ethicists have used their experience analyzing medical-ethical dilemmas in the context of hospital ethics consultations to propose systematic processes for analyzing and resolving these cases. I briefly discuss several of the most useful systems.

Fletcher's Method

In his monograph, the philosopher and clinical ethicist John Fletcher proposed one of the most popular approaches.[11] Fletcher's approach was selected by the American Academy of Neurology (AAN) Ethics, Law and

Humanities Committee (on which John Fletcher formerly served as a consultant) as the standard tool to systematically analyze each of the cases in the neurology residents' ethics casebook *Ethical Dimensions of Neurologic Practice* published by the AAN in 2000.[12] This casebook has been rewritten, expanded, and now is titled *Practical Ethics in Clinical Neurology*. It is co-published by the AAN and Lippincott Williams & Wilkins and is cross-referenced to this book.[13] Readers can review the cases and their analyses in this accompanying casebook to inspect the clinical application of this analytic model. Fletcher's analysis poses the following questions grouped by category, including medical, social, and ethical factors.

A. Assessment

   1. What is the patient's medical condition?
   2. What treatment options exist?
   3. What is the predicted outcome of each treatment?
   4. Who is the appropriate decision maker?
   5. What are the patient's preferences?
   6. What are the preferences of the family or surrogate decision makers?
   7. Are there interests other than, and potentially conflicting with, those of the patient that need to be considered?
   8. Are there institutional, legal, or other factors that need to be considered? (For example, what is the legal status of surrogates?)

B. Identification of the Ethical Problem

   9. What are the ethical problems in the case? (If appropriate, rank by magnitude.)
   10. What ethical considerations are most relevant?
   11. Are there analogous cases?
   12. What are the relevant guidelines for clinicians regarding the problem(s)?

C. Decision Making and Implementation

   13. What are the ethically acceptable options?
   14. What is the ethically preferred resolution of the case? What justification can be given for it?
   15. How is a satisfactory resolution of the case to be accomplished?
   16. Is a recommendation by ethics consultants or an ethics committee necessary or desirable?
   17. Is judicial review necessary or desirable?[14]

The neurologist David Goldblatt proposed adding three questions at the beginning under a section he called "Ethics Chief Complaint" to supplement Fletcher's analysis and to make it more useful as a guide to perform hospital ethics consultation: (1) What is the problem for which ethics consultation was requested? (2) Did the request come from a source that holds a legitimate interest in the outcome of the consultation? (3) If the person requesting consultation wishes not to be identified, has that person's wish for privacy been determined and respected?[15]

Lo's Method

Bernard Lo's method mirrors the practical clinical approach of John Fletcher. He provides a procedural analysis in three sequential stages: gathering information, clarifying the ethical issues, and resolving the dilemma.[16]

A. Gather information

   1. What is the medical situation?
   2. If the patient is competent, what are her preferences?
   3. If the patient lacks decision-making capacity, have advance directives been provided?
   4. If the patient lacks decision-making capacity, who should act as the surrogate?
   5. What are the views of the health-care team?
   6. What pragmatic issues complicate the case?

B. Clarify the ethical issues

    7. What are the pertinent ethical issues?

    8. Articulate the ethical guidelines participants are using.

    9. What are the reasons for and against alternative plans of care?

C. Resolve dilemmas

    10. Meet with the health-care team and the patient or surrogate.

    11. List the alternatives for care.

    12. Negotiate a mutually acceptable decision.

Siegler's Method

Mark Siegler's approach involves the sequential consideration of four important categories. First, the clinician should identify all medical indications, including the diagnosis, prognosis, and recommended treatment. These issues are the sole domain of the physician. Second, the physician should interpret his recommendation within the context of the patient's preferences, based on the concept of patient self-determination. Third, the physician and patient jointly should consider the patient's present and future quality of life in their decision-making process. Finally, the physician should consider such external factors as the family's wishes and needs, the costs of medical care, the allocation of limited resources, the research and teaching needs of the medical profession, and the safety and well-being of society. In his popular textbook on clinical ethics, Siegler illustrated the use of his method to study and resolve common clinical ethical dilemmas.[17]

American College of Physicians Method

The American College of Physicians in their current *Ethics Manual* provides a sequential case method to assist with clinical-ethical decision making, comprising the following steps with an example illustrating its usage.[18]

  1. *Define the ethics problem as an "ought" or "should" question.* For example, should we withhold ventilatory therapy from a patient with advanced AIDS when his parents request it?

  2a. *List significant facts and uncertainties relevant to the question.* The patient has a dedicated partner for the past decade and has been estranged from his parents and siblings.

  2b. *Include physiologic facts.* The patient is permanently unconscious and incapacitated.

  2c. *Include significant medical uncertainties, such as prognosis with and without treatment.* He may be able to be weaned from the ventilator but his life expectancy is 6 to 9 months.

  2d. *Include the benefits and harms of the treatment options.* The respirator will prolong his life but is burdensome and invasive.

  3. *Identify a decision maker.* The patient has no formal advance directives but has a loving and dedicated partner.

  4. *Give understandable, relevant, desired information to the decision maker and dispel myths and misconceptions.* The ventilator and antibiotics can prolong his life but will not cure his underlying condition. If the respirator is begun, it can be discontinued if no response. If it is not begun, he can be given palliative care to maintain comfort.

  5. *Solicit values of the patient that are relevant to the question.* The patient valued privacy and quality of life over prolonging life at any cost. He had refused further anti-retroviral therapies and told his partner that we wanted no life-sustaining treatments.

  6. *Identify health professional values.* Physicians generally should respect and follow the health-care values of their patients to the extent they can be known.

  7. *Propose and critique solutions, including multiple options for treatment and alternative providers.* The physician could provide palliative care without intubation, or transfer the patient to another physician willing to intubate and ventilate him.

  8. *Identify and remove or address constraints on solutions (such as reimbursement, unavailability of services, laws, or legal myths).* The physicians are not required to provide ventilator therapy requested by his parents simply because they are his parents and request it.

CLINICAL PRAGMATISM

The method of clinical pragmatism has roots in the American pragmatic tradition of Oliver Wendell Holmes and William James, but was most profoundly inspired by the writings of the American philosopher John Dewey (1859–1952). In an analytic, inductive approach he called pragmatism, Dewey fused theory and practice by using empirical observations and the scientific method to inform normative questions. He viewed ethical principles not as absolute truths but as ongoing hypotheses to be tested and retested in light of the empirical facts determining context. He emphasized an analytical process, akin to the scientific process, to study the facts under consideration that leads to the delineation of ethical positions.[19]

The application of Dewey's philosophical pragmatism to medical-ethical dilemmas ("clinical pragmatism") addresses clinical problems with the same approach of relevant data gathering. It then attempts to achieve an "ethically acceptable consensus" through a democratic deliberative process that allows all involved parties to participate in determining the solution.[20] Clinicians guide the process by providing a forum in which the opinions of all involved parties can be heard and addressed, where the goals of care and the preferences of the patient are understood, and where moral principles are discussed but are not solely relied upon in justifying possible conclusions.

Clinical pragmatism is the process used by most ethics consultants and committees in their attempts to settle clinical-ethical disputes in the care of hospitalized patients as described in practice in chapter 5. It is a logical and common-sense approach that has great intuitive appeal. Critics of the method of clinical pragmatism claim it has three shortcomings that stem from its lack of rigor in moral analysis: it is inadequate to solve moral problems experimentally, it undervalues the role of judgment in clinical ethics, and it understates the importance of moral principles.[21]

A leading advocate of the method of clinical pragmatism, Joseph Fins, described how clinical pragmatism can satisfactorily address the medical-ethical issues arising in the care of patients with impaired consciousness resulting from traumatic brain injury.[22] Fins proposed the following steps to use clinical pragmatism to achieve a "palliative neuroethics" for the care of brain-injured patients. I summarize his approach using his example of traumatic brain injury (TBI).

I.   *Recognition of the problematic situation and the need for inquiry*   The assumption should be challenged that no therapy can help the TBI patient to recover. Decision making should take into account the limitations of a statistical prognosis. Clinicians should be patient and anticipate improvement.[23]

II. *Data Collection: medical, narrative, contextual*

   A.   *Medical facts*   The precise diagnosis and prognosis of the TBI patient may be difficult to clarify. Clinicians should consider the limitations of our knowledge about the conscious life of a TBI patient who appears unresponsive.[24]

   B.   *Patient/surrogate preferences*   Most TBI patients are young and previously healthy, and have not executed advance directives. Parents or other surrogate decision makers need medical information to provide the proper context in which to implement the patient's preferences. They should try to represent their best understanding of the patient's preferences for life-sustaining therapy, as they understand them given the limitations of accuracy of the diagnosis and prognosis.

   C.   *Family dynamics*   Clinicians need to understand the role played in clinical decision making by family stress and anticipated emotional and financial burdens on family members.

   D.   *Institutional arrangements*   The family dynamic is often played out in an institutional setting. Some institutional views of what constitutes "futile care" should be clarified because they may obstruct attempts at further treatment or rehabilitation.[25]

E. *Broader societal issues and norms* The recent case of Theresa Schiavo brought into public scrutiny the tension between two important goals: preserving a patient's right to refuse life-sustaining treatment and affirming a patient's right to have continued medical care.[26] Both family and staff members may have attitudes molded by this case that impact on decision making in TBI patients.

III. *Interpretation (ethics differential diagnosis)* The ethics "differential diagnosis" (a medical metaphor because diagnosis is not the essential issue) is between continuing life-sustaining treatment and discontinuing it. The patient's diagnosis, prognosis, and previously expressed treatment preferences should be combined to reach the decision. Fins proposed the term "palliative neuroethics" to epitomize that the palliative care ethos represents the best metaphor for the care of these patients.

IV. *Negotiation* The plan of care is negotiated among clinicians, surrogates, and family members on the basis of the foregoing facts.

V. *Intervention* In the setting of prognostic uncertainty, it may be desirable to perform a time-limited trial of therapy to see if there is improvement or until the prognosis is further clarified.

VI. *Periodic review/experiential learning* reassessment is important to examine decisions and modifications of a course of action. Collecting and analyzing the observations from individual cases can inform medical practice standards and public policy.

BIOMEDICAL ETHICS AND EXPERTISE

There is not universal agreement that bioethical analysis is definitive or objective. The authority and objectivity of bioethicists have been questioned on two grounds: (1) What kind and extent of expertise can bioethicists rightfully claim? (2) How objective is bioethical opinion and how much of it is determined politically? I end this chapter with brief responses to both questions.

Over the past generation, the field of biomedical ethics has become both a defined discipline and an industry employing practicing "bioethicists" and bioethics scholars. The field now offers its own texts, scholarly journals, conferences, professional organizations, credentials, professional standards, jargon, and a growing body of practitioners and teachers. Biomedical ethicists enter the field from various backgrounds in medicine, nursing, law, philosophy, religion, social work, and other disciplines. Some prominent bioethicists have become regarded as experts in the field of bioethics. Their opinions are influential and sought after, they are called upon to sit on powerful governmental and professional society advisory bodies, and they are retained as experts to testify in courtroom proceedings by virtue of their prominence and expertise in the discipline. While experienced bioethicists are knowledgeable about bioethics writings and may become skilled in techniques of moral analysis, clinical ethics consultation, and conflict resolution, it does not necessarily follow that possessing this knowledge and these skills justifies them in asserting any special claim on moral insight or authority.[27]

The debate about whether bioethicsts can rightfully claim special expertise in ethical matters has raged for over a quarter century. In 1982, Cheryl Noble argued that philosophers who practice as bioethicists have no justification for any unique claim on moral expertise.[28] A decade later, Giles Scofield launched a similar attack on the moral authority and expertise of bioethicists.[29] Both attacks were defended by prominent bioethicist-philosophers who denied that they and their colleagues ever claimed to be "moral experts."[30] But at least one bioethicist defended the claim that philosopher-ethicists are indeed moral experts.[31] After studying the debate, Scott Yoder argued that the disagreement is fruitless because it is founded on three erroneous assumptions: (1) ethics expertise results from possessing objective moral facts and knowledge; (2) ethics expertise is univocal across disciplinary boundaries; and (3) ethics expertise requires specialization because depth of moral knowledge and experience is more important than breadth.[32]

My impression is that bioethics, as currently described and practiced, is a loosely defined discipline with ambiguous credentialing and vague standards of expertise.[33] Bioethicists achieve prominence and influence through their writings and respect from their clinical peers by their insights on difficult problems and their success in conducting clinical ethics consultations. I believe that bioethicists can achieve a level of expertise from an understanding of moral philosophy and from experience gained by practicing clinical ethics. Knowledge of moral philosophy permits them to systematically and usefully analyze an ethical dilemma by using one of the methods discussed above. Knowledge of the scholarly literature of bioethics and competence in using a system for resolving ethical dilemmas justify the claim that bioethicists have expertise in resolving bioethical issues and disputes. But I agree with the skeptics that bioethicists have no justified grounds to assert any greater claim on moral authority to know the "right" answer to moral questions than anyone else.[34]

BIOMEDICAL ETHICS AND POLITICS

The final issue is whether bioethical opinion can be objective or is inherently subjective because it derives from individual political beliefs. It is generally accepted that concepts of distributive justice (one of the four "principles" of biomedical ethics in the Beauchamp-Childress account [35] described in chapter 1) are inherently political. For example, the disagreement between egalitarians like John Rawls and libertarians like Robert Nozick about the meaning of fairness in distributive justice is essentially political. Rawls adherents claim that principles of justice require society to devise means to further the equality of all citizens, despite obvious differences of birth, luck, ability, and accomplishment that create inequalities, by redistributing benefits to maintain equal opportunity.[36] Nozick adherents counter that while citizens are equal in their most fundamental moral rights; thereafter, their rights are unjustifiably compromised

when society requires them to sacrifice their personal goods for the benefit of others without their consent.[37] Because of their different concepts of justice, they disagree on whether societal rules to redistribute wealth, such as inheritance taxes, are ethical. Eric Cohen recently argued that the principal difference between liberal and conservative bioethicists centers on their moral ideal of equality.[38]

Differing political views can color the understanding of moral ideas in addition to those involving distributive justice. In some contemporary bioethics writings, the extreme emphasis afforded to respect for personal autonomy (another Beauchamp-Childress "principle") represents a classic libertarian ideal: each citizen should be free to pursue her own concept of happiness and the best way to live a life unfettered by societal interference.[39] A similarly strong emphasis on respect for autonomy and self-determination may lead some bioethicists to question validity of the grounds for paternalism inherent in governmental regulations that prohibit individuals from consenting as research subjects in certain circumstances.[40] Daniel Callahan expressed the "libertarian proposition" as, "If someone wants something that medicine can give them, they have a right to it unless immediate and demonstrable harm to others can be proved."[41] To some extent, the way a bioethicist resolves the intrinsic tension between respecting unfettered patient autonomy and advocating beneficent paternalism results from her political orientation.[42]

My colleague, Bernard Gert, argues that common morality (described in chapter 1) is universal and that most moral conflicts stem from disagreements about factual matters. He rejects the idea that morality is relativistic and culturally determined. He points out that his project is merely to make explicit consensual moral intuition that is universal. Of course, he acknowledges the existence of unresolvable moral disagreement (say, over the morality of abortion or euthanasia) and believes that these relatively few areas of disagreement have four primary sources: (1) persons' differences in the ranking of evils and harms, e.g., if death is preferable to suffering a lingering painful illness; (2) who is protected by morality and how are they protected, e.g., if fetuses and animals are protected; (3) what would be the consequences of everyone knowing they are allowed to violate a moral rule, e.g., if doctors were permitted to euthanize patients at their request; and (4) the interpretation of a moral rule, e.g., does stopping a ventilator count as killing when the patient refuses it? Gert concludes that in these relatively few instances, political deliberation is the proper forum in which to decide how to resolve disagreements.[43]

Although common morality is universal, much of published biomedical ethical discourse is inherently political.[44] Many commentators and most experienced bioethicists agree that the prevailing political strain among American bioethicists is liberal.[45] Many influential bioethicists are college professors in philosophy departments or law schools that advocate liberal positions. On bioethical issues as diverse as health-care access,[46] voluntary euthanasia,[47] and accepting advances in biotechnology,[48] opinions from the bioethics community are largely liberal and permissive. Many of the pronouncements of prestigious ethics policy groups similarly have a liberal political orientation.[49] Only recently has bioethics emerged as a priority for the American right wing.[50] Recent appointments to George W. Bush's President's Council on Bioethics have given conservative bioethics opinions greater visibility and power.[51]

One of the most respected conservative bioethics scholars, Leon Kass, distinguished himself by his cautionary position on the ethical issues of emerging biotechnologies. In two influential books [52] and through his work chairing the President's Council on Bioethics,[53] Kass has eloquently warned of the dehumanization that he predicts will result from society's acceptance of new biotechnologies as unqualified goods without an adequate appreciation of their attendant dangers. He cited Aldous Huxley's dystopian novel *Brave New World* to exemplify his concern that technology-induced dehumanization occurs in increments. Because it evolves gradually with the acceptance and accommodation of each new biotechnological advance, people are unaware of the dehumanization it has produced until it is too late. Although I disagree with several of his conclusions, Kass's writings deserve a careful reading by more liberal and permissive bioethicists.[54] Physicians and scientists who disagree with his conclusions or politics would be wrong to dismiss him summarily.

Beginning with the Belmont report[55] and the reports of the President's Commission for the Study of Ethical Problems in Medicine and Biomedical and Behavioral Research,[56] the field of bioethics has provided a public face in addition to its scholarly one. Elevating bioethical discourse to the public policy level has been controversial primarily because of the political bias implicit in bioethical opinion. Our pluralistic society embraces diverse cultural, religious, and philosophical traditions. Bioethicists functioning in public policy roles need to understand and wisely accommodate this pluralism in their public pronouncements.[57]

A prerequisite for the development of acceptable public policy on potentially divisive bioethical issues—particularly those with obvious political overtones—is the achievement of consensus.[58] Public consensus is obviously difficult on ethically divisive issues such as abortion, physician-assisted suicide, and human embryonic stem cell research. If consensus can be achieved, it must be based on carefully argued, balanced positions that incorporate diverse ethical, legal, and cultural factors.[59] Only a balanced position derived from fair and impartial accounts of each side of the debate can be acceptable and deflect criticism that public policy bioethics recommendations are political, not ethical.

NOTES

1. Lo B. *Resolving Ethical Dilemmas*, 3rd ed. Philadelphia: Lippincott Williams & Wilkins, 2005.
2. Hamric AB, Davis WS, Childress MD. Moral distress in health care professionals: what is it and what can we do about it? *The Pharos* 2006;69(1):17–23.
3. See Corley MC. Nurse moral distress: a proposed theory and research agenda. *Nurs Ethics* 2002;9:636–650.
4. Hamric AB, et al. *The Pharos* 2006:20.

5. For a brief and lucid explanation of Gert's method for justifying a moral rule violation, see Gert B. *Common Morality*. New York: Oxford University Press, 2004:55–76.

6. I defend classifying this act as "allowing to die" and discuss appropriate palliative care in chapter 8.

7. The value of the principle of double effect has been debated at length by clinical ethics scholars. For accounts advocating its value in ethical analysis, see Sulmasy DP, Pellegrino ED. The rule of double effect: clearing up the double talk. *Arch Intern Med* 1999;159:545–550; and Sulmasy DP. Commentary: double effect—intention is the solution, not the problem. *J Law Med Ethics* 2000;28:26–29. For criticism of its value, see Quill TE, Dresser R, Brock DW. The rule of double effect—a critique of its role in end-of-life decision making. *N Engl J Med* 1997;337:1768–1771; and Nuccetelli S, Seay G. Relieving pain and foreseeing death: a paradox about accountability and blame. *J Law Med Ethics* 2000;28:19–25.

8. The acceleration of death resulting from proper palliative opioid treatment is an overstated worry. It rarely happens in clinical practice. See Foley KM. Misconceptions and controversies regarding the use of opioids in cancer pain. *Anticancer Drugs* 1995;April 6, Suppl 3:4–13 and the further discussion of this point in chapters 7 and 8.

9. Clouser KD, Gert B. A critique of principlism. *J Med Philosophy* 1990;15:219–236.

10. For a scholarly history and analysis of the practice of casuistry, see Jonsen AR, Toulmin S. *The Abuse of Casuistry. A History of Moral Reasoning*. Berkeley: University of California Press, 1988:5–20. For the limits of casuistic analysis, see Englehardt HT Jr. *The Foundations of Bioethics*, 2nd ed. New York: Oxford University Press, 1996:43–46.

11. Fletcher JF, Hite CA, Lombardo PA, Marshall MF (eds). *Introduction to Clinical Ethics*. Hagerstown, MD: University Publishing Group, 1995. In the third edition of Fletcher's textbook, Edward Spencer expanded Fletcher's methodical checklist to more than 80 items. I chose not to include it here because of its length. Interested readers can consult it for greater analytic depth. See Spencer EM. A case method for consideration of moral problems (Appendix 2) in Fletcher JC, Spencer EM, Lombardo PA (eds). *Fletcher's Introduction to Clinical Ethics*, 3rd ed. Hagerstown, MD: University Publishing Group, 2005.

12. American Academy of Neurology Ethics, Law & Humanities Committee. *AAN Ethics Casebook*. St Paul, MN: American Academy of Neurology, 2000.

13. Reimschisel TE, Williams MA (eds). *Practical Ethics in Clinical Neurology*. Philadelphia: Lippincott Williams & Wilkins, 2008 (in press).

14. Fletcher JF, Hite CA, Lombardo PA, Marshall MF (eds). *Introduction to Clinical Ethics*. Hagerstown, MD: University Publishing Group, 1995.

15. David Goldblatt, M.D. Personal communication, October 28, 2006.

16. Lo B. *Resolving Ethical Dilemmas*, 3rd ed. Philadelphia: Lippincott Williams & Wilkins, 2005.

17. Siegler M. Decision-making strategy for clinical ethical problems in medicine. *Arch Intern Med* 1982;142:2178–2179. See also Jonsen AR, Siegler M, Winslade WJ. *Clinical Ethics*, 1986:6–9.

18. Snyder L, Leffler C. Ethics Manual, 5th edition. *Ann Intern Med* 2005;142:560–582. I used the example provided in the Manual but redrafted and shortened the discussion of each item.

19. Fins JJ. Clinical pragmatism and the care of brain damaged patients: toward a palliative neuroethics for disorders of consciousness. *Prog Brain Res* 2005;150:565–582.

20. Miller FG, Fins JJ, Bachetta MD. Clinical pragmatism: John Dewey and clinical ethics. *J Contemp Health Law Policy* 1996;13:27–51 and Fins JJ, Bachetta MD, Miller FG. Clinical pragmatism: a method of moral problem solving. *Kennedy Inst Ethics J* 1997;7:129–145. Clinical pragmatism and related methods of ethical analysis are discussed in Martin PA. Bioethics and the whole: pluralism, consensus, and the transmutation of bioethical methods into gold. *J Law Med Ethics* 1999;27:316–327. Clinical pragmatism also forms the basis for analysis in the most recent edition of John Fletcher's textbook. See Fletcher JC, Spencer EM, Lombardo PA (eds). *Fletcher's Introduction to Clinical Ethics*, 3rd ed. Hagerstown, MD: University Publishing Group, 2005.

21. Jansen LA. Assessing clinical pragmatism. *Kennedy Inst Ethics J* 1998;8:23–36. Joseph Fins and colleagues answered these criticisms in Fins JJ, Miller FG, Bacchetta MD. Clinical pragmatism: bridging theory and practice. *Kennedy Inst Ethics J* 1998;8:37–42.

22. Fins JJ. *Prog Brain Res* 2005;150:569.

23. I discuss the diagnosis and prognosis of patients in a vegetative state or minimally conscious state in Bernat JL. Chronic disorders of consciousness. *Lancet* 2006;367:1181–1192 and in chapter 12.

24. The limitations of the neurological examination to determine awareness are discussed in chapter 12.

25. The concept of medical futility is discussed in chapter 10.

26. For a factual account of the controversial, sad case of Theresa Schiavo with a balanced analysis of the ethical issues involved, see Hook CC, Mueller PS. The Terri Schiavo saga: the making of a tragedy and lessons learned. *Mayo Clin Proc* 2005;80:1449–60 and the discussion in chapter 12.

27. Casarett DJ, Daskal F, Lantos J. Experts in ethics? The authority of the clinical ethicist. *Hastings Cent Rep* 1998;28(6):6–11.

28 Noble CN. Ethics and experts. *Hastings Cent Rep* 1982;12(3):7–9.

29. Scofield GR. Ethics consultation: the least dangerous profession? *Camb Q Healthc Ethics* 1993;2:417–426.

30. For bioethicists' defenses against Noble's attack, see Wikler D. Ethicists, critics, and expertise. *Hastings Cent Rep* 1982;12(3):12–13 and Beauchamp TL What philosophers can offer. *Hastings Cent Rep* 1982;12(3):13–14. For bioethicists' defenses against Scofield's attack, see Fletcher JF. Commentary: constructiveness where it counts. *Camb Q Healthc Ethics* 1993;2:426–434 and Jonsen AR. Commentary: Scofield as Socrates. *Camb Q Healthc Ethics* 1993;2:434–438.

31. Meyers C. A defense of the philosopher-ethicist as moral expert. *J Clin Ethics* 2003;14:259–269.

32. Yoder SD. Experts in ethics? The nature of ethical expertise. *Hastings Cent Rep* 1998;28(6):11–19.

33. See the discussion in chapter 5 explaining why the American Society of Bioethics and Humanities decided not to formally credential bioethicists. American Society for Bioethics and Humanities. *Core Competencies for Health Care Ethics Consultation.* Glenview, IL: American Society for Bioethics and Humanities, 1998.

34. My colleague, Professor Bernard Gert of the Philosophy Department at Dartmouth College, is amused when physicians ask him to decide whether a particular course of action in patient care is morally correct. He usually turns the question around and asks them their opinion. Because Gert's system of morality strives to make common, consensual morality explicit, he denies that he has any special insight into questions of moral correctness other than providing clarity in analyzing the moral issues involved. See Gert B. *Common Morality.* New York: Oxford University Press, 2004.

35. Beauchamp TL, Childress JF. *Principles of Biomedical Ethics,* 5th ed. New York: Oxford University Press, 2001.

36. Rawls J. *A Theory of Justice.* Cambridge, MA: Harvard University Press, 1971.

37. Nozick R. *Anarchy, State, and Utopia.* New York: Basic Books, 1974.

38. Cohen E. Conservative bioethics and the search for wisdom. *Hasting Cent Rep* 2006;36(1):44–56. Eric Cohen and other scholars agree that facile political labels such as "liberal" and "conservative" mask the nuance and complexity of most bioethical dialogue. Nevertheless, there is some value in retaining these familiar terms in their commonly understood meanings.

39. May T. Bioethics in a liberal society—political not moral. *Int J Applied Philos* 1999;13(1):1–19.

40. Kuczewski M. Two models of ethical consensus, or what good is a bunch of bioethicists? *Camb Q Healthc Ethics* 2002;11:27–36.

41. Callahan D. Communitarian bioethics: a pious hope. *The Responsive Community* 1996;6(4):28.

42. This point is carefully argued in Dworkin G. *The Theory and Practice of Autonomy.* Cambridge: Cambridge University Press, 1988.

43. Gert B. Another view on ethics and politics. *Lahey Clinic Medical Ethics* 2007;14(1):6–7.

44. Powers M. Bioethics as politics: the limits of moral expertise. *Kennedy Inst Ethics J* 2005;15:305–322.

45. For the evidence that the majority of "mainstream" bioethicists are politically liberal and a discussion of the problem of misleading and oversimplified political labels, see Macklin R. The new conservatives in bioethics: who are they and what do they seek? *Hastings Cent Rep* 2006;36(1):34–43.

46. Daniels N. *Just Health Care.* New York: Cambridge University Press, 1995. For an argument for universal access to health care from a conservative viewpoint, see Menzel P, Light DW. A conservative case for universal access to health care. *Hastings Cent Rep* 2006;36(4):36–45.

47. See, for example, Daniel Brock's permissive stance on voluntary euthanasia in Brock DW. Voluntary active euthanasia. *Hastings Cent Rep* 1992;22(2):10–22.

48. See, for example, Ronald Green's ethical arguments defending the research of the company Advanced Cell Technology on human embryonic stem cell cloning in Green RM, DeVries KO, Bernstein J, et al. Overseeing research on therapeutic cloning: a private ethics board responds to its critics. *Hastings Cent Rep* 2002;32(3):27–33.

49. For example, the National Bioethics Advisory Commission impaneled by President Clinton contained leading bioethicists and scholars but no members who opposed human embryonic stem cell cloning. See http://bioethics.georgetown.edu/nbac/about/nbacroster.htm (Accessed June 17, 2007).

50. Levin Y. The paradox of conservative bioethics. *New Atlantis* 2003;1:53–65.

51. Charo RA. Passing on the right: conservative bioethics is closer than it appears. *J Law Med Ethics* 2004; 32:307–314.

52. Kass LR. *Toward a More Natural Science: Biology and Human Affairs*. New York: Free Press, 1985 and Kass LR. *Life, Liberty and the Defense of Dignity: The Challenge for Bioethics*. San Francisco: Encounter Books, 2002.

53. Leon Kass was the founding chairman of the President's Council on Bioethics, currently chaired by Edmund Pellegrino. Under Kass's chairmanship, the Council published several reports warning of the dangers introduced by new biotechnologies, such as human embryonic stem cell research and cloning. See www.bioethics.gov/reports (Accessed June 17, 2007).

54. I have explained the political basis for the rejection of Kass's claims in Bernat JL. Book Review: Kass LR. Life, Liberty and the Defense of Dignity: The Challenge for Bioethics. *Neurology Today* 2003;3(2):22–23.

55. The National Commission for the Protection of Human Subjects of Biomedical and Behavioral Research. *The Belmont Report: Ethical Principles and Guidelines for the Protection of Human Subjects of Research*. US Department of Health, Education and Welfare, DHEW Publication No. (OS) 78-0012, 1978.

56. The President's Commission, impaneled by President Carter and chartered by the United States Congress in 1978, published 12 influential reports on bioethics topics from 1981–1983. These works are summarized in President's Commission for the Study of Ethical Problems in Medicine and Biomedical and Behavioral Research. *Summing Up: The Ethical and Legal Problems in Medicine and Biomedical and Behavioral Research*. Washington, DC: US Government Printing Office, 1983.

57. Turner L. Bioethics in pluralistic societies. *Med Health Care Philos* 2004;7:201–208.

58. Moreno JD. *Deciding Together: Bioethics and Moral Consensus*. New York: Oxford University Press, 1995.

59. For an example of an ideally balanced synthesis of ethical, legal, and cultural factors, see Dworkin R. *Life's Dominion: An Argument about Abortion, Euthanasia, and Individual Freedom*. New York: Alfred A. Knopf, 1993.

ETHICAL ISSUES
IN DEATH AND DYING

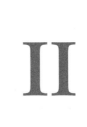

Dying and Palliative Care

7

The management of the dying patient is the focus of many ethical issues in medicine in general and neurology in particular. Ethical issues arise frequently in the care of dying and critically ill patients because technological advances in life-sustaining therapies have introduced new questions, particularly how, when, and for whom these therapies should be administered. Life-saving technologies are marvelous when they succeed in restoring a critically ill patient's health and function. But when they fail, paradoxically they may worsen the care of dying patients, especially when they interfere with the provision of good palliative care.

In this chapter, I consider ethical issues surrounding management of the dying patient and focus on how to optimize the patient's palliative care. I discuss the goal of a "good death," explain how the principles of palliative care can achieve it, and discuss the barriers preventing physicians from implementing it. I conclude with a discussion of palliative sedation, the principal ethical controversy in palliative care. I discuss the related subjects of refusal of life-sustaining therapy, patient refusal of hydration and nutrition, physician-assisted suicide, euthanasia, and medical futility in subsequent chapters in this section.

THE DEMOGRAPHICS OF DYING

During the past century in the United States, we have witnessed enormous changes in the demographics of dying. In the 19th century, most Americans died at home under the care of family members, as a result of acute illnesses, particularly infections. Today, by contrast, most Americans die in hospitals or nursing homes, isolated from their families. They usually die as a result of a progressive, chronic illness following a period of failing health. The change in the demographics of dying results partly from the marked increase in the average life expectancy of Americans over the past century, steadily increasing from approximately 49 years at the turn of the 20th century to approximately 77 years at the turn of the 21st century. The increase in mean longevity is a consequence of fewer deaths in infancy; improvements in public health, preventive health, and nutrition; successful treatment of infections and other acute illnesses; and advances in workplace safety. Most Americans now can look forward to a long life terminated by a chronic illness.[1]

The change in the demographics of dying in America also reflects a profound sociological phenomenon: the growth of the technological, professional, and institutional process of the care of the dying.[2] In our time, the care of dying patients largely has been relegated to institutions and away from families and homes. Thus, approximately 80% of Americans now die in hospitals or nursing homes whereas a century ago an institutional location for death was uncommon.[3]

The reasons for this phenomenon reflect the prevailing American societal attitudes about dying. First, we embrace a technological and interventionalist imperative: we value the use of technology to extend our lives as long as possible. This attitude is evidenced in the greater utilization of diagnostic testing, surgery, intensive care unit treatment, chronic hemodialysis, chemotherapy, and other life-sustaining interventions by Americans as compared to other cultures.[4] One cultural explanation for the technological imperative is the quintessential American heroic-positivist philosophy of medicine that celebrates the intrinsic value of action and preferentially values "doing something" rather than nothing, even if that something is not beneficial or even harmful.[5]

Second, our culture is "death-denying." Daniel Callahan observed that our culture treats death "as a kind of accident, a contingent event that greater prevention, proven technology, and further research could do away with." He notes further that Americans, compared to people in other cultures, show "an unwillingness to let nature take its course" that in many cases tragically leads to "death in a technological cocoon."[6] In her famous book *On Death and Dying*, Elizabeth Kubler-Ross outlined some of the psychological reasons for the contemporary phenomenon of denying death.[7] Robert Burt explained how American cultural factors also shape our public policies about death and dying.[8]

Third, our prevailing attitude is that death should be "medicalized." We believe that the messy process of dying and the frightening event of death are handled best by trained professionals within institutions, not by family members at home.[9] Although there is evidence that these attitudes now are changing with the rise of the palliative care and hospice movements,[10] the care of the dying patient remains largely consigned to institutions. Despite our institutionalization of death and dying, polls of Americans of all ages consistently reveal that 90% of people say they would prefer to be cared for at home during the last six months of their lives.[11] One study, however, surveying community-dwelling elderly patients about their preferred site of death found 48% chose the hospital, 43% preferred home, and 9% were unsure.[12] These findings may indicate that the proximity of death in the elderly generates a more realistic concern about stresses on family members caring for a dying

patient at home. This concern may lead some patients to prefer to die in the hospital. Family members of patients who died at home report more favorable dying experiences than family members of institutionalized dying patients, who are more likely to report unmet needs for symptom control, physician communication and emotional support.[13] Programs have been established to optimize palliative care within long-term institutions.[14]

Prevailing practices in hospitals largely shape the end of life for dying inpatients. In an ethnographic study of dying in American hospitals, Sharon Kaufman found that hospitals organized dying through acculturated behaviors that shaped medical practices. She found that shared medical rhetoric frames decision making about dying patients and cultural factors shape the way death occurs in the hospital, even governing which patients whom physicians and nurses consider to be dying. Today, death usually is orchestrated by professionals in hospitals and no longer is waited for, a transition that has markedly shortened the "waiting time" for dying. Hospital procedures and bureaucracy produced an imperative to "move things along," mandating health-care professionals to expedite decision making and produce the conditions for death. The American hospital system and the social processes of American hospital subculture shape the end of life for dying inpatients.[15]

THE PHYSIOLOGY OF DYING

Implicit in the optimal care of the dying patient is an understanding of the physiology of dying. Some of the conceptual errors made by lay people and the treatment errors made by medical professionals stem from their failure to understand the important physiological differences between the dying patient and the healthy patient. The physiology of dying has not been the subject of many recent investigations but enough scientific information is known to make a few rational recommendations.

Involution of thirst and hunger is a normal part of the dying process. The reduction in thirst and hunger drives result from a gradual reduction in gastrointestinal peristalsis and a decrease in intravascular volume.[16] A well-meaning but poorly informed physician who observes that a patient dying of widely metastatic cancer is not eating and drinking "normally" (in comparison to what would be expected for a healthy person) may consider treating the patient by inserting a nasogastric feeding tube and infusing tube feedings, or inserting an intravenous line and infusing crystalloid hydration. However, these measures could create discomfort to the patient in addition to the direct discomfort of the tubes themselves. Forced nutrition in the presence of diminished peristalsis produces nausea and vomiting. Forced hydration in the presence of a diminished plasma volume produces fluid overload, pulmonary edema, and dyspnea. Thus, well-meaning but misdirected attempts to compensate for the normal reduction of food or fluid intake in dying patients paradoxically increase their discomfort.

Indeed, studies of patients dying in hospices who have refused food and water clearly show that, despite progressive dehydration, inanition, and weight loss, dying patients experience little or no suffering from feeling parched nor do they have a marked sensation of thirst or hunger.[17] Proper mouth care to keep the lips moist helps preserve mouth comfort in dying patients.[18] Understanding these few physiological principles helps guide physicians providing palliative care to prescribe only those measures that will contribute to dying patients' comfort.

FACILITATING A "GOOD" DEATH

Several studies and case reports of the quality of dying in hospitals [19] and published personal anecdotes by affected family members recounting the horrors of the deaths of hospitalized loved ones[20] attest to the unfortunate reality that the dying experience of many hospitalized patients is far from ideal. Many patients receive unwanted life-sustaining treatment and other aggressive therapy, but fail to receive adequate palliative care. Similarly, most children who die in the hospital die in the intensive care unit (ICU) following a prolonged hospitalization during which they received aggressive rather than palliative therapy.[21] These studies and anecdotes portray dying hospitalized patients trapped in a medical system that ignores their wishes and victimizes and degrades them, while failing to provide basic human contact and comfort. These studies and anecdotes clearly reveal cases of bad deaths. What then constitutes a good death?

To answer this question, Karen Steinhauser and colleagues conducted a series of focus groups with health-care workers, dying patients, and family members of recently deceased patients. They identified six common components of a good death as perceived by these interviewees. First, there should be adequate management of pain and other distressing symptoms of dying. The confidence of dying patients that they will not suffer adds immeasurable comfort to their final days. Second, to the fullest extent possible, the patients should remain in control of decision making with their thinking unclouded by medications. The assurance that physicians will permit them to remain in control also is comforting. Third, they should be adequately prepared for the event of death. They need to know what to expect so they can plan accordingly. Fourth, they need the opportunity for personal completion. Completion encompasses spirituality and meaning at the end of life, life review, spending time with family, resolving disagreements, and saying good-bye. Fifth, they need the opportunity to contribute to the well-being of others. This contribution can be in the form of a gift, time spent, knowledge and wisdom imparted, or volunteered participation in a clinical trial or other research study for the good of others. Sixth, they need affirmation as a whole and unique person. They want to be treated not as a disease but as a person in the context of their lives, values, and preferences.[22]

In a similar vein, Daniel Callahan offered a personal reflection on the qualities of a peaceful death. It should be meaningful. The dying patient should be treated with respect and sympathy. The patient's death should matter to others. Patients should not be abandoned by family or friends. The patient should not be an undue burden on others. Our society should not dread death but accept it. The patient should remain conscious as long as possible. The death should occur quickly and not be drawn out. There should be minimal pain and suffering.[23] These two sets of characteristics of a good death create reasonable goals for a program of palliative care of the dying patient.

Elizabeth Vig and colleagues surveyed terminally ill men about their views on good and bad deaths. They found consensus in the obvious desire to avoid suffering and die in one's sleep if possible, but variability in their responses about whether other people should be present and where patients prefer to die. The authors advocated an individualized approach: each patient's view of what constitutes a "good death" should be used to plan terminal arrangements to assure that they conform with the patient's wishes.[24]

A BRIEF HISTORY OF PALLIATIVE CARE

The modern history of palliative care is relatively short. Until the 20th century, the diagnosis and treatment of the dying patient always had been part of traditional medicine. For example, in his famous text, *The Principles and Practice of Medicine* (1892), Sir William Osler described in detail the recognition of the terminal stages of various diseases and their management. Over a decade later, Osler published a series of 486 sequential deaths he personally studied at the Johns Hopkins Hospital, detailing the symptoms and signs of death and treatments that helped comfort the dying patient.[25] As the 20th century progressed, however, and medical textbooks became increasingly scientific, there was a commensurate reduction in the emphasis on the diagnosis and treatment of the dying patient. Until recently, most contemporary textbooks of internal medicine and neurology contained little mention of the care of the dying patient.[26] Similarly, medical society treatment practice guidelines for life-limiting diseases offered little guidance in end-of-life care.[27] Some physicians continue to record their personal experiences treating dying patients[28] including dying physicians.[29]

Although some institutions dedicated to care of the dying patient have operated for a millennium, the modern palliative care movement began in 1967 with the founding of St. Christopher's Hospice in London by Dame Cicely Saunders.[30] The first freestanding American hospice was founded in Connecticut in 1974. Hospice philosophy, according to Saunders, is holistic, encompassing adequate symptom control, care of the patient and family as a unit, the use of an interdisciplinary approach, the use of volunteers, providing a continuum of care including home care and continuity of care across different settings, and follow-up on family members after death.[31]

Hospice philosophy quickly spread across the United Kingdom, the United States, Canada, and other developed countries. In 1982 in the United States, Medicare began offering a hospice benefit through Medicare Part A that reimbursed approved hospices for care of dying patients. A Medicare beneficiary electing the hospice benefit must be diagnosed as terminally ill, which means the patient's life expectancy is judged by a physician to be under six months.[32] The Medicare hospice benefit includes a range of noncurative medical benefits and medical and support services, many of which would not be covered otherwise, including physicians' services, nursing care, pharmaceuticals, medical appliances, short-term hospitalization, services of homemakers and health aides, physical, occupational, and speech therapy, psychological counseling, and social services.[33] Physicians continue mostly to refer dying cancer patients to hospice; approximately 89% of enrolled hospice patients have cancer.[34] By 2004, more than 3,200 hospice programs in the United States cared for more than 900,000 patients.[35]

Although Dame Cicely Saunders was a physician, much of the hospice movement was developed by nurses and volunteers. In a parallel development, much of hospice's philosophy and many of its goals were incorporated into a new branch of medicine called palliative medicine. Physicians in England and Canada spearheaded this movement and developed palliative care services in hospitals primarily treating dying cancer patients. The pioneering palliative care service at the Royal Victoria Hospital in Montreal was opened in 1975 by Dr. Balfour Mount, who coined the term "palliative medicine." Currently, over 20% of American hospitals have palliative care units or services.[36]

Palliative medicine comprises most but not all elements of hospice philosophy.[37] The two disciplines differ in their patient domains. Hospice provides palliative care to dying patients. Palliative medicine widens its focus to also include patients suffering from chronic illnesses to attempt to reduce their symptom burden and improve their quality of life. In neurology, palliative medicine has been applied not just to patients dying of ALS and malignant gliomas but also to patients chronically ill with multiple sclerosis, Parkinson's disease, Alzheimer's disease, muscular dystrophy, and epilepsy.[38] One palliative practice merits particular attention because of its ethical and legal implications: the opioid treatment of patients with chronic pain not caused by cancer.[39] The American Academy of Neurology Ethics, Law & Humanities Committee published a practice advisory for neurologists asserting that treatment of such patients falls within the scope of neurological practice and outlining the ethical responsibilities neurologists have to diagnose and treat such patients properly.[40]

The palliative care movement now is an established branch of organized medicine.[41] There are numerous textbooks on palliative medicine,[42] five journals specializing in palliative medicine or palliative care,[43] numerous courses at medical society meetings teaching palliative medicine, and courses on palliative medicine directed to medical students[44] and house officers. Palliative medicine is an accredited medical specialty in the United States.

Within the field of neurology, special issues of the *Journal of Neurology* [45] and *Neurologic Clinics*[46] have been devoted to palliative care in neurology and a comprehensive textbook on that topic was published by Oxford University Press.[47] The American Medical Association developed a training program in palliative medicine called Education for Physicians on End-of-Life Care (EPEC) that

functions as a "train the trainer" course. The goal of EPEC is to educate every practicing physician in the United States on the principles of palliative medicine. EPEC has been converted to an independent organization organized through Northwestern University that charges a fee for its educational services.[48] Similar excellent teaching information is available at several free websites.[49] In 2008, the American Board of Medical Specialties plans to offer a subspecialty certificate in hospice and palliative medicine to neurologists through the American Board of Psychiatry and Neurology.

THE PRINCIPLES OF PALLIATIVE MEDICINE

The World Health Organization defined palliative care in 1982 as "the active total care of patients whose disease is not responsive to curative treatment. Control of pain, of other symptoms, and of psychological, social and spiritual problems is paramount. The goal of palliative care is achievement of the best quality of life for patients and their families."[50] In a similar vein, one of the leaders of the field, Neil MacDonald, defined palliative medicine in 1991 as "the study and management of patients with active, progressive, far advanced disease, for whom the prognosis is limited and the focus of care is the quality of life."[51] In 2002, the World Health Organization amended their definition to "Palliative care is an approach which improves quality of life of patients and their families facing life-threatening illness, through the prevention and relief of suffering by means of early identification and impeccable assessment and treatment of pain and other problems, physical, psychosocial, and spiritual."[52]

Palliative care addresses the quality of life, not its quantity. Palliative care affirms life and strives to help patients live as actively as possible until death. The intent of palliative care is neither to lengthen nor shorten life but to allow the patient's inevitable death to occur with the least suffering and the greatest meaning. The goal of palliative care, in short, is to maximize the quality of the patient's remaining life and to permit a good death, as outlined previously. The principal distinction between palliative medicine and hospice care is that whereas the latter is generally limited to dying patients, the former is applicable also to patients with progressive, incurable illnesses.[53] Thus, most of the principles of palliative medicine are applicable to the majority of patients living with chronic neurological diseases.[54]

I identify 10 cardinal principles of palliative medicine and palliative care:

1. *Palliative care, like hospice, is not a building, department, or program but is an* approach *to patient care embodying an* attitude *to improve the quality of the patient's remaining life.* This principle highlights one difficulty in its implementation: that physicians need to alter their conceptualization of their professional responsibility to dying patients by replacing the traditional curative model of treatment with a palliative care model.[55] Thus, physicians need to accept that they have an important professional responsibility in managing the dying patient and actively helping their patient experience a good death. They need to learn to value the time they spend on improving their patient's quality of life by attending to small details that may seem clinically inconsequential (bowel care, for example) but can produce great improvements in the patient's quality of life. They also should try to learn to derive satisfaction from knowing that their medical intervention improved the quality of the patient's remaining life and death.

2. *Physicians need to acquire a working technical knowledge of opiate, benzodiazepine, and barbiturate pharmacology, and training in the ordering of pharmacological and other measures to suppress distressing symptoms in dying patients.* Palliative medicine requires knowledge of the right drug, in the right dosage, with the right dosage interval, and through the right route of administration. Physicians need to understand pharmacological concepts such dose-response curves, time-action curves, and the development of tolerance to drugs. For management of patients on ventilators, this pharmacological knowledge should include the use of neuromuscular blocking drugs to induce paralysis. Treatment of pain is of particular importance. Physicians needs to know that, contrary to opinion, oral or parenteral dosages of opioid drugs that are adequate to palliate pain do not accelerate the moment of death.[56] Textbooks of palliative medicine can be consulted for specific treatment regimens recommended to suppress other unpleasant symptoms of dying patients, such as nausea[56a], cough, hiccups, dyspnea,[57] agitation, confusion,[58] anxiety, anorexia, fatigue,[59] constipation, and xerostomia.[60]

3. *Physicians need to address the psychological, emotional, and spiritual needs of the dying patient.* Depression and anxiety require identification and treatment in a palliative care plan. Depression is common in dying patients[61] and along with demoralization (morbid existential distress)[62] frequently contributes to their decisions to withdraw treatment or request physician-assisted suicide.[63] The issue of dying patients' spiritual needs usually encompasses their search for the meaning of their lives in the face of death. Many dying patients can make their lives whole by completing this spiritual journey, and thereafter face their death with serenity and peace.[64] This process of spiritual growth during dying can be transcendently meaningful.[65] Chaplains, families, and friends can help provide spiritual support. Alan Astrow and colleagues pointed out that to care for a person, the physician must first learn to be a person, thus physicians should cultivate and deepen their own spiritual lives.[66]

4. *Physicians should try to identify and relieve all sources of suffering, in addition to those produced by pain, depression, and anxiety.* Suffering is an intensely personal, existential experience that also encompasses anguish, fear, apprehension, helplessness, hopelessness, despondency, dependency, and meaninglessness. In his monograph, Eric Cassell pointed out that the treatment of patients' suffering is the primary goal of medicine. Suffering is the final common pathway of all negative physical,

psychological, and spiritual human experiences. The essence of suffering is the perception of a threat to the integrity of the person.[67] Other common sources of suffering in dying patients include exhaustion, anhedonia, cachexia, unpleasant odors, helplessness, and loss of dignity.[68] Max Chochinov described what he calls "dignity-conserving care" as the essence of palliative care.[69] He and his colleagues found that dying patients' perceived loss of dignity was correlated to their psychological and symptom distress, heightened dependency, and loss of the will to live.[70] Although existential suffering may not be immediately amenable to palliative care, not all patients' existential concerns cause suffering.[71]

5. *Palliative medicine uses a team approach to the care of the patient.* In many hospitals, palliative care is provided by an interdisciplinary care team led by a palliative care physician. The team should freely request consultations from colleagues in other fields who can contribute specialized knowledge. Thus, for example, anesthesiologists and neurosurgeons may be helpful in suppressing intractable pain while maintaining normal consciousness by using indwelling intraspinal opiate pumps. Physical, occupational, and speech therapists can help improve motor and communicative function. Social workers can help optimize interactions with the family. Chaplains can address spiritual and religious needs. Nurses can address the needs of the whole patient and help integrate the care team. Despite the desirability of a team approach, each member of the team should retain a personal ethical responsibility and accountability to the patient.

6. *The patient-family dyad comprises the unit of palliative care.* It is almost always family members who care for the patient, pay for the costs, and undergo the stress of illness. Family members provide the principal psychosocial support structure for the patient. Therefore, the needs of family caregivers are directly relevant to those of the patient and should be addressed in a comprehensive palliative care plan. These needs include good information, education, training, support and counseling, assistance in communication, practical and financial support, around-the-clock availability of medical support, and support during grief and bereavement.[72] A recent study of the caregivers of terminally ill patients remaining at home found that the majority were female family members and paid assistants, with few volunteers.[73] The major burdens on family caregivers are time and logistical stresses, physical tasks, financial costs, emotional burdens and mental health risks, and physical health risks.[74]

7. *Communication with dying patients and their families is essential to understand the needs of patients, to teach them and their families what to expect, and to clarify the medical decisions that must be made.*[75] In an article explaining how physicians can discuss palliative care with patients, Bernard Lo and colleagues outlined the essential communication strategies. Physicians can employ open-ended questions about end-of-life care, such as, "What concerns you most about your illness?" and "How is the treatment going?" Physicians can explore spirituality with questions such as, "Is your faith (religion, spirituality) important to you in this illness?" or "Do you have someone to talk to about religious matters?" If necessary, physicians can employ more direct questions such as, "What do you still hope to accomplish during your life?" or "What do you want your children and grandchildren to remember about you?"[76] Yet, at least one study of terminally ill outpatients showed that the majority of palliative treatment office visit time was devoted to medical-technical issues and not quality of life concerns.[77] Communication strategies can be learned to help clinicians achieve the delicate balance between being honest about prognosis yet not discouraging hope.[78] Anthony Back and colleagues suggest that physicians help dying patients to achieve this balance by "hoping for the best, while preparing for the worst."[79] Physicians also should say "goodbye" to the patient near

death to acknowledge the closure of the patient-physician relationship.[80]

8. *Patients and caregivers should plan in advance for the process of dying and the event of death.*[81] The setting of death is determined by patient or family preference, patient need, and available resources. Choices include the hospital, nursing home, at home with hospice assistance, or at home without hospice assistance. Often, a dying patient will need to spend time at more than one site. A comprehensive palliative care plan provides coordination across all these settings. Advance care planning involves discussions with the patient and family of the specific nature of desired and undesired medical interventions in anticipation of their possible need.[82] For example, most patients with agonal symptoms during the last few hours of life wish to avoid being treated by emergency medical technicians and sent to emergency rooms. Adequate planning includes education of family members about what to expect and how to treat common agonal problems, and planning for the provision of trained personnel and medications for on-site terminal care.[83]

9. *Physicians should write explicit palliative care orders on inpatients and not rely on the vague order "comfort measures only."* Vague orders thrust upon the nursing staff the responsibility to determine whether a particular therapy is appropriate for palliative purposes, an unfair transfer of responsibility. Many institutions have created pre-printed palliative care order forms to remind physicians to anticipate patients' palliative needs for each common symptom likely to occur.[84] The test for whether a given therapy is appropriate for a palliative care plan is the extent to which it will contribute to the goal of comfort. A clear focus on the palliative goals of care should be maintained to permit an analysis of which types of treatment to provide in emergency circumstances, such as seizures, aspiration, choking, and delirium. A structured approach includes consideration of the patient's physical, psychological, and spiritual needs and appropriate patient-specific goals.[85]

10. *While the aims of palliative care are admirable, physicians and other team members should be watchful not to elevate it to an ideology.* Edmund Pellegrino warned not to cherish it as "the only right and true way to die." Raising palliative care to an ideology runs the risk of medicalizing and professionalizing a process that depends at least as much on human feelings as on technical expertise. Family members and friends may be more responsive to the personal needs of the patient than the medical professionals. Pellegrino warned that making palliative care an ideology may paradoxically discourage the desirable attention of family and friends in favor of the prerogatives of the treatment team.[86]

Palliative medicine is one of the components of ideal end-of-life care for dying patients. The overall principles of end-of-life care were outlined by Christine Cassel and Kathleen Foley on the basis of a conference endorsed by representatives from 14 medical specialty societies (including the American Academy of Neurology) and the Joint Commission on the Accreditation of Healthcare Organizations (JCAHO), and sponsored by the Milbank Memorial Fund. They reached consensus on 11 core principles for end-of-life care. They concluded that: "Clinical policy of care at the end of life and the professional practice it guides should:

1. Respect the dignity of both patient and caregivers;

2. Be sensitive to and respectful of the patient's and family's wishes;

3. Use the most appropriate measures that are consistent with the patient's choices;

4. Encompass alleviation of pain and other physical symptoms;

5. Assess and manage psychological, social, and spiritual/religious problems;

6. Offer continuity (the patient should be able to continue to be cared for, if so desired, by his/her primary care and specialist providers);

7. Provide access to any therapy which may realistically be expected to improve the patient's quality of life; including alternative or nontraditional treatments;

8. Provide access to palliative care and hospice care;

9. Respect the right to refuse treatment;

10. Respect the physician's professional responsibility to discontinue some treatments when appropriate, with consideration for both patient and family preferences; and

11. Promote clinical and evidence-based research on providing care at the end of life."[87]

THE PALLIATIVE CARE SERVICE

The practice of palliative care within hospitals has been operationalized using two principal models: the inpatient palliative care or hospice unit and the palliative care consultation service. There are advantages and disadvantages to both models and experience has been published from their implementation in a number of hospitals.

The inpatient palliative care unit, based on the analogy to a hospice unit, was the first model employed. These units are staffed by physicians and nurses trained in palliative care and accept dying patients from other services for terminal care.[88] In some hospitals, the palliative care unit is primarily a nursing unit and the care of the patient is retained by the attending physician. Many units have designed preprinted palliative care admission order sheets that stipulate exactly which treatments will be given and which will not, and provide medications and other remedies to treat the full range of symptoms likely to be experienced by dying patients.[89] Some of the units can be structurally integrated with ICUs to accept dying patients more efficiently once the decision has been reached that only palliative care will be given.[90] The United States Centers for Medicare and Medicaid Services (formerly the Health Care Financing Administration or HCFA) provides an ICD-9 code for palliative care to reimburse treatment on these units. This provision reflects a determined effort to improve palliative care by eliminating the barrier of inadequate reimbursement.[91]

Other institutions have created palliative care consultation services. These services are multidisciplinary teams composed of physicians, nurses, socials workers, pharmacists, chaplains, and others who are called to see hospitalized dying patients and who make recommendations for optimal palliative care.[92] One advantage of organizing the service as a consultation service and having the patient's attending physician retain responsibility for care is that the consultation process educates the attending physician in palliative medicine. Once the physician has requested several consultations and has observed the orders and treatments suggested, the physician can internalize that information and thereafter provide good palliative care to other patients without the need to request further consultations except in difficult cases. Thus, as in ethics consultation, palliative care consultation provides an educational process for physicians to continuously improve their care of patients.

Palliative care programs are increasing in numbers in American hospitals. A study of American Hospital Association data showed a linear increase in the prevalence of palliative care programs, from 632 (15% of hospitals) in 2000 to 1,027 (25% of hospitals) in 2003. Predictors associated with an increased likelihood of a hospital's having a palliative care program were greater number of hospital beds, greater number of critical care beds, geographic region, academic medical center, V.A. medical center, Catholic church affiliation, and the presence of a hospital-owned hospice program.[93]

PALLIATIVE CARE FOR CHILDREN

The provision of palliative care for dying children has now been explored in nearly as great detail as for dying adults.[94] Dying children experience the same range of pain and suffering as adults and require the same needs for palliative care. But children have additional needs based on their unique fears and their development-related capacity to understand. Further, parents may wish to protect them from bad news and create barriers for communication that impair ideal care. Most children dying gradually from a terminal disease have cancer.[95]

Joanne Wolfe and colleagues reported a detailed account of the symptoms, signs, and palliative care of children dying of cancer treated at the Boston Children's Hospital and the Dana-Farber Cancer Center.[96] They found that 80% of children died of the direct effects of the disease and 20% of the complications of treatment. Half of the children died in the hospital and half of this group died in the ICU. By the parents' rating, 89% of the children suffered "a lot" or "a great deal" during their last month of life, with fatigue, dyspnea, and pain representing the major symptoms. They found a discord between the physicians' rating of the child's symptoms and the parents' ratings. In most cases, the parents graded the child's suffering as greater than did the physician, a finding suggesting that physicians may under-recognize the sources of suffering in dying children. They also found that an earlier discussion of hospice was associated with greater calm and peace of the child in the final month of life. They concluded that children dying of cancer experienced significant suffering that could be ameliorated by greater attention to symptom control. As in adults, the duty to palliate is both medical and ethical.[97]

In an accompanying editorial, Elaine Morgan and Sharon Murphy pointed out that one reason for these findings is that children are not just "little adults" and that many caregivers lack specific training in the palliative care of children.[98] There are features distinguishing both the medical treatment and the palliative care of children from that of adults. First, many parents and physicians are less likely to "give up" on children and persist with aggressive (and often painful) treatment beyond the point at which they would stop in adults, often to the very moment of death. This position of aggressive treatment may deprive patients, family members, and caregivers from giving sufficient consideration to comfort care. Second, certain supportive measures, such as blood transfusions and supplemental feeding, are continued

longer in children with the unfounded expectation that they will contribute to their well-being. Finally, parents may feel guilty about "giving up" and discontinuing life-sustaining therapy that they believe it is their duty to continue in their role as the child's protector. They may be unwilling to admit failure in this valiant effort by subscribing only to palliative care. However, when they do finally accept the prognosis, they become more willing to advocate for palliative care.[99]

Communication about death and dying with children differs from that in adults. The content of communication with children depends on the child's age and ability to comprehend their circumstance. Children aged 2 to 7 years should not be separated from their parents if possible and should be reassured that their illness was not punishment for bad thoughts or actions. Children aged 7 to 12 years should be given details about treatment and permitted to maintain control over certain activities. Teenagers should be allowed to ventilate anger, given privacy, and given access to peers and support groups.[100] The optimal structure of conferences to present bad news to families of children and examples of conversations that promote hope and establish goals of care have been described.[101]

The question of whether terminally ill children should be explicitly told of their impending death was addressed in a survey study of parents following their children's deaths from cancer. None of the parents who had discussed death with their child expressed any regrets about the conversation, but 27% of the parents who did not discuss death with their child regretted not having the conversation.[102] It is clear that even very young children can conceptualize death.[103] Parents should be encouraged to explain death to their terminally ill children and to work with pediatric palliative care experts to implement developmentally specific care.[104]

BARRIERS TO PALLIATIVE CARE

Medical society publications and position statements over the past decade have admonished physicians about the critical importance of providing effective palliative care.[105] Additionally, as I noted earlier, palliative care textbooks, courses, and curricula have become widespread and easily available to practicing physicians. Yet, despite this recognition and emphasis, a number of studies have shown that most practicing physicians are not providing proper palliative care.[106] This mismatch of supply and demand raises the question: what are the barriers preventing physicians from implementing effective palliative care?[107]

In a thoughtful review of this topic, Diane Meier and colleagues identified three groups of barriers to palliative care: deficiencies in physician knowledge and skills, improper physician attitudes, and inadequacies in the health-care system.[108] To improve physician knowledge and skills, Meier and colleagues suggested that, in addition to including palliative care in medical curricula at various levels, these topics should be placed on board certification examinations and included in residency review requirements. Most importantly, faculty development should be funded to provide mentors in palliative medicine for physicians-in-training to learn from and emulate. Physicians should follow expert guidelines for initiating timely and effective discussions with dying patients about palliative care and hospice.[109]

Practice guidelines and quality improvement programs have been developed for palliative care.[110] The Ethics Committee of the American Geriatrics Society identified 14 quality indicators for end-of-life care suitable for inclusion in clinical programs and research studies.[111] The American College of Physicians-American Society of Internal Medicine End-of-Life Care Consensus Panel recommended that clinical teams conduct the iterative "Plan, Do, Study, and Act" cycle to improve the quality of palliative care in hospitals and nursing homes.[112]

To address improper physician attitudes, Meier and colleagues suggested further education of practicing physicians on fundamental ethical and legal issues in the care of the dying patient, such as how to use advance directives, how to distinguish between decisions to terminate life-sustaining treatment and active euthanasia, and how to separate palliative sedation and euthanasia. They suggested that professional organizations establish standards on medical futility through consensus. To be

able to derive professional satisfaction from easing the suffering of dying patients, physicians also need to learn to convert their professional expectations from cure to care

Improving end-of-life care requires an approach from a policy and population perspective in addition to the clinical one.[113] The revisions of the health-care system suggested by Meier and colleagues include having the JCAHO develop and enforce standards for end-of-life care, encouraging hospitals to develop palliative care units or consultation services and including end-of-life quality standards in managed care organizations. Onerous state regulations requiring the recording of physicians' prescriptions for controlled substances that have the effect of promoting under-treatment of pain and suffering should be revised to eliminate that perverse incentive.[114] Hospital risk management standards should be revised to promote palliative care and assure that patients' wishes are respected. A recent study revealed that the problem of implementing optimal palliative care is not restricted to small or community hospitals. In studying a group of 77 prestigious academic medical centers, the investigators found a marked variation in their use of hospice and palliative care services as well as ICU care during the last six months of patients' lives.[115]

PALLIATIVE SEDATION

The principal ethical controversy in palliative medicine is palliative sedation, the purposeful sedation of the suffering, dying patient to unconsciousness or near-unconsciousness by administering barbiturates or benzodiazepines, when doing so becomes the only means of achieving comfort care.[116] "Terminal sedation," the former name of this practice, should be discarded in favor of "palliative sedation" to emphasize that the physician's intent and medication orders are entirely palliative: they are neither intended nor designed to kill the patient. Palliative sedation is an accepted element of palliative care that can be used when necessary: when no other means of palliation is successful. Palliative sedation remains controversial for two reasons. First, patients cannot eat or drink when so heavily sedated. Unlike other forms of palliative therapy, including nearly all appropriate opioid treatment to suppress pain or dyspnea, palliative sedation accelerates the moment of death. Second, some have justified active euthanasia by calling it palliative sedation. The distinction can be difficult at times but is important ethically and legally.[117]

Analyses of the morality of palliative sedation using the principle of double effect (see chapter 2) conclude that it is morally permissible, largely because the intent is to palliate and not kill the patient. First, the act of sedation for comfort is moral. Second, the death of the patient may be a foreseen consequence but is not the intended consequence; only pain relief is intended. Third, the relief of pain does not require the death of the patient to be effective. Fourth, there is no reasonable alternative. And fifth, the act is performed for a proportionately serious reason, namely preventing suffering.[118] The patient's informed consent or that of a surrogate decision maker is necessary.

The technical details of administering palliative sedation have been reviewed.[119] Some patients can achieve comfort during light sedation; others require heavy sedation to the point of full unconsciousness. Palliative sedation is often used during the withdrawal of life-sustaining therapy, especially when withdrawing ventilator-dependent patients from the ventilator.[120] It may be necessary also as the only effective palliative measure in some patients with intractable pain.

However, it is unnecessary and undesirable to prescribe palliative sedation when lesser degrees of sedation are sufficient to provide symptom relief. Some physicians have performed active euthanasia under a guise of palliative sedation (see chapter 9) when doing so was unnecessary for palliative care. In addition to its illegality, such an act is not morally justified by the principle of double effect because the intended consequence is to kill the patient and there are alternatives available for palliative care that do not require killing. One reason palliative sedation remains controversial is that some physicians have used it as an excuse for active euthanasia rather than as an appropriate element of palliative care.

Another controversy in palliative sedation surrounds the use of neuromuscular blocking drugs to contribute to palliative care when removing patients from ventilators after they or their surrogates have refused life-sustaining therapy on their behalf. A patient treated with neuromuscular blockade cannot breathe and will quickly die, creating a situation that can be plausibly construed as active euthanasia irrespective of intent. In a balanced analysis, Robert Truog and colleagues concluded that neuromuscular blocking drugs should not be introduced at the time of removal from the ventilator and usually should be discontinued upon withdrawal of the ventilator. The only exception is when the death is expected to be rapid and certain, regardless of the presence of neuromuscular blocking drugs, and when the burdens to the patient and family of waiting for the drugs to wear off before extubation are greater than the potential benefits.[121]

The separation of palliative sedation from euthanasia involves examining three factors: (1) the intent of treatment; (2) the drugs prescribed; and (3) the dosages administered. In palliative sedation, the intent should be to provide comfort, not to kill the patient. The drugs prescribed should be those with accepted palliative indications, such as opioids, benzodiazepines, and barbiturates, and not neuromuscular blocking drugs which lack a palliative purpose. The dosages administered should be those appropriate for palliative purposes and not excessively higher dosages. Seemingly high dosages of opioid and benzodiazepine drugs may be necessary for patients who have become tolerant to these agents as a result of previous usage.[122] If physicians prescribe drugs without known palliative indications, or drugs with known palliative indications at dosages exceeding those necessary for palliation, a plausible claim of active euthanasia can be made.[123] Physicians considering prescribing palliative sedation should follow published practice guidelines.[124]

LEGAL ISSUES

Strong legal support for palliative care in America was voiced by the justices in the U.S. Supreme Court *Cruzan* decision in 1990.[125] Although the principal broad ruling of the

Cruzan court was the finding of a constitutionally protected right of all citizens to refuse life-sustaining therapy, including artificial hydration and nutrition, the court also strongly endorsed the benefit of palliative treatment of the dying patient. It clarified that medications given to reduce pain and suffering were not euthanasia or physician-assisted suicide. Of course, if a physician were to prescribe an unnecessarily large dose of opiates, benzodiazepines, or barbiturates for the express purpose of killing a patient, a plausible case could be made that the act qualified as active euthanasia. As discussed in chapter 9, such an act may be considered criminal homicide. Assuming that the medications and their prescribed dosages are appropriate for symptom palliation, palliative sedation is a lawful practice.[126]

Prescription laws are a well-known legal obstacle for providing adequate analgesia. Legal and regulatory policies governing controlled substances attempt to prevent diversion of the substances for illegal purposes. Laws requiring triplicate prescriptions have been implemented in some jurisdictions to help law enforcement authorities monitor the usage of controlled substances. Physicians practicing in these jurisdictions must submit one copy of each opiate prescription to the state Drug Enforcement Agency (DEA) office. Irrespective of the criminal law merits of this regulation, it clearly has had a dampening effect upon the prescribing patterns of physicians because of their understandable fear that they could become the subject of a criminal investigation if the local DEA officer suspects they have been over-prescribing opioid drugs.[127] There is evidence that such laws contribute to physicians' practices of widespread opioid under-treatment of pain in cancer outpatients.[128]

Physician attitudes have been surveyed regarding legal constraints on palliative care. Oncologists clearly believe that triplicate prescription regulations impair the provision of palliative care of cancer patients.[129] Many neurologists remain confused about legal issues in palliative care. For example, in a survey of American neurologist members of the American Academy of Neurology, 38% of respondents wrongly believed that it was illegal to prescribe pain killers in doses that risk respiratory depression to the point of death and 40% wrongly believed that treating a dying ALS patient with morphine sufficient to decrease respiratory drive was euthanasia.[130]

In a similar vein, Alan Meisel and colleagues identified seven alleged "legal barriers" to end-of-life care that actually were only myths and misunderstandings by physicians about how the legal system governs patient care and decision making. They found the following myths: (1) that physicians must know the actual wishes of incompetent patients before acting; (2) that withholding or withdrawing AHN is illegal; (3) that risk management personnel must be contacted before withdrawing LST; (4) that advance directives must be executed on specific forms and oral directives are unenforceable; (5) that if a physician prescribes medication to treat discomfort and the patient dies, the physician will be criminally prosecuted; (6) that there are no legally permissible options to ease suffering if palliative care fails; and (7) that the 1997 U.S. Supreme Court decision (discussed in chapter 9) outlawed physician-assisted suicide.[131] Because some of these myths were based on "grains of truth," the importance of improving physician education in the legal dimensions of end-of-life care is obvious.

Physicians are not alone in their ignorance of law governing decisions at the end of life: patients are equally ignorant. In a recent study of 1,000 terminally ill outpatients, Silveira and colleagues found that 69% correctly understood the legality of refusal of LST, but only 46% understood the legality of withdrawal of LST, 32% understood the legality of euthanasia, and 23% understood the legality of assisted suicide.[132] Educating patients on the legality of end-of-life options is another necessary step to help implement effective palliative care.

Criminal charges have infrequently been brought against physicians for palliative treatment. There have been several reported cases in which physicians were charged with homicide (euthanasia) for allegedly administering excessive dosages of opioid or benzodiazepine drugs to dying patients.[133] As in the palliative sedation issue discussed earlier, the separation of proper palliative care from euthanasia in such cases turns on two technical questions: (1) Were the administered drugs appropriate for palliative purposes? (2) Were the dosages administered appropriate for palliative purposes? If appropriate drugs were given in appropriate dosages, proper palliative care was given. If drugs were administered with no known palliative purposes (such as neuromuscular blocking drugs) or if the dosages of appropriate drugs such as opioids were ordered far in excess of those necessary for palliative purposes, a plausible claim of euthanasia may be sustained. In general, physicians will be well protected if they practice within the proper standards of medical care and medical practice guidelines established for palliative care of the dying patient.[134]

NOTES

1. Lynn J. Living long in fragile health: the new demographics shape end of life care. *Hastings Cent Rep Special Report* 2005;35(6):S14–S18. In the United States in 2005, life expectancy from birth was 75 years for men and 80 years for women. There also has been an increase in life expectancy at age 65, which in 2005 was 17 years for men and 20 years for women. See National Center for Health Statistics. *Health, United States 2005 with Chartbook on Trends in the Health of Americans.* Hyattsville, MD, 2005.

2. National Academy of Sciences Institute of Medicine. *Approaching Death: Improving Care at the End of Life.* Washington, DC: National Academy Press, 1997:33–49.

3. *Approaching Death*: 39–41. However, there is variability of these rates in different parts of the United States. In Oregon, for example, only 31% of deaths occur in the hospital. See Tolle SW, Rosenfeld AG, Tilden VP, Park Y. Oregon's low in-hospital death rates: what determines where people die and satisfaction with decisions on place of death. *Ann Intern Med* 1999;130:681–685.

4. These data are described in Aaron HJ, Schwartz WB. Rationing health care: the choice before us. *Science* 1990;247:418–422. The reasons for the American technological imperative in diagnosis and treatment are discussed in Nahm FKD. Neurology, technology, and the diagnostic imperative. *Perspectives Biol Med* 2001;44:99–1207 and Cassell EJ. The sorcerer's broom: medicine's rampant technology. *Hastings Cent Rep* 1993; 23(6):32–39.

5. Gruman GJ. Ethics of death and dying: historical perspective. *Omega* 1978;9:203–237.

6. Callahan D. Frustrated mastery: the cultural context of death in America. *West J Med* 1995;163:226–230.

7. Kubler-Ross E. *On Death and Dying.* New York: Macmillan, 1969. A recent empirical study on grief rebutted the stages asserted by Kubler-Ross and found that acceptance was a common initial reaction and that yearning remained present for many years. See Maciejewski PK, Zhang B, Block S, Prigerson HG. An empirical examination of the stage theory of grief. *JAMA* 2007;297:716–723.

8. Burt RA. *Death is That Man Taking Names: Intersections of American Medicine, Law, and Culture.* Berkley, CA: University of California Press, 2002.

9. The term "medicalization" of death was coined in Aries P. *The Hour of Our Death.* New York: Vintage Books, 1981 and explained in McCue JD. The naturalness of dying. *JAMA* 1995;273:1039–1043.

10. For example, a recent study showed a much greater percentage of children with complex chronic conditions who now die at home than was the case 14 years previously. See Feudtner C, Feinstein JA, Satchell M, Zhao H, Kang TI. Shifting place of death among children with complex chronic conditions in the United States, 1989–2003. *JAMA* 2007;297:2725–2732

11. Seidlitz L, Duberstein PR, Cox C, Conwell Y. Attitudes of older people to suicide and assisted suicide: an analysis of Gallop Poll findings. *J Am Geriatr Soc* 1995;43:993–998.

12. Fried TR, van Doorn C, O'Leary JR, Tinetti ME, Drickamer MA. Older persons' preferences for site of terminal care. *Ann Intern Med* 1999;131:109–112.

13. Teno JM, Clarridge BR, Casey V, et al. Family perspectives on end-of-life care at the last place of care. *JAMA* 2004;291:88–93.

14. Hanson LC, Ersek M. Meeting palliative care needs in post-acute care settings. "To help them live until they die." *JAMA* 2006;295:681–686.

15. Kaufman SR . . . *And a Time to Die. How American Hospitals Shape the End of Life.* New York: Scribner, 2005. Portions of this paragraph were modified from my review of this book in *N Engl J Med* 2005;352: 1500–1501.

16. My colleagues and I summarized several of the studies on the physiology of death and the effects of dehydration in Bernat JL, Mogielnicki RP, Gert B. Patient refusal of hydration and nutrition: an alternative to physician-assisted suicide or voluntary active euthanasia. *Arch Intern Med* 1993;153:2723–2728.

17. See, for example, Miller RJ, Albright PG. What is the role of nutritional support and hydration in terminal cancer patients? *Am J Hospice Care* 1989;6:33–38 and Lichter J. The last 48 hours of life. *J Palliat Care* 1990;6:7–15.

18. For example, see the description of mouth care in Waller A, Caroline NL. *Handbook of Palliative Care in Cancer*, 2nd ed. Boston: Butterworth-Heinemann, 2000:135–148.

19. For studies of dying in hospitals, see Mogielnicki RP, Nelson WA, Dulca J. A study of the dying process in elderly hospitalized males. *J Cancer Ed* 1990;5:135–145 and Goodlin SJ, Winzelberg GS, Teno JM, Whedon M, Lynn J. Death in the hospital. *Arch Intern Med* 1998;158:1570–1572. For medical case reports of "bad deaths," see Morrison RS, Meier DE, Cassell CK. When too much is too little. *N Engl J Med* 1996;335:1755–1759 and Quill TE. You promised me I wouldn't die like this! Bad death as a medical emergency. *Arch Intern Med* 1995;155:1250–1254. Data from the widely publicized SUPPORT study, showing many of the shortcomings of the treatment of hospitalized critically ill and dying patients, are discussed in chapter 8.

20. See, for example, Hansot E. A letter from a patient's daughter. *Ann Intern Med* 1996;125:149–151. The experience of dying recorded in literature was reviewed in Bone RC. As I was dying: an examination of classic literature and dying. *Ann Intern Med* 1996;124:1091–1093.

21. Ramnarayan P, Craig F, Petros A, Pierce C. Characteristics of deaths occurring in hospitalised children: changing trends. *J Med Ethics* 2007;33:255–260. This study of 1127 childhood deaths occurring in hospitals in the UK found that 86% took place in ICUs with a significant increase in the percentage dying in ICUs over the 7-year study period (80% in 1998 to 91% in 2004). It is unclear if similar findings are present in the United States.

22. Steinhauser KE, Clipp EC, McNeilly M, Christakis NA, McIntyre LM, Tulsky JA. In search of a good death: observations of patients, families, and providers. *Ann Intern Med* 2000;132:825–832. For a related publication of these data, see Steinhauser KE, Christakis NA, Clipp EC, McNeilly M, McIntyre L, Tulsky JA. Factors considered important at the end of life by patients, family, physicians, and other care providers. *JAMA* 2000;284:2476–2482.

23. Callahan D. Pursuing a peaceful death. *Hastings Cent Rep* 1993;23(4):33–38. This topic also is discussed at length in Byock I. *Dying Well: The Prospect for Growth at the End of Life.* New York: Riverhead Books, 1997.

24. Vig EK, Pearlman RA. Good and bad dying from the perspective of terminally ill men. *Arch Intern Med* 2004;164:977–981.

25. Osler W. *Science and Immortality.* New York: Riverside Press, 1908. For a full account of Osler's attitudes about death, see Hinohara S. Sir William Osler's philosophy on death. *Ann Intern Med* 1993;118:638–642.

26. The distressingly small number of pages in leading internal medicine and neurology textbooks dedicated to the management of the dying patients was quantified in Carron AT, Lynn J, Keaney P. End-of-life care in medical textbooks. *Ann Intern Med* 1999;130:82086 and Rabow MW, Fair JM, Hardie GE, McPhee SJ. An evaluation of the end-of-life care content in leading neurology textbooks. *Neurology* 2000;55:893–894.

27. Mast KR, Salama M, Silverman GK, Arnold RM. End-of-life content in treatment guidelines for life-limiting diseases. *J Palliat Med* 2004;7:754–773.

28. Parker RA. Caring for patients at the end of life: reflections after 12 years of practice. *Ann Intern Med* 2002;136:72–75.

29. Fromme E, Billings JA. Care of the dying doctor. On the other end of the stethoscope. *JAMA* 2003; 290:2048–2055.

30. Clark D. Religion, medicine, and community in the early origins of St. Christopher's Hospice. *J Palliat Med* 2001;4:353–360.

31. Rhymes J. Hospice care in America. *JAMA* 1990;264:369–372.

32. The National Hospice and Palliative Care Organization has published criteria for determining prognosis in patients with selected non-cancer diseases. See the table in Lynn J. Serving patients who may die soon and their families: the role of hospice and other services. *JAMA* 2001;285:925–932.

33. Christakis NA, Escarce JJ. Survival of Medicare patients after enrollment in hospice programs. *N Engl J Med* 1996;335:172–178.

34. Kaur JS. Palliative care and hospice programs. *Mayo Clin Proc* 2000;75:181–184.

35. Foley KM. The past and future of palliative care. *Hastings Cent Rep Special Report* 2005;35(6):S42–S46. For a current review of hospice programs, eligibility, rules, and care, see Gazelle G. Understanding hospice—an underutilized option for life's final chapter. *N Engl J Med* 2007;357:321–327.

36. Foley KM. *Hastings Cent Rep Special Report* 2005;35(6):S42–S46.

37. Byock I. Hospice and palliative care: a parting of ways or a path to the future? *J Palliat Med* 1998; 1:165–176.

38. For discussions on how palliative medicine has been applied to specific diseases in neurology, see Voltz R, Bernat JL, Borasio GD, Maddocks I, Oliver D, Portenoy RK (eds). *Palliative Care in Neurology*. Oxford: Oxford University Press, 2004.

39. Jacobson PL, Mann JD. Evolving role of the neurologist in the diagnosis and treatment of chronic non-cancer pain. *Mayo Clin Proc* 2003;78:80–84.

40. American Academy of Neurology Ethics, Law & Humanities Committee. Ethical considerations for neurologists in the management of chronic pain. *Neurology* 2001;57:2166–2167.

41. For a brief, authoritative review of palliative medicine, see Morrison RS, Meier DE. Palliative care. *N Engl J Med* 2004;350:2582–2590.

42. The most comprehensive textbook of palliative medicine is Doyle D, Hanks G, Cherny N, Calman K (eds). *Oxford Textbook of Palliative Medicine*, 3rd ed. Oxford: Oxford University Press, 2005. See also Foley KM, Back A, Bruera E, Coyle N, Loscalzo MJ, Shuster JL, Teschendorf B, Von Roenn JH (eds). *When the Focus is on Care: Palliative Care and Cancer*. Atlanta, GA: American Cancer Society, 2005.

43. Four of the journals are listed in the *Index Medicus*. They are *Palliative Medicine*, the *Journal of Palliative Care*, *The American Journal of Hospice and Palliative Care*, and the *Journal of Pain and Symptom Management*.

44. Billings JA, Block S. Palliative care in undergraduate medical education: status report and future directions. *JAMA* 1997;278:733–738.

45. Borasio GD, Doyle D (eds). Proceedings of the satellite symposium "Palliative Care in Neurology." *J Neurol* 1997;244(Suppl 4):S1–S29.

46. Carver AC, Foley KM (eds). Palliative care in neurology. *Neurol Clin* 2001;19(4).

47. Voltz R, Bernat JL, Borasio GD, Maddocks I, Oliver D, Portenoy RK (eds). *Palliative Care in Neurology*. Oxford: Oxford University Press, 2004.

48. Education in Palliative and End-of-Life Care. http://www.epec.net/EPEC/Webpages/index.cfm (Accessed June 9, 2007).

49. End of Life/Palliative Education Resource Center http://www.eperc.mcw.edu/ (Accessed June 9, 2007) and Center to Advance Palliative Care http://www.capc.org/ (Accessed Jun 9, 2007).

50. World Health Organization. *Cancer Pain Relief and Palliative Care*. WHO Technical Report Series 804. Geneva: World Health Organization, 1990:11.

51. MacDonald N. Palliative care—the fourth phase of cancer prevention. *Cancer Detect Prev* 1991;3:253–255.

52. Foley KM. The past and future of palliative care. *Hastings Cent Rep Special Report* 2005;35(6):S42–S46.

53. For an example of how the practice of palliative medicine applies to the care of non-terminally-ill older adults with chronic medical problems, see Boockvar KS, Meier. Palliative care for frail older adults. "There are things I can't do anymore that I wish I could . . ." *JAMA* 2006;296:2245–2253.

54. American Academy of Neurology Ethics and Humanities Subcommittee. Palliative care in neurology. *Neurology* 1996;46:870–872.

55. Fox E. Predominance of the curative model of medical care: a residual problem. *JAMA* 1997; 278:761–763. See also Jecker NS, Self DJ. Separating care and cure: an analysis of historical and contemporary images of nursing and medicine. *J Med Philosophy* 1991;16:285–306.

56. Portenoy RK, Sibirceva U, Smout R, et al. Opioid use and survival at the end of life: a survey of a hospice population. *J Pain Symptom Manage* 2006;32:532–540 and Sykes N, Thorns A. The use of opioids and sedatives at the end of life. *Lancet Oncol* 2003;4:312–318. A recent study showed no respiratory suppression in cancer patients receiving parenteral opioid therapy. See Estfan B, Mahmoud F, Shaheen P, et al. Respiratory function during parenteral opioid titration for cancer pain. *Palliative Med* 2007;21:81–86.

56a. Wood GJ, Shega JW, Lynch B, Von Roenn JH. Management of intractable nausea and vomiting in patients at the end of life: "I was feeling nauseous all of the time . . . nothing was working." *JAMA* 2007; 298:1196–1207.

57. Luce JM, Luce JA. Management of dyspnea in patients with far-advanced lung disease. "Once I lose it, it's kind of hard to catch it . . ." *JAMA* 2001;285;1331–1337.

58. Casarett DJ, Inouye SK. Diagnosis and management of delirium near the end of life. *Ann Intern Med* 2001;135:32–40.

59. Yennurajalingam S, Bruera E. Palliative management of fatigue at the close of life: "it feels like my body is just worn out." *JAMA* 2007;297:295–304.

60. For details of symptom management, see Doyle D, Hanks G, Cherny N, Calman K (eds). *Oxford Textbook of Palliative Medicine*, 3rd ed. Oxford: Oxford University Press, 2005.

61. Chochinov HM, Wilson KG, Enns M, Lander S. The prevalence of depression in the terminally ill: effects of diagnostic criteria and symptom threshold judgments. *Am J Psychiatry* 1994;151:537–540.

62. Kissane DW. The contribution of demoralization to end of life decisionmaking. *Hastings Cent Rep* 2004;34(4):21–31.

63. Block S, Billings JA. Patient requests for euthanasia and assisted suicide in terminal illness: the role of the psychiatrist. *Psychosomatics* 1995;36:445–457 and Breitbart W, Rosenfeld B, Pessin H, et al. Depression, hopelessness, and desire for hastened death in terminally ill patients with cancer. *JAMA* 2000;284:2907–2911.

64. A number of articles explored the spiritual dimensions of medical care in general and of the care of the dying patient in particular. Puchalski CM, Romer AL. Taking a patient's spiritual history allows clinicians to understand patients more fully. *J Palliat Med* 2000;30:40–47; Kuczewski MG. Talking about spirituality in the clinical setting: can being professional require being personal? *Am J Bioethics* 2007;7(7):4–11; Post SG, Puchalski CM, Larson DB. Physicians and patient spirituality: professional boundaries, competency, and ethics. *Ann Intern Med* 2000;132:578–583; Daaleman TP. Placing religion and spirituality in end-of-life care. *JAMA* 2000;284:2514–2517. One study found a positive correlation between ALS patients' levels of spirituality and religion and their use of life support. Murphy PL, Albert SM, Weber CM, Del Bene ML, Rowland LP. Impact of spirituality and religiousness on outcomes in patients with ALS. *Neurology* 2000;55:1581–1584.

65. Block SD. Psychological considerations, growth, and transcendence at the end of life. The art of the possible. *JAMA* 2001;285:2898–2905.

66. Astrow AB, Puchalski CM, Sulmasy DP. Religion, spirituality, and health care: social, ethical, and practical considerations. *Am J Med* 2001;110:283–287.

67. Cassell EJ. *The Nature of Suffering and the Goals of Medicine.* New York: Oxford University Press, 1991:30–65. Examples of suffering in dying patients caused by existential distress, including problems involving the meaning of life, human relations, personal autonomy, guilt, and human dignity, were described in Bolmsö I. Existential issues in palliative care? interviews with cancer patients. *J Palliat Care* 2000;16(2):20–24. The author emphasized the importance of permitting dying patients to discuss these issues with someone to help relieve their existential suffering.

68. Portenoy RK, Thaler HT, Kornblith AB, et al. Symptom prevalence, characteristics, and distress in a cancer population. *Qual Life Res* 1994;3:183–189.

69. Chochinov HM. Dignity-conserving care–a new model for palliative care. Helping the patient feel valued. *JAMA* 2002;287:2253–2260.

70. Chochinov HM, Hack T, Hassard T, Kristjanson LJ, McClement S, Harlos M. Dignity in the terminally ill: a cross-sectional, cohort study. *Lancet* 2002;360:2026–2030.

71. Blinderman CD, Cherny NI. Existential issues do not necessarily result in existential suffering: lesson from cancer patients in Israel. *Palliative Med* 2005;19:371–380.

72. Waller A, Caroline NL. *Handbook of Palliative Care in Cancer*, 2nd ed. Boston: Butterworth-Heinemann, 2000:xxi–xxii. For a review of the management of bereavement, see Casarett D, Kutner JS, Abrahm J. Life after death: a practical approach to grief and bereavement. *Ann Intern Med* 2001;134:208–215 and Prigereson HG, Jacobs SC. Caring for bereaved patients. "All the doctors just suddenly go." *JAMA* 2001;286:1369–1376.

73. Emanuel EJ, Fairclough DL, Slutsman J, Alpert H, Baldwin D, Emanuel LL. Assistance from family members, friends, paid caregivers, and volunteers in the care of terminally ill patients. *N Engl J Med* 1999;341:956–963.

74. Rabow MW, Hauser JM, Adams J. Supporting family caregivers at the end of life. "They don't know what they don't know." *JAMA* 2004;291:483–491. Similar findings were reported in Wolff JL, Dy SM, Frick KD, Kasper JD. End-of-life care: findings from a national survey of informal caregivers. *Arch Intern Med* 2007;167:40–46.

75. For communication strategies, see Larson DG, Tobin DR. End-of-life conversations: evolving practice and theory. *JAMA* 2000;284:1573–1578; Quill TE. Initiating end-of-life discussions with seriously ill patients: addressing the "elephant in the room." *JAMA* 2000;284:2502–2507; and von Guten CF, Ferris FD, Emanuel LL. Ensuring competency in end-of-life care: communication and relational skills. JAMA 2000;284:3051–3057.

76. Lo B, Quill T, Tulsky J, et al. Discussing palliative care with patients. *Ann Intern Med* 1999;130:744–749.

77. Detmar SB, Muller MJ, Wever LDV, Schornagel JH, Aaronson NK. Patient-physician communication during outpatient palliative treatment visits: an observational study. *JAMA* 2001;285:1351–1357.

78. Wenrich MD, Curtis JR, Shannon SE, Carline JD, Ambrozy DM, Ramsey PG. Communicating with dying patients within the spectrum of medical care from terminal diagnosis to death. *Arch Intern Med* 2001; 161:868–874. The role of nurses is helping dying patients achieve the balance of hope and reality was discussed in Murray MA, Miller T, Fiset V, O'Connor A, Jacobsen MJ. Decision support: helping patients and families to find a balance at the end of life. *Int J Palliat Nurs* 2004;10:270–277.

79. Back AL, Arnold RM, Quill TE. Hope for the best, and prepare for the worst. *Ann Intern Med* 2003; 138:439–443.

80. Back AL, Arnold RM, Tulsky JA, Baie WF, Fryer-Edwards KA. On saying goodbye: acknowledging the end of the patient-physician relationship with patients who are near death. *Ann Intern Med* 2005;142:682–685. The value of saying goodbye is illustrated beautifully in Byock I. *The Four Things That Matter Most: A Book about Living.* New York: Free Press, 2004:173–216.

81. Lynn J. Serving patients who may die soon and their families: the role of hospice and other services. *JAMA* 2001;285:925–932.

82. Gillick MR. A broader role for advance medical planning. *Ann Intern Med* 1995;123:621–624 and Miles SH, Koepp R, Weber EP. Advance end-of-life treatment planning: a research review. *Arch Intern Med* 1996; 156:1062–1068. Access to palliative care and hospice among nursing home residents may be limited. See Zerzan J, Stearns S, Hanson L. Access to palliative care and hospice in nursing homes. *JAMA* 2000;284: 2489–2494.

83. Hallenbeck J. Palliative care in the final days of life. "They were expecting it at any time." *JAMA* 2005; 293:2265–2271.

84. For an example of an inpatient palliative care order page, see O'Toole EE, Youngner SJ, Juknialis BW, Daly B, Bartlett ET, Landefeld CS. Evaluation of a treatment limitation policy with a specific treatment-limiting order page. *Arch Intern Med* 1994;154:425–432.

85. Weissman DE. Decision making at a time of crisis near the end of life. *JAMA* 2004;292:1738–1743.

86. Pellegrino ED. Emerging ethical issues in palliative care. *JAMA* 1998;279;1521–1522.

87. Cassel CK, Foley KM. *Principles for Care of Patients at the End of Life: An Emerging Consensus among the Specialties of Medicine.* New York: Milbank Memorial Fund, 1999.

88. For an early report on such a service, see Carlson RW, Devich L, Frank RR. Development of a comprehensive supportive care team for the hopelessly ill on a university hospital medical service. *JAMA* 1988; 259:378–383.

89. O'Toole EE, Youngner SJ, Juknialis BW, Daly B, Bartlett ET, Landefeld CS. Evaluation of a treatment limitation policy with a specific treatment-limiting order page. *Arch Intern Med* 1994;154:425–432.

90. Miller KG, Fins JJ. A proposal to restructure hospital care for dying patients. *N Engl J Med* 1996; 334:1740–1742.

91. Cassel CK, Vladeck BC. ICD-9 code for palliative or terminal care. *N Engl J Med* 1996;335:1232–1234.

92. Bascom PB. A hospital-based comfort care team: consultation for seriously ill and dying patients. *Am J Hospice Palliat Care* 1997(March/April):57–60.

93. Morrison RS, Maroney-Galin C, Kralovec PD, Meier DE. The growth of palliative care programs in United States Hospitals. *J Palliat Med* 2005;8:1127–1134.

94. Himelstein BP, Hilden JM, Boldt AM, Weissman D. Pediatric palliative care. *N Engl J Med* 2004;350: 1752–1762.

95. Goldman A. ABC of palliative care: special problems of children. *Br Med J* 1998;316:49–52.

96. Wolfe J, Grier HE, Klar N, et al. Symptoms and suffering at the end of life in children with cancer. *N Engl J Med* 2000;342:326–333.

97. Wolfe J. Suffering in children at the end of life: recognizing an ethical duty to palliate. *J Clin Ethics* 2000;11:157–163 and Walco GA, Cassidy RC, Schechter NL. Pain, hurt, and harm: the ethics of pain control in infants and children. *N Engl J Med* 1994;331:541–544.

98. Morgan ER, Murphy SB. Care of children who are dying of cancer. *N Engl J Med* 2000;342:347–348. See also Frager G. Pediatric palliative care: building the model, bridging the gap. *J Palliat Care* 1996;12:9–12.

99. Wolfe J, Klar N, Grier HE. Understanding of prognosis among parents of children who died of cancer: impact on treatment goals and integration of palliative care. *JAMA* 2000;284:2469–2475.

100. Wass H. Concepts of death: a developmental perspective. In, Wass H, Corr CA (eds). *Childhood and Death.* Washington, DC: Hemisphere Publishing, 1984.

101. Hurwitz CA, Duncan J, Wolfe J. Caring for the child with cancer at the close of life. "There are people who make it, and I'm hoping I'm one of them." *JAMA* 2004; 292:2141–2149.

102. Kreicbergs U, Valdimarsdóttir U, Onelöv E, Henter J-I, Steineck G. Talking about death with children who have severe malignant disease. *N Engl J Med* 2004;351:1175–1186.

103. Wolfe L. Should parents speak with a dying child about impending death? *N Engl J Med* 2004; 351:1251–1253.

104. A detailed account of the elements of pediatric palliative care was presented in Himelstein BP, Hilden JM, Boldt AM, Weissman D. Pediatric palliative care. *N Engl J Med* 2004;350:1752–1762.

105. For a few examples, see American Medical Association Council on Scientific Affairs. Good care of the dying patient. *JAMA* 1996;275:474–478; Sachs GA, Ahronheim JC, Rhymes JA, Volicer L, Lynn L. Good care of dying patients: the alternative to physician-assisted suicide and euthanasia. *J Am Geriatr Soc* 1995; 43:553–562; American Academy of Neurology Ethics and Humanities Subcommittee. Palliative care in neurology. *Neurology* 1996;46:870–872; and Bernat JL, Goldstein ML, Viste KM Jr. The neurologist and the dying patient. *Neurology* 1996;46:598–599.

106. These studies are summarized in American Medical Association Council on Scientific Affairs. Good care of the dying patient. *JAMA* 1996;275:474–478 and in McCue JD. The naturalness of dying. *JAMA* 1995;273:1039–1043. See also the analysis of the SUPPORT study discussed in chapter 8.

107. For a collection of essays addressing the barriers to improving palliative care, see Jennings B, Kaebnick GE, Murray TH (eds). Improving end of life care: why has it been so difficult? *Hastings Cent Rep Special Report* 2005;35(6):S1–S60.

108. Meier DE, Morrison RS, Cassel CK. Improving palliative care. *Ann Intern Med* 1997;127:225–230.

109. Casarett DJ, Quill TE. "I'm not ready for hospice": strategies for timely and effective hospice discussions. *Ann Intern Med* 2007;146:443–449.

110. For example, see Singer PA, Martin DK, Kelner M. Quality end-of-life care: patient perspectives. *JAMA* 1999;281:163–168; American Pain Society Quality Care Committee. Quality improvement guidelines for the treatment of acute pain and cancer pain. *JAMA* 1995; 274:1874–1880; and Latimer E. Auditing the hospital care of dying patients. *J Palliat Care* 1991;7:12–17.

111. Wenger NS, Rosenfeld K. Quality indicators for end-of-life care in vulnerable elders. *Ann Intern Med* 2001;135:677–685.

112. Lynn J, Nolan K, Kabcenell A, Weissman D, Milne C, Berwick DM. Reforming care for persons near the end of life: the promise of quality improvement. *Ann Intern Med* 2002;137:117–122.

113. Murray TH, Jennings B. The quest to reform end of life care: rethinking assumptions and setting new directions. *Hastings Cent Rep Special Report* 2005;35(6):S52–S57.

114. The legal and regulatory barriers to the effective treatment of pain were addressed in a special edition of the *Journal of Law Medicine and Ethics*. See Symposium: appropriate management of pain: addressing the clinical, legal, and regulatory barriers. *J Law Med Ethics* 1996;24:285–364.

115. Wennberg JE, Fisher ES, Stukel TA, Skinner JS, Sharp SM, Bronner KK. Use of hospitals, physician visits, and hospice during the last six months of life among cohorts loyal to highly respected hospitals in the United States. *BMJ* 2004;328:607–610.

116. For reviews of palliative sedation, see Smith GP II. Terminal sedation as palliative care: revalidating a right to the good death. *Camb Q Healthc Ethics* 1998;7:382–387; Rousseau P. Terminal sedation in the care of dying patients. *Arch Intern Med* 1996;156:1785–1786; Quill TE, Byock IR. Responding to intractable terminal suffering: the role of terminal sedation and voluntary refusal of food and fluids. *Ann Intern Med* 2000;132:408–414; and National Ethics Committee, Veterans Health Administration. The ethics of palliative sedation as a therapy of last resort. *Am J Hosp Palliat Med* 2007;23:483–491.

117. The vexing decision between treating pain and accelerating death in palliave sedation has been called "the devil's choice." See Magnusson RS. The devil's choice: re-thinking law, ethics, and symptom relief in palliative care. *J law Med Ethics* 2006;559–569.

118. Sulmasy DP. The use and abuse of the principle of double effect. *Clin Pract* 1996;3:86–90.

119. Truog RD, Berde CB, Mitchell C, Grier HE. Barbiturates in the terminally ill. *N Engl J Med* 1992;327:1678–1682 and Cherny NI, Portnoy RK. Sedation in the management of refractory symptoms: guidelines for evaluation and treatment. *J Palliat Care* 1994;10:31–38.

120. Brody H, Campbell ML, Faber-Langendoen K, Ogle KS. Withdrawing intensive life-sustaining treatment—recommendations for compassionate clinical management. *N Engl J Med* 1997;336:652–657 and Wilson WC, Smedira NG, Fink C, McDowell JA, Luce JM. Ordering and administration of sedatives and analgesics during the withholding and withdrawal of life support from critically ill patients. *JAMA* 1992;267:949–953. See chapter 8 for further discussion of management of the patient being withdrawn from life-sustaining therapy.

121. Truog RD, Burns JP, Mitchell C, Johnson J, Robinson W. Pharmacologic paralysis and withdrawal of mechanical ventilation at the end of life. *N Engl J Med* 2000;342:508–511.

122. Lo B, Rubenfeld G. Palliative sedation in dying patients. "We turn to it when everything else hasn't worked." *JAMA* 2005;294:1810–1816.

123. The distinction between palliative sedation and voluntary active euthanasia has been most extensively blurred in the Netherlands where voluntary active euthanasia is legally permissible. Dutch physicians state that their clear intent in giving palliative sedation is to hasten death. See Rietjens JAC, van der Heide A, Vrakking AM, Ontwuteaka-Philipsen BD, van der Mass PJ, van der Wal G. Physician reports of terminal sedation without hydration or nutrition for patients nearing death in the Netherlands. *Ann Intern Med* 2004;141:178–185. Dutch euthanasia practices are considered further in chapter 9.

124. See, for example, Rousseau PC. Palliative sedation. *Am J Hospice Palliat* Care 2002;19:295–297 and Lo B, Rubenfeld G. Palliative sedation in dying patients. *JAMA* 2005;294:1810–1816.

125. *Cruzan v. Director, Missouri Department of Health*, 497 US 261, 268 (1990). This ruling is discussed further in chapter 8.

126. The legal basis for the conclusion "Terminal sedation is a legally justifiable practice, supported by established jurisprudence" is presented in McStay R. Terminal sedation: palliative care for intractable pain, post *Glucksberg* and *Quill. Am J Law Med* 2003;29:45–76.

127. For an account of how regulatory reform of controlled substance law could improve palliative care, see Hyman CS. Pain management and disciplinary action: how medical boards can remove barriers to effective treatment. *J Law Med Ethics* 1996;24:338–343 and Joranson DE, Gilson AM. Improving pain management through policy making and education for medical regulators. *J Law Med Ethics* 1996;24:344–347.

128. Cooper JR, Czechowicz DJ, Petersen RC, Molinari SP. Prescription drug diversion control and medical practice. *JAMA* 1992;268:1306–1310.

129. von Roenn JH, Cleeland CS, Gonin R, et al. Physician attitudes and practice in cancer pain management: a survey from the Eastern Cooperative Oncology Group. *Ann Intern Med* 1993;119:121–126.

130. Carver AC, Vickrey BG, Bernat JL, Keran C, Ringel SP, Foley KM. End of life care: a survey of U.S. neurologists' attitudes, behavior, and knowledge. *Neurology* 1999;53:284–293.

131. Meisel A, Snyder L, Quill T. Seven legal barriers to end-of-life care: myths, realities, and grains of truth. *JAMA* 2000;284;2495–2501.

132. Silveira MJ, DiPiero A, Gerrity MS, Feudtner C. Patients' knowledge of options at the end of life: ignorance in the face of death. *JAMA* 2000;284:2483–2488.

133. Alpers A. Criminal act or palliative care? Prosecutions involving the care of the dying. *J Law Med Ethics* 1998;26:308–331. The recent criminal homicide charges brought against Dr. Anna Maria Pou and two nurses who prescribed and administered intravenous morphine and midazolam to four dying patients in the evacuated and isolated hospital after hurricane Katrina struck New Orleans were discussed in Curiel TJ. Murder or mercy? Hurricane Katrina and the need for disaster training. *N Engl J Med* 2006; 355:2067–2069. In June 2007, the charges against the nurses were dropped. In August 2007, an Orleans Parish grand jury declined to indict Dr. Pou.

134. Pestaner JP. End-of-life care: forensic medicine v. palliative medicine. *J Law Med Ethics* 2003;31:365–376. For a review of international laws governing palliative and end-of-life care, see Mendelson D, Jost TS. A comparative study of the law of palliative care and end-of-life treatment. *J Law Med Ethics* 2003;31:130–143.

Refusal of Life-Sustaining Treatment

8

A defining characteristic of Western medicine over the past three decades is the formalization of the right of patients to refuse unwanted medical therapy including life-sustaining treatment (LST). In the United States, the decision to withhold or withdraw LST has evolved from being physician-centered to being patient-centered.[1] Until around 1990, the issue was conceptualized by defining those circumstances in which a physician was ethically and legally permitted to discontinue a patient's LST. Currently, however, the topic is conceptualized as informed refusal: the application of the doctrine of informed consent that permits all patients to refuse tests or treatments they wish to forego, even if they will die as a result of their refusal. In nearly every instance, the physician must discontinue the unwanted treatments, including LST, once a patient has validly refused them. Thus, it is no longer accurate to consider the topic as the physician-centered "termination of LST" but rather as the patient-centered "refusal of LST," acknowledging that the decision to forego LST ultimately is the patient's to make and, when valid, the physician's to carry out.

ETHICAL AND MEDICAL ISSUES

The ethical basis of the right to refuse LST arises from our respect of patients' autonomy and self-determination. Only patients ultimately know and are authorized to decide what treatments best satisfy their health values and goals. The doctrine of self-determination respects the fact that

values and goals of treatment may differ between physicians and patients, and may vary among patients. It is the patient's own values and goals of treatment that should be granted primacy.[2] The patient's ethical right to consent to or refuse therapy is not extinguished if the patient loses the cognitive or communicative capacity to make a medical decision. The right endures and is transferred to a surrogate decision maker to exercise on behalf of the patient.

The patient's right to refuse therapy is operationalized through the doctrine of informed consent, as explained in chapter 2. The criteria of informed refusal are identical with those of consent. First, adequate information— information that a reasonable person would need to know to be able to consent or refuse— must be conveyed by the physician to the patient. Patients deciding to accept or refuse LST need to know their diagnosis and prognosis, the available treatments, their likely beneficial and harmful effects and outcomes, the physician's treatment recommendation, and the reason for the recommendation. As is true in any consent discussion, consent is a process, not an event. Proper informed consent and refusal requires thoughtful dialogue that proceeds over time, ideally in a calm, unhurried environment, with the proper ambience for patients' and families' questions and fears to be adequately addressed.

Second, the patient should possess the cognitive and communicative capacities to understand, achieve, and communicate a decision to consent or refuse. Many critically ill and dying patients lack either the cognitive capacity to

171

provide consent or the ability to communicate a decision. If the patient lacks these capacities, the physician should conduct an identical conversation with the patient's lawful surrogate decision maker, a third party who has been granted the authority to consent or refuse on behalf of the patient. Informed consent or refusal becomes a more difficult process when the patient loses capacity because the physician and the surrogate both must attempt to divine and carry out the true wishes of the patient.

Third, although physicians are permitted to make strong treatment recommendations, they should not coerce patients or surrogates into accepting medical treatment. The line between a strong recommendation and coercion at times may be hard to draw. Physicians should not threaten patients or surrogates, not exaggerate facts, and not communicate nonfactual circumstances which no person reasonably could resist.[3]

The physician and the competent patient create a decision-making dyad in a process called shared decision making. In the shared decision-making model, the clinician contributes specialized knowledge, training, and experience regarding medical diagnosis, prognosis, and treatment options and their outcomes; the patient contributes a unique knowledge of personal values, preferences, and health-care goals. Together, they reach a mutually agreeable medical care plan that represents the best treatment for that patient. The shared decision-making model does not abdicate complete control of health-care decisions to patients; it merely acknowledges that only patients can define what treatment options ultimately are best for themselves.[4]

When the patient loses cognitive or communicative capacities, the patient's lawful surrogate decision maker joins the patient-physician dyad to form a decision-making triad. As discussed in chapter 4, there are accepted standards for surrogate decision making. The surrogate decision maker should strive faithfully to represent the wishes and values of the patient. First, the surrogate should communicate the expressed wishes of the patient, if known, including those in valid written advance directives.[5] If the patient's specific wishes are unknown, the surrogate should attempt to reproduce that decision the patient would have made, by employing the preferences and values of the patient using the doctrine of substituted judgment. If the surrogate does not know the values of the patient, the surrogate should balance the burdens and benefits of treatment to the patient and render a best interest judgment.[6]

Physicians should identify barriers to proper decision making and attempt to surmount them to enhance the quality of patients' and surrogates' decisions. A patient's desire no longer to be a burden to loved ones is a common motivation for refusing LST.[7] Many critically ill and dying patients experience potentially reversible degrees of depression that may influence their decisions to consent to or refuse LST. Not surprisingly, the presence of psychological distress, including depression, has been found to be responsible for decisions of dying patients to terminate LST and to request physician-assisted suicide.[8] The longer survival of non-depressed than depressed ALS patients is at least partially the result of the latter's earlier refusal of LST.[9] The question of whether severe depression invalidates a patient's refusal of LST is difficult because the severity of depression comprises a continuum and not all depressed dying patients are thinking irrationally when they wish to die sooner.[10] Physicians' diagnosis and treatment of reversible depression can improve the quality of life and decision making of terminally ill patients.[11]

Not all ostensibly rational decisions reached by patients or surrogates to continue or discontinue LST are completely rational. This fact imposes an ethical duty on physicians to try to identify sources of irrational thinking and to help correct them. Denial represents the principal irrational thought process of dying patients. The dying patient's acceptance of the inevitability of impending death takes time and can be assisted by compassionate counseling from physicians. It is often difficult for physicians to strike the ideal balance between maintaining hope and providing accurate prognostic information.[12] Physicians should try to understand and respond to patients' fears. Most patients need reassurance that they will not suffer and that their physician will loyally care for and not abandon them as they become sicker. Physicians also can reassure them that their treatment preferences and wishes will be carried out faithfully.

Some patients dying of neurological diseases continue to maintain intact cognition but suffer severe paralysis or other physical impairments that interfere with efficient communication. This is a common situation in the ALS patient as discussed in chapter 14. Neurologists should try to enhance patients' communication capacities to permit them to continue to participate maximally in clinical decisions. Assistance from occupational therapists trained in computer communications technology can be requested to design an efficient communication system.[13]

Many physicians express more difficulty stopping LST that already has been started than not providing LST in the first place because they conceptualize discontinuing ongoing LST as "killing" the patient. Although the psychological grounds for this difficulty are understandable because of the intuitive distinction between the omission and commission of an act, it is not a defensible ethical distinction. A broad consensus holds that there is no important ethical or legal difference between withholding and withdrawing LST. Once LST has been refused by a competent patient or by the lawful surrogate of an incompetent patient, physicians generally must not start it, or must stop it if it has been started.[14]

Do-Not-Resuscitate Orders

The earliest permissible withholding of life-sustaining treatment was the Do-Not-Resuscitate order. Closed-chest cardiopulmonary resuscitation (CPR) was described in 1960 as an emergency treatment designed to save the lives of patients who had suffered cardiopulmonary arrest.[15] Within a decade, CPR techniques had become standardized and were taught to physicians as a routine part of medical care. The American Heart Association and other groups helped teach CPR to laymen so they could initiate and continue the therapy until the patient with an out-of-hospital cardiac arrest reached medical attention.[16]

Hospitals organized resuscitation teams to respond rapidly to cardiac arrest "codes" in the hospital and perform CPR. By the late 1980s, it was estimated that CPR was being attempted on one-third of patients dying in American hospitals and on countless people who collapsed outside of hospitals.[17]

Cardiopulmonary resuscitation became routine medical treatment because of the obvious benefits of restoring heartbeat and breathing and thus rescuing the lives of patients suffering sudden cardiopulmonary arrest. The intent was to restore patients to their previous health. CPR was neither developed nor intended to prolong the lives of patients who were dying inexorably of terminal illness. Yet the routine, mandatory nature of performing CPR led physicians and others to perform it in a rote manner in instances of obvious terminal illness for which it was neither intended nor effective.

Beginning in the late 1960s, physicians became increasingly aware of the uselessness and undesirability of performing CPR on irreversibly dying patients. But because performing CPR had become obligatory treatment, physicians were required to attempt it when a patient suffered a cardiopulmonary arrest. The knowledge that CPR was futile in these cases led physicians to perform "slow codes" (half-hearted attempts to perform CPR), while realizing that it was ineffective and senseless. In these cases, the resuscitation team went through the motions of CPR out of a sense of obligation rather than from a belief that it would produce any therapeutic benefit to the patient or was appropriate.[18]

Thereafter, the concept was advanced that it was wrong to attempt CPR on all patients suffering cardiac arrest. Certain patients could be identified in advance who were clearly so ill and irreversibly dying that CPR would almost certainly fail. When physicians identified such patients upon admission to the hospital, or during a hospitalization, they could write Do-Not-Resuscitate (DNR) orders to prevent them from receiving futile and medically inappropriate CPR attempts. Some institutions preferred to call them Do-Not-Attempt-Resuscitation (DNAR) orders to clarify what the order actually signified.[19]

The drafting and implementation of hospital policies permitting physicians to formally write DNR orders lagged behind the need for these policies. In hospitals in which DNR orders were not permitted, physicians communicated the DNR decision verbally to nurses who then annotated the decision on the chart in pencil (thus permitting its easy erasure) or employed one of a series of other informal mechanisms to signify DNR status, such as noting the decision in chalk on a blackboard or placing a colored dot on the patient's medical record.[20] Not until a decade later had most hospitals implemented DNR policies permitting physicians to formally and openly write DNR orders.

Thereafter, the issue of providing explicit consent or refusal for CPR began to receive attention.[21] As is true in other instances of emergency medical care, consent for CPR is presumed. Currently, for cardiopulmonary arrests occurring in the hospital, CPR is performed by default unless there is a specific DNR order prohibiting it. Only competent patients and the lawful surrogate decision makers of incompetent patients can authorize physicians to write DNR orders. Unlike most treatments that require a patient or surrogate's valid consent to receive them, CPR requires a valid refusal or it will be performed automatically under the doctrine of presumed consent. This inversion of the consent process is responsible for some of the confusion and unique clinical-ethical issues of DNR orders. The special problems of DNR orders in children have been explored in ethical and legal detail.[22]

Patients who suffer out-of-hospital cardiac arrests have a 3% to 14% chance of survival to hospital discharge whereas patients who suffer in-hospital cardiac arrests have a 10% to 20% chance of survival to hospital discharge.[23] Embedded within these figures, however, are important variables: CPR success rates vary as a function of the type and severity of the patient's underlying illness. In two of the largest published studies of in-hospital CPR encompassing over 26,000 attempted cases, 16% of patients survived to be discharged from the hospital.[24] However, the 16% figure was a mean of all recovered cases including those for which the prior probability of CPR success was high and other cases for which it was low. For example, in two studies of CPR success rates, none of the patients with metastatic cancer, acute stroke, sepsis, or pneumonia on whom CPR was attempted survived to hospital discharge.[25] Similar finding have been observed in other studies.[26] There is a debate about whether advanced age is an independent risk factor for CPR success.[27]

In addition to survival as an end-point of CPR outcome studies, quality of life has been examined. Of those patients surviving hospital discharge after CPR, 93% were found to be alert and oriented, 11% to 44% had evidence of "neurologic impairment,"[28] and less than 3% had gross impairment of mental status. Most patients, however, had diminished global function compared to pre-hospital functional status.[29] The majority of patients with poor outcomes did not survive until hospital discharge.

Nearly all hospitals now have DNR policies based on local practices and DNR guidelines published by national bodies.[30] The remaining ethical and practical questions in writing DNR orders include: (1) When can physicians write DNR orders unilaterally—without consent of patient or surrogate, or even against the patient's or surrogate's wishes—on the grounds of medical futility? I discuss this issue in chapter 10. (2) How do partial DNR orders fit in a limited aggressive therapy order? (3) Should physicians temporarily suspend DNR orders when patients require general anesthesia and surgery? (4) How can hospital DNR orders be maintained during home care following discharge to prevent unwanted CPR?[31]

A DNR order in most hospitals prohibits chest compressions, defibrillation, endotracheal intubation, mechanical and mouth-to-mouth ventilation, and the administration of vasopressor and cardiac stimulant drugs. In some cases, patients and surrogates do not want blanket DNR but wish to permit one or more of these therapies in case of cardiopulmonary arrest. For example, some patients expressly refuse intubation but will permit defibrillation and the administration of cardiac drugs. They may request a "Do-Not-Intubate" order, which is a common partial DNR order. It is best not to regard DNR automatically as a blanket order but to discuss the separate elements of CPR with patients and surrogates to permit a tailored order that prohibits all or part of the array of CPR techniques. Some scholars have called this a "limited aggressive therapy order"[32] or a partial DNR order.[33] Ideally, the partial or full DNR order will arise from an individualized care plan negotiated with the patient or surrogate that is correlated with the patient's health-care goals and preferences for resuscitative treatment.

DNR orders indicate only that the elements of CPR will not be performed. Yet, there is widespread misunderstanding among lay persons and some professionals that once a patient is labeled "DNR" the overall aggressiveness of treatment should be lessened. Although this belief is technically erroneous, it has been found to be true in practice. In several studies, the presence of a DNR order was correlated with an overall lack of aggressiveness of treatment.[34] Most hospitals have developed limitation of therapy orders or palliative care orders to accomplish limiting aggressive therapy in addition to DNR orders. These orders should be used if the plan is to limit treatment and the DNR order reserved solely to refuse CPR.

Occasionally, patients with DNR orders require surgery and general anesthesia. For example, a patient with widely metastatic cancer may require an emergency operation for acute cholecystitis or bowel obstruction. The decision to proceed with surgery in such cases usually is based on the palliative goals of surgery: the procedure will promote comfort in the remaining weeks or months of life [35] General anesthesia usually requires endotracheal intubation and mechanical ventilation, which otherwise is forbidden by a blanket DNR order. Surgeons and anesthesiologists may ask the patient or surrogate temporarily to suspend parts of the DNR order during the peri-operative period to permit the successful completion of the procedure.[36] There should be additional discussions over whether an intraoperative cardiac arrest will be treated or whether prolonged mechanical ventilation will be performed if needed.[37]

There are generally accepted guidelines to settle these questions and negotiate a temporary suspension or modification of the DNR order during the peri-operative period. The guidelines require the surgeon or anesthesiologist to conduct a pre-operative conversation with the patient or surrogate during which the goals of treatment are discussed and the means to achieve those goals are agreed upon. The patient or surrogate may or may not grant permission for the DNR order to be modified or rescinded temporarily. If a suspension or modification of the DNR order is made, the terms and time limit of the suspension are agreed upon and further agreement is reached over whether intra-operative cardiac arrest will be treated or prolonged ventilation provided.[38] In most cases in my experience, the patient or surrogate permits mechanical ventilation during and within a few hours of the surgical procedure but refuses consent for both intra-operative cardiac resuscitation and prolonged mechanical ventilation.

Although the DNR order was developed for inpatient use in hospitals and other institutions, there is no compelling reason for limiting it to them. Many patients want their DNR orders to remain in force during their outpatient care to prevent unwanted CPR by emergency medical service (EMS) personnel that otherwise would be required by their regulations if they determined that a patient needs CPR. As of 2006, at least 42 states had provided a legal mechanism for outpatient DNR orders that would be respected by EMS personnel called to treat them.[39] Many states have created DNR wristbands, forms, or registries to identify valid outpatient DNR orders. In Oregon, Physician Orders for Life-Sustaining Treatment (POLST) now have become routine,[40] noteworthy in a state in which an impressive 78% of decedents have written advance directives.[41] In King County, Washington, a new guideline permits EMS personnel to withhold CPR from terminally ill patients if a family member or caregiver at the scene notifies them that the patient requested DNR status, even in the absence of a completed DNR form or bracelet.[42]

Withholding and Withdrawing Life-Sustaining Treatment in the Intensive Care Unit

Over the past century in the United States, there has been a striking change in how and where people die. Whereas, 100 years ago, most people died at home, now most people die in hospitals or nursing homes.[43] And whereas formerly most people died of untreatable acute or chronic illnesses, today an increasing percentage of patients in hospitals die from refusal of LST. This phenomenon is particularly common in intensive care units (ICUs). Critically ill patients are admitted to ICUs with the hope of rescue therapy, but many do not recover. A large, recent epidemiologic study showed that as many as one in five Americans die in an ICU or shortly after they have received ICU care.[44] Another recent population-based study showed that ICU admission rates strikingly increase with advancing age and the burden of coexisting chronic illnesses. The ICU admission rate is 75 times higher for patients over age 85 than for patients 18 to 44 years old and 900 times higher in persons with five or more chronic conditions than in those with none.[45]

Not only do many patients now die in ICUs but the mode of their demise is not entirely natural. Many or most ICU patients now die as a result of decisions made to limit treatment. In recent surveys, 40% to 65% of ICU deaths are the direct consequence of termination of LST resulting from patient or surrogate treatment refusals. Indeed, 74% of patients dying in ICUs have had at least some form of treatment withheld or withdrawn.[46]

The principles by which patients can refuse LST and the standards by which physicians must accede to these refusals have been asserted by a number of authorities over the past two decades.[47] Physicians should explain the patient's diagnosis and prognosis. Prognostic certainty often is impossible but the physician should make an evidence-based prognosis and communicate it with whatever confidence level is possible.[48] The physician then should outline the acceptable treatment options and offer treatment alternatives that are medical and ethically appropriate, including maintaining or withdrawing LST. The physician should explain the concept of palliative care and that the patient will be made comfortable if LST is refused and withdrawn. The physician should offer a treatment recommendation based on the diagnosis, prognosis, and patient's values and treatment goals, but the patient or surrogate has the authority to accept it or reject it.[49]

Despite this consensus, there remain cultural and geographic differences in the acceptance of these principles. A series of international conferences held at Appleton, Wisconsin between 1987 and 1991 developed a set of universally accepted principles for withholding and withdrawing LST, with only a few dissenters from the fifteen participating countries.[50] Specific principles and practices of withholding and withdrawing LST reflecting national normative practices have been published from the Netherlands,[51] Israel,[52] Canada,[53] and France.[54]

Three studies compared end-of-life practices in ICUs among European countries. The Ethicus Study of 37 ICUs in 17 European countries found that limiting LST in European countries was common but variable, and correlated with advancing age, severity of diagnoses, length of ICU stay, and geographic and religious factors.[55] In another study of six European countries, the percentage of deaths preceded by end-of-life family decisions ranged from 23% in Italy to 51% in Switzerland.[56] The European End-of-Life Consortium found great variation among countries, with Belgium, the Netherlands, and Switzerland forgoing treatment more often than Denmark, Italy, and Sweden.[57]

An essential ingredient in the discussion with the patient and surrogate is the identification of and agreement on the goals of medical treatment. In the case of an unequivocally dying patient, the goal may be purely palliation. When there is more than a trivial chance of saving the patient's life, the goal may be both life-saving and palliation. When the prognosis is ambiguous, many patients and physicians agree on a time-limited trial of therapy. The patient consents to aggressive LST for an agreed-upon interval hoping for improvement. If improvement does not occur by the end of this interval, the aggressive LST is discontinued and purely palliative care is provided.

A vexing situation arises when the critically ill ICU patient has lost decision-making capacity and there is neither family member nor surrogate decision maker on whom to rely for informed consent or refusal of LST. These patients who, in urban medical centers, often are homeless have been termed "unbefriended."[58] Douglas White and colleagues reported this circumstance in 16% of patients admitted to an ICU in San Francisco.[59] They found that physicians generally based decisions to limit life support on their understanding of the patient's diagnosis and prognosis and their determination of appropriate treatment. Notably, they requested neither further institutional nor judicial review in most cases. In a similar study of ICU deaths in seven medical centers, the same investigators found that 5.5% of cognitively incapacitated patients dying in the ICUs lacked both surrogate decision makers and advance directives.[60] They observed a wide variability in physician practices and hospital policies about who was authorized to make decisions in such cases. Physicians managing such patients should follow their hospital's decision-making policies.[61]

Holding a family conference is a common practice to maintain communication about treatment options and to solicit the family's preferences for the treatment of critically ill patients.[62] Families are told the diagnosis, prognosis with and without available treatments including palliative care, and their advice is sought to represent the patient's wishes. These meetings often are productive but may yield conflict when family members disagree.[63] Ethics consultants may help lead the meetings when conflict is anticipated.

Once patients or surrogates have made the decision to refuse LST, physicians should discuss with them exactly which treatments will be given and which will not. Following the principles of palliative care (chapter 7), I use a test I have found useful in such cases. If the treatment will contribute to the comfort of the patient, it will be provided; if not, it will be withdrawn or withheld. The goal of care in the setting of refusal of LST becomes to enhance the quality but not address the quantity of remaining life.

Once the decision has been agreed upon about the appropriate level of treatment, the physician should write explicit orders for medical and nursing care. These orders should be accompanied by explanations to the nursing staff that the orders follow the expressed wishes of the competent patient or of the incompetent patient as communicated by the surrogate. Most often the orders will be to limit the aggressiveness of LST. The exact language of any orders to limit therapy should make explicit which treatments will be provided and which will not. Some hospitals have developed specific treatment-limiting order pages with full palliative care orders.[64]

Physicians may enhance patients' and families' understanding by stratifying levels of treatment into descriptive classes that patients may accept or refuse. Level 1 is high-technology, high-expense, and high-invasiveness care, such as respirators, dialysis, cardiopulmonary resuscitation, and pacemakers. Level 2 is medications, such as vasopressors and antibiotics. Level 3 is hydration and nutrition. Level 4 is basic nursing care necessary to maintain hygiene, dignity, and comfort that should be maintained at all times.[65]

Studies of patients in intensive care units confirm that, in practice, the orders to limit treatment usually begin with omitting level 1, then encompass level 2, and finally include level 3. In an intensive care unit study of termination of LST, Smeidera and colleagues found that therapies were eliminated roughly in the following frequency and order: CPR, vasopressors, ventilators, supplemental oxygen, blood transfusions, antibiotics, antiarrhythmic drugs, dialysis, neurosurgery, intravenous fluids, and total parenteral nutrition.[66]

Physicians have personal biases that govern which therapies they are willing to discontinue and in what situations. One survey study found that physicians preferred to withdraw therapies: (1) from organs that failed from natural rather than iatrogenic causes; (2) that had been started recently, as opposed to those that had been of long duration; (3) that would result in the patient's immediate death rather than in delayed death; and (4) that would result in delayed death when the physician was unsure of the diagnosis.[67]

Deborah Cook and colleagues studied the factors associated with Canadian critical care physicians' decisions to withdraw ventilation from critically ill ICU patients in anticipation of their death. They found that, more than severity of illness or degrees of organ dysfunction, the strongest predictors for withdrawal were: (1) physicians' perceptions that patients would not want life support; (2) physicians' predictions of low likelihood of survival irrespective of treatment; and (3) high likelihood of poor cognitive outcome.[68]

Steven Mayor and Sharon Kossoff reported their experience of withdrawal of LST in a neurological ICU. Brain-dead patients were excluded. Forty-three percent of dying patients were terminally extubated; the mean duration of survival following extubation was 7.5 hours. Morphine or fentanyl was administered to combat labored breathing in two-thirds. A subsequent survey of surrogate decision makers revealed that 88% were comfortable and satisfied with the process of withdrawing LST.[69] Douglas White and colleagues showed that unfortunately, the ideal of shared decision making usually is not practiced in end-of-life decisions in ICUs, particularly among less educated families.[70]

Thomas Prendergast and Kathleen Puntillo reviewed families' reasons to refuse to consider a physician's recommendation to withdraw LST. They found four principal reasons: (1) mistrust of medical professionals resulting from lack of a prior relationship, perceived lack of empathy, or cultural or economic factors; (2) poor communication by medical personnel causing families to fail to understand the medical facts and clinicians' reluctance to acknowledge dying; (3) guilt by family members over personal responsibility for the patient's death or resulting from fractured past interpersonal relationships; and (4) families' cultural, religious, or scientific views outside the mainstream such as considering withdrawal of LST as euthanasia or finding meaning in continuing non-cognitive life.[71] Alexandre Lautrette and colleagues showed

that implementing a proactive communication strategy with family members, including the use of specially designed brochures, lessened the burdens of subsequent bereavement.[72]

Physicians should strive to practice ideal palliative care (chapter 7) when withdrawing LST as outlined in detail by the Ethics Committee of the Society of Critical Care Medicine.[73] The patient should be kept comfortable at all times through the judicious use of opiates, benzodiazepines, and barbiturates.[74] Timothy Gilligan and Thomas Raffin showed that for the patient in whom the ventilator is being withdrawn, rapidly dialing down the ventilator settings was less uncomfortable for patients than extubation or prolonged terminal weaning.[75] Reports from ICUs reveal that, in practice, nearly all noncomatose patients undergoing withdrawal of LST are given adequate doses of opiates and benzodiazepines, but there is no evidence that these medications when administered during ventilator weaning accelerate the moment of death.[76] Some patients require continuous use of benzodiazepine and barbiturate sedation, a practice known as palliative sedation.[77] Neuromuscular blocking drugs usually should be stopped.[78]

Several barriers impede the provision of ideal palliative care in the ICU. Many physicians continue to dichotomize therapeutic goals into curative and palliative. As long as the goal is curative, they may pay less attention to palliative issues. This phenomenon was shown clearly in the SUPPORT study (see below). In a survey of physician and nursing directors of 600 ICUs in the United States, Judith Nelson and colleagues identified several other barriers: (1) unrealistic family expectations causing unreasonable demands for more aggressive treatment; (2) the inability of most patients to participate directly in decision making about themselves; (3) lack of advance directives; (4) inadequate physician training in communication skills; (5) inadequate time for physicians to engage families in discussions; (6) inadequate space in the ICU for family meetings; and (7) lack of a palliative care service.[79] Success in surmounting these barriers has formed the basis of defining quality indicators for end-of-life care in ICUs.[80]

A survey of practicing neurologists revealed the extent of their misunderstanding of the ethical and legal dimensions of patient refusal of LST and physician withholding and withdrawal of LST. In a survey administered by the American Academy of Neurology to American member neurologists, 40% wrongly believed that they needed to consult legal counsel before withdrawing a patient's LST and 38% wrongly were concerned that they might be charged with a crime for withdrawing LST.[81] The need for further education here is obvious.

The Artificial Hydration and Nutrition Question

Some physicians continue to express concern over whether they are permitted to discontinue artificial hydration and nutrition (AHN) along with other medical therapies once AHN has been validly refused by a patient or surrogate, or if laws, ethics, and medical standards require them to maintain it. The controversy centers on the question of whether AHN counts as a form of medical therapy or whether it comprises a unique class of treatment because it represents a basic nonmedical requirement for the maintenance of life. By AHN, I refer to hydration and nutrition provided through a nasogastric, gastrostomy, or jejunostomy tube, or intravenously. The term "artificial" in this context and its distinction from "natural" has been criticized recently as ethically irrelevant because patients also have the right to refuse oral hydration and nutrition[82] "Medically administered hydration and nutrition" is a more exact term than AHN.[83]

One camp of opinion holds that AHN is not a medical therapy: it is simply food and water. According to this argument, AHN is not synthetic, mechanical, technologic, pharmacologically active, or therapeutic. Proponents of this position point out that, whereas some people can live without penicillin or digitalis, no one can live without hydration and nutrition. Therefore, a physician's act to terminate AHN *causes* death as directly as actively killing. They believe that it is inhumane and is morally wrong to stop AHN, according to Judeo-Christian teachings. Finally, they warn that

permitting physicians to terminate a patient's AHN (even in response to a patient's refusal to receive it) is the first step on a slippery slope toward euthanasia and the general devaluation and degradation of human life.[84]

The opposing camp holds that AHN is a medical treatment for a dying or critically ill, technologically supported patient. In an awake, alert person, eating and drinking obviously cannot be construed as medical therapies, but patients requiring AHN, who cannot eat or drink, must be nourished and hydrated by medical means. Maintaining their hydration and nutrition requires technology, such as surgical placement of a feeding gastrostomy tube and calibration of hourly quantities of tube feedings and hydration based upon nutritional and fluid demands. This technologic hydration and nutrition is ordered by physicians and administered by nurses along with medications and other treatments. It is only within the past two generations that these technologies have been perfected to permit keeping such patients alive. Were it not for the vigilant application of these technologies, patients requiring AHN would die. For these reasons, AHN in such patients can be considered as a form of medical therapy to which patients may consent or refuse.[85]

On balance, I believe it is most coherent to view AHN as a form of medical therapy.[86] Patients have the autonomy-based right to refuse all medical therapies, including AHN. American patients have a constitutional right to refuse AHN as explained below. This right can be exercised by executing advance directives for medical care and can be carried out by patients' surrogate decision makers on their behalf. Patients should not be required to be kept alive by AHN against their previously stated wishes because of physicians' unwillingness to stop AHN based on the questionable assertions that it is not a medical therapy or that stopping it is unethical. The majority of surveyed physicians agree that AHN is a medical therapy that can refused by patients and their surrogate decision makers.[87]

Once a dying patient refuses AHN and, in response, a physician orders its cessation, the physician has a duty to provide proper palliative care to assure that the patient will not suffer if that capacity is retained. David Casarett and colleagues recently emphasized the elements of palliative care that are appropriate in this situation, including mouth care, management of delirium, and attention to the patient's emotional and spiritual issues.[88] Molly McMahon and colleagues additionally provided a useful checklist for physicians when ordering long-term enteral tube feeding or ordering its cessation. The list included relevant medical, nutritional, and ethical considerations.[89]

The SUPPORT Study

The Study to Understand Prognoses and Preferences for Outcomes and Risks of Treatment (SUPPORT) was the largest and most comprehensive study of physicians' practices of withdrawing LST from critically ill and dying patients. SUPPORT was a carefully planned and executed four-year, two-phase study of over 9,000 hospitalized, seriously ill patients. The goals of the study were to measure the quality of end-of-life decision making and the frequency of unnecessarily painful or prolonged death in the hospital, and to attempt to improve the quality of terminal care. Phase I of SUPPORT showed that there were serious shortcomings in the care of critically ill and dying patients: many patients did not receive DNR orders until two days before death; less than half of physicians knew their patients' CPR preferences; and half of conscious patients suffered pain before they died.

Phase II of SUPPORT showed that an intervention by trained nurses to communicate to physicians the patient's up-to-date prognosis failed to influence the physicians in their treatment behaviors.[90] Since the original publication of SUPPORT data in 1995, a series of related research reports have been published as a result of further analysis of the wealth of data accumulated by SUPPORT.[91]

When SUPPORT was published, the popular press and the academy excoriated the medical community for their insensitivity and arrogance in the care of dying patients. For example, the medicolegal scholar George Annas fumed, "Physicians simply have never taken the rights of hospitalized patients seriously . . . the only

realistic way to improve the care of dying patients in the short run is to get them out of the hospital . . ." Annas then suggested that a reasonable corrective strategy would be for our society to establish a system of law firms, connected to hospitals by a hotline, whose sole purpose would be to routinely sue physicians who refused to grant patients their right to refuse life-prolonging therapy.[92]

Despite the disheartening findings of SUPPORT that physicians did not listen to patients' wishes and generally ignored their prognoses, the public overreaction to SUPPORT revealed a misunderstanding of the important distinction between critical and terminal illness, and the reality of the clinical context in which sick patients must make treatment choices. Patients were enrolled in SUPPORT who were in the advanced stages of one or more of nine serious illnesses and most were admitted to ICUs for treatment. SUPPORT was a study of physicians' treatment of critically ill but not necessarily terminally ill patients. Indeed, three-fourths of the study patients later were discharged from the hospital and two-thirds of those discharged remained alive six months later.

That a critically ill patient also is terminally ill is a determination often made more accurately in retrospect. Despite the fact that trained nurses provided the study physicians with prognostic data from computerized models, a serious and possibly insurmountable barrier prevented both physicians and patients from incorporating these statistical data into their life-or-death treatment decisions.

That barrier was the patient's intermediate prognosis for survival. It is easy for patients and physicians to make the correct decision when the prognosis is clear that a patient will either live or die. It is the group of critically ill patients with an intermediate prognosis for survival for whom decision making is most vexing. Would most patients with a critical illness who are given a 60% chance of cure and a 50% chance of surviving an additional six months (approximately the mean prognosis for SUPPORT patients) choose to receive LST or choose withdrawal of LST with only palliative care?

I agree with other experienced clinicians that most patients and families given those odds would choose a time-limited trial of life-sustaining treatment, at least until it became clear later that the patient's prognosis was poor.[93] Unfortunately, patients, families, and physicians must make life-or-death treatment decisions on critically ill patients in the face of a continuum of changing statistical outcome probabilities. The true lessons of SUPPORT are that physicians should try to establish prognoses as accurately as possible, they should provide proper palliative care whether or not a patient is terminally ill, and patients should be encouraged to complete advance directives and discuss them with their physicians, who should honor them.

Physicians should offer evidence-based prognoses. An important pitfall for physicians to avoid when rendering a prognosis is the fallacy of the self-fulfilling prophecy. In this fallacy, physicians cite outcome data from published series in which many of the critically ill patients had undergone termination of LST because of their purportedly poor prognoses. The poor prognoses reported in such studies then become grounds for recommending cessation of LST in new cases with similar disorders.[94] Importantly, these studies do not record the history of the disorders in question when they have been aggressively treated, but only the experiential history resulting from various levels of support.

For example, in the study by Kyra Beker and colleagues of withdrawal of LST in patients with large intracerebral hemorrhages (ICH), physicians based a recommendation to surrogates to discontinue the patient's LST on statistical prognoses that may have been incorrect because they were derived from studies containing patients who underwent termination of LST.[95] Indeed, several of the purportedly moribund patients in Becker's study who were treated aggressively had favorable outcomes. The physicians recommending withdrawal of LST in some of these patients may have committed the fallacy of making a self-fulfilling prophesy.

These issues are common. In a recent study of mortality in patients with ICH, the most common cause of death (in 68% of patients) was withdrawal of LST.[96] A large community hospital study of patients admitted with ICH found that early DNR orders and other orders to limit treatment were associated with a doubling of mortality irrespective of other factors associated with increased mortality.[97] Similarly, Claude Hemphill and colleagues found that early DNR orders in patients with ICH predicted death more accurately than did patients' clinical characteristics.[98] Another recent study showed favorable outcomes after surgery to remove massive anticoagulation-induced ICH, even in purportedly moribund patients with signs of uncal herniation.[99] The perceived prognosis of patients rendered comatose after cardiac arrest predicts whether LST will be withdrawn.[100] Physicians should make evidence-based prognoses and try to avoid the fallacy of the self-fulfilling prophecy.[101] A 2007 ICH clinical practice guideline recommends careful consideration of aggressive, full care during the first 24 hours after ICH onset and postponement of new DNR orders during that period.[102]

Refusal of Life-Sustaining Treatment for Children

Children have the same ethical and legal rights as adults to refuse LST. The principal difference in practice is that the child is not authorized independently to refuse LST, therefore the child's parents must serve as surrogate decision makers. Infants and younger children fall into the category of the "never-competent"; thus, the parents cannot employ a substituted judgment standard of decision making and must rely on a best interest standard. Parents must make painful decisions for their children using the same elements of informed consent and refusal as would any other surrogate decision maker. Older children and adolescents can contribute their values and treatment preferences to the decision according to the principles of assent in childhood discussed in chapter 2. The related subject of withholding and withdrawing LST from neonates is discussed in chapter 13.

Empirical studies on children dying in pediatric ICUs reveal that, in a large percentage of deaths, physicians had ordered limitation or termination of LST after a discussion of the child's diagnosis and prognosis with the surrogate decision maker. These data are similar to those from adult ICUs and suggest that most hopelessly ill children are not being inappropriately overtreated in pediatric ICUs. For example, in a survey of 16 pediatric ICUs, Marcia Levetown and colleagues found that 38% of all deaths resulted from withdrawal of LST.[103] In another large single-institution study, Richard Mink and Murray Pollack found that 32% of pediatric ICU deaths were from withdrawal of LST.[104] In a similar but smaller single-institution study, Donald Vernon and colleagues found that 58% of the pediatric ICU deaths were from withdrawing LST.[105]

The decision to withdraw AHN from children is particularly vexing. While the relevant principles for children are identical to those of adults, the symbolic meaning of parental duty to assure continued hydration and nutrition adds a layer of psychological difficulty. Lawrence Nelson and colleagues and Judith Johnson with Christine Mitchell have offered thoughtful ethical and legal analyses of this painful subject.[106]

Overruling Patients' Treatment Refusals

There are only very rare instances in which physicians are ethically justified in overruling patients' refusals of LST and continuing to treat them against their will. As discussed in chapter 2, the ethical justification for such a paternalistic act would require that: (1) the patient's refusal of LST was seriously irrational; (2) the evils the paternalistic act would prevent are objectively greater than those without it; and (3) the physician must be willing to state publicly that overruling the patient's refusal was the correct course of action and one that should be advocated as the correct action in all similar cases. In the case of a dying patient who refuses LST, it is hard to sustain the argument that refusal of LST is a seriously irrational act because the patient inevitably will die soon from the terminal illness. It is similarly hard to sustain a claim that the evils avoided are great.

The only plausible case in which it might be ethically justified for a physician to overrule a dying patient's refusal of LST is one in which

the patient is seriously depressed and wishes to die as a result. An argument could be made that it might be in the patient's best interest to try to treat the depression before acceding to the irreversible consequences of withdrawing LST. However, such cases must be individualized to rigorously test if paternalism can be justified, as discussed in chapter 2. In my experience, paternalistic overruling of a dying patient's refusal of LST usually cannot be ethically justified, even in patients with depression.

A more common and difficult ethical problem arises when the lawful surrogate decision maker of an incompetent patient insists that LST be withdrawn against the recommendation of the physician. The physician in such cases may believe that the therapy should be continued because of a favorable prognosis with treatment or because the physician understood from previous discussions that the patient wished continued LST. Such disagreements produce serious conflicts between physicians and the surrogates. The hospital ethics committee can be consulted to help resolve such conflicts.[107]

LEGAL ISSUES

Physicians should be knowledgeable about the extent to which the law governs their actions to implement decisions to withhold or withdraw LST. In the United States, legal constraints on physicians' actions can be classified into the following five areas of law: (1) state criminal statutes; (2) the evolving corpus of case law resulting from high court judicial decisions; (3) state civil statutes; (4) state and federal administrative regulations; and (5) medical malpractice law.[108] I consider each of these areas except the administrative regulations, which I discuss in chapter 13. I discuss general medicolegal issues in chapter 4.

In the more than three decades since the *Quinlan* decision, there have been scores of important judicial rulings from high courts addressing the broad or narrow legal issues of withholding or withdrawing medical treatment. Courts have attempted to settle several questions. Do patients have a constitutional right to refuse unwanted medical treatment, even if they will die as a direct result? If physicians order cessation of LST and the patient dies as a direct result, have they committed homicide or euthanasia? Can the decision to withdraw or withhold medical treatment be made by a surrogate? What are the standards for decision making by surrogates? Can patients or surrogates refuse life-sustaining artificial hydration and nutrition? These questions have been answered in a more or less consistent manner by high courts in several influential judicial decisions, culminating in the U.S. Supreme Court *Cruzan* decision of 1990.

The Right to Refuse Medical Therapy

Beginning with *Quinlan* in the mid-1970s and continuing through *Cruzan* in 1990, courts have underscored the right of patients to refuse unwanted medical therapy. Karen Ann Quinlan was a young woman in a persistent vegetative state (PVS) due to hypoxic-ischemic brain damage following a presumed aspiration-induced asphyxia. After she had remained on a ventilator in a PVS for many months and it became clear that she would not recover awareness, her father, Joseph Quinlan, asked her neurologist, in writing, to "discontinue all extraordinary measures, including the use of a respirator." Her neurologist was reluctant to accede to this request because he believed that doing so would be inconsistent with accepted medical practice. Joseph Quinlan therefore sued the neurologist and hospital and asked that the court name him as her guardian for the purpose of removing her from the ventilator. When the lower court refused the request, arguing that such questions should be left to physicians, he appealed to the New Jersey Supreme Court which agreed to hear the case.

The New Jersey Supreme Court's 1976 *Quinlan* decision stands as one of the landmark American rulings in cases of refusal of medical treatment. Among other conclusions, the *Quinlan* court reversed the decision of the lower court, finding that Karen's constitutionally protected right of privacy encompassed her right to refuse medical therapy, a right that her father could exercise on her behalf. The *Quinlan* court balanced this right against the state's interest in preserving her life and concluded: "We think that the State's interest weakens and the individual's right to privacy grows as the degree of bodily invasion increases and the prognosis dims. Ultimately there comes a point at which the individual's rights overcome the State's interest."[109]

The ironic postscript to *Quinlan* was that by the time the decision was handed down and she was extubated, she no longer was dependent on the ventilator and did not die as the result of its long-awaited withdrawal. Although her neurologist knew this information and informed the judge, it apparently was not communicated adequately to the press which reported her continued breathing as a medical surprise.[110] She remained in a PVS for an additional nine years and died of sepsis in 1985.[111]

A number of high courts later also concurred that both incompetent and competent patients have a right to refuse therapy. Many of these rulings were grounded in citizens' common law rights of autonomy and self-determination, such as the freedom to retain bodily integrity and the freedom from unwanted interference from others. A few rulings were grounded in the so-called "penumbral" constitutional right of privacy, usually citing the argument in *Quinlan*.

The most influential ruling was *Cruzan* in 1990, concerning the fate of another young woman in a PVS. Nancy Beth Cruzan suffered a hypoxic-ischemic brain injury from cardiopulmonary arrest when she was thrown from the car she was driving and landed face down on the ground. She suffered cardiopulmonary arrest and hypoxic-ischemic neuronal damage. When she failed to recover awareness and remained in a PVS for over three years, her parents, as court-appointed guardians, requested that she no longer receive the tube feedings that had been keeping her alive. Before approving the request, the hospital administrator required her parents to obtain a court order to discontinue her tube feedings. A county probate court willingly issued the order. However, in the ensuing publicity, the state of Missouri appealed the probate court decision and it was later reversed by the Missouri Supreme Court.

The Missouri Supreme Court ruled that in cases in which a patient is incompetent but not terminally ill, the state required that a subjective standard of evidence must be satisfied, clearly showing that the patient would have refused LST and AHN, before physicians were permitted to terminate them. The subjective standard required "clear and convincing evidence" that, while competent, Cruzan had indicated specifically that she would not want her tube feedings continued were she ever in a PVS.

Nancy's parent's provided evidence from her previous conversations with them that she would not want to continue to live in a PVS if there was no hope for recovery of consciousness. The Missouri Supreme Court assessed this evidence as not satisfying the clear and convincing standard. The Court clarified that a clear and convincing standard could be satisfied only if she had provided written evidence through a living will or a similar written directive addressing discontinuation of AHN. The parents appealed the decision to the U.S. Supreme Court which granted *certiorari*, an event noteworthy because it was the first time the Supreme Court agreed to hear a state "right to die" case.

In the narrow dimension of its ruling, the *Cruzan* decision of 1990 upheld the state of Missouri's right to stipulate the standard of evidence of an incompetent patient's wishes, including a clear and convincing standard, before permitting termination of medical treatment. It agreed that the evidence supplied by Nancy's parents failed to achieve the state's clear and convincing standard. Of more importance, however, was the broad dimension of the *Cruzan* ruling. The Court found a constitutionally protected right for competent or incompetent citizens to refuse any form of medical therapy, including AHN. Unlike the *Quinlan* court which found this right in the doctrine of privacy, the *Cruzan* court derived the constitutional right from the Due Process clause of the Fourteenth Amendment that guarantees liberty rights.

Cruzan was welcomed as an important precedent that once and for all underscored the constitutional basis for the right of people to refuse all forms of medical treatment.[112] However, the ruling had several limitations. It rejected the decision-making standard of substituted judgment on the basis that family members cannot be "disinterested parties." It underscored the primacy of the state's interest in "the protection and preservation of human life" by its willingness to permit impractical standards of evidence such as the clear and convincing standard that few cases would ever satisfy.[113] Justice Stevens issued a dissenting opinion that highlighted the practical limitations of the *Cruzan* decision: "An innocent person's constitutional right to be free from unwanted medical treatment is thereby categorically limited to those patients who had the foresight to make an unambiguous statement of their wishes while competent. The Court's decision affords no protection to children, to young people who are victims of unexpected accidents or illnesses, or to the countless thousands of elderly persons who either fail to decide, or fail to explain, how they want to be treated if they should experience a similar fate."[114]

The fate of Nancy Beth Cruzan, like that of Karen Ann Quinlan, was ironic. Following the U.S. Supreme Court decision, the parents again approached the local probate court to request removal of the feeding tube, citing new evidence from one of Nancy's friends of a conversation she had shared during which Nancy had commented that she never wanted to be kept alive in a meaningless state. Again the probate court ordered removal of the feeding tube but this time the state of Missouri chose not to oppose the order, concluding that the clear and convincing standard now had been satisfied. Despite physical interference from protestors, her feeding tube was removed and she died 11 days later. Almost immediately thereafter, the state of Missouri enacted a health-care power of attorney statute that empowered surrogates to withhold AHN if authorized by the patient. Of greater national significance, Missouri Senator John Danforth led a federal legislative effort culminating in the Patient Self-Determination Act of 1991, discussed in chapter 4.

Liability for Homicide

Many physicians fear that if they withhold or withdraw LST and the patient dies as a direct result, they may be liable for homicide.[115]

Although state statutes have varying definitions of homicide, most statutes contain language such as "unlawful conduct (e.g., action with malicious intent or negligent disregard for the safety or interests of others) leading to a person's death." Insofar as intentional killing usually counts as homicide, there exists at least the possibility that physicians ordering withdrawal of LST could incur liability to homicide. Primarily because the physician is following the valid refusal of a patient or authorized surrogate and secondarily because of the absence of malice or negligence and the presence of a compassionate motive, courts have rejected homicide liability for physicians who order cessation of LST. This uniform rejection of homicide does not necessarily apply, however, to physicians performing active euthanasia (see chapter 9).

The *Quinlan* court considered the question of physician liability for homicide if Karen were to die as the result of removal from the ventilator. The neurologist who refused to comply with Joseph Quinlan's request to extubate his daughter did not cite, as one of his reasons, his concern about liability for homicide. Nevertheless, the court presumed the existence of such a concern and ruled that were Karen to die as the direct result of removal of the ventilator, the physician would not be liable for homicide. They ruled that, if she died, her death would be the direct result of her pre-existing illness, anoxic encephalopathy.

Subsequent court rulings similarly rejected physician liability for homicide.[116] The question was again most directly addressed by the *Barber* court. In *Barber*, a man suffered hypoxic-ischemic brain damage as the result of perioperative cardiopulmonary arrest. After the patient had been unconscious for several days his attending physicians ordered cessation of LST including AHN on the basis of his presumed hopeless prognosis. A prosecutor charged the physicians with homicide, but the charges were dropped by a municipal court judge. The charges later were reinstated and the case was heard by the California Court of Appeals. The *Barber* court ruled that although the physicians' discontinuation of AHN directly led to the patient's death, it did not

count as murder under the California homicide statute because his prognosis was so poor that his treating physicians had no legally enforceable duty to sustain his life.[117]

Legal reviews of withholding and withdrawing LST found no cases of physician liability for homicide when physicians followed the treatment refusals of patients and surrogates. There have been a few cases in which aggressive palliative care of the dying with analgesics and sedatives has been construed as homicide,[118] but a survey of district attorneys shows that a large majority would not prosecute cases falling within the accepted medical practices of refusal of LST and palliative treatment. State criminal prosecutors generally have been unwilling to prosecute physician-assisted suicide even when it is illegal in their jurisdiction.[119]

Surrogate Decision Making

Many courts have addressed the question of surrogate decision making for the incompetent patient. In nearly every instance, courts have ruled that surrogates can be authorized to make judgments for incompetent patients. Only in the idiosyncratic and impractical *Saikewicz* ruling was it suggested that these cases routinely should be referred to courts for judicial review.[120]

While courts have agreed that surrogates may decide, there has been disagreement on the decision-making doctrines that surrogates should employ. The *Cruzan* court relied upon a subjective doctrine requiring clear and convincing evidence before a surrogate could stop LST. The states of Missouri, New York, and Maine routinely employ this high evidentiary standard. Most other states use either the substituted judgment or best interest doctrines.[121] For example, the *Quinlan* court held that Joseph Quinlan was lawfully authorized to exercise his daughter's right to refuse therapy by the doctrine of substituted judgment. The *Barber* court, conversely, articulated a best interest doctrine in its analysis of whether the burdens of continued treatment outweighed the benefits. They wrote: ". . . a treatment course which is only minimally painful or intrusive may nonetheless be considered disproportionate to the potential benefits if the prognosis is virtually hopeless for any significant improvement in condition."[122]

Legal scholars have made additional contributions to this discussion. Nancy Rhoden argued that because it is unrealistic to achieve the standards of substituted judgment and best interest, less reliance should be placed on the subjective and objective tests traditionally used by courts. She pointed out that total objectivity in such matters was neither possible nor desirable. As an alternative, she suggested that physicians should follow the decisions of family members or close friends, or else be required to convince a court that such decisions are unreasonable. Under this scheme, the physician can overrule the surrogate only if there is evidence that the surrogate is not deciding altruistically.[123] This idea has become the basis for legislatures' enacting health-care surrogacy acts. (See chapter 4.)

Withdrawing Artificial Hydration and Nutrition

Many states have enacted statutes permitting physicians to discontinue AHN or limiting their authority to do so unless the patient had left specific written instructions.[124] Additionally, a number of state courts and the U.S. Supreme Court have considered whether AHN could be discontinued as part of cessation of LST. In *Brophy*, a Massachusetts trial court refused the petition of the wife of a middle-aged man to remove his AHN after he remained in a PVS for several years following unsuccessful surgery for a ruptured basilar artery aneurysm. His wife produced evidence that he never wanted to be kept alive on machines and that he wished to be permitted to die in this circumstance. The lower court accepted the evidence as indicating Brophy's preference but, nevertheless, found that the state's interest in preserving his life was more compelling than his right to be permitted to die. It found that a feeding tube was not "highly invasive or intrusive" and that it did "not subject him to pain and suffering."

Upon appeal, the Massachusetts Supreme Judicial Court reversed the lower court ruling in a split decision with strongly worded dissents. Citing the primacy of self-determination, the

higher court ruled that the feeding tube should be removed because it was in accordance with Brophy's clearly stated wishes. They weighed his tangible rights of self-determination as more compelling than the state's abstract interest in maintaining his life.[125] As they later did in *Cruzan*, also, the American Academy of Neurology, the American Medical Association, and other medical societies submitted briefs of *amicus curiae* to argue for reversal of the lower court decision.

Most influentially, the *Cruzan* court ruled that AHN was indistinguishable from other medical therapies and could be refused by patients or surrogates and withheld or withdrawn by physicians. In her concurring opinion, Justice Sandra Day O'Connor wrote: "Artificial feeding cannot readily be distinguished from other forms of medical treatment . . . Accordingly, the liberty guaranteed by the Due Process Clause must protect, if it protects anything, an individual's deeply personal decision to reject medical treatment, including the artificial delivery of food and water."[126] The *Cruzan* precedent was cited as the legal basis for the lawful surrogate of Theresa Schiavo to refuse AHN on her behalf, as discussed in chapter 12.

Despite the clarity of American law on this matter, some physicians and nurses in the United States have been slow to understand this development and to incorporate it into their practices. Alan Meisel presented data and explained why many physicians practicing in nursing homes may decide not to permit AHN to be discontinued even when it has been validly refused. Although some physicians misunderstand the law, other fear citations by state departments of health.[127] Mildred Solomon and colleagues showed that many physicians and nurses do not follow accepted practices and national guidelines because they disagree with them or are unaware of them.[128] Our own data from the American Academy of Neurology survey of neurologists' attitudes and practices in end-of-life care reveal similar misunderstandings.[129] Neurologists should be knowledgeable about the statutes governing withholding or withdrawing AHN in the states in which they practice. The American Academy of Neurology recently reaffirmed its support for incapacitated patients to accept or refuse AHN, exercised by surrogates, without unreasonable interference by state or federal legislation that presumes to prescribe their preferences.[130]

Medical Malpractice

Liability for medical malpractice exists if a decision to terminate LST is based on a physician's inadequate assessment of the patient's diagnosis and prognosis that falls below the standard of care. (See chapter 4.) The standard of medical practice in decisions to terminate treatment requires a reasonably considered prognosis based upon an adequate assessment of the patient by history, physical examination, and laboratory tests. But how often is fear of committing malpractice a relevant factor in physicians' actions to withhold or withdraw LST?

A survey of members of the American Society of Law and Medicine and the Society of Critical Care Medicine disclosed that physicians' fear of legal liability was an important external factor in their decisions whether or not to terminate patients' medical treatment. This factor became of paramount importance in those cases in which the patient's preferences were not known.[131]

In the *Barber* case, once the criminal homicide charges were dropped, the attending physicians were sued for malpractice. The lawsuit was based upon the allegation that they had performed an inadequate assessment of the patient before deciding to withdraw all therapy. In the ensuing litigation, neurologists testified that four days of observation usually was an inadequate time to prognosticate recovery from a vegetative state with sufficient confidence to order cessation of LST.

Physicians can protect themselves from the small potential risk of malpractice liability in decisions to terminate LST by arriving at a diagnosis as the result of a careful assessment by repeated neurological examinations, by formulating an evidence-based prognosis, and by following the treatment decisions of competent patients and the lawful surrogates of incompetent patients.

Advance Directive Statutes

During the past two decades, all states have enacted laws providing formal recognition of advance directives for health care. As discussed in chapter 4, advance directives can be executed in the form of documents such as the living will, or in the form of appointments of surrogate decision makers such as the Durable Power of Attorney for Health Care. The written directives have the advantage of providing clear and convincing evidence of a person's treatment preferences but usually have the disadvantage of being drafted in overly general language of ambiguous applicability to specific clinical situations.

For example, the typical living will provides that a person refuses "life-prolonging therapy" if he is "terminally ill." But is the persistent vegetative state a terminal illness, given that patients may survive in for decades? And is AHN a form of life-prolonging therapy? The answers to these questions may vary from one person to another. Unless the person had clarified these ambiguities in a written directive, the application of a typical living will to withdrawing AHN in PVS may be unclear.

The surrogate appointment directives have the advantage of greater flexibility, in that a surrogate can apply his general knowledge of a patient's values to make a novel choice in a specific unanticipated clinical situation. The disadvantage is that the surrogate's attempt to decide using the standard of substituted judgment may fail to make the choice the patient would have made. The failure to reproduce the patient's decision may not matter if the patient simply is willing to defer complete responsibility to the surrogate to decide what course of action is best. Physicians have the ethical duty to encourage their competent patients to execute advance directives and the legal duty to follow those directives when choosing a medical treatment plan.[132]

Health-care surrogate laws (discussed in chapter 4) may be an additionally useful legislative solution to overcome the problems resulting when advance directives have not been executed. In those states with health-care surrogate laws, the law automatically names a relative or friend from a statutorily determined list to serve as the legally authorized surrogate for patients without advance directives who qualify by illness condition.[133]

The Role of the Hospital Ethics Committee

The *Quinlan* court and the President's Commission, among others, called for the development of hospital ethics committees to oversee decisions when termination of LST was ordered for incompetent patients. As discussed in chapter 5, the committee should not be authorized to make clinical decisions; this authority should remain in the hands of the attending physician. In principle, the committee should act as an impartial third party to inspect the process of decision making and try to assure that proper procedures have been followed to protect the patient. The committee's role thus should be limited to procedural oversight rather than substantive decision making.

In practice, the committee should ascertain that physicians have reached a clear diagnosis and prognosis; that advance directives, if available, are followed; and that the previous wishes of the patient and the present wishes of the family or surrogate are known and followed. The President's Commission opined that if hospital ethics committees were available and functioning successfully, the need to refer these cases routinely for formal judicial review would be minimized.[134] The ethics consultant called to assist decisions concerning termination of LST generally should restrict participation to providing procedural oversight.

GUIDELINES FOR WITHHOLDING AND WITHDRAWING LIFE-SUSTAINING THERAPY

A series of guidelines epitomizes the principles discussed in this chapter. Treating the competent patient is relatively straightforward because the physician follows the patient's valid consent or refusal of LST. Guidelines are necessary in the more difficult instance in which the patient is incompetent. Clinicians should individualize the specific aspects of each case in applying these guidelines.

General

1. *Communicate with the family and surrogate decision maker.* Adequate communication with family members and the surrogate is essential to be reasonably confident that the physician is following the wishes of the patient. The theme of the communication should be that the hospital staff and family are jointly struggling to do the right thing, namely make that decision that the patient would make were he able. Adequate communication is time consuming. It should be as unhurried and open as possible.[135] To diminish their inevitable feelings of guilt, the physician should reassure the family or surrogate that, by using the substituted judgment or best interests standard, they are making the right choice because that is what the patient would want.

2. *Communicate with the hospital staff.* The nursing and ancillary hospital staff, as well as the house staff in teaching hospitals, should clearly understand the treatment plans and goals and how and why they have been chosen. They should be willing to carry out the treatment plan because following the patient's wishes is the ethically correct course of action.

3. *Document decisions in the medical record.* Notes in the medical record should reflect the reasons the specific treatment plan has been chosen and the process of decision making. Orders to nurses should be consistent with this plan. The types of therapy to be administered or withheld should be made explicit in a series of orders.

4. *Follow hospital bylaws.* Physicians should follow their hospital's bylaws that pertain to decisions to withdraw or withhold LST.

5. *Follow state laws.* Physicians should be knowledgeable and ready to follow applicable state laws pertaining to termination of LST, including advance directive statutes. For example, several states have statutes permitting withdrawal of LST but forbidding withdrawal of AHN unless the patient had so stipulated specifically.[136]

Specific

1. *Establish the correct diagnosis.* Diagnosis is a prerequisite for prognosis.

2. *Establish the correct prognosis.* Prognosis may not be known to a high degree of certainty, but physicians should strive to make an evidence-based prognosis and share the extent of their understanding of it with the patient and surrogate.

3. *Identify the patient's preferences.* The physician should attempt to discover the patient's previously expressed wish for continuing or discontinuing LST. This information may be learned from advance directives or from statements of family members or friends. The decision about treatment of the incompetent patient should be made by a surrogate using the standards of expressed wishes when possible; substituted judgment; or, when this is impossible, best interest.

4. *Identify the family's preference.* In the ideal situation, the surrogate and family will agree on the treatment plan. It is desirable for the family to have achieved consensus on the grounds that the treatment plan is ethically correct because it follows the patient's wishes. If consensus cannot be reached, family meetings with physicians, nurses, chaplains, and social workers may help. A common and vexing problem is caused by the family member who arrives from out of town and summarily disagrees with the consensus that had been reached among the other family members, often out of guilt or because he has another agenda.[137] If the family remains divided intractably despite the best efforts of other professionals and after family meetings, the case should be referred to the hospital ethics committee for review. In some cases in which the family is divided and there is no legally authorized surrogate, it may be desirable to refer the matter to court for formal appointment of a legally authorized surrogate.

5. *Choose appropriate level of treatment.* After establishing diagnosis, prognosis, and preferences, the physician and surrogate should agree on a level of treatment that is consistent with the previous wishes of the patient. This treatment plan may include provision or withdrawal of LST, medications, and AHN. The physician should write orders explicitly describing which therapies will be provided and which will not. Nursing care to maintain dignity and hygiene always should be maintained.

6. *Provide ideal palliative care.* As discussed in chapter 7, the patient for whom LST has been discontinued should be kept comfortable and free from suffering by the judicious use of opiates, benzodiazepines, and barbiturates, with attention also directed to emotional and spiritual needs.

7. *Request oversight by the hospital ethics committee.* The physician should consider asking the hospital ethics committee to review the decision-making process for any patient who is not terminally ill for whom orders have been written terminating LST. This review primarily protects the patient by insuring due process and secondarily helps the physician by demonstrating that he has followed the proper procedure in his decision. If the committee feels that proper procedures have not been followed, the orders to terminate LST should be suspended until proper procedures are established. In the absence of a functioning hospital ethics committee, another physician can provide the oversight role.

8. *Refer to court for judicial review in certain circumstances.* If the preceding guidelines are followed, judicial oversight or formal proxy appointment should be necessary only rarely. However, it should be considered in several circumstances: (1) when suggested by the hospital attorney or provided in hospital regulations; (2) when there is an intractable substantive disagreement within the family and no formal surrogate has been appointed; (3) when there is evidence that a surrogate is deciding for reasons that are not altrusitic; and (4) in those instances in which the prognosis remains uncertain and there is neither advance directive nor surrogate available to guide the physician.

NOTES

1. The concept of patient-centered medicine and its evolution from physician-centered medicine are explained in Laine C, Davidoff F. Patient-centered medicine: a professional evolution. *JAMA* 1996; 275:152–156.

2. Bernat JL, Cranford RE, Kittredge FI Jr, Rosenberg RN. Competent patients with advanced states of permanent paralysis have the right to forgo life-sustaining therapy. *Neurology* 1993;43:224–225.

3. For a rigorous analysis of informed consent and refusal, see Gert B, Culver CM, Clouser KD. *Bioethics: A Return to Fundamentals*, 2nd ed. New York: Oxford University Press, 2006:213–282. See also their earlier, shorter works: Culver CM, Gert B. Basic ethical concepts in neurologic practice. *Semin Neurol* 1984;4:1–8; Gert B, Culver CM. Moral theory in neurologic practice. *Semin Neurol* 1984;4:9–13; and Gert B, Nelson WA, Culver CM. Moral theory and neurology. *Neurol Clin* 1989;7:681–696. See also President's Commission for the Study of Ethical Problems in Medicine and Biomedical and Behavioral Research. *Making Health Care Decisions: The Ethical and Legal Implications of Informed Consent in the Patient-Practitioner Relationship*. Washington, DC, US Government Printing Office, 1982. The criteria and references for informed consent and refusal are explained further in chapter 2.

4. King JS, Moulton BW. Rethinking informed consent: the case for shared medical decision-making. *Am J Law Med* 2006;32:429–501 and Brock DW. The ideal of shared decision making between physicians and patients. *Kennedy Inst Ethics J* 1991;1:28–47.

5. Bernat JL. Plan ahead: how neurologists can enhance patient-centered medicine. *Neurology* 2001; 56:144–145.

6. The standards for surrogate decision making are discussed further in chapter 4.

7. Gunderson M. Being a burden: reflections on refusing medical care. *Hastings Cent Rep* 2004;34(5):37–43.

8. Chochinov HM, Wilson KG, Enns M, et al. Desire for death in the terminally ill. *Am J Psychiatry* 1995; 152:1185–1191.

9. McDonald ER, Wiedenfeld SA, Hillel A, et al. Survival in amyotrophic lateral sclerosis: the role of psychological factors. *Arch Neurol* 1994;51:17–23.

10. See Sullivan MD, Youngner SJ. Depression, competence, and the right to refuse life-sustaining treatment. *Am J Psychiatry* 1994;151:971–978; Young EWD, Corby JC, Johnson R. Does depression invalidate competence? Consultants' ethical, psychiatric, and legal considerations. *Cambridge Q Healthcare Ethics* 1993; 2:505–515; and Ganzini L, Lee MA, Heintz RT, et al. Depression, suicide, and the right to refuse life-sustaining treatment. *J Clin Ethics* 1993;4:337–340.

11. Block SD. Assessing and managing depression in the terminally ill patient. *Ann Intern Med* 2000; 132:209–218.

12. Back AL, Arnold RM, Quill TE. Hope for the best, and prepare for the worst. *Ann Intern Med* 2003; 138:439–443.

13. The physician's ethical duties are discussed in American Academy of Neurology Ethics and Humanities Subcommittee. Position statement: certain aspects of the care and management of profoundly and irreversibly paralyzed patients with retained consciousness and cognition. *Neurology* 1993;43:222–223. See also the discussion of this topic in chapter 14.

14. Wanzer SH, Adelstein SJ, Cranford RE, et al. The physician's responsibility toward hopelessly ill patients. *N Engl J Med* 1984;310:955–959; President's Commission for the Study of Ethical Problems in Medicine and Biomedical and Behavioral Research. *Deciding to Forego Life-Sustaining Treatment: Ethical, Medical and Legal Issues in Treatment Decisions*. Washington, DC: US Government Printing Office, 1983; Hastings Center. *Guidelines on the Termination of Life-Sustaining Treatment and the Care of the Dying*. Briarcliff Manor, NY: Hastings Center, 1987:130–131.

15. Kouwenhoven WB, Jude JR, Knickerbocker GG. Closed-chest cardiac massage. *JAMA* 1960;173:94–97.

16. For international standards for CPR, see American Heart Association. Guidelines 2000 for cardiopulmonary resuscitation and emergency cardiovascular care. *Circulation* 2000;102(suppl 8):I1–I384. The changes in these guidelines from the previous 1992 guidelines are detailed in Kern KB, Halperin HR, Field J. New guidelines for cardiopulmonary resuscitation and emergency cardiac care: changes in the management of cardiac arrest. *JAMA* 2001;285:1267–1269.

17. Schiedermayer DL. The decision to forgo CPR in the elderly patient. *JAMA* 1988;260:2096–2097.

18. Gazelle G. The slow code—should anyone rush to its defense? *N Engl J Med* 1998;338:467–469.

19. See, for example, Smith GB, Poplett N, Williams D. Staff awareness of a 'Do Not Attempt Resuscitation' policy in a district general hospital. *Resuscitation* 2005;65:159–163.

20. The history of informal DNR orders is presented in Rothman DJ. Medicine at the end of life. *Neurology* 1987;37:1079–1083.

21. For example, see Bedell SE, Pelle D, Maher PL, et al. Do-not-resuscitate orders for critically ill patients in the hospital: how are they used and what is their impact? *JAMA* 1986;256:233–237; Charlson ME, Sax FL, MacKenzie CR, et al. Resuscitation: how do we decide? A prospective study of physicians' preferences and the clinical course of hospitalized patients. *JAMA* 1986;255:1316–1322; and Youngner SJ. Do-not-resuscitate orders: no longer secret, but still a problem. *Hastings Cent Rep* 1987;17(1):24–33.

22. Kimberly MB, Forte AL, Carroll JM, Feudtner C. Pediatric Do-Not-Attempt-Resuscitation orders and public schools: a national assessment of policies and laws. *Am J Bioethics* 2005;5:59–65.

23. Choudhry NK, Choudhry S, Singer PA. CPR for patients labeled DNR: the role of the limited aggressive therapy order. *Ann Intern Med* 2003;138:65–68.

24. These data were combined from two studies: DeBard ML. Cardiopulmonary resuscitation—analysis of six years' experience and review of the literature. *Ann Emerg Med* 1981;147:37–38 and McGrath RB. In-house cardiopulmonary resuscitation—after a quarter of a century. *Ann Emerg Med* 1987;16:1365–1368.

25. Bedell SE, Delbanco TL, Cook EF, et al. Survival after cardiopulmonary resuscitation in the hospital. *N Engl J Med* 1983;309:569–576 and Taffet GE, Teasdale TA, Lucho RJ. In-hospital cardiopulmonary resuscitation. *JAMA* 1988;260:2069–2072.

26. For a review of outcome studies in CPR, see Moss AH. Informing the patient about cardiopulmonary resuscitation: when the risks outweigh the benefits. *J Gen Intern Med* 1989;4:349–355. More recent studies of outcomes of CPR among hospitalized patients reveal higher rates of survival because, with the increase in prevalence of DNR orders, resuscitation is not being attempted on many of the sicker hospitalized patients. See Ballew KA, Philbrick JT, Caven DE, Schorling JB. Predictors of survival following in-hospital cardiopulmonary resuscitation. *Arch Intern Med* 1994;154:2426–2432.

27. Initial studies suggested age was an independent risk factor for poor CPR outcome: Murphy DJ, Murray AM, Robinson BE, et al. Outcomes of cardiopulmonary resuscitation in the elderly. *Ann Intern Med* 1989; 111:199–205. Later studies have refuted this association. See Tresch D, Heudebert G, Kutty K, et al. Cardiopulmonary resuscitation in elderly patients hospitalized in the 1990s: a favorable outcome. *J Am Geriatr Soc* 1994;42:137–141.

28. Choudhry NK, Choudhry S, Singer PA. CPR for patients labeled DNR: the role of the limited aggressive therapy order. *Ann Intern Med* 2003;138:65–68.

29. Bedell SE, Delbanco TL, Cook EF, et al. Survival after cardiopulmonary resuscitation in the hospital. *N Engl J Med* 1983;309:569–576.

30. See, for example, American Medical Association Council on Ethical and Judicial Affairs. Guidelines for the appropriate use of do-not-resuscitate orders. *JAMA* 1991;265:1868–1871 and American College of Physicians Ethics Manual, 4th ed. *Ann Intern Med* 1998;128:576–594. For the most current ethical guidelines on CPR and DNR orders, see American Heart Association. Part 2: Ethical issues. *Circulation* 2005;112 (Suppl):IV-6–IV-11.

31. Burns JP, Edwards J, Johnson J, Cassem NH, Truog RD. Do-not-resuscitate order after 25 years. *Crit Care Med* 2003;31:1393–1395.

32. Choudhry NK, Choudhry S, Singer PA. CPR for patients labeled DNR: the role of the limited aggressive therapy order. *Ann Intern Med* 2003;138:65–68.

33. Berger JT. Ethical challenges of partial Do-Not-Resuscitate orders. *Arch Intern Med* 2003;163:2270–2275.

34. Wenger NS, Pearson ML, Desmond KA, Brook RH, Kahn KL. Outcomes of patients with do-not-resuscitate orders. Toward an understanding of what do-not-resuscitate orders mean and how they affect patients. *Arch Intern Med* 1995;155:2063–2068; Beach MC, Morrison RS. The effect of do-not-resuscitate orders on physician decision making. *J Am Geriatr Soc* 2002;50:2057–2061; and Sulmasy DP, Sood JR, Ury WA. The quality of care plans for patients with do-not-resuscitate orders. *Arch Intern Med* 2004;164:1573–1578.

35. Margolis JO, McGrath BJ, Kussin PS, Schwinn DA. Do not resuscitate (DNR) orders during surgery: ethical foundations for institutional policies in the United States. *Anesth Analg* 1995;80:806–809.

36. Cohen CB, Cohen PJ. Do-not-resuscitate orders in the operating room. *N Engl J Med* 1991;325:1879–1882 and Bernat JL, Grabowski EW. Suspending do-not-resuscitate orders during anesthesia and surgery. *Surg Neurol* 1993;40:7–9.

37. Truog RD. "Do-not-resuscitate" orders during anesthesia and surgery. *Anesthesiology* 1991;74:606–608.

38. American College of Surgeons. Statement on Advance Directives by Patients: "Do Not Resuscitate" in the Operating Room. *Bull Am Coll Surg* 1994;79(9):29 and Truog RD, Waisel DB, Burns JP. DNR in the OR: a goal-directed approach. *Anesthesiology* 1999;90:289–295. For guidelines on suspending peri-operative DNR orders

in children, see Fallat ME, Deshpande JK and the Section on Surgery, Section on Anesthesia and Pain Medicine, and Committee on Bioethics of the American Academy of Pediatrics. Do-not-resuscitate orders for pediatric patients who require anesthesia and surgery. *Pediatrics* 2004;114:1686–1692.

39. Kellermann A, Lynn J. Withholding resuscitation in prehospital care. *Ann Intern Med* 2006;144:692–693.

40. Tolle SW, Tilden VP, Nelson CA, Dunn PM. A prospective study of the efficacy of the physician order form for life-sustaining treatment. *J Am Geriatr Soc* 1998;46:1097–1102. The order form and educational material are available at Physician Orders for Life-Sustaining Treatment Paradigm. http://www.ohsu.edu/ethics/polst/ (Accessed July 10, 2007).

41. Tilden VP, Tolle SW, Drach LL, Perrin NA. Out-of-hospital death: advance care planning, decedent symptoms, and caregiver burden. *J Am Geriatr Soc* 2004;52:532–539.

42. Feder S, Matheny RL, Loveless RS Jr, Rea TD. Withholding resuscitation: a new approach to prehospital end-of-life decisions. *Ann Intern Med* 2006;144:634–640.

43. Institute of Medicine. *Approaching Death: Improving Care at the End of Life.* Washington, DC: National Academy Press, 1997:39–41.

44. Angus DC, Barnato AE, Linde-Zwirble WT, et al. Robert Wood Johnson Foundation ICU End-of Life Peer Group. Use of intensive care at the end of life in the United States: an epidemiologic study. *Crit Care Med* 2004;32:638–643.

45. Seferian EG, Afessa B. Adult intensive care unit use at the end of life: a population-based study. *Mayo Clin Proc* 2006;81:896–901.

46. The 40% to 65% figure is from Raffin TA. Withdrawing life support: how is the decision made? *JAMA* 1995;273:738–739. The 74% figure was from a survey of 5,910 patients cared for in 136 ICUs. See Prendergast TJ, Claessens MT, Luce JM. A national survey of end-of-life care for critically ill patients. *Am J Respir Crit Care Med* 1998;158:1163–1167.

47. For example, see President's Commission. *Deciding to Forego Life-Sustaining Treatment: Ethical, Medical and Legal Issues in Treatment Decisions,* 1982; Hastings Center. *Guidelines on the Termination of Life-Sustaining Treatment and the Care of the Dying,* 1987; Weir RF. *Abating Treatment with Critically Ill Patients: Ethical and Legal Limits to the Medical Prolongation of Life.* New York: Oxford University Press, 1989; Emanuel EJ. A review of the ethical and legal aspects of terminating medical care. *Am J Med* 1988;84:291–301; Beresford HR. Legal aspects of termination of treatment decisions. *Neurol Clin* 1989;7:775–788; Weir RF, Gostin L. Decisions to abate life-sustaining treatment for nonautonomous patients: ethical standards and legal liability for physicians after *Cruzan. JAMA* 1990;264:1846–1853; American Thoracic Society. Withholding and withdrawing life-sustaining therapy. *Ann Intern Med* 1991;115:478–485; and Faber-Langendoen K, Lanken PN. Dying patients in the intensive care unit: forgoing treatment, maintaining care. *Ann Intern Med* 2000;133:886–893.

48. Bernat JL. Ethical aspects of determining and communicating prognoses in critical care. *Neurocrit Care* 2004;1:107–118.

49. Bernat JL. Areas of consensus in withdrawing life-sustaining treatment in the neurointensive care unit. *Neurology* 1999;52:1538–1539.

50. Stanley JM (ed). The Appleton International Conference: developing guidelines for decisions to forgo life-prolonging medical treatment. *J Med Ethics* 1992;18(suppl):1–22.

51. Pijenborg L, van der Maas PJ, Kardaun JWPF, Glerum JJ, van Delden JJM, Looman CWN. Withdrawal or withholding of treatment at the end of life: results of a nationwide survey. *Arch Intern Med* 1995;155:286–292.

52. Glick SM. Unlimited human autonomy—a cultural bias? *N Engl J Med* 1997;336:954–956.

53. Cook DJ, Guyatt GH, Jaeschke R, et al. Determinants in Canadian health care workers of the decision to withdraw life support from the critically ill. *JAMA* 1995;273:703–708.

54. Ferrand E, Robert R, Ingrand P, Lemaire F. Withholding and withdrawal of life support in intensive care units in France: a prospective study. *Lancet* 2001;357:9–14.

55. Sprung CL, Cohen SL, Sjokvist P, et al. End-of-life practices in European intensive care units. The Ethicus Study. *JAMA* 2003;290:790–797.

56. van der Heide A, Deliens L, Faisst K, et al. End-of-life decision-making in six European countries: a descriptive study. *Lancet* 2003;362:345–350.

57. Bosshard G, Nilstun T, Bilsen J, et al. Forgoing treatment at the end of life in 6 European countries. *Arch Intern Med* 2005;165:401–407.

58. Kushel MB, Miaskowski C. End of life care for homeless patients: "she says she is there to help me in any situation." *JAMA* 2006;296:2959–2966.

59. White DB, Curtis JR, Lo B, Luce JM. Decisions to limit life-sustaining treatment for critically ill patients who lack both decision-making capacity and surrogate decision-makers. *Crit Care Med* 2006;34: 2053–2059.

60. White DB, Curtis JR, Wolf LE, et al. Life support for patients without a surrogate decision maker: who decides? *Ann Intern Med* 2007;147:34–40.

61. For an example of such a hospital policy, see Hyun I, Griggins C, Weiss M, Robbins D, Robichaud A, Daly B. When patients do not have a proxy: a procedure for medical decision making when there is no one to speak for the patient. *J Clin Ethics* 2006;17:323–330.

62. Curtis JR, Patrick DL, Shannon SE, Treece PD, Engelberg RA, Rubenfeld GD. The family conference as a focus to improve communication about end-of-life care in the intensive care unit: opportunities for improvement. *Crit Care Med* 2001;29(2 Suppl):N26–N33 and Curtis JR, Engelberg RA, Wenrich MD, Shannon SE, Treece PD, Rubenfeld GD. Missed opportunities during family conferences about end-of-life care in the intensive care unit. *Am J Respir Crit Care Med* 2005;171:844–849.

63. Wijdicks EFM, Rabinstein AA. The family conference: end-of-life guidelines at work for comatose patients. *Neurology* 2007;68:1092–1094.

64. For an example of a successful hospital order form conveying orders to limit treatment, see O'Toole EE, Youngner SJ, Juknialis BW, Daly B, Bartlett ET, Landefeld CS. Evaluation of a treatment limitation policy with a specific treatment-limiting order page. *Arch Intern Med* 1994;154:425–432.

65. Cranford RE. Termination of treatment in the persistent vegetative state. *Semin Neurol* 1984;4:36–44.

66. Smedira NG, Evans BH, Grais LS, et al. Withholding and withdrawal of life support from the critically ill. *N Engl J Med* 1990;322:309–315. That termination of medical treatment is a gradual process rather than a discrete event also was found in the study by Faber-Langendoen K, Bartels DM. Process of forgoing life-sustaining treatment in a university hospital: an empirical study. *Crit Care Med* 1992;20:570–577. The increasing incidence of termination of LST in ICUs over the past decade was found in Prendergast TJ, Luce JM. Increasing incidence of withholding and withdrawal of life support from the critically ill. *Am J Respir Crit Care Med* 1997;155:15–20 and Koch KA, Rodefer HD, Wears RL. Changing patterns of terminal care management in an intensive care unit. *Crit Care Med* 1994;22:233–243.

67. Christakis NA, Asch DA. Biases in how physicians choose to withdraw life support. *Lancet* 1993; 342:642–646. The same investigators found physicians to be more likely to withdraw therapies related to their own specialty. See Christakis NA, Asch DA. Medical specialists prefer to withdraw familiar technologies when discontinuing life support. *J Gen Intern Med* 1995;10:491–494. For a discussion of the unique issues in discontinuing oxygen, see Halpern SD, Hansen-Flaschen J. Terminal withdrawal of life-sustaining supplemental oxygen. *JAMA* 2006;296;1397–1400.

68. Cook D, Rocker G, Marshall J, et al. Withdrawal of mechanical ventilation in anticipation of death in the intensive care unit. *N Engl J Med* 2003;349:1123–1132.

69. Mayer SA, Kossoff SB. Withdrawal of life support in the neurological intensive care unit. *Neurology* 1999;52:1602–1609.

70. White DB, Braddock CH III, Bereknyei S, Curtis JR. Toward shared decision making at the end of life in intensive care units: opportunities for improvement. *Arch Intern Med* 2007;167:461–467.

71. Prendergast TJ, Puntillo KA. Withdrawal of life support: intensive caring at the end of life. *JAMA* 2002;288:2732–2740. So-called "medical futility" disputes with families over continuing LST are considered further in chapter 10.

72. Lautrette A, Darmon M, Megarbane B, et al. A communication strategy and brochure for relatives of patients dying in the ICU. *N Engl J Med* 2007;356:469–478.

73. Truog RD, Cist AFM, Brackett SE, et al. Recommendations for end-of-life care in the intensive care unit: the Ethics Committee of the Society of Critical Care Medicine. *Crit Care Med* 2001;29:2332–2348.

74. The theory and technique of withdrawing LST are described in Brody H, Campbell ML, Faber-Langendoen K, Ogle KS. Withdrawing intensive life-sustaining treatment—recommendations for compassionate clinical management. *N Engl J Med* 1997;336:652–657 and Daily BJ, Thomas DT, Dyer MA. Procedures used in withdrawal of mechanical ventilation. *Am J Crit Care* 1996;5:331–338.

75. Gilligan T, Raffin TA. Withdrawing life support: extubation and prolonged terminal weans are inappropriate. *Crit Care Med* 1996;24:352–353.

76. Wilson WC, Smedira NG, Fink C, McDowell JA, Luce JM. Ordering and administration of sedatives and analgesics during the withholding and withdrawal of life support from critically ill patients. *JAMA* 1992; 267:949–953.

77. See, for example, Truog RD, Berde CB, Mitchell C, Grier HE. Barbiturates in the care of the terminally ill. *N Engl J Med* 1992;327:1678–1682 and Rousseau P. Terminal sedation in the care of dying patients. *Arch Intern Med* 1996;156:1785–1786. This topic is considered further in chapter 7.

78. Truog RD, Burns JP, Mitchell C, Johnson J, Robinson W. Pharmacologic paralysis and withdrawal of mechanical ventilation at the end of life. *N Engl J Med* 2000;342:508–511.

79. Nelson JE, Angus DC, Weissfeld LA, et al. End-of-life care for the critically ill: a national intensive care unit survey. *Crit Care Med* 2006;34:2547–2553.

80. Byock I. Improving palliative care in intensive care units: identifying strategies and interventions that work. *Crit Care Med* 2006;34(Suppl):S302-S305 and Levy MM, McBride DL. End-of-life care in the intensive care unit: state of the art in 2006. *Crit Care Med* 2006;34(Suppl):S306-S308.

81. Carver AC, Vickrey BG, Bernat JL, Keran C, Ringel SP, Foley KM. End of life care: a survey of U.S. neurologists' attitudes, behavior, and knowledge. *Neurology* 1999;53:284–293.

82. Truog RD, Cochrane TI. Refusal of hydration and nutrition: irrelevance of the "artificial" versus "natural" distinction. *Arch Intern Med* 2005;165:2574–2576. See the discussion in chapter 9 on how physicians should respond to a patient's refusal of oral hydration and nutrition.

83. For example, the 2007 New Hampshire Advance Directive statute used the term "medically administered hydration and nutrition."

84. For compelling accounts of why physicians should not withhold hydration and nutrition from patients, see Derr PG. Why food and fluids can never be denied. *Hastings Cent Rep* 1986;16:28–30; Meilaender G. On removing food and water: against the stream. *Hastings Cent Rep* 1984;14(6):11–13; Siegler M, Weisbard AJ. Against the emerging stream. Should fluids and nutritional support be discontinued? *Arch Intern Med* 1985;145:129–131; and Rosner F. Why nutrition and hydration should not be withheld from patients. *Chest* 1993;104:1892–1896.

85. See Cantor NL. The permanently unconscious patient, non-feeding, and euthanasia. *Am J Law Med* 1989;15:381–437; Lynn J, Childress JF. Must patients always be given food and water? *Hastings Cent Rep* 1983;13(5):17–21; Steinbrook R, Lo B. Artificial feeding—solid ground, not a slippery slope. *N Engl J Med* 1988;318:286–290; Slomka J. What do apple pie and motherhood have to do with feeding tubes and caring for the patient? *Arch Intern Med* 1995;155:1258–1263; and Winter SM. Terminal nutrition: framing the debate for the withdrawal of nutritional support in terminally ill patients. *Am J Med* 2000;109:723–726.

86. Bernat JL, Beresford HR. The controversy over artificial hydration and nutrition. *Neurology* 2006;66:1618–1619.

87. These data are reviewed in Hodges MO, Tolle SW, Stocking C, Cassel CK. Tube feeding: internists attitudes regarding ethical obligations. *Arch Intern Med* 1994;154:1013–1020.

88. Casarett D, Kapo J, Caplan A. Appropriate use of artificial nutrition and hydration—fundamental principles and recommendations. *N Engl J Med* 2005;353:2607–2612.

89. McMahon MM, Hurley DL, Kamath PS, Mueller PS. Medical and ethical aspects of long-term enteral tube feeding. *Mayo Clin Proc* 2005;80:1461–1476.

90. SUPPORT Principal Investigators. A controlled trial to improve care for seriously ill hospitalized patients. The Study to Understand Prognoses and Preferences for Outcomes and Risks of Treatment (SUPPORT). *JAMA* 1995;274:1591–1598.

91. Some of the more noteworthy publications from SUPPORT include Knaus WA, Harrell FE Jr, Lynn J, et al. The SUPPORT model: objective estimates of survival for seriously ill hospitalized adults. *Ann Intern Med* 1995;122:191–203; Phillips RS, Wenger NS, Teno J, et al. Choices of seriously ill patients about cardiopulmonary resuscitation; correlates and outcomes. *Am J Med* 1996;100:128–137; Rosenfeld KE, Wenger NS, Phillips RS, et al. Factors associated with change in resuscitation preference of seriously ill patients. *Arch Intern Med* 1996;156:1558–1564; Haykim RB, Teno J, Harrell FE Jr, et al. Factors associated with do-not-resuscitate orders: patients' preferences, prognoses, and physicians' judgments. *Ann Intern Med* 1996;125:284–293; Hamel MB, David RB, Teno J, et al. Older age, aggressiveness of care, and survival for seriously ill, hospitalized adults. *Ann Intern Med* 1999;131:721–728; and Teno J, Lynn J, Phillips RS, et al. Do formal advance directives affect resuscitation decisions and the use of resources for seriously ill patients? *J Clin Ethics* 1994;5:23–30. For commentaries on the SUPPORT findings, see the essays in Moskowitz EH, Nelson JL (eds). Dying well in the hospital: the lessons of SUPPORT. *Hastings Cent Rep* 1995;25(6 suppl):S1–S36.

92. Annas GJ. How we lie. *Hastings Cent Rep* 1995;25(6 suppl):S12–S14.

93. Lo B. Improving care near the end of life. Why is it so hard? *JAMA* 1995;274:1634–1636 and Prendergast TJ. The SUPPORT project and improving care for seriously ill patients. *JAMA* 1996;275:1227.

94. Shewmon DA, DiGiorgio CM. Early prognosis in anoxic coma: reliability and rationale. *Neurol Clin* 1989;7:823–843.

95. Becker KJ, Baxter AB, Cohen WA, et al. Withdrawal of support in intracerebral hemorrhage may lead to self-fulfilling prophecies. *Neurology* 2001;56:766–772.

96. Zurasky JA, Aiyagari V, Zazulia AR, Shackelford A, Diringer MN. Early mortality following spontaneous intracerebral hemorrhage. *Neurology* 2005;64:725–727.

97. Zahuranec DB, Brown DL, Lisabeth LD, et al. Early care limitations independently predict mortality after intracerebral hemorrhage. *Neurology* 2007;68:1651–1657.

98. Hemphill JC III, Newman J, Zhao S, Johnston SC. Hospital usage of early do-not-resuscitate orders and outcome after intracerebral hemorrhage. *Stroke* 2004;35:1130–1134.

99. Rabinstein AA, Wijdicks EFM. Determinants of outcome in anticoagulation-associated cerebral hematoma requiring emergency evacuation. *Arch Neurol* 2007;64:203–206.

100. Geocadin RG, Buitrago MM, Torbey MT, Chandra-Strobos N, Williams MA, Kaplan PW. Neurologic prognosis and withdrawal of life support after resuscitation from cardiac arrest. *Neurology* 2006;67:105–108.

101. I discussed this and other ethical issues in making prognoses on critically ill patients in Bernat JL. Ethical aspects of determining and communicating prognoses in critical care. *Neurocrit Care* 2004;1: 107–118.

102. Broderick J, Connolly S, Feldmann E, et al. Guidelines for the management of spontaneous intracerebral hemorrhage in adults. 2007 Update. A guideline from the American Heart Association/American Stroke Association Stroke Council, High Blood Pressure Research Council, and the Quality of Care and Outcomes in Research Interdisciplinary Working Group. *Stroke* 2007;38:2001–2023.

103. Levetown M, Pollock MM, Cuerdon TT, Ruttimann UE, Glover JJ. Limitations and withdrawals of medical intervention in pediatric critical care. *JAMA* 1994;272:1271–1275.

104. Mink RB, Pollack MM. Resuscitation and withdrawal of therapy in pediatric intensive care. *Pediatrics* 1992;89:961–963.

105. Vernon DD, Dean JM, Timmons OD, et al. Modes of death in the pediatric intensive care unit: withdrawal and limitation of supportive care. *Crit Care Med* 1993;21:1798–1802.

106. Nelson LJ, Rushton CH, Cranford RE, Nelson RM, Glover JJ, Truog RD. Forgoing medically provided nutrition and hydration in pediatric patients. *J Law Med Ethics* 1995;23:33–46 and Johnson J, Mitchell C. Responding to parental requests to forgo pediatric nutrition and hydration. *J Clin Ethics* 2000;11:128–135.

107. A number of disturbing cases of conflicts between surrogates and physicians that are hard to resolve have been reported. See Schneiderman LJ, Teetzel H, Kalmanson AG. Who decides who decides? When disagreement occurs between the physician and the patient's appointed proxy about the patient's decision making capacity. *Arch Intern Med* 1995;155:793–796; Spike J, Greenlaw J. Ethics consultation: refusal of beneficial treatment by a surrogate decision maker. *J Law Med Ethics* 1995;23:202–204; Gillick MR, Fried T. The limits of proxy decision making: undertreatment. *Cambridge Q Healthcare Ethics* 1995; 4:172–177; and Terry PB, Vettese M, Song J, et al. End-of-life decision making: when patients and surrogates disagree. *J Clin Ethics* 1999;10:286–293.

108. For the most authoritative and encyclopedic source on American laws governing decisions to withhold or withdraw treatment, see Meisel A, Cerminara KL. *The Right to Die: The Law of End-of-Life Decisionmaking*, 3rd ed. Aspen Publishers, Inc, 2004.

109. *In re Quinlan*, 70 NJ 10, 355 A2d 647, *cert denied sub nom. Garger v New Jersey*, 429 US 922 (1976).

110. Personal communication. Fred Plum, April 27, 1989.

111. There has been much learned commentary interpreting the *Quinlan* ruling for physicians. See, especially, Beresford HR. The Quinlan decision: problems and legislative alternatives. *Ann Neurol* 1977;2:74–81. For a thorough biography of the Quinlan story, see *In the Matter of Karen Quinlan*, 2 vol. Frederick MD: University Publications of America, 1977. For Quinlan's autopsy report, see Kinney HC, Korein J, Panigrahy A, Dikkes P, Goode R. Neuropathological findings in the brain of Karen Ann Quinlan. The role of the thalamus in the persistent vegetative state. *N Engl J Med* 1994;330:1469–1475.

112. Of the voluminous medicolegal commentary on *Cruzan*, useful works include Meisel A. A retrospective on *Cruzan*. *Law Med Health Care* 1992;20:340–353; Capron AM (ed). Medical decision-making and the "right to die" after *Cruzan*. *Law Med Health Care* 1991;19:1–104; White BD, Siegler M, Singer PA, et al. What does *Cruzan* mean to the practicing physician? *Arch Intern Med* 1991;151:925–928; Orentlicher D. The right to die after *Cruzan*. *JAMA* 1990;264:2444–2446; Annas GJ. Nancy Cruzan and the right to die. *N Engl J Med* 1990;323:670–673; Lo B, Steinbrook R. Beyond the Cruzan case: The U.S. Supreme Court and medical practice. *Ann Intern Med* 1991;114:895–901; and Weir RF, Gostin L. Decisions to abate life-sustaining treatment for nonautonomous patients: ethical standards and legal liability for physicians after *Cruzan*. *JAMA* 1990;264: 1846–1853.

113. The scope of a state's legitimate interests in preserving life includes the protection of incompetent subjects, maintaining the integrity of the medical profession, and the prevention of suicide. See Blake DC. State interest in terminating medical treatment. *Hastings Cent Rep* 1989;19(3):5–13.

114. *Cruzan v. Harmon*, 760 SW 2d 408 (Mo 1988) (en banc); *Cruzan v. Director, Missouri Dept. of Health*, 110 S Ct 2841, 1990.

115. In the American Academy of Neurology survey, 38% of respondent neurologists held this view. See Carver AC, Vickrey BG, Bernat JL, Keran C, Ringel SP, Foley KM. End of life care: a survey of U.S. neurologists' attitudes, behavior, and knowledge. *Neurology* 1999;53:284–293.

116. See, especially, *Eichner v. Dillon*, 426 NYS 2d 517, modified in, *In re Storar*, 420 NE 2d 64 NY Ct App, 1981.

117. *Barber v. Superior Ct*, 147 Call App 3d 1006, 195 Cal Rptr 414, 1983.

118. Alpers A. Criminal act or palliative care? Prosecutions involving care of the dying. *J Law Med Ethics* 1998;26:308–331.

119. Meisel A, Jernigan JC, Youngner SJ. Prosecutors and end-of-life decision making. *Arch Intern Med* 1999;159:1089–1095.

120. *Superintendent of Belchertown School v. Saikewicz*, 373 Mass 728, 370 NE 2d 417, 1977. This decision was discussed and critiqued in Curran WJ. The Saikewicz decision. *N Engl J Med* 1978;298:499–500 and Relman AS. The Saikewicz decision: judges as physicians. *N Engl J Med* 1978;298:508–509.

121. For a scholarly review of case laws and decision making doctrines in different states, see Meisel A. *The Right To Die*, 2nd ed. New York: John Wiley & Sons, 1995.

122. *Barber v. Superior Ct*, 147 Call App 3d 1006, 195 Cal Rptr 414, 1983.

123. Rhoden NK. Litigating life and death. *Harvard Law Rev* 1988;102:375–446. A similar suggestion was made in Lo B, Rouse F, Dornbrand L. Family decision making on trial. Who decides for incompetent patients? *N Engl J Med* 1990;322:1228–1232.

124. For a clinically useful review of state laws governing physicians' orders to withhold or withdraw artificial hydration and nutrition in terminally ill and permanently unconscious patients, see Larriviere D, Bonnie RJ. Terminating artificial nutrition and hydration in persistent vegetative state patients: current and proposed state laws. *Neurology* 2006;66:1624–1628.

125. *Brophy v. New England Sinai Hospital, Inc*, 398 Mass 417, 497 NE 2d 626, 1986.

126. *Cruzan v. Director, Missouri Dept. of Health*, 110 S Ct 2841, 1990.

127. Meisel A. Barriers to forgoing nutrition and hydration in nursing homes. *Am J Law Med* 1995; 21:335–382.

128. Solomon MZ, O'Donnell L, Jennings B, et al. Decisions near the end of life: professional views on life-sustaining treatments. *Am J Public Health* 1993;83:14–23. An excellent set of medical and legal guidelines that, despite its target audience, is better known by judges than by physicians is Hafemeister TL, Hannaford PL. *Resolving Disputes Over Life-Sustaining Treatment: A Health Care Provider's Guide*. Williamsburg, VA: National Center for State Courts, 1996.

129. Although 98% of neurologists responded that a competent, terminally ill patient has the right to refuse life-sustaining treatment, including hydration and nutrition, 53% asserted that withdrawing a treatment is ethically different from withholding or not starting it. See Carver AC, Vickrey BG, Bernat JL, Keran C, Ringel SP, Foley KM. End of life care: a survey of U.S. neurologists' attitudes, behavior, and knowledge. *Neurology* 1999;53:284–293. These findings are distressing given the clear statements of practice standards published earlier in relevant *Neurology* journal articles, such as Rothman DJ. Medicine at the end of life. *Neurology* 1987;37:1079–1083 and editorials such as Bernat JL, Goldstein ML, Viste KM Jr. The neurologist and the dying patient. *Neurology* 1996;46:598–599 and Bernat JL, Cranford RE, Kittredge FI Jr, Rosenberg RN. Competent patients with advanced states of permanent paralysis have the right to forgo life-sustaining therapy. *Neurology* 1993;43:224–225.

130. Bacon D, Williams MA, Gordon J. Position statement on laws and regulations concerning life-sustaining treatment, including artificial nutrition and hydration, for patients lacking decision-making capacity. *Neurology* 2007;68:1097–1100.

131. Perkins HS, Bauer RL, Hazuda HP, et al. Impact of legal liability, family wishes, and other "external factors" on physicians' life-support decisions. *Am J Med* 1990;89:185–194.

132. Goldblatt D. A messy, necessary end: health care proxies need our support. *Neurology* 2001;56:148–152 and Bernat JL. Plan ahead: how neurologists can enhance patient-centered medicine. *Neurology* 2001; 56:144–145.

133. Menikoff JA, Sachs GA, Siegler M. Beyond advance directives—health care surrogate laws. *N Engl J Med* 1992;327:1165–1169.

134. President's Commission. *Deciding to Forego Life-Sustaining Treatment*: 1983:160–165 and President's Commission. *Making Health Care Decisions*. 1982:187–188.

135. For examples of conversations with patients' families in which physicians present treatment or non-treatment options, see Miller DK, Coe RM, Hyers TM. Achieving consensus on withdrawing or withholding care for critically ill patients. *J Gen Intern Med* 1992;7:475–480.

136. See Larriviere D, Bonnie RJ. Terminating artificial nutrition and hydration in persistent vegetative state patients: current and proposed state laws. *Neurology* 2006:66:1624–1628.

137. Molloy DW, Clarnette RM, Braun EA, et al. Decision making in the incompetent elderly: "the daughter from California syndrome." *J Am Geriatr Soc* 1991;39:396–399.

Physician-Assisted Suicide and Voluntary Active Euthanasia

9

In the preceding chapter, I showed that over the past three decades, Western society has accepted the ethical and legal rights of terminally ill patients to refuse life-sustaining therapy. This acceptance has led some advocates of the "death with dignity" movement to make the further claim that terminally ill patients who are not receiving life-sustaining therapy, but who wish to die sooner than would occur otherwise, have a right to receive a physician's assistance to kill them or to help them kill themselves. By the early 21st century, this claim had not been accepted most of by Western society. Both the morality of and ideal public policy regarding physician-assisted suicide (PAS) and voluntary active euthanasia (VAE) remain topics of ongoing debate.

In this chapter, I review the history of PAS and VAE in the United States. I summarize the arguments for and against explicitly legalizing PAS and VAE on moral, legal, and pragmatic grounds. I report on the findings in the Netherlands and in the state of Oregon where some of these activities are licit, and discuss current professional and lay opinion about these practices. I conclude that PAS and VAE may be morally defensible in rare instances in which a patient's suffering cannot be controlled with optimal palliative care. But I believe the public interest would be better served if PAS and VAE were not explicitly legalized and if the resources expended by advocates of legalization were instead devoted to improving the provision of palliative care. I end by discussing how physicians should address patients' requests for PAS and VAE.

I show that, if all other palliative measures fail, a patient's voluntary refusal of hydration and nutrition remains a preferable ethical and legal alternative to legalizing PAS and VAE.[1]

HISTORY

In Western society over the past two decades, the question of legalizing PAS or VAE has been discussed widely by the media, the academy, and the polity. This contemporary public debate represents only the most recent chapter in the history of euthanasia.[2] Although euthanasia was practiced by Greek and Roman physicians, it was explicitly outlawed by the Hippocratic Oath that forbade physicians from "giving a deadly drug to a patient." The general opposition of organized medicine to euthanasia has continued to present times. Modern attention to euthanasia began in the late 19th century in England, where it became the topic of speeches at medical societies and was discussed in scholarly articles in medical journals. A bill to legalize euthanasia, introduced in the Ohio legislature in 1906, sparked considerable debate but ultimately was defeated.[3]

In Germany in 1920, psychiatry professor Alfred Hoche and Chief Justice of the Reich Karl Binding reintroduced the topic in their infamous book *The Permission to Destroy Life Unworthy of Life.*[4] They argued that the lives led by certain unfortunate people, such as the institutionalized mentally retarded, mentally ill, and incurably ill, were "lives unworthy of life" (*lebensunwerten Lebens*) and their "merciful" killing by physicians constituted "healing treatment." Further, because these unworthy lives drained the state's finite resources and contaminated the German gene pool, killing them also represented a social good. Hoche and Binding's book and earlier works from the *Rassenhygiene* (racial hygiene) movement, such as the widely read text by Alfred Ploetz,[5] served as the theoretical basis for the German sterilization plan begun in the early 1930s and followed quickly by the involuntary euthanasia program. As is now well known, within just a few years, these programs evolved into the Nazi death camp mass killings of the Holocaust. Less well appreciated is how the acceptance of the theories of racial hygiene and lives unworthy of life convinced many German physicians practicing in the Third Reich to actively participate in both programs in their deranged belief that "healing by killing" followed medical ethics and represented good citizenship.[6]

Debate on legalizing euthanasia was renewed in England in the 1930s. British physicians formed the Voluntary Euthanasia Legalization Society and unsuccessfully attempted to pass a bill in Parliament legalizing euthanasia.[7] The discovery shortly thereafter of the horrors of the Holocaust and the willing participation of some German and Austrian physicians in the mass killings quelled interest in legalizing euthanasia for several decades thereafter.

In the United States, aside from a few scholarly works in the 1950s on the pros and cons of legalizing euthanasia,[8] attention to this subject was not rekindled until the 1980s, when reports from the Netherlands on their program of permissible PAS and VAE were publicized (see later). In 1988, *JAMA* published the provocative vignette of casual euthanasia of a young woman with cancer in a short piece entitled "It's over, Debbie" which sparked a tremendous and heated response from physicians on both sides of the debate.[9] Later, publication of Timothy Quill's case of PAS performed more cautiously on "Diane," similarly evoked much reaction from the professional community and culminated in a grand jury investigation that refused to hand down a murder indictment to Quill.[10] Scholarly journals such as the *Hastings Center Report*, the *Journal of Medicine and Philosophy*,

and the *Cambridge Quarterly of Healthcare Ethics* featured special issues dedicated to discussions of the theoretical and practical aspects of legalizing PAS and VAE.[11] Numerous scholarly books and edited conferences, debating various aspects of PAS and VAE, continue to be published.[12]

The popular press in the United States continues to kindle public fascination with the question of legalizing PAS and VAE. Articles about the activities of assisted suicide advocate Dr. Jack Kevorkian were a staple of news reports throughout the 1990s until his conviction and incarceration for 2nd degree murder in 1999 for performing VAE on Thomas Youk, a man with ALS who requested his assistance.[13] The Hemlock Society, under the leadership of Derek Humphry and, more recently, Faye Girsh, has conducted a well-funded grass roots national campaign to legalize PAS. *Final Exit*, the Hemlock Society's suicide manual for the terminally ill, remains a best-seller.[14] Numerous polls have indicated that an increasing proportion of United States citizens favors the legalization of PAS and VAE.[15] Although Washington state's Initiative 119, which would have legalized PAS, was narrowly defeated,[16] Oregon voters in 1994 and again in 1997 approved by referendum the legalization of PAS.[17] (See below.)

Several factors are responsible for intense public and scholarly interest in PAS and VAE. Many people fear that they will suffer needlessly during the course of a terminal illness because their physicians will institute inappropriately aggressive life-sustaining treatments they do not want that will prolong their dying process. Yet, despite receiving aggressive life-support, many people also fear they will not receive adequate treatment for pain and suffering while dying.[18] They further fear they will lose control over their lives, making their final days personally degrading. Finally, many people fear that their terminal illnesses will bankrupt them and their families.

Over the past decade, scholarly attention to PAS and VAE shows signs of waning. A year-by-year tabulation of published journal articles on PAS and VAE shows a bell-shaped curve. The output of scholarly articles peaked in the mid-1990s. The number of articles in published in 2003 was only one-fifth the number published in 1993.[19] As is true in other controversies such as medical futility (chapter 10), this decline in scholarship volume does not reflect a growing consensus so much as the reality that the essential points of the arguments have been made and only reports of new data justify publication. In the case of PAS, it also may reflect a growing sense of its inconsequentiality because the Oregon data (see below) show that PAS is used in only about one in a thousand deaths.[20]

Some scholars and legislators have concluded that the explicit legalization of PAS or VAE for terminally ill patients would best prevent dying patients' fears. In the idealized PAS model, a physician would be permitted to write a prescription for a lethal dose of a barbiturate at a patient's request. The physician would instruct the patient how to take the drug for a successful suicide. The patient later could consume the drug when and where she wished to die. In the idealized VAE model, the dying patient would ask her physician to kill her mercifully. After satisfying appropriate preconditions, the physician would administer a lethal parenteral injection. Both these models carry the theoretical advantage of empowering patients to control the time and mode of their death, thus giving them the option to allay fears of suffering a prolonged, painful, degrading, and expensive death. But, aside from the moral issues, they create a number of serious problems that lead me to conclude that their legalization is undesirable public policy.

DEFINITIONS

First, it is necessary to precisely define the terms used in this debate because some of the disagreement stems from definitional ambiguity.[21] Physician-assisted suicide ("assisted killing") refers to the act wherein, at the request of a competent patient, a physician provides the necessary medical means for the patient to commit suicide, and the patient subsequently follows the physician's instructions to employ these medical means to take her own life. A suicide is physician-assisted if the physician's participation is a necessary but not a sufficient component of the suicide. For

example, a physician becomes a necessary component of a dying patient's suicide if she complies with a patient's request to prescribe 100 pentobarbital tablets, for the express purpose of committing suicide. If the patient later swallows the medication to commit suicide, the physician would be considered an assistant to this act for providing the medication and explaining its use for suicide.

The physician who merely notifies a dying patient interested in committing suicide that books have been published on this subject has not committed PAS. Because this information is widely available, the physician's participation is an unnecessary component of the suicide. Similarly, physicians who warn patients that unadvisedly taking an overdose of a properly prescribed medication may be lethal have not performed PAS because it is customary medical practice to caution patients about the effects of medication overdosage. Providing properly prescribed palliative treatment to alleviate a dying patient's pain and suffering is not PAS or VAE, even if the patient dies sooner as an unintended consequence, if the intent was to prevent suffering and the medication type and amount were appropriate for the goal of palliation.

Voluntary active euthanasia ("mercy killing") refers to an act that a physician performs at the request of a competent dying patient, most commonly a lethal injection, to directly kill the patient. Death usually follows immediately after the injection is completed. In VAE, the physician's act is both necessary and sufficient to produce the patient's death. The patient's underlying medical condition does not contribute to causing her death in VAE but only provides the context to make it acceptable. For example, a physician performs VAE if she complies with a dying patient's request to end the patient's life mercifully with a lethal intravenous injection of Pentothal.

Voluntary passive euthanasia ("allowing to die") is an archaic term used to describe the death of a patient following the withdrawing or withholding of life-sustaining therapy (LST). This term arose in the physician-centered era in which physicians determined when and for whom LST would be discontinued. When they decided and stopped LST and the patient died as a result, a plausible claim could be made that they had committed "passive euthanasia."

However in today's patient-centered environment, patients or their lawful surrogates refuse LST and the physician generally must stop LST once it has been refused. (See chapter 8.) Now it is misleading to use the term "passive euthanasia" if the patient dies as a consequence of stopping LST because the patient has a disease that is fatal in the absence of LST and the patient has the right and authority to refuse LST. Take, for example, the case of a physician who complies with the rational refusal of a ventilator-dependent patient with amyotrophic lateral sclerosis (ALS) to continue further positive-pressure ventilatory support and the patient dies from ALS-induced respiratory failure as the result of extubation. Labeling such an act as euthanasia is incorrect. The physician has not euthanized the patient by terminating LST. The patient has died of her underlying disease (ALS) after validly refusing LST that the physician, therefore, was required to withhold. In this situation, unlike in PAS or VAE, the underlying disease is both necessary and sufficient to cause the patient's death, in the absence of the LST that the patient has validly refused. The term "passive euthanasia" should be abandoned in this context.

Palliative care of the dying patient includes the relief of pain and other causes of suffering, as described in chapter 7. Physicians have the duty to provide palliative care to the best of their ability. If providing adequate palliative care has the unintended secondary effect of accelerating the moment of death (which rarely occurs), such an occurrence is not considered PAS or VAE because the medical treatment is designed and intended to prevent suffering, not to kill the patient. This foreseen but unintended "double effect" is simply the price of providing patients with adequate palliative care.[22]

"Physician aid-in-dying" is a term that has been used to refer to any or all of the different activities defined in this section. Although the term was developed as a euphemism for physician-assisted suicide, presumably to make it more publicly acceptable, the term should be abandoned because it is inherently ambiguous

and misleading.[23] Other euphemisms such as "assisted dying" and "assisted death" also should be abandoned because they are misleading and can be confused with palliative care of the dying patient.

There are critical differences between the morality and legality of PAS, VAE, withholding therapy, and palliative care. Despite the fact that suicide is not unlawful in any American jurisdiction, PAS is unlawful in most jurisdictions. There is a current controversy about the morality of PAS in certain circumstances. Presently, VAE is classified as homicide and is illegal in every jurisdiction in the United States and in nearly every jurisdiction in the world. [24] Like PAS, the morality of VAE in certain circumstances remains a subject of heated controversy. By contrast, withholding and withdrawing LST are morally acceptable and widely permitted (or required) legally as a consequence of a patient's valid treatment refusal. Palliative care should always be provided.

THE DISTINCTION BETWEEN PATIENT REFUSALS AND PATIENT REQUESTS

Some philosophers and physicians have had difficulty making the conceptual distinction between PAS (or VAE) and withdrawing or withholding of LST because they failed to understand the important moral difference between a patient's right to refuse therapy and a patient's right to request therapy or some other act.[25] Physicians are morally and legally required to honor a competent patient's rational refusal of LST, even if the patient's death results directly from the underlying disease in the absence of LST. This requirement arises from the powerful moral and legal prohibition against depriving a person of freedom and the corollary liberty-based rights of a person to be left alone. In the medical context, this right of freedom requires that a patient provide valid consent before a physician can perform medical tests or treatments. Valid refusal is an implicit component of valid consent (chapter 2).[26]

The moral and legal requirement to honor a patient's treatment refusal does not imply a correlative duty to honor a patient's request for specific therapy or another act. Rather, a physician can base a decision whether or not to honor a patient's request on his or her professional judgment about the legal, moral, or medical appropriateness of the request.[27] For example, patients commonly request antibiotics for viral respiratory infections, but physicians can refuse to comply with this request if they judge antibiotics to be inappropriate therapy. Physicians do not have the same duty to honor to a request for therapy that they have to honor a valid treatment refusal. A patient may request—or even demand—treatment, but has no right to specific treatment.

Confusion can be created when a patient's refusal is framed misleadingly in terms that resemble a request. For example, a patient's "request" for a Do-Not-Resuscitate order is actually a refusal of consent for resuscitation. This inversion occurs because, whereas most therapies can be given only after consent, cardiopulmonary resuscitation is routinely provided on the basis of implied consent unless a person has explicitly refused. Similarly, written advance directives "requesting" that other treatments be stopped or omitted are actually refusals to consent to treatment. Some writers have added to the confusion by referring to a patient's "choice" to forego therapy as if there were no morally significant distinction between refusing and requesting.[28]

Whether a patient's expressed verbal wish or advance directive is a refusal or request can be clarified by paraphrasing it. If the treatment wish, however it is communicated, can be paraphrased to mean "stop doing that to me," the patient has made a refusal. If her wish cannot be paraphrased in this way, the communication was a request.[29]

The distinction between requests and refusals is of critical importance in understanding the moral distinction between withdrawal or withholding therapy (letting die) and PAS (assisted killing) or VAE (killing). Competent patients' rational refusals must be honored even when physicians know death will result from the underlying disease. There is no concomitant moral requirement to honor patient requests at all and particularly when physicians know that death will result from the requested act; there also may be legal prohibitions against doing so.

Some scholars have rejected the important moral distinction between PAS or VAE as "killing" and cessation of LST as "letting die." They argue that if a malicious person disconnected LST from a patient who wanted to live, the malicious person could not defend himself on the grounds that he did not kill the patient because the patient died from her underlying disease.[30] This argument misses the point. The most relevant moral difference between killing and letting die is not the specific act of the physician; it is that the patient has refused LST and the physician, therefore, must comply. The physician has no similar moral requirement to comply with a request for performing PAS or VAE.[31]

THE MORALITY OF PAS AND VAE

PAS and VAE has been debated at both moral and public policy levels. Are acts of assisted suicide or patient killing at a patient's request morally justified? If so, is the legalization of these acts desirable public policy for society? In this section, I present arguments that have been advanced to defend the morality of PAS and VAE. In the next section, I consider arguments advanced to defend the immorality of these acts. Following these discussions, I highlight the pros and cons of implementing PAS and VAE as public policy.[32] I consider both PAS and VAE together in these discussions because, despite their obvious differences, they share many of the same relevant characteristics regarding morality and suitability for public policy.[33]

All arguments accept the premise that VAE is deliberate killing and PAS is deliberate assisted killing. Five arguments seek to justify the morality of deliberate killing or assisted killing by showing that: (1) these acts yield fewer net harms than the alternative of letting dying patients suffer; or (2) they fulfill physicians' duties to suffering patients.[34]

Respecting the right of patient self-determination is the primary moral argument used to defend PAS and VAE. According to this argument, patients should be granted full control in determining the manner and time of their death; therefore, they should have the right to request PAS or VAE. Granting them this control parallels the control they are permitted by rights of self-determination in other avenues of life. Only the dying person herself can determine that time when the burdens of her life exceed the benefits and when her life is no longer worth living. Our respect for human dignity requires that persons possess the rights of full self-determination throughout adult life, and those rights include the ability to control the time and mode of their demise.[35]

Second, physicians have a professional duty to alleviate suffering of their dying patients. When physicians no longer can cure their patients or prevent them from dying of a terminal illness, their duty shifts to that of preventing pain and suffering. Because some dying patients suffer intractably with symptoms so refractory to medical treatment, death may represent the only solution to alleviate suffering. Under these circumstances, physicians have the responsibility to accede to their patients' requests to end their lives mercifully or help them to do so themselves. Not doing so would violate the physician's moral and professional duty to prevent suffering.[36]

Third, PAS and VAE are compassionate and beneficent acts. Physicians should have compassion for patients and for their suffering. They cannot stand by idly and permit patients to suffer when technological attempts fail to provide adequate palliation. In this circumstance, not to accede to the patient's wish for assisted suicide or mercy killing would be to consign the patients to a death of suffering that could have been prevented. Moreover, we exhibit sufficient compassion to euthanize our dying pet animals to prevent their suffering. Why then can we not apply this same humane and compassionate behavior toward our suffering patients?[37]

Fourth, PAS and VAE minimize harms to the patient and others. The concept of nonmaleficence and the duty not to cause pain or to disable can be satisfied by acceding to a dying patient's wish for PAS or VAE. Although a physician violates the moral rule "Do not kill" in acquiescing to these wishes of a patient, there are some experiences that are worse than death. According to this argument, assisting in a suffering patient's suicide or killing the patient at

her request is a morally justified breach of the moral rule not to kill, and it respects the concept of nonmaleficence because it minimize the net harm to the patient.[38]

Fifth, permitting these acts corresponds to current medical reality and medical responsibility. Life-sustaining and resuscitative technology now permits physicians to prolong the lives of patients, many of whom otherwise would have died earlier. Unfortunately, when rescue therapy fails to restore health, some patients are left in a state of "prolonged dying," an end-stage of chronic illness accompanied by suffering. Physicians share a responsibility for the patient's present suffering because, in the most relevant sense, they facilitated it with technology by interrupting the natural progression of illness and prevented the patient's earlier death. This responsibility imparts a special moral duty for a physician to permit a patient to complete the dying process that the physician interrupted, thereby to escape the suffering for which the physician is partially responsible.[39]

THE IMMORALITY OF PAS AND VAE

There are an equal number of arguments that PAS and VAE are immoral acts inimical to the ethical foundation of the practice of medicine.[40] In a rebuttal of the self-determination argument supporting PAS and VAE, Edmund Pellegrino pointed out its weakness: when a patient opts for VAE or PAS, she uses her freedom to relinquish her freedom and autonomy. By killing herself, the patient loses control over a range of options that she cannot foresee but forever become precluded. Further, if the patient's suffering is so intense that there is no choice except PAS or VAE, then, ironically, that choice no longer is free and autonomous because there are no alternatives.[41]

Second, PAS and VAE distort and corrupt the healing relationship between patient and physician and thereby violate the moral purposes of medicine. By its very nature, medicine is a healing profession. It intends to restore patients' health. When cure is not possible, the goal of medicine is to help patients cope with disability or death. Medicine is grounded in trust, an essential ingredient for treating a patient rendered vulnerable by illness. If euthanasia became an option and the healing profession approved of killing, the physician would breach this relationship of trust. Rather than working with patients to help them cope with their disability or reduce their suffering to enable them to live meaningfully, killing them becomes an option for physicians. How can a trusting relationship survive if patients feel uncertain about their physician's intentions? Will the physician attempt every means to reduce a patient's suffering when it would be easier simply to promote PAS or VAE? How can the fiduciary relationship between patient and physician survive if the patient fears that the physician no longer pursues her best interests?[42]

Third, PAS and VAE damage the traditional role of physicians as counselors and healers by misdirecting their emphasis in the care of the dying patient. Rather than physicians directing their attention to their traditional roles of providing palliative treatment for the dying patient, comforting her and her family, and easing her passing, they have the moral right to end the patient's life or help her to end her own life. The power to kill is an awesome and corrupting responsibility that distorts the traditional role of physicians in a damaging way. Why should physicians bother to pursue the difficult task of learning and practicing optimal palliative care? If PAS or VAE were acceptable options, physicians could influence their patients' choices by explicitly or implicitly suggesting that patients consider these solutions to the problem of dying.[43] Then the profession of medicine would advocate killing rather than healing.

Fourth, the goals of beneficence and compassion are not served only by euthanizing a suffering patient. There is some benefit in suffering to some degree because the human condition can grow even with negative experiences. Patients may see themselves most starkly at the moment of their death. To amputate this experience prematurely may be to deny a patient the opportunity to gain profound final insights about herself and the meaning of her life.[44]

Finally, the goals of nonmaleficence and patient self-determination are bounded by the accuracy of the physician's clinical determination and the rationality of the patient's decision to choose PAS or VAE. There is an irreducible degree of uncertainty in determining a terminal prognosis, which is a prerequisite for euthanasia. By the errors intrinsic to the practice of medicine, some patients who may not be terminally ill will be euthanized. Similarly, there is inescapable error in determining a patient's competency, another prerequisite for PAS or VAE. The effects of concomitant depression on a patient's "autonomous" decision for PAS or VAE may not be clearly discernable. Thus, potentially treatable conditions may remain untreated and the patient may be euthanized unnecessarily because of the limits of medical diagnosis and prognosis.[45]

PAS AND VAE SHOULD BE LEGALIZED

Many scholars advocating the morality of PAS and VAE also hold that these practices should be legalized. Advocates claim that decriminalizing these acts in the states in which they are now felonies, and legalizing them by statute in jurisdictions in which they are neither lawful nor unlawful presently, will empower physicians with the ability to offer a new variety of desirable medical services to their dying patients. The numerous legal and constitutional issues involved in drafting laws to permit or prohibit PAS and VAE have been the subject of several reviews.[46]

Polls of public opinion have yielded data showing that the majority of the American population favors legalizing PAS.[47] However, many of these data are of questionable validity. The confounding effects of improper framing, poor question design, false dichotomies, and leading questions have contaminated the interpretation of many of the surveys. The fact that most people cannot discriminate between VAE or PAS and the refusal of medical treatment confounds the interpretation of an alleged preference to legalize PAS. Further, most people are not aware of the alternatives to VAE; therefore, they incorrectly conceptualize their choice as being between VAE or PAS and prolonged suffering.[48]

Roger Magnusson pointed out that, despite its illegality, covert PAS and VAE are being conducted in the United States. Dying patients are licitly obtaining and hoarding opioid and depressant medications that they later use to commit suicide. Physicians and nurses are conducting clandestine active euthanasia, with and without patients' permission. He argued that the failure of medical bodies to regulate this covert activity is a "scandal" that would be solved by explicitly legalizing PAS and having it performed properly in the open according to medically accepted standards. He pointed out that scholars opposed to legalizing VAE from a "harm minimization" perspective also should consider the harm produced by permitting the current practice of clandestine PAS and VAE.[49] Stephen Smith reached a similar conclusion that the problems of explicitly legalizing euthanasia would probably be fewer than those currently resulting from its covert practice by the euthanasia "underground."[50]

All those advocating legalization of PAS and VAE agree that clinical practice guidelines and procedural safeguards must be carefully drafted and enforced to prevent abuses.[51] In this regard, the seven criteria proposed by Timothy Quill, Christine Cassel, and Diane Meier for the legalization of PAS have received the greatest attention and acceptance.[52] In their proposed statute, all seven preconditions must be satisfied before the physician can provide PAS.

First, the patient must have an incurable condition that causes profound suffering, but it is not necessary for the patient to be in imminent danger of death. If there is doubt about the diagnosis or prognosis, the patient must seek a second opinion. The patient must understand the prognosis and available alternative options for palliative treatment.

Second, the physician must ascertain that all reasonable attempts to provide palliative care have been tried and have failed or, at least, have been discussed with the patient. The patient's request for PAS cannot result from inadequate treatment; the request truly must be a last resort. The strict satisfaction of this condition will markedly limit the valid candidates for PAS.

Third, the patient's request for PAS must be purely voluntary. Family members or others should not induce the request. It must represent the patient's free and autonomous choice.

Fourth, the physician should ascertain that the patient's judgment is not impaired and that the decision for PAS is rational. The physician can test its rationality by examining the patient's reasons for wanting to commit suicide. To wish to die sooner from a terminal illness and thereby avoid days, weeks, or months of suffering generally counts as a rational decision.[53] Consistent, repeated requests with full support of the family also help assure the physician that the decision was not merely an impulsive response to the illness. The presence of potentially reversible depression must be ruled out with caution, although this determination is admittedly difficult in patients dying of terminal illnesses.[54]

Fifth, PAS should be performed within the context of a stable and continuous physician-patient relationship. Only the physician caring for the patient can determine the rationality of a request for PAS. In this way, the physician can confirm that she and the patient have fulfilled all preconditions. In this context, the impersonal and mechanical PAS-by-arrangement as practiced by Jack Kevorkian can be censured as immoral.

Sixth, all preconditions should be reviewed by another physician to confirm that they have been fulfilled properly. Seventh, all preconditions and decisions should be documented fully, including the signing of a consent form. The physicians and family members participating must receive adequate assurance that they will not be liable for criminal prosecution if the preceding preconditions are satisfied.[55]

PAS AND VAE SHOULD NOT BE LEGALIZED

All persons who hold that PAS and VAE are immoral, and many who hold that PAS and VAE may be moral under certain circumstances, believe that the practices should not be legalized. Generally, they fear that explicit legalization of PAS and VAE would impose harmful effects on society, patients, and the practice of medicine that would outweigh the totality of benefits they offer. Changing public policy to legalize PAS creates a new and troubling set of problems that are different from those that result merely from accepting the moral permissibility of PAS in individual isolated circumstances. Keeping PAS illegal would prevent these problems.

Legalization of a practice that has been strictly forbidden previously by society removes a longstanding taboo. Laws regulating the permissibility of a previously forbidden practice may be drafted carefully and in a highly specific manner, thereby theoretically eliminating the possibility of abuse. However, once the societal taboo has been broken, it is simply a consequence of human nature for people to extend the boundaries of the practice ineluctably beyond those stipulated by law. By doing so, harms are produced that, while not permitted by the law, could have been anticipated as a consequence of the new law, and certainly are the direct result of changing the law.[56] Any proposal to break a longstanding taboo, even one containing provisions that have been drafted carefully to prevent abuses, is doomed to foster those abuses because of the tendency of people to "push the envelope." As discussed in the following section, VAE is now permitted under certain circumstances in the Netherlands. Unfortunately, involuntary euthanasia, which is strictly forbidden by Dutch law, also is being practiced on the infirm and elderly because the taboo against medical killing has been broken. (See below.)

A number of harms that otherwise would be avoided could be produced by legalizing PAS and VAE. Legalization could damage public confidence in the medical profession because physicians would be regarded as killers in addition to healers. Could patients continue to trust implicitly that their physician always would try to improve their health if they had the power to kill? Loss of public confidence would reduce the public's trust in physicians and produce irreparable harm to the patient-physician relationship, subsequently harming all patients.

An example of loss of public confidence in physicians already has occurred in the Netherlands where VAE is lawful under certain circumstances. According to several on-site commentators, some handicapped and elderly patients are frightened to enter Dutch hospitals and nursing homes for fear of becoming subjects of VAE.[57] Public trust in the medical profession to look out for patients' best interests is a precious but precarious commodity. It must not be jeopardized by unwisely and unnecessarily altering the role of physicians and the meaning of medicine.

Legalization of PAS or VAE would likely create unintended and harmful social pressures and place high expectations on patients. Many elderly, disabled, or chronically ill patients might feel "the duty to die." They would request euthanasia not on the basis of a free, personal choice but because they perceived that their families considered them an emotional or financial burden and expected them to agree to die and get out of the way.[58] In a similar vein, patients might sense subtle pressure from their physicians to consider VAE or PAS as an alternative because the physician was tired of struggling to provide them with adequate palliative care. In the end, they would request it because they believed that the physician must know what was best for them. The meaning of the prerequisite "voluntary" in a euthanasia statute could be corrupted, causing the elderly and chronically ill to become victimized.[59]

Explicit legalization of PAS in a fragmented health system, such as that currently existing in the United States, potentially could victimize members of lower socioeconomic classes. Patients without insurance or access to the full complement of health care may lack access to palliative care. If PAS were legalized and widely available by law, some lower socioeconomic class patients might be steered to choose it over palliative care by this direct availability.[60]

Legalization of PAS or VAE could require the creation of a network of cumbersome legal safeguards to protect patients from abuse and misunderstanding or miscommunication. Safeguards would require the involvement of courts, lawyers, and bureaucrats. New legal requirements could have the effect of delaying the patient's death and generating unnecessary administrative complexity and expense.[61] Even if the bureaucratic machinery were in place, it might not be able to prevent the systematic practice of involuntary euthanasia, such as is occurring now in the Netherlands.

The policy issue of quantifying the cost savings resulting from the legalization of PAS was analyzed by Ezekiel Emanuel and Margaret Battin. Using the Netherlands data on PAS utilization and United States data on end-of-life costs, they estimated that the legalization of PAS in the United States would save approximately $627 million in 1998 dollars, or 0.07% of total health-care expenditures. They concluded that these cost savings should not be a major factor in the policy debate about legalizing PAS.[62]

EUTHANASIA AND PHYSICIAN-ASSISTED SUICIDE IN THE NETHERLANDS

Scholars and politicians debating the effects on society of legalizing PAS or VAE need only examine the experience over the past few decades in the Netherlands, a country that Edmund Pellegrino called the "great social laboratory for euthanasia."[63] In 1985, the State Commission on Euthanasia endorsed a series of judicial rules that permitted Dutch physicians conducting PAS and VAE to avoid prosecution if they followed them.[64] Although until 2001, PAS and VAE were not explicitly "legal" in the Netherlands, because of their prohibition under Article 293 of the Dutch Penal Code, they were permissible in the Netherlands and practiced widely by physicians who followed the judicial rules.[65] In November 2000, the Dutch Parliament voted to explicitly legalize the practices of PAS and VAE that had been conducted widely for the previous 15 years. The bill, incorporating guidelines accepted by the Royal Dutch Medical Association, was signed into a law in 2001 that became effective in February 2002 known as the Euthanasia Act. Although the law explicitly legalizing PAS and VAE was not enacted until 2002, it simply codified what already had become normative medical practice. Raphael Cohen-Almagor analyzed the historical and sociological reasons why this practice began in the Netherlands.[66] In 2002, Belgium also legalized VAE but there are inadequate data to assess its impact.[67]

The original Dutch euthanasia guidelines mandated that four criteria be satisfied: (1) the patient must be competent; (2) the act must be voluntary and requested repeatedly by the patient; (3) the patient must experience unbearable suffering with no prospect of relief other than death; and (4) the physician must obtain a corroborating consultation that the preconditions have been met and that the patient's request is appropriate. The cause of death must be reported accurately to state authorities.[68] The 2001 law provided six criteria granting physicians legal immunity for performing euthanasia: a physician must (1) be convinced that the patient's request was voluntary, well considered, and lasting; (2) be convinced that the patient's suffering was prospectless and unbearable; (3) have informed the patient about his situation as well as about his prognosis; (4) be convinced, together with the patient, that there was no reasonable alternative solution for his situation; (5) have consulted at least one other independent physician who has seen the patient and has formed an opinion in writing about the requirements of due care described in (1) through (4); and (6) have terminated the patient's life with due medical care.[69]

Dr. P.V. Admiraal, one of euthanasia's most vocal proponents, explained the bedside medical techniques of VAE to Dutch physicians in a monograph in great detail. His euthanasia manual for physicians provides the dosages, routes of administration, and other technical details necessary to perform successful VAE by lethal injection of benzodiazepines, barbiturates, opiates, neuromuscular blocking agents, or insulin.[70]

As a result of the acceptance of this program, data have been generated on the frequency of VAE, who performs it, and the diseases for which it has been used. One figure for 1990 indicated that VAE was responsible for 4,000 to 6,000 deaths annually in the Netherlands—that is, between 3.0% and 4.5% of all deaths.[71] In the official study based on questionnaire and death certificate data, commissioned by Jan Remmelink, VAE by lethal injection was estimated to be responsible for 2,300 deaths or 1.8% of all deaths in the Netherlands in 1990.[72] In a similarly commissioned subsequent study in

1995, 2.4% of deaths were found to be from VAE and 0.2% from PAS.[73] Dutch physicians granted euthanasia in somewhat less than half of requested instances. VAE was performed mostly by family physicians and general practitioners.[74]

The most recent and complete survey conducted by Agnes van der Heide and colleagues found that in 2005, 1.7% of all deaths in the Netherlands were the result of VAE and 0.1% were the result of PAS. Combining the two practices, VAE accounts for 94% of cases and PAS for 6%. Interestingly, these percentages were lower than in 2001 when 2.6% of all deaths were from VAE and 0.2% from PAS. Additionally, 7.1% of all deaths in the Netherlands were the result of continuous deep sedation (increased from 5.6% in 2001) in which the intent may have been to hasten death.[75]

The underlying diseases in patients requesting VAE were cancer (70%), chronic degenerative neurological disorders (10%), chronic obstructive pulmonary disease (10%), and others (10%). The principal reason patients gave for requesting VAE was unbearable suffering, both physical and emotional. Patient's sources of suffering included more than intractable pain. Many patients endured intractable nausea and vomiting; some had incontinence; others had foul odors and advanced cachexia; and many could not face the progressive disintegration of their body and loss of their bodily functions.[76] Requests for VAE for psychiatric reasons, such as depression, were common but were granted only rarely.[77] Dutch physicians rarely refer prospective PAS and VAE patients for psychiatric evaluation.[78] Recent reports from the Netherlands document a few patients requesting and receiving PAS or VAE in the early stages of Alzheimer's disease.[79]

Dutch physicians take their responsibilities for conducting PAS and VAE seriously. A qualitative study of 30 Dutch physicians showed the extent to which they performed extensive self-reflection on each case of PAS or VAE. They spent weeks to months debating whether VAE would be appropriate and examined their feelings, emotions, and reactions. They concluded that they had upheld their duty to their patients in their patients' time of need.[80] Another large questionnaire study of Dutch

physicians revealed the complexity of decision making and how much care was taken in each case before proceeding.[81]

However, abuses of the strictly delineated rules of one critical and recurring type have been reported. These reports allege that physicians are conducting active euthanasia on unwilling individuals in the absence of voluntary requests. Despite de Wachter's admonition that voluntariness was so essential to the concept of euthanasia in the Netherlands that the term voluntary euthanasia was a tautology and the term involuntary euthanasia an oxymoron,[82] the feared outcome of involuntary euthanasia has been realized, at least in some reported cases.

Physicians have reported that incompetent adults and children in coma or a persistent vegetative state or with dementia, mental retardation, or other forms of chronic illness are being involuntarily euthanized in Dutch hospitals, nursing homes, and institutions for the mentally retarded.[83] Euthanasia of hopelessly ill newborns currently is practiced in the Netherlands under the "Groningen Protocol."[84] In some instances, physicians justified this action by rationalizing that patients would have consented to be euthanized if they had the capacity to consent, rather than to continue living in their present miserable state. Thus, these physicians were merely carrying out the patients' implied wishes, perhaps acting on a variation of the substituted judgment or best interest standards. The similarity of this justification to the infamous Nazi philosophy of *lebensunwerten Leben* (lives unworthy of life) is disturbing.[85]

The extent to which physicians carry out this illegal act of involuntary active euthanasia in the Netherlands is not precisely known; however, a recent study has provided some data. On the basis of physician interviews and questionnaires, Pijnenborg and colleagues reported in 1993 that a total of 0.8% of all deaths in the Netherlands resulted from a life-terminating act performed by a physician without the explicit request of the patient.[86] In the most recent study of deaths in 2005, the figure was 0.4%.[87] Many of these cases involved imminently dying patients whose death was induced by a large bolus of intravenous morphine or patients treated with continuous deep sedation with the intent of hastening death. The extent of involuntary euthanasia on hospitalized patients or nursing home residents with stable, chronic illnesses or disabilities remains unknown.

Another issue of concern in the Dutch practices of VAE and PAS is the extent to which physicians suggest them to patients. A 1990 study found that VAE was suggested to patients by 50% of Dutch physicians.[88] This finding raises serious questions about whether the requirement that patients' requests are strictly voluntary is being satisfied.[89] Further, studies have shown that 59% of Dutch physicians failed to report cases of PAS and VAE [90] even though there have been measurable improvements in the notification procedures.[91]

One study analyzed the complications of performing PAS and VAE in the Netherlands. In 23% of the PAS cases, complications arose necessitating that physicians convert the unsuccessful PAS to VAE by administering a lethal injection. The most common problem was that the patient did not die quickly after ingesting the purportedly lethal dose of depressant drugs and thus later had to be actively euthanized by the physician.[92] Another study of consent complications showed that 26% of patients' requests for PAS or VAE were not accomplished because the patient died before it could be performed or did not finalize the request before dying; 13% later withdrew the request, and in 12% of cases the physician refused to comply with the request.[93]

The experience in the Netherlands shows that even a carefully crafted program of purely voluntary euthanasia is destined to be corrupted by apparently well-intentioned physicians who wish to extend the benefits of euthanasia to others. Once society has lifted the taboo on physician killing, involuntary active euthanasia inevitably follows. There is no technical solution to prevent this abuse.[94] There are cultural reasons to believe that the risk of involuntary euthanasia is lower in Oregon than in the Netherlands.[95] Philosophers are debating the desirability of permitting VAE by advance directive, but this idea has the same drawbacks discussed previously.[96]

I conclude that the best interests of society and its citizens are served if VAE and PAS remain illegal. Although all experienced physicians can recall instances of intractable suffering in which they believed that PAS or VAE might have been morally justified,[97] legalizing these acts makes poor public policy because the totality of the negative effects of doing so exceeds the positive ones. Public policy should not be dictated by individual heart-wrenching cases.[98] A legalized program of VAE or PAS is not desirable because the inevitable side effect of involuntary euthanasia is intolerable.[99]

THE OREGON DEATH WITH DIGNITY ACT

In the United States, Oregon is the only state that explicitly legalized PAS. In November 1994, Oregon voters, on ballot referendum, approved the Death with Dignity Act, or "Measure 16." The act removed criminal penalties against physicians for helping terminally ill patients commit suicide by writing a prescription for a lethal dose of medication upon their request.[100] Measure 16 permitted qualifying patients to "legally request and obtain medication from a physician to achieve a humane and dignified death." Previous similar measures had failed in the states of Washington (Initiative 119) and California (Proposition 161) and in other states.[101] Measure 16 immediately became the target of lawsuits questioning its constitutionality and a federal district court issued an injunction delaying its implementation until the constitutional issues could be resolved. Following the 1997 U.S. Supreme Court ruling (discussed below), the Act was returned to Oregon voters who again approved it in November 1997, at which time injunctions against it were removed and it became law.[102]

The Oregon Death with Dignity Act provides terminally ill patients the right to request and receive prescriptions for a lethal dose of medications to self-administer to commit suicide. To be eligible, patients must be "capable," that is, have the ability to make and communicate a request. They must make one written and two oral requests to the physician, separated by at least 15 days. The patient's primary physician and a consultant must concur that the patient is terminally ill, that the patient is capable, and that the patient's judgment is not impaired by a psychological disorder. If the patient's judgment is impaired, the patient must be referred for counseling. The physician must inform the patient about alternatives, such as pain control and hospice care. Physicians then must report all prescriptions they write for PAS to the Oregon Health Division (OHD), the state agency monitoring the law.[103]

The OHD has reported its experience with legalized PAS during the first nine years of the law.[104] Through January 1, 2007, a total of 292 patients had committed suicide under the Act; 54% were men and 58% were aged 65 to 84. PAS patients' underlying diseases were malignant neoplasms in 81%, ALS in 8%, chronic lung disease in 4%, HIV/AIDS in 2%, and a miscellany of diseases in the remaining 5%. In 2006, the PAS cohort accounted for approximately 1.5 of each 1,000 deaths in Oregon. However PAS is practiced disproportionately by patients with ALS and HIV/AIDS. Over the nine-year period, PAS accounted for 27 per 1,000 deaths among ALS patients and 23 per 1,000 deaths among HIV/AIDS patients. The nine-year PAS patient group had the following further characteristics: 86% were enrolled in hospice, 13% were referred for psychological evaluation, 94% died at home, 99% were prescribed lethal dosages of secobarbital or pentobarbital, 94% had no complications, and the median duration between medication ingestion and death was 25 minutes. Four end-of-life concerns were cited by over 50% of PAS patients: loss of autonomy, diminished ability to engage in activities making life enjoyable, loss of dignity, and loss of control of bodily functions. Concern over pain control was cited in only 26% of patients.[105]

Over the past four years, the number of patients requesting PAS prescriptions has been stable at an annual mean of 62 and the number of patients consuming the prescriptions for a successful suicide had remained at a stable annual mean of 39, though 46 patients committed suicide under the Act in 2006. The 2006 data show fewer psychiatric referrals (4%).[106] A questionnaire study of Oregon physicians revealed that they granted only one

in six patient requests for PAS and that only one in 10 requests eventually resulted in suicide.[107] Another physician questionnaire showed that since the passage of the Oregon Death with Dignity Act, Oregon physicians were 30% more likely to refer terminally ill patients to hospice; 76% of physicians reported that they had made efforts to improve their knowledge of the use of pain medications in terminally ill patients.[108]

The Oregon Medical Association has taken an ambivalent and evolving position in this debate. Reflecting conflicted physician opinion on legalizing PAS, they were neutral on the 1994 referendum but expressed mild and reserved opposition to the 1997 referendum. They now have expressed a willingness to comply with the provisions of the new law. The Oregon Nurses Association requested legal clarification on what assistance, if any, a nurse can give a patient who is attempting PAS. Can they, for example, help weak patients place the medication in their mouths, or does this constitute illegal VAE? Similarly, the Oregon Board of Pharmacy has sought clarification of the exact role of pharmacists who fill PAS prescriptions because of the lethal dosages.[109] Hospice nurses and social workers commonly care for the Oregon PAS patients. A survey of hospice nurses and social workers showed that 45% had cared for a PAS patient. The most commonly cited reason for the patient's action was desire for control of his or her fate.[110]

In November 2001, U.S. Attorney General John Ashcroft ruled that the Oregon Death with Dignity Act violated the federal Controlled Substances Act of 1970 and authorized the Drug Enforcement Administration to take legal action against Oregon physicians who prescribed lethal dosages of medication for PAS under Oregon law.[111] Physicians and medical societies immediately criticized this action as a harmful and unjustified intrusion of the federal government into the practice of medicine and predicted chilling effects on appropriate palliative care practices if the order survived judicial appeal.[112] In May 2004, the U.S. Court of Appeals for the Ninth Circuit struck down Ashcroft's order as unlawful because it violated the language of the Controlled Substances Act (CSA) and overstepped his statutory authority. In January 2006, in *Gonzalez v. Oregon*, the U.S. Supreme Court upheld this ruling asserting that the CSA does not prohibit Oregon physicians from prescribing under the Death with Dignity Act.[113]

Critics have identified several shortcomings of the Death with Dignity Act. Alexander Capron pointed out that, even though the Act legalizes only PAS and not VAE, it will be impossible for any coherent law to restrict VAE in the future. Why, he asks, should the law not provide a remedy for the patient who lacks the physical capacity to place the medication in his mouth and swallow it? Why should disabled patients be deprived of the "right" to PAS enjoyed by other terminally ill Oregon citizens? Capron argues that there is no coherent legal mechanism to prevent broadening the scope of the act to encompass VAE for the patient lacking the capacity to commit the act without assistance.[114] Sherwin Nuland wondered why Dutch physicians reported complications of PAS in nearly a quarter of attempted cases but none were reported in Oregon.[115]

In another critique, Kathleen Foley and Herbert Hendin identified several weaknesses of the Act and its monitoring by the Oregon Health Division. They first asked how OHD could be so certain that the patients using PAS had received adequate end-of-life care when the data they collected were purely epidemiologic. Second, although physicians are required to point out alternatives to PAS, such as palliative care, the law does not require them to be knowledgeable about how to use palliative care. Third, although OHD concluded that economic factors were irrelevant in patients' decisions to request PAS, the Act did not require them to inquire about financial circumstances. Fourth, although the Act required physicians to refer for counseling any patient suspected of having a psychiatric impairment, it did not mandate psychiatric evaluation despite the fact that many physicians cannot reliably diagnose depression. Fifth, unlike the law in the Netherlands, the Oregon law stipulates only that the patient must be terminally ill. Intolerable and unrelievable suffering is not an eligibility requirement. Finally, Foley and Hendin criticized OHD for a conflict of interest because, while they administer the law and analyze its effect, they have adopted a

strong position of public advocacy for PAS. This advocacy has caused them to overstate what they know about how the law is being used. Foley and Hendin recommended the appointment of an independent task force of professionals knowledgeable in palliative care, psychiatry, and medicine to review and analyze the Oregon PAS cases.[116]

At this intermediate stage of the law's implementation, a few further conclusions are possible. PAS is being used highly selectively and only rarely. Most of the dire problems critics had feared apparently have not occurred. Whether the acceptance of PAS will lead to legalization of VAE remains to be seen. Because PAS is being used by only about one-tenth of one percent of dying patients in Oregon, such a rarely used option cannot be the sole answer to the problems of the dying patient. Purely from a pragmatic perspective, improving systems of palliative care that benefit all dying patients comprises a more sensible public policy than legalizing PAS. The Oregon experience should continue to be studied in depth as other states consider enacting similar laws.

PHYSICIAN-ASSISTED SUICIDE AND THE CONSTITUTION

In parallel and nearly contemporaneous rulings in 1996 that state laws banning PAS were unconstitutional, two federal appeals courts ruled that citizens have a constitutional right to PAS for the same reason they have a constitutional right to refuse LST. The U.S. Court of Appeals for the Second Circuit ruled that the New York state ban on PAS violated the 14th amendment to the constitution guaranteeing equal protection under the law. They opined that only by guaranteeing a right to PAS could terminally ill patients not dependent on LST receive equal protection of the "right to die" granted to terminally ill patients dependent on LST.[117] In a related line of argument, the U.S. Court of Appeals for the Ninth Circuit ruled that Washington state's ban on PAS was unconstitutional because the right to determine the time and manner of death is a liberty right protected under the due process clause of the 14th amendment. The court found "no ethical or constitutionally cognizable difference between a doctor's pulling the plug on a respirator and his prescribing drugs which will permit a terminally ill patient to end his own life."[118] Surprisingly, both courts dismissed the commonly held and common-sense moral distinction between patients' refusals and requests that I have previously emphasized.[119]

The following year, the U.S. Supreme Court reversed both these decisions, ruling that there is no constitutionally protected right to receive PAS and that state laws banning PAS violate neither the due process clause nor the equal protection clause of the 14th amendment.[120] The concurring justices offered various rationales for their opinions, but implicit in them all was finding an important distinction between the constitutionally protected right to be left alone that underlies the right to refuse LST and a purported "right" to receive medication or other services from a physician upon request. The former right is constitutionally protected under the 14th amendment while the latter is not. The Supreme Court ruling made no change in a state's authority to outlaw or decriminalize PAS.[121] The Court's finding that PAS can continue to be regulated by state law was the basis for permitting the Oregon Death with Dignity Act to become law later in 1997.

The slogan "the right to die" is cited frequently as the purported constitutional basis for the legalization of PAS by its proponents. However, the U.S. Supreme Court found no such constitutionally protected right in the United States. They asserted that the only relevant constitutionally protected right is the right to refuse therapy.[122] Laws governing PAS and VAE in other countries have been reviewed.[123]

EMPIRICAL DATA

Physician attitudes toward practicing PAS and VAE and the current prevalence of covertly practiced PAS and VAE have been studied in a number of surveys. Diane Meier and colleagues found that 11% of American physicians currently were willing to perform PAS and 7% were willing to perform VAE despite their illegality. These figures increased to 36%

and 24% respectively in the hypothetical situation that they became legal. They found that 18% of physicians had received patient requests for PAS and 11% for VAE. Of this group, 16% (3% of the total group) reported that they had complied at least once with PAS and 5% of the total reported that they had administered at least one lethal injection.[124]

In a similar national survey of oncologists, Ezekiel Emanuel and colleagues found that 22.5% supported the use of PAS and 6.5% supported VAE for a terminally ill patient with unremitting pain. They found that about 11% reported conducting PAS at least once and 4.8% had performed VAE.[125] Similar data have been recorded from state surveys of physicians in Washington,[126] Oregon,[127] and Michigan,[128] and in earlier, smaller, national surveys.[129] A survey of practicing physicians in Connecticut found that those physicians who endorsed PAS made no meaningful distinction between PAS and VAE.[130]

In a survey of neurologists belonging to the American Academy of Neurology, Alan Carver and colleagues found that under current law, 13% of respondent neurologists said they would participate in PAS and 4% in VAE. However, if PAS and VAE were legalized, 44% would participate in PAS and 28% in VAE. One-third of respondents believed that physicians have the same ethical duty to honor a terminally ill patient's request for PAS as they do to honor the terminally ill patient's refusal of LST.[131]

Diane Meier and colleagues reported a large survey of United States physicians who received and honored PAS requests. Of 1,902 respondents (63% of those surveyed), 379 reported 415 cases in which they refused the most recent request and 80 cases in which they honored the most recent request. The large majority of patients requesting PAS were near death from terminal illness and "had a significant burden of pain and physical discomfort." Nearly half the patients were thought to be depressed. Physicians were more likely to grant PAS requests if the patients were in severe pain, had a life expectancy of less than one month, and were not believed to be depressed at the time of the request.[132]

A highly publicized survey of critical care nurses found that among nurses who practiced exclusively in adult ICUs, 17% had received requests from patients or family members for PAS or VAE. A surprising 16% reported that they had engaged in one or both practices and an additional 4% responded that they had hastened a patient's death by only pretending to provide LST ordered by a physician. The method of VAE used most commonly was administering an unnecessarily high dose of an opioid drug to a terminally ill patient.[133]

The attitudes of terminally ill patients toward PAS and VAE also have been surveyed. Linda Ganzini and colleagues found that 56% patients with ALS in Washington and Oregon said they would consider PAS and 79% of this group would request a prescription for PAS if it were legal. Only one patient would have used the prescription immediately and most of the others would have kept it for future use.[134]

In a study of 988 terminally ill patients and their caregivers, Ezekiel Emanuel and his colleagues found that 60% of the patients supported PAS and VAE in theory but only 11% considered it seriously for themselves. Of note, at a follow-up interview, about half the patients had changed their minds. Ultimately, only one patient (0.4% of the group) died of PAS or VAE, one attempted suicide, and one repeatedly requested that physicians end her life. (This plea was refused by her family and physicians.)[135]

In a qualitative interview study of PAS patients' and family members of patients' motivations for choosing PAS, Robert Pearlman and colleagues found that before proceeding, nearly all patients deliberated for a considerable time, repeatedly debating its benefits and burdens. They concluded that most patients chose PAS after following a thoughtful deliberative process and not impulsively.[136]

MEDICAL SOCIETY POSITIONS

Nearly all medical societies that have expressed an official position on PAS and VAE have stated opposition. The American Medical Association (AMA) stated that PAS was "totally incompatible with the nature and purposes of the healing arts and sciences."[137] The American College of Physicians-American Society of Internal Medicine "does not support the legalization of physician-assisted suicide."[138] The British Medical Association and the British House of Lords Select Committee on Medical Ethics reaffirmed their stand against legalizing PAS and VAE.[139] The American Academy of Neurology said that it joins other societies in "vigorously opposing physician-assisted suicide, euthanasia, and any other actions by neurologists that are directly intended to cause the death of patients."[140] The New York State Task Force on Life and the Law published a book opposing the legalization of PAS and VAE.[141] The European Association of Palliative Care stated that "the provision of euthanasia and physician-assisted suicide should not be part of the responsibility of palliative care."[142] The American Nurses Association published a complex policy attempting to balance nurses' conflicting duties given the likelihood that PAS would become legal in some jurisdictions. The policy allows that PAS is "part of a continuum of end-of-life choices" of patients but stated that PAS was "outside the historic tradition and normative framework of nursing practice." They cautioned nurses to "react with compassion, rather than judgment" in such cases.[143]

Two physician-scholars who are prominent in end-of-life care recommended that, in light of the contentiousness of the PAS debate and the documented limitations of palliative care to alleviate all end-of-life suffering, medical societies should maintain "studied neutrality" on the question of legalizing PAS.[144] In a questionnaire survey, Simon Whitney and colleagues found that while the majority of members of the AMA House of Delegates opposed legalizing PAS (as does their official policy), rank-and-file AMA members were evenly divided on this issue. Both groups agreed it would be best if there were no laws governing PAS at all.[145]

RESPONDING TO A PATIENT'S REQUEST FOR ASSISTED SUICIDE OR EUTHANASIA

The preceding data show that despite the illegality of PAS and VAE, some patients request these procedures from their physicians. How should physicians respond to such requests?

First, the physician should explore the reasons for the patient's request and try to understand the sources of suffering. There are some empirical data relevant to this question in addition to those from Oregon already discussed. Several researchers found that the request for PAS correlated with depression, but these studies used questionnaires with forced-choice answers that may have biased the responses.[146] Another reason commonly cited in several surveys was to prevent being a burden on other people.[147] James Lavery and colleagues used open-ended interviews to study qualitatively the reasons for patients with HIV/AIDS gave for requesting PAS. They found that the reason most commonly expressed was to prevent personal disintegration. Loss of normal functioning, loss of community, and loss of relationships brought about this sense of personal disintegration.[148]

Second, the physician should attempt to provide ideal palliative therapy with medications and other available means as discussed in chapter 7. Physicians should be trained to practice "aggressive palliative care" in order to suppress the sources of suffering in dying patients by employing the same attitude of aggressiveness with which they were trained to treat life-threatening disease in other patients. The physician should pledge not to abandon the patient but to treat and comfort the patient to the fullest extent possible. Toward this end, the physician should remain ever vigilant to identify and treat reversible depression. Psychiatrists can assist this process.[149]

Maintaining an open dialogue with patients who request PAS permits exploration of their expectations and fears, sources of suffering, and knowledge of end-of-life care options.[150] Susan Block and Andrew Billings outlined the subject areas that should be explored by physicians when a patient requests PAS or VAE. They should address the adequacy of symptom control and assure that all possible palliative measures are being used. They should explore the patient's relationships with family, friends and coworkers, and pursue especially the patient's fear of being a burden. They should assess the patient for psychological disturbances, particularly grief, depression, and delirium, and make necessary psychiatric referrals for diagnosis and treatment. They should explore the meaning of suffering and death to the patient. Physicians also should consider their personal feelings about requests to hasten death and the extent to which fulfilling such requests might relieve or produce their own anxiety.[151]

Linda Emanuel proposed a sequential eight-step approach to patient requests for PAS or VAE that can be learned by physicians as a skill set. (1) Assess for depression and treat if present. (2) Assess for decision-making capacity. If it is impaired and cannot be improved with treatment, seek a surrogate. (3) Engage in a structured deliberation including advance care planning and palliative care, and provide the requested care. (4) Establish and treat the root causes of the requests, including the physical, personal, and social issues uncovered. (5) Ensure that the patient has received full information on consequences, risks, and responsibilities, and attempt to dissuade from PAS. (6) If this fails to stop the request, involve consultants such as a hospital ethics committee. (7) Review adherence to all goals and reevaluate the palliative care plan. (8) If the request continues, discuss legally and ethically acceptable alternatives to PAS and VAE.[152] Such possible alternatives include voluntary refusal of hydration and nutrition (discussed below) and palliative sedation (discussed in chapter 7).[153]

Jeffery Kohlwes and associates studied the question of how physicians in practice respond to patients' requests for PAS. They found that the physicians surveyed followed a similar approach, first inquiring, "Why do you want to die now?" The physicians reported three classes of answers to this question: unendurable physical symptoms, psychological symptoms, and existential suffering. They responded to these concerns by enhancing palliative care and treating depression. Physicians who subsequently provided PAS did so most often because of their inability to help their patients' existential suffering.[154] Existential suffering in dying patients results from concerns about the meaning of life, human relations, personal autonomy, guilt, and human dignity. Physicians treating existential suffering can assist their patients in discussing their concerns with friends or spiritual counselors.[155]

PATIENT REFUSAL OF HYDRATION AND NUTRITION

If, after the physician has made a thorough attempt to treat the patient's sources of suffering, the patient continues to express a wish to die sooner, the physician can inform the patient of the right to refuse enteral or parenteral hydration and nutrition. The patient can be informed that she may refuse food, tube feedings, and intravenous hydration or nutrition and that her physician will help her to carry out her refusal in a way that minimizes her suffering. My colleagues and I called this practice "patient refusal of hydration and nutrition" (PRHN). It empowers dying patients in a manner that is both ethically acceptable and lawful.[156]

Until the past 15 years, the euthanasia debate failed to include PRHN as an alternative for two reasons. The important moral distinction between a patient's right to refuse treatment (including hydration and nutrition) and the right to request PAS and VAE was not sufficiently appreciated. More significant was the erroneous but widely held assumption that thirst and hunger remain strong drives in terminal illness and that unmanageable suffering inevitably accompanies the lack of hydration and nutrition.

It is the consensus of experienced physicians and nurses that terminally ill patients dying of dehydration or lack of nutrition usually do not suffer if given proper palliative care. Maintaining physiological hydration and adequate nutrition can be difficult in dying and seriously ill patients because intrinsic thirst and hunger drives usually are diminished or absent. For many years, physicians and nurses have observed that dying patients lose hunger and thirst drives and experience peaceful and apparently comfortable deaths although they neither request nor receive hydration or nutrition.[157]

Reports from hospice nurses indicate that the large majority of hospice deaths resulting from lack of hydration and nutrition can be managed in such a manner that the patients remain comfortable.[158] In a 1990 survey of 826 members of the Academy of Hospice Physicians, 89% of the hospice nurses and 86% of the hospice physicians said that their terminal patients who refused hydration and nutrition experienced peaceful and comfortable deaths.[159] Dry mouth, the major symptom of dehydration, can be relieved adequately by ice chips, methyl cellulose, artificial saliva, or small sips of water insufficient to reverse progressive dehydration.[160] Oregon hospice nurses, who attended the deaths of over 100 patients dying of PRHN, reported that nearly all patients experienced a very good death. The mean score of the PRHN group was eight on a 0–9 scale where zero was a very bad death and nine was a very good death.[161]

The idea that dying patients can accelerate the moment of death by refusing hydration and nutrition is not new. Variations on this practice have been recorded by many cultures throughout history. The oldest carefully recorded experience of PRHN is the Jainist method of *bhaktapratyakhyana*, or fasting and meditating until death.[162] That such practices can be conducted commonly without suffering also has been documented in poignantly described personal accounts.[163] Contemporary reviews of the management options available to terminally ill patients now consider PRHN as a major option.[164]

As a public policy, there are several tangible benefits of offering PRHN over legalizing PAS and VAE. Unlike PAS and VAE, PRHN is consistent with traditional medical, moral, and legal practices because patients have the right to refuse life-sustaining therapies, including hydration and nutrition.[165] PRHN does not compromise public confidence in the medical profession because, unlike PAS and VAE, it does not require physicians to assume any new role or responsibility that could alter their roles as healers, caregivers, and counselors. It places proper emphasis on the duty of physicians to care for dying patients, because these patients need care and comfort measures during the dying period. It encourages physicians to engage in educational discussions with patients and families about dying and the desirability of formulating clear advance directives.[166]

It is unlikely that patients who refuse hydration and nutrition will feel that they have the same "duty to die" as patients who choose PAS or VAE. Because of the duration of the PRHN process and the opportunity therein for reconsideration and family interaction, it is improbable that physicians or other health-care professionals would pressure dying patients into taking such a course.[167]

Unlike PAS and VAE, PRHN is lawful in most jurisdictions. Refusal of hydration and nutrition is a common option in most statutory advance directives. Because communication errors, misunderstandings, and abuses are less likely for inpatients who choose PRHN, unwanted earlier deaths are less likely to result. The patient who chooses PRHN clearly demonstrates the seriousness and consistency of her desire to die. During the interval before the patient becomes unconscious, she has time to reconsider her decision and her family has time to accept that she clearly wishes to die. Further, the process can begin immediately without the patient's or physician's having first to obtain legal approval or other bureaucratic requirements. Ironically, PRHN may permit the patient to die faster than PAS or VAE, given the waiting periods mandated by the latter.[168]

Once a dying patient has refused hydration and nutrition, the physician has the continued responsibility to maintain her comfort. Comfort measures include proper mouth care, suppression of dyspnea, and provision of adequate analgesia. Physicians should provide whatever dosages of morphine or benzodiazepines are necessary to suppress the patient's pain and suffering.[169] The goal of therapeutics in this setting is not to kill the patient but to permit her to experience as painless a death as

possible. If physicians were sufficiently attentive to the suffering of dying patients, the demand for PAS and VAE probably would lessen.[170]

Dying from PRHN does not appeal to all dying patients but represents a "palliative option of last resort" that to some patients may be an acceptable alternative to PAS or VAE.[171] Interestingly, in Oregon, PRHN has proved more popular than PAS. Oregon hospice nurses report that PRHN was used more than twice as frequently as PAS despite the explicit legalization of PAS with its attendant publicity. Patients who preferred PRHN to PAS were older, more likely to have a neurological disorder, less likely to want to control the circumstances of their death, and less likely to have been evaluated by a mental health professional.[172]

Physicians should educate their patients and each other that PRHN is an acceptable alternative to PAS and VAE. Medical schools should improve their teaching of the principles of excellent terminal care, including the palliation of common symptoms and the benefits of hospice programs. All physicians should become skilled in providing optimal and aggressive palliative care and should be willing to prescribe adequate medications to reduce the suffering of the dying patient. Physicians should work to dispel the widespread myth that dehydration and lack of nutrition produce unmanageable suffering in dying terminally ill patients.[173] Adopting these measures likely will reduce patient demand for PAS and VAE and remove the call for their legalization from its prominent place on the public agenda.

NOTES

1. Sections of this chapter were modified with permission, as cited, from Bernat JL, Gert B, Mogielnicki RP. Patient refusal of hydration and nutrition: an alternative to physician-assisted suicide or voluntary active euthanasia. *Arch Intern Med* 1993;153:2723–2728 (©1993, American Medical Association).
2. The history of euthanasia has been carefully analyzed in Emanuel EJ. Euthanasia: historical, ethical, and empirical perspectives. *Arch Intern Med* 1994;154:1890–1901 and Emanuel EJ. The history of euthanasia debates in the United States and Britain. *Ann Intern Med* 1994;121:793–802. I draw on these accounts for the history of euthanasia prior to 1980.
3. Emanuel EJ. *Arch Intern Med* 1994:1891–1892 and Emanuel EJ. *Ann Intern Med* 1994:793–796.
4. Hoche A, Binding K. *Die Friegabe der Vernichtung lebensunwerten Lebens*. Leipzig: F Meiner, 1920.
5. Ploetz A. Die Tuchtigkeit unserer Rasse und der Schutz der Schwacken. In PloetzA. *Grundlinien einer Rassenhygiene*. Vol 1. Berlin: S Fischer, 1895, as discussed in Proctor R. *Racial Hygiene: Medicine Under the Nazis*. Cambridge, MA: Harvard University Press, 1988.

6. See the discussion of the influence of Hoche and Binding on the German medical profession in Lifton RJ. *The Nazi Doctors: Medical Killing and the Psychology of Genocide.* New York: Basic Books, 1986. The participation of German and Austrian physicians in the Nazi programs of involuntary sterilization, euthanasia, and killing also was discussed in Caplan AL ed. *When Medicine Went Mad: Bioethics and the Holocaust.* Totowa, NJ: Human Press, 1992. The influence of the German racial hygiene movement is discussed in Barondess JA. Medicine against society: lessons from the Third Reich. *JAMA* 1996;276:1657–1661 and Barondess JA. Care of the medical ethos: reflections on social Darwinism, racial hygiene, and the Holocaust. *Ann Intern Med* 1998;129:891–898.

7. Editorial. Voluntary euthanasia: the new society states its case. *Br Med J* 1935;2:1168–1169. See the discussion of this society in Emanuel EJ. *Arch Intern Med* 1892 and Emanuel EJ. *Ann Intern Med* 1994:796–797.

8. For example, see Kamisar Y. Some non-religious views against proposed 'mercy killing' legislation. *Minn Law Rev* 1958;42:969–1042 and Williams G. 'Mercy killing' legislation—a rejoinder. *Minn Law Rev* 1958;43:1–12.

9. Anonymous. A piece of my mind. It's over, Debbie. *JAMA* 1988;259:272; Letters to the editor. It's over, Debbie. *JAMA* 1988;259:2094–2098; Gaylin W, Kass LR, Pellegrino ED, et al. Doctors must not kill. *JAMA* 1988;259:2139–2140; and Lundberg GD. "It's over, Debbie" and the euthanasia debate. *JAMA* 1988; 259: 2142–2143.

10. Quill TE. Death and dignity: a case of individualized decision making. *N Engl J Med* 1991;324:691–694.

11. Crigger BJ, ed. Dying well? A colloquy on euthanasia and assisted suicide. *Hastings Cent Rep* 1992; 22(2):6–55; Campbell CS, Crigger BJ, eds. Mercy, murder, and morality: perspectives on euthanasia. *Hastings Cent Rep* 1989;19(suppl 1):1–32; Battin MP, Bole TJ III, eds. Legal euthanasia: ethical issues in an era of legalized aid in dying. *J Med Philosophy* 1993;18:237–341; Euthanasia and physician-assisted suicide: murder or mercy? *Cambridge Q Healthcare Ethics* 1993;2(special section):9–62; and Snyder L, Caplan AL eds. Assisted suicide: finding common ground. *Ann Intern Med* 2000;132:467–499.

12. Two more recent volumes constitute an excellent point-counterpoint for readers wishing to consider the best arguments from each side of the PAS debate. See Foley K, Hendin H (eds). *The Case Against Assisted Suicide: For the Right to End-of-Life Care.* Baltimore: Johns Hopkins University Press, 2002 and Quill TE, Batten MP (eds). *Physician-Assisted Dying: The Case for Palliative Care & Patient Choice.* Baltimore, Johns Hopkins University Press, 2004.

13. An analysis of 69 of the persons whose suicides Kevorkian assisted was reported in Roscoe LA, Malphurs JE, Dragovic LJ, Cohen D. Dr. Jack Kevorkian and cases of euthanasia in Oakland County, Michigan, 1990–1998. *N Engl J Med* 2000;343:1735–1736. The story of the public rise of Jack Kevorkian, abetted by his pugnacious attorney Geoffrey Fieger, was told in Betzold J. The selling of Doctor Death. *The New Republic* May 26,1997:22–28. Kevorkian published his philosophy in Kevorkian J. *Prescription: Medicide: The Goodness of Planned Death.* Buffalo, NY: Prometheus Books, 1991. Kevorkian was released from prison in 2007 after serving eight years of a 10 to 25 year sentence.

14. Humphry D. *Final Exit: The Practicalities of Self-Deliverance and Assisted Suicide for the Dying.* Eugene, OR: Hemlock Society, 1991. Not only are people reading this book, they are also following its advice. See Marzuk PM, Tardiff K, Hirsch CS, et al. Increase in suicide by asphyxiation in New York City after the publication of Final Exit. *N Engl J Med* 1993;329:1508–1510.

15. Blendon RJ, Szalay US, Knox RA. Should physicians aid their patients in dying? The public perspective. *JAMA* 1992;267:2658–2662.

16. See Misbin RI. Physicians' aid in dying. *N Engl J Med* 1991;325:1307–1311; Carson R. Washington's I-119. *Hastings Cent Rep* 1992;22(2):7–9; and McGough PM. Washington State Initiative 119: the first public vote on legalizing physician-assisted death. *Cambridge Q Healthcare Ethics* 1993;2:63–67.

17. Alpers A, Lo B. Physician-assisted suicide in Oregon: a bold experiment. *JAMA* 1995;274:483–487.

18. The public is probably correct on this point. As discussed in chapters 7 and 8, studies and surveys have shown that many physicians either are ignorant of or unwilling to provide adequate analgesia for their terminally ill, dying patients. See Solomon MS, O'Donnell L, Jennings B, et al. Decisions near the end of life: professional views on life-sustaining treatments. *Am J Public Health* 1993;83:14–23 and Von Roenn JH, Cleeland CS, Gonin R, et al. Physician attitudes and practices in cancer pain management: a survey from the Eastern Cooperative Oncology Group. *Ann Intern Med* 1993;119:121–126.

19. Shalowitz D, Emanuel E. Euthanasia and physician-assisted suicide: implications for physicians. *J Clin Ethics* 2004;15:232–236.

20. Denny CC, Emanuel EJ. "Physician-assisted suicide among Oregon cancer patients: a fading issue. *J Clin Ethics* 2006;17:39–42.

21. These definitions are modified, with permission, from Bernat JL, Gert B, Mogielnicki RP. *Arch Intern Med* 1993;153:2723–2724 (©1993, American Medical Association).

22. See the discussion of the principle of double effect in chapters 1 and 6.

23. The misleading term "physician aid-in-dying" was coined by, or at least used most prominently in, the State of Washington's Initiative 119. The voters of Washington were asked on ballot: "Shall adult patients who are in a medically terminal condition be permitted to request and receive from a physician aid-in-dying?" Presumably, the term physician aid-in-dying was chosen by its proponents for its euphemistic value. Who could argue with the desirability of a physician giving aid to a dying patient? It is likely that many people voted for Initiative 119 as a result of this language, despite lacking a clear understanding of its meaning. The debate on the morality and legalization of PAS and VAE is sufficiently complex without unnecessarily confusing the issues by employing misleading and ambiguous terminology coined or exploited for political purposes.

24. Despite the illegality of VAE in all American jurisdictions and the illegality of PAS in most of them, prosecutors have pressed criminal charges against very few physicians for performing them. See Ziegler SJ. Physician-assisted suicide and criminal prosecution: are physicians at risk? *J Law Med Ethics* 2005;33:349–358.

25. This section is adapted, with permission, from Bernat JL, Gert B, Mogielnicki RP. *Arch Intern Med* 1993;153:2724 (©1993, American Medical Association).

26. See the discussion on valid consent in chapter 2.

27. For examples of physicians refusing patients' requests on medical grounds, see Brett AS, McCullough LB. When patients request specific interventions: defining the limits of the physician's obligation. *N Engl J Med* 1986;315:1347–1351.

28. In an otherwise lucid essay, the American Medical Association Council on Ethical and Judicial Affairs slipped into equating patient requests with their refusals. See American Medical Association Council on Ethical and Judicial Affairs. Decisions near the end of life. *JAMA* 1992;267:2229–2233.

29. Gert B, Bernat JL, Mogielnicki RP. The moral distinction between patient refusals and requests. *Hastings Cent Rep* 1994;24(4):13–15.

30. Rachels J. Active and passive euthanasia. *N Engl J Med* 1975;292:78–80. See also Hopkins PD. Why does removing machines count as "passive" euthanasia? *Hastings Cent Rep* 1997;27(3):29–37.

31. The important moral distinction between killing and allowing to die has been defended in Sulmasy DP. Killing and allowing to die: another look. *J Law Med Ethics* 1998;26:55–64 and Miller FG, Fins JJ, Snyder L. Assisted suicide compared with refusal of treatment: a valid distinction? *Ann Intern Med* 2000;132:470–475.

32. A fair balance of the dialectical moral arguments has been offered in Thomasma DC. An analysis of the arguments for and against euthanasia and assisted suicide: part one. *Camb Q Healthc Ethics* 1996;5:62–76 and Thomasma DC. Assessing the arguments for and against euthanasia and assisted suicide: part two. *Camb Q Healthc Ethics* 1998;7:388–401.

33. Dixon N. On the difference between physician-assisted suicide and active euthanasia. *Hastings Cent Rep* 1998;28(5):25–29.

34. I concentrate on two philosophical defenses of the morality of PAS and VAE: Weir RF. The morality of physician-assisted suicide. *Law Med Health Care* 1992;20:116–126 and Brock DW. Voluntary active euthanasia. *Hastings Cent Rep* 1992;22(2):10–22. For similar views, see Brody H. Assisted death—A compassionate response to a medical failure. *N Engl J Med* 1992;327:1384–1388; Quill TE. Doctor, I want to die. Will you help me? *JAMA* 1993;270:870–873; and Miller PJ. Death with dignity and the right to die: sometimes doctors have a duty to hasten death. *J Med Ethics* 1987;13:81–85.

35. Brock DW. *Hastings Cent Rep* 1992:11 and Weir RF. *Law Med Health Care* 1992:123–124.

36. Weir RF. *Law Med Health Care* 1992:124 and Brock DW. *Hastings Cent Rep* 1992:14–16. For a variation on this theme, emphasizing the physician's professional integrity, see Miller FG, Brody H. Professional integrity and physician-assisted death. *Hastings Cent Rep* 1995;25(3):8–17.

37. Weir RF. *Law Med Health Care* 1992:124 and Brock DW. *Hastings Cent Rep* 1992:16.

38. Weir RF. *Law Med Health Care* 1992:124.

39. Weir RF. *Law Med Health Care* 1992:123.

40. I concentrate on three philosophical arguments that advance the immorality of PAS and VAE: Pellegrino ED. Doctors must not kill. *J Clin Ethics* 1992;3:95–102; Kass LR. Neither for love nor money: why doctors must not kill. *Public Interest* 1989;94:25–46; and Dinwiddie SH. Physician-assisted suicide: epistemological problems. *Med Law* 1992;11:345–352. For similar views, see Callahan D. When self-determination runs amok. *Hastings Cent Rep* 1992;22(2):52–55; Singer PA, Siegler M. Euthanasia—a critique. *N Engl J Med* 1990;322:1881–1883; and American Medical Association Council on Ethical and Judicial Affairs. Decisions near the end of life. *JAMA* 1992;267:2229–2233.

41. Pellegrino ED. *J Clin Ethics* 1992:96–97. The same point later was made in greater detail by Safranek JP. Autonomy and the assisted suicide: the execution of freedom. *Hastings Cent Rep* 1998;28(4):32–36.

42. Pellegrino ED. *J Clin Ethics* 1992:97; Kass LR. *Public Interest* 1989:25–46; and Singer PA, Siegler M. *N Engl J Med* 1990:1883.

43. For the effect of countertransference on the patient-physician relationship and the emotional harm to physicians by conducting PAS or VAE, see Stevens KR Jr. Emotional and psychological effects of physician-assisted suicide and euthanasia on participating physicians. *Issues Law Med* 2006;21:187–200.

44. Pellegrino ED. *J Clin Ethics* 1992:97. Pellegrino discusses a statement by the philosopher Miguel de Unamuno: "Suffering is the substance of life and the root of personality. Only suffering makes us persons."

45. Dinwiddie SH. *Med Law* 1992:347–350.

46. Kamisar Y. Are laws against assisted suicide unconstitutional? *Hastings Cent Rep* 1993;23(3):32–41; Sedler RA. The constitution and hastening inevitable death. *Hastings Cent Rep* 1993;23(5):20–25; Gostin LO. Drawing a line between killing and letting die: the law, and law reform, on medically assisted dying. *J Law Med Ethics* 1993;21;94–101; CeloCruz MT. Aid-in-dying: should we decriminalize physician-assisted suicide and physician-committed euthanasia? *Am J Law Med* 1992;18:369–394; and Lewis P. Rights discourse and assisted suicide. *Am J Law Med* 2001;27:45–99. For a comprehensive source, see Meisel A, Cerminara KL. *The Right to Die: The Law of End-of-Life Decisionmaking*, 3rd ed. Aspen Publishers, Inc, 2004.

47. Blendon RJ, Szalay US, Knox RA. Should physicians aid their patients in dying? The public perspective. *JAMA* 1992;267:2658–2662.

48. Pellegrino ED. *J Clin Ethics* 1992:97–98.

49. Magnusson RS. "Underground euthanasia" and the harm minimization debate. *J Law Med Ethics* 2004;32:486–495.

50. Smith SW. Some realism about end of life: the current prohibition and the euthanasia underground. *Am J Law Med* 2007;33:55–95.

51. For the role of guidelines and safeguards in PAS, see Benrubi GI. Euthanasia—the need for procedural safeguards. *N Engl J Med* 1992,326:197–199 and Caplan AL, Snyder L, Faber-Langendoen K. The role of guidelines in the practice of physician-assisted suicide. *Ann Intern Med* 2000;132:476–481.

52. Quill TE, Cassel CK, Meier DE. Care of the hopelessly ill: proposed clinical criteria for physician-assisted suicide. *N Engl J Med* 1992;327:1380–1384.

53. The rationality of suicide under any circumstances remains controversial. For discussions of whether "rational suicide" exists, see Childress JF, Roehinger RL, Siegler M, Thorup OA Jr. Voluntary exit: is there a case for rational suicide—a panel discussion. *Pharos* 1982;45(4):25–31; Mayo DJ. The concept of rational suicide. *J Med Philosophy* 1986;11:143–155; Conwell Y, Caine ED. Rational suicide and the right to die: reality and myth. *N Engl J Med* 1991;325:1100–1103; and Clarke DM. Autonomy, rationality and the wish to die. *J Med Ethics* 1999;25:457–462.

54. Sullivan MD, Ganzini L, Youngner SJ. Should psychiatrists serve as gatekeepers for physician-assisted suicide? *Hastings Cent Rep* 1998;28(4):24–31. The relationship of depression to requests for PAS is considered later in the chapter.

55. Quill TE, Cassel CK, Meier DE. *N Engl J Med* 1992:1381–1382.

56. Callahan D. *Hastings Cent Rep* 1992:54. The legal slippery slope problem introduced by eliminating a long-standing taboo is discussed in Gunderson M, Mayo DJ. Altruism and physician assisted death. *J Med Philosophy* 1993;18:281–295. For an entertaining and frightening depiction of future medical care if PAS or VAE were legalized, see Jonsen AR. Living with euthanasia: a futuristic scenario. *J Med Philosophy* 1993;18: 241–251.

57. Fenigson R. A case against Dutch euthanasia. *Hastings Cent Rep* 1989;19(1):522–530 and Fenigson R. Euthanasia in the Netherlands. *Issues Law Med* 1990;6:229–245.

58. The claim that harms of legalized PAS would fall disproportionately on disabled patients is rebutted in Mayo DJ, Gundereson M. Vitalism revitalized: vulnerable populations, prejudice, and physician-assisted death. *Hastings Cent Rep* 2002;32(4):14–21.

59. Hendin H, Klerman G. Physician-assisted suicide: the dangers of legalization. *Am J Psychiatry* 1993;150:143–145. See also Hardwick J. Is there a duty to die? *Hastings Cent Rep* 1997;27(2):34–42 and Humber JM, Almeder RF eds. *Is There a Duty to Die?* (Biomedical Ethics Review, vol 17). Totowa, NJ: Humana Press, 2000.

60. For a vigorous debate on this theoretical assertion, see Lindsay RA. Should we impose quotas? Evaluating the "disparate impact" argument against legalizing assisted suicide. *J Law Med Ethics* 2002;30:6–16 and Coleman CH. The "disparate impact" argument reconsidered: making room for justice in the assisted suicide debate. *J Law Med Ethics* 2002; 30:17–23.

61. The preceding two paragraphs were adapted, with permission, from Bernat JL, Gert B, Mogielnicki RP. *Arch Intern Med* 1993;153:2726 (©1993, American Medical Association).

62. Emanuel EJ, Battin MP. What are the potential cost savings from legalizing physician-assisted suicide? *N Engl J Med* 1998;339:167–172.

63. Pellegrino ED. *J Clin Ethics* 1992:99.

64. de Wachter MAM. Euthanasia in the Netherlands. *Hastings Cent Rep* 1992;22(2):23–30. See also Final report of the Netherlands State Commission on Euthanasia: An English summary. *Bioethics* 1987;1:163–174; de Wachter MAM. Active euthanasia in the Netherlands. *JAMA* 1989;262:3316–3319; and Pence GE. Do not go slowly into that dark night: mercy killing in Holland. *Am J Med* 1988;84:139–141.

65. For an analysis of the remarkable evolution of Dutch opinion to accept euthanasia, see van der Maas PJ, Pijnenborg L, van Delden JJM. Changes in Dutch opinions on active euthanasia, 1966 through 1991. *JAMA* 1995;273:1411–1414.

66. Cohen-Almagor R. Why the Netherlands? *J Law Med Ethics* 2002;30:95–104.

67. Quill TE. Legal regulation of physician-assisted death—the latest report cards. *N Engl J Med* 2007;356:1911–1913.

68. de Wachter MAM. *Hastings Cent Rep* 1992:23.

69. These criteria and other features of the current Dutch euthanasia law are discussed in Welie JVM. Why physicians? Reflections on the Netherlands' new euthanasia law. *Hastings Cent Rep* 2002;32(1):42–44.

70. Admiraal PV. *Justifiable Euthanasia. A Manual for the Medical Profession.* Amsterdam: Nederlandse Vereniging voor Vrijwillige Euthanasie, 1980.

71. Quoted in de Wachter MAM. *Hastings Cent Rep* 1992:24.

72. van der Maas PJ, van Delden JJM, Pijnenborg L, et al. Euthanasia and other medical decisions concerning the end of life. *Lancet* 1991;338:669–674.

73. van der Maas PJ, van der Wal G, Haverkate I, et al. Euthanasia, physician-assisted suicide, and other medical practices involving the end of life in the Netherlands, 1990–1995. *N Engl J Med* 1996;335:1699–1705.

74. ten Have HAMJ, Welie JVM. Euthanasia: normal medical practice? *Hastings Cent Rep* 1992;22(2):34–38.

75. van der Heide A, Onwuteaka-Philipsen BD, Rurup ML, et al. End-of-life practices in the Netherlands under the Euthanasia Act. *N Engl J Med* 2007;356:1957–1965.

76. de Wachter MAM. *Hastings Cent Rep* 1992:24.

77. Nevertheless, 64% of Dutch psychiatrists believe that PAS is acceptable for patients suffering only a psychiatric disorder and no physical or terminal illness. See Groenewoud JH, van der Maas PJ, van der Wal G, et al. Physician-assisted death in psychiatric practice in the Netherlands. *N Engl J Med* 1997;336:1795–1801. That chronic depression ever should be used as a justification for PAS is decried in Ganzini L, Lee MA. Psychiatry and assisted suicide in the United States. *N Engl J Med* 1997;336:1824–1826. The complexities of psychiatric assessment in such cases are explained in Sullivan MD, Ganzini L, Youngner SJ. Should psychiatrists serve as gatekeepers for physician-assisted suicide? *Hastings Cent Rep* 1998;28(4):24–31.

78. Groenewoud JH, van der Heide A, Tholen AJ, et al. Psychiatric consultation with regard to requests for euthanasia or physician-assisted suicide. *Gen Hosp Psychiatry* 2004;26:323–330.

79. Hertogh CMPM, de Boer ME, Dröes RM, Eefsting JA. Would we rather lose our life than lose our self? Lessons from the Dutch debate on euthanasia for patients with dementia. *Am J Bioethics* 2007;7(4):48–56.

80. Obstein KL, Kimsma G, Chambers T. Practicing euthanasia: the perspective of physicians. *J Clin Ethics* 2004;15:223–231.

81. Jansen-can der Weide MC, Onwuteaka-Philipsen BD, van der Wal G. Granted, undecided, withdrawn, and refused requests for euthanasia and physician-assisted suicide. *Arch Intern Med* 2005;165:1698–1704.

82. de Wachter MAM. *Hastings Cent Rep* 1992:23.

83. These activities are described comprehensively in Fenigson R. *Hastings Cent Rep* 522–530; and Fenigson R. *Issues Law Med* 1990;6:229–245. See also van der Sluis I. The practice of euthanasia in the Netherlands. *Issues Law Med* 1989;4:455–465 and Bostrom B. Euthanasia in the Netherlands: a model for the United States? *Issues Law Med* 1989;4:467–486.

84. Verhagen E, Sauer PJJ. The Groningen Protocol—euthanasia in severely ill newborns. *N Engl J Med* 2005; 352:959–962. For a thoughtful essay arguing that the Groningen Protocol is unethical and unjustified, see Chervenak FA, McCullough LB, Arabin B. Why the Groningen Protocol should be rejected. *Hastings Cent Rep* 2006;36(5):30–33.

85. The valid comparison of involuntary euthanasia currently practiced in the Netherlands to that practiced in Weimar and Nazi Germany was discussed in Derr PG. Hadamar, Hippocrates, and the future of medicine: reflections on euthanasia and the history of German medicine. *Issues Law Med* 1989;4:487–495 and Hentoff N. Contested terrain: the Nazi analogy in bioethics. *Hastings Cent Rep* 1988;18(4):29–30. For a more general background, see Lifton RJ. *The Nazi Doctors: Medical Killing and the Psychology of Genocide.* New York: Basic Books, 1986 and Caplan AL, ed. *When Medicine Went Mad: Bioethics and the Holocaust.* Totowa. NJ: Humana Press, 1992.

86. Pijnenborg L, van der Maas PJ, van Delden JJM, et al. Life-terminating acts without explicit request of patient. *Lancet* 1993;341:1196–1199.

87. van der Heide A, Onwuteaka-Philipsen BD, Rurup ML, et al. End-of-life practices in the Netherlands under the Euthanasia Act. *N Engl J Med* 2007;356:1957–1965.

88. van der Maas PJ, van Delden JJM, Pijnenborg L. *Euthanasia and Other Medical Decisions Concerning the End of Life.* New York: Elsevier, 1992.

89. Hendin H. Euthanasia and physician-assisted suicide in the Netherlands (letter). *N Engl J Med* 1997; 336:1385.

90. Hendin H, Rutenfrans C, Zylicz Z. Physician-assisted suicide and euthanasia in the Netherlands: lessons from the Dutch. *JAMA* 1997;277:1720–1722.

91. van der Wal G, van der Maas PJ, Bosma JM, et al. Evaluation of the notification procedure for physician-assisted death in the Netherlands. *N Engl J Med* 1996;335:1706–1711.

92. Groenewoud JH, van der Heide A, Onwuteka-Philipsen BD, Willems DL, van der Maas PJ, van der Wal G. Clinical problems with the performance of euthanasia and physician-assisted suicide in the Netherlands. *N Engl J Med* 2000;342:551–556.

93. Jansen-can der Weide MC, Onwuteaka-Philipsen BD, van der Wal G. Granted, undecided, withdrawn, and refused requests for euthanasia and physician-assisted suicide. *Arch Intern Med* 2005;165:1698–1704.

94. Battin M. Voluntary euthanasia and the risks of abuse: can we learn anything from the Netherlands? *Law Med Health Care* 1992;20:133–143.

95. Patel K. Euthanasia and physician-assisted suicide policy in the Netherlands and Oregon: a comparative analysis. *J Health Soc Policy* 2004;19:37–55.

96. Francis LP. Advance directives for voluntary euthanasia: a volatile combination? *J Med Philosophy* 1993;18:297–322.

97. Poignant vignettes of individual cases of suffering, for which PAS or VAE seem a plausible solution, continue to be published. For example, see Poenisch C. Merian Frederick's story. *N Engl J Med* 1998;339:996–998.

98. Steinbock B. The case for physician-assisted suicide: not (yet) proven. *J Med Ethics* 2005;31:235–241.

99. This conclusion is drawn forcefully and convincingly in Hendin H. *Seduced by Death: Doctors, Patients, and Assisted Suicide.* New York: W. W. Norton, 1998. For a critique of the slippery slope argument of inevitably evolving from voluntary to involuntary euthanasia, see Lewis P. The empirical slippery slope from voluntary to non-voluntary euthanasia. *J Law Med Ethics* 2007;35:197–210.

100. Alpers A, Lo B. Physician-assisted suicide in Oregon: a bold experiment. *JAMA* 1995;274:483–487.

101. For legal commentaries on this measure, see Annas GJ. Death by prescription: the Oregon initiative. *N Engl J Med* 1994;331:1240–1243 and Capron AM. Sledding in Oregon. *Hastings Cent Rep* 1995;25(1):34–35. A measure with the same provisions as the Oregon law was voted down in 2007 by the Vermont legislature. A similar bill is pending in California.

102. Chin AE, Hedberg K, Higginson GK, Fleming DW. Legalized physician-assisted suicide in Oregon—the first year's experience. *N Engl J Med* 1999;340:577–583.

103. Chin, et al. *N Engl J Med* 1999:577.

104. These data were abstracted from Oregon Department of Human Services. *Ninth Annual Report on Oregon's Death with Dignity Act.* March 2007 available at http://egov.oregon.gov/ DHS/ph/pas/ar-index.shtml and www.deathwithdignity.org (Accessed March 31, 2007). Earlier annual reports contain additional information and also are available on these websites. Earlier data from these reports are presented and discussed in Sullivan AD, Hedberg K, Fleming DW. Legalized physician-assisted suicide in Oregon—the second year. *N Engl J Med* 2000;342:598–604; Sullivan AD, Hedberg K, Hopkins D. Legalized physician-assisted suicide in Oregon, 1998–2000. *N Engl J Med* 2001;344:605–607; Hedberg K, Hopkins D, Southwick K. Legalized physician-assisted suicide in Oregon, 2001. *N Engl J Med* 2002;346:450–452; and Hedberg K, Hopkins D, Kohn M. Five years of legal physician-assisted suicide in Oregon. *N Engl J Med* 2003;348:961–964.

105. Oregon Department of Human Services. *Ninth Annual Report on Oregon's Death With Dignity Act.* March 2007.

106. Oregon Department of Human Services. *Ninth Annual Report on Oregon's Death With Dignity Act.* March 2007.

107. Ganzini L, Nelson HD, Schmidt TA, Kraemer DF, Delorit MA, Lee ME. Physicians' experience with the Oregon Death with Dignity Act. *N Engl J Med* 2000;342:557–563.

108. Ganzini L, Nelson HD, Lee MA, Kraemer DF, Schmidt TA, Delorit MA. Oregon physicians' attitudes with end-of-life care since passage of the Oregon Death with Dignity Act. *JAMA* 2001;285:2363–2369.

109. Woolfrey J. What happens now? Oregon and physician-assisted suicide. *Hastings Cent Rep* 1998;28(3): 9–17.

110. Ganzini L, Harvath TA, Jackson A, Goy ER, Miller LL, Delorit MA. Experience of Oregon nurses and social workers with hospice patients who requested assistance with suicide. *N Engl J Med* 2002;347:582–588.

111. Steinbrook R. Physician-assisted suicide in Oregon—an uncertain future. *N Engl J Med* 2002;346: 460–464.

112. See, for example, Lowenstein E, Wanzer SH. The U.S. Attorney General's intrusion into medical practice. *N Engl J Med* 2002;346:447–448.

113. Hilliard B. The politics of palliative care and the ethical boundaries of medicine: *Gonzales v. Oregon* as a cautionary tale. *J Law Med Ethics* 2007;35:158–174.

114. Capron AM. Sledding in Oregon. *Hastings Center Rep* 1995;25(1):34–35. See also the discussion on this point in Emanuel EJ, Daniels E. Oregon's physician-assisted suicide law: provisions and problems. *Arch Intern Med* 1995;156:825–829. In a similar vein, it may become impossible to maintain the restriction of physician-assisted suicide to terminally ill patients, despite pleas to do so. See Gunderson M, Mayo DJ. Restricting physician-assisted suicide to the terminally ill. *Hastings Cent Rep* 2000;30(6):17–23. For a thoughtful and balanced account of whether PAS ever can be adequately regulated by law, see Orentlicher D, Snyder L. Can assisted suicide be regulated? *J Clin Ethics* 2000;11:358–366.

115. Nuland SB. Physician-assisted suicide and euthanasia in practice. *N Engl J Med* 2000;342:583–584. Nuland's skepticism over the accuracy of the reported Oregon data was justified. The OHD later reported that regurgitation of the ingested medications occurred in 5% of Oregon PAS attempts.

116. Foley K, Hendin H. The Oregon report: don't ask, don't tell. *Hastings Cent Rep* 1999;29(3):37–42.

117. *Quill v. Vacco*, 80 F3d 716 (2nd Cir), *cert granted* 135 LE2d 1127 (1996).

118. Compassion in Dying v. Washington, 79 F3d 790 (9th Cir), cert granted sub nom, Washington v. Glucksberg, 135 LED2d 1128 (1996).

119. There is a voluminous literature rejecting the equivalence of PAS and refusal of LST and disagreeing with the two federal circuit court opinions. For example, see Alpers A, Lo B. Does it make clinical sense to equate terminally ill patients who require life-sustaining interventions with those who do not? *JAMA* 1997;277:1705–1708; Capron AM. Liberty, equality, death! *Hastings Cent Rep* 1996;26(3):23–24; and Miller FG, Fins JJ, Snyder L. Assisted suicide compared with refusal of treatment: a valid distinction? *Ann Intern Med* 2000;132:470–475.

120. *Washington v. Glucksberg*, 117 S. Ct. 2302 (1997) and *Vacco v. Quill*, 117 S. Ct. 2293 (1997).

121. For legal analyses of the U.S. Supreme Court PAS decisions, see Annas GJ. The bell tolls for a constitutional right to physician-assisted suicide. *N Engl J Med* 1997;l337:1098–1103; Gostin LO. Deciding life and death in the courtroom: from *Quinlan* to *Cruzan, Glucksberg*, and *Vacco*—a brief history and analysis of constitutional protection of the 'right to die.' *JAMA* 1997;278:1523–1528; and Capron AM. Death and the court. *Hastings Cent Rep* 1997; 27(5):25–29.

122. For penetrating critiques of the slogan "the right to die," see Kass LR. Is there a right to die? *Hastings Cent Rep* 1993;23(1):34–42 and Emanuel E. Whose right to die? *Atlantic Monthly*. March 1997:73–79.

123. Phillips P. Views of assisted suicide from several nations. *JAMA* 1997;278:969–970.

124. Meier DE, Emmons CE, Wallenstein S, Quill T, Morrison RS, Cassel CK. A national survey of physician-assisted suicide and euthanasia in the United States. *N Engl J Med* 1998;338:1193–1201.

125. Emanuel EJ, Fairclough D, Clarridge BC, et al. Attitudes and practices of U.S. oncologists regarding euthanasia and physician-assisted suicide. *Ann Intern Med* 2000;133:527–532.

126. Back AL, Wallace JI, Starks HE, Pearlman RA. Physician-assisted suicide and euthanasia in Washington state: patient requests and physician responses. *JAMA* 1996;275:919–925.

127. Lee MA, Nelson HD, Tilden VP, Ganzini L, Schmidt TA, Tolle SW. Legalizing assisted suicide—views of physicians in Oregon. *N Engl J Med* 1996;334:310–315.

128. Bachman JG, Alcser KH, Doukas DJ, Lichtenstein RL, Corning AD, Brody H. Attitudes of Michigan physicians toward legalizing physician-assisted suicide and voluntary euthanasia. *N Engl J Med* 1996; 334:303–309.

129. Shapiro RS, Derse AR, Gottlieb M, Schiedermayer D. Willingness to perform euthanasia: a survey of physician attitudes. *Arch Intern Med* 1994;154:575–584; Caralis PV, Hammond JS. Attitudes of medical students, house staff, and faculty physicians toward euthanasia and termination of life-sustaining treatment. *Crit Care Med* 1992;20:683–690; Kinsella TD, Verhoef MJ. Alberta euthanasia survey: 1. Physicians' opinions about the morality and legalization of active euthanasia. *Can Med Assoc J* 1993;148:1921–1926. Verhoef MJ, Kinsella TD. Alberta euthanasia survey: 2. Physicians' opinions about the acceptance of active euthanasia as a medical act and the reporting of such practice. *Can Med Assoc J* 1993;148:1929–1933; and Shapiro RS, Derse AR, Gottlieb M, et al. Willingness to perform euthanasia: a survey of physician attitudes. *Arch Intern Med* 1994;154:575–584.

130. Schwartz HI, Curry L, Blank K, Gruman C. Physician-assisted suicide or voluntary euthanasia: a meaningless distinction for practicing physicians. *J Clin Ethics* 2001;12:51–63.

131. Carver AC, Vickrey BG, Bernat JL, Keran C, Ringel SP, Foley KM. End of life care: a survey of U.S. neurologists' attitudes, behavior, and knowledge. *Neurology* 1999;53:284–293.

132. Meier DE, Emmons C-A, Litke A, Wallenstein S, Morrison RS. Characteristics of patients requesting and receiving physician-assisted death. *Arch Intern Med* 2003;163:1537–1542.

133. Asch DA. The role of critical care nurses in euthanasia and assisted suicide. *N Engl J Med* 1996;334: 1374–1379.

134. Ganzini L, Johnston WS, McFarland BH, Tolle SW, Lee MA. Attitudes of patients with amyotrophic lateral sclerosis and their care givers toward assisted suicide. *N Engl J Med* 1998;339:967–973.

135. Emanuel EJ, Fairclough DL, Emanuel LL. Attitudes and desires related to euthanasia and physician-assisted suicide among terminally ill patients and their caregivers. *JAMA* 2000;284:2460–2468.

136. Pearlman RA, Hsu C, Starks H, et al. Motivations for physician-assisted suicide. *J Gen Intern Med* 2005;20:234–239.

137. American Medical Association Council on Ethical and Judicial Affairs. *JAMA* 1992;267:2229–2233.

138. Snyder L, Sulmasy DP. Physician-assisted suicide. *Ann Intern Med* 2001;135:209–216.

139. *Euthanasia: Report of a Working Party to Review the British Medical Association Guidelines on Euthanasia.* London: British Medical Association, 1988 *and Report of the House of Lords Select Committee on Medical Ethics.* London: Her Majesty's Stationery Office, 1994.

140. American Academy of Neurology Ethics and Humanities Subcommittee. Assisted suicide, euthanasia, and the neurologist. *Neurology* 1998;50:596–598.

141. New York State Task Force on Life and the Law. *When Death Is Sought: Assisted Suicide and Euthanasia in the Medical Context.* New York: New York State Task Force on Life and the Law, 1994.

142. Materstvedt LJ, Clark D, Ellershaw J, et al. Euthanasia and physician-assisted suicide: a view from an EAPC ethics task force. *Palliative Med* 2003;17:97–101.

143. Price DM, Murphy PA. Assisted suicide: new ANA policy reflects difficulty of issue. *J Nursing Law* 1994;2(2):53–62.

144. Quill TE, Cassel CK. Professional organizations' position statement on physician-assisted suicide: a case for studied neutrality. *Ann Intern Med* 2003;138:208–211.

145. Whitney SN, Brown BW Jr, Brody H, Alcser KH, Bachman JG, Greely HT. Views of United States physicians and members of the American Medical Association House of Delegates on physician-assisted suicide. *J Gen Intern Med* 2001;16:290–296.

146. The depression data are summarized and critiqued in Back AL, Pearlman RA. Desire for physician-assisted suicide: requests for a better death? *Lancet* 2001;358:344–345.

147. The burden data are discussed in Gunderson M. Being a burden: reflections on refusing medical care. *Hastings Cent Rep* 2004;34(5):37–43.

148. Lavery JV, Boyle J, Dickens BM, MacLean H, Singer PA. Origins of the desire for euthanasia and assisted suicide in people with HIV-1 or AIDS: a qualitative study. *Lancet* 2001;358:362–367.

149. Muskin PR. The request to die: role for a psychodynamic perspective on physician-assisted suicide. *JAMA* 1998;279:323–328. Depression and hopelessness are common reasons for terminally ill patients' desire to die more quickly. See Breitbart W, Rosenfeld B, Pessin H, et al. Depression, hopelessness, and desire for hastened death in terminally ill patients with cancer. *JAMA* 2000;284:2907–2911.

150. Bascom PB, Tolle SW. Responding to requests for physician-assisted suicide: "these are uncharted waters for both of us . . . " *JAMA* 2002;288:91–98.

151. Block SD, Billings JA. Patient requests to hasten death: evaluation and management in terminal care. *Arch Intern Med* 1994;154:2039–2047.

152. Emanuel LL. Facing requests for physician-assisted suicide: toward a practical and principled skill set. *JAMA* 1998;280:643–647.

153. Quill TE, Meier DE, Block SD, Billings JA. The debate over assisted suicide: empirical data and convergent views. *Ann Intern Med* 1998;128:552–558. For the approach of physicians practicing in jurisdictions where PAS is legal in response to a request for PAS, see Tulsky JA, Ciampa R, Rosen EJ. Responding to legal requests for physician-assisted suicide. *Ann Intern Med* 2000;132:494–499.

154. Kohlwes RJ, Koepsell TD, Rhodes LA, Pearlman RA. Physicians' responses to patients' requests for physician-assisted suicide. *Arch Intern Med* 2001;161:657–663.

155. Bolmsö I. Existential issues in palliative care—interviews with cancer patients. *J Palliat Care* 2000;16(2):20–24.

156. This section was adapted, with permission, from Bernat JL, Gert B, Mogielnicki RP. *Arch Intern Med* 1993:153:2725–2727 (©1993, American Medical Association). Some scholars agree with our assertion that there is little moral significance in the "artificial" vs. "natural" distinction as applied to hydration and nutrition once a competent patient has validly refused it. See Truog RD, Cochrane TI. Refusal of hydration and nutrition: irrelevance of the "artificial" vs "natural" distinction. *Arch Intern Med* 2005;165:2574–2576.

157. These data are reviewed in Andrews M, Levine A. Dehydration in the terminal patient: perception of hospice nurses. *Am J Hospice Care* 1989;3:31–34 and Printz LA. Terminal dehydration, a compassionate treatment. *Arch Intern Med* 1992;152:697–700.

158. Miller RJ, Albright PG. What is the role of nutritional support and hydration in terminal cancer patients? *Am J Hospice Care* 1989;6:33–38; Lichter I, Hunt E. The last 48 hours of life. *J Palliative Care* 1990;6(4):7–15; Schmitz P. The process of dying, with and without feeding and fluids by tube. *Law Med Health Care* 1991;19:23–26; Miller RJ. Hospice care as an alternative to euthanasia. *Law Med Health Care* 1992;20:127–132; and Sullivan RJ. Accepting death without artificial nutrition or hydration. *J Gen Intern Med* 1993;8:220–224.

159. Miller RJ. Nutrition and hydration in terminal disease. (unpublished manuscript). That dehydration in terminal illness in some cases can cause restlessness and added discomfort that requires specific management was pointed out in Fainsinger RL, MacDonald SM. Letter to the editor. *J Gen Intern Med* 1994;9:115–116.

160. McCann RM, Hall WJ, Groth-Juncker A. Comfort care for terminally ill patients: the appropriate use of nutrition and hydration. *JAMA* 1994;272:1263–1266.

161. Ganzini L, Goy ER, Miller LL, Harvath TA, Jackson A, Delorit MA. Nurses' experiences with hospice patients who refuse food and fluids to hasten death. *N Engl J Med* 2003;349:359–365.

162. The history and method of *bhaktapratyakhyana* are beautifully described in Settar S. *Pursuing Death: Philosophy and Practice of Voluntary Termination of Life.* Dharwad, India: Karnatak University Institute of Indian Art History, 1990.

163. For highly personalized accounts of the experience of patient refusal of hydration and nutrition, see Nearing H. *Loving and Leaving the Good Life.* Post Mills, Vt: Chelsea Green Publishing Co, 1992 and Eddy DM. "A conversation with my mother." *JAMA* 1994;272:179–181.

164. Quill TE, Lo B, Brock DW. Palliative options of last resort: a comparison of voluntarily stopping eating and drinking, terminal sedation, physician-assisted suicide, and voluntary active euthanasia. *JAMA* 1997;278:2099–2104; Miller FG, Meier DE. Voluntary death: a comparison of terminal dehydration and physician-assisted suicide. *Ann Intern Med* 1998;128:559–562; and Quill TE, Lee BC, Nunn S. Palliative treatments of last resort: choosing the least harmful alternative. *Ann Intern Med* 2000;132:488–493.

165. Not all authors agree that PRHN is entirely free of moral controversy. See Jansen LA, Sulmasy DP. Sedation, alimentation, hydration, and equivocation: careful conversation about care at the end of life. *Ann Intern Med* 2002;136:845–849.

166. Bernat JL, et al. *Arch Intern Med* 1993:2726.

167. Bernat JL, et al. *Arch Intern Med* 1993:2726.

168. Bernat JL, et al. *Arch Intern Med* 1993:2726–2727.

169. For example, guidelines for providing proper analgesia in chronically ill and terminally ill cancer patients have been published. See Jacox A. Carr DB, Payne R. New clinical-practice guidelines for the management of pain in patients with cancer. *N Engl J Med* 1994;330:651–656. See the discussion of palliative medicine in chapter 7.

170. Foley KM. The relationship of pain and symptom management to patient requests for physician-assisted suicide. *J Pain Symptom Management* 1991;6:289–297.

171. Quill TE, Lo B, Brock DW. Palliative options of last resort: a comparison of voluntarily stopping eating and drinking, terminal sedation, physician-assisted suicide, and voluntary active euthanasia. *JAMA* 1997;278:2099–2104.

172. Ganzini L, Goy ER, Miller LL, Harvath TA, Jackson A, Delorit MA. Nurses' experiences with hospice patients who refuse food and fluids to hasten death. *N Engl J Med* 2003;349:359–365.

173. Even physicians are poorly informed about the phenomenon of dying from lack of hydration and nutrition. See Ahronheim JC, Gasner MR. The sloganism of starvation. *Lancet* 1990;335:278–279.

Medical Futility

10

The concept of medical futility continues to provoke bioethical controversy although scholarly debate about it has diminished over the past decade. A requested therapy may be said to be medically futile when there is reasonable evidence to believe that it will not improve a patient's medical condition.

A determination of medical futility has practical importance in medical decision making because once a possible treatment is determined to be futile, physicians no longer have an ethical duty to provide it to patients, even if patients, family members, or other surrogates ask for it. Determining medical futility has become an important and, at times, a necessary step toward withholding or withdrawing a particular medical treatment that the physician believes cannot help, especially when family members or surrogates plead for it. Some scholars have argued further that physicians have an ethical obligation based on concepts of justice not to prescribe futile therapies.[1]

Despite its ambiguity and controversy, the term "medical futility" remains widely used in medical-ethical discourse, hospital policies, commission reports, medical society opinions, scholarly writings, statutory law, and judicial rulings. For example, the President's Commission cited futility as one condition for withholding and withdrawing medical treatment.[2] The United States Department of Health and Human Services "Baby Doe" regulations used futility as a condition for terminating medical treatment on hopelessly ill newborns.[3] The American Medical Association and the American Heart Association mentioned futility as one condition for eliminating the requirement to obtain consent from a patient or surrogate for a Do-Not-Resuscitate order.[4] Moreover, countless hospitals have cited medical futility in their policies as one condition for justifying a physician's order to withhold or withdraw medical treatment. The scholarly output in the medical futility debate is declining. Paul Helft and colleagues described the "rise and fall of the futility movement" pointing out that the concept of futility was nearly unrecognized prior to 1987, published articles about it in scholarly journals peaked in 1995, and interest in it had waned by the turn of the 21st century. The reason for the reduction in scholarly output remains unclear but Helft and colleagues wondered if it was because, in a series of legal rulings, courts failed to uphold its validity.[5] Interest in it did not decline because the controversies surrounding futility had been resolved. I suspect that fewer articles now are being written about medical futility because the salient arguments on all sides of the controversy have been made and guidelines to prevent and resolve futility disputes have been drafted and generally accepted.

In this chapter, I critically analyze the concept of futility to define it and identify its criterion. I give examples how physicians have used the definition and criterion in practice by discussing paradigmatic clinical scenarios in neurology: discontinuing ventilator treatment in brain death; writing Do-Not-Resuscitate orders for seriously-ill patients; and withdrawing life-sustaining treatment from patients with persistent vegetative state, anencephaly, or severe dementia with multi-organ failure. I explain the causes of futility disputes and stress the importance of communicating effectively with patients and families as the best way to prevent and resolve them. I discuss the design of proposed hospital and regional policies and state laws to resolve futility disputes. I end by discussing the ethical duties of physicians to provide demanded but futile treatment in the context of society's finite healthcare resources.[6]

THE DEFINITION AND CRITERION OF MEDICAL FUTILITY

Despite the categorical ring of the word "futility" and its ostensible explicitness, its underlying concept is subtle and complex.[7] Like the concept of death discussed in chapter 11, the concept of futility, rigorously explicated, requires the difficult tasks of seeking a definition and a criterion. Yet, when we attempt to define medical futility precisely, we discover that the concept has been applied to at least two distinct phenomena: physiologic effect and therapeutic benefit. Further, when we try to determine the criterion by which a particular therapy or clinical situation is considered medically futile, we discover that futility must be determined along a continuum of outcome probabilities in which it seems arbitrary to stipulate a single point of uselessness.

Robert Truog and colleagues observed that the difficulty in precisely defining medical futility is analogous to the difficulty in defining pornography, as famously stated by U.S. Supreme Court Justice Potter Stewart "But I know it when I see it."[8] Indeed, the term "medical futility" conveys different meanings to different physicians.[9] An adequate definition of futility should attempt to capture the meaning implicit in our ordinary and consensual usage of the word. Then we can seek a criterion for futility that shows the definition has been fulfilled and stipulates how futility can be determined in practice.[10]

The Definition of Futility

Although explicating the definition of medical futility is a contemporary problem, the concept of futility has an ancient heritage. Classical Greek physicians recognized diseases whose outcomes they were powerless to change. Greek physicians believed not only that they had no ethical obligation to attempt to cure an incurable disease, but that they had the obligation not even to attempt to treat it.[11] Hippocrates, for example, admonished physicians to "refuse to treat those who are overmastered by their diseases, realizing that in such cases medicine is powerless."[12]

Similarly, ancient Jewish law required physicians to try to save life in all circumstances except in the state of *gesisah*. A patient is in a state of *gesisah* if the patient is incipiently dying and death seems inevitable within 72 hours, irrespective of treatment. As was true for the Greeks, medical treatment for *gesisah* not only is not required, it is not permitted, because treatment is viewed as interfering with the peaceful departure of the soul from the imminently dying person.[13]

Christian ethics contains a similar recognition that ordinary ethical obligations to treat are suspended in states of medical futility. In Roman Catholic doctrine, patients may refuse treatments that "would not offer a reasonable hope of benefit to the patient" and physicians are not required to provide "extraordinary treatment." Similarly, Protestant writings indicate that patients may refuse life-sustaining treatment when that treatment only "prolongs the dying process."[14]

Futility is defined in the Oxford English Dictionary (OED) as "inadequacy to produce a result or bring about a required end; ineffectiveness; uselessness." The word "futile" is derived from the Latin word *futilis* meaning leaky. The OED defines a futile action as "leaky, hence untrustworthy, vain; failing utterly of the desired end through intrinsic defect; useless."[15] The relationship of the words "leaky" and "futile" is based on the Greek myth of the 50 daughters of Danaus. As punishment for murdering their husbands, 49 of the 50 Danaïdes were condemned in Hades to carry water to fill a leaky jar. No matter how hard they tried, their attempt was futile because the water leaked out. Thus, from its original use, "futility" implies that the desired ends cannot be accomplished no matter how hard one tries or how often one's act is repeated.[16]

The term "futility" is used in contemporary medical literature to refer generally to the uselessness and unsuccessfulness of certain treatments to provide desired benefits. However, the term "futile," like many quantitative verbal expressions in medicine, including "rare," "unusual," "common," and "infrequent," has varying quantitative connotations to different physicians. For example, some physicians regard a treatment as futile only if its success rate is 0% whereas other physicians consider treatments futile despite success rates as high as 13%.[17] A study of the concordance of ICU futility determinations by critical care physicians and nurses disclosed disagreements about at least one of the daily futility judgments concerning 63% of dying patients.[18] A qualitative study of outpatients' concerns about the utility or futility of end-of-life intensive treatment showed that, although patients did not use those precise words, they exhibited a perception of the concepts of utility and futility of treatment by expressing concern with quality of life, emotional and financial costs of treatment, likelihood of treatment success, and effect of treatment on their longevity.[19]

It is useful to distinguish futility from related concepts to delineate its boundaries more precisely. Futility should not be used to describe biological acts that are physically or logically impossible, such as a man running a mile in 30 seconds. Neither should futility be used to describe biological acts that are possible but implausible because of current technological limitations, such as trying to revive a decapitated head. Futility should be distinguished from hopelessness. Hopelessness describes a subjective attitude whereas futility refers to an objective quality of an action. Thus, it is possible to say that I realize that an action I am proposing is futile, yet I have hope it will succeed.[20]

Some physicians have abused the concept of futility by invoking it in an incorrect, inappropriate, and self-serving manner. They glibly justify their decisions to withdraw or withhold treatment misleadingly under the guise of futility when, for a variety of other reasons, they do not wish to provide further aggressive care for a patient. Or, without studying outcome data for the treatment of a particular condition, they summarily but ignorantly declare it to be futile. That some physicians have carelessly and erroneously cited futility as a rationalization for discontinuing treatment they do not wish to provide has led others to recommend a complete moratorium on using futility as the basis for any decision to withdraw or withhold treatment.[21]

I believe that the concept of medical futility, although difficult, remains useful when it is employed in a precise and consistent manner. I follow the erudite analysis of this topic provided by Lawrence Schneiderman and colleagues.[22] The essence of futility is overwhelming improbability in the face of possibility. An act is futile if the desired outcome, while empirically possible, is so unlikely that its exact probability may be incalculable. The fact that a few isolated successes have occurred against a background of thousands of past failures does not disprove futility. Indeed, the rare successes prove that the desired outcome is possible, a prerequisite for a concept of futility.[23]

Medical futility exists when a treatment of hoped-for benefit may, on the best evidence available, be predicted not to help a patient's medical condition. The therapy may not be able to provide benefit to the patient either because it is highly unlikely to produce the desired physiologic effect or because it produces a physiologic effect that does not confer benefit to the patient.

The Criterion of Futility

Futility has quantitative and qualitative dimensions both of which are necessary and sufficient to satisfy the definition. The quantitative dimension is the absolute numerical probability of the occurrence of an event, expressed as a fraction or decimal. The qualitative component is the extent to which the outcome event produces benefit to the patient.[24]

Determining futility is analogous to analyzing a clinical decision. In decision analysis, the force of a medical decision to proceed with a treatment is directly proportional to the product of two independent variables: the numerical probability of its success and its utility. In this context, utility refers to the quality of the outcome produced by the treatment. A determination of futility, therefore, can result either from an exceedingly small probability of success or from a very poor quality of the outcome. As either the quantity or the quality of the outcome approaches zero, their product approaches zero, hence the act becomes futile. Both the quantitative and qualitative components must be calculated in a determination of futility.[25]

The best criterion of a medically futile action is one in which either of the following conditions is present: (a) the ability to achieve the desired result is possible, but is one which reasoning or experience suggests is highly improbable and cannot be produced systematically; or (b) a physiological effect may occur, but the physiologic effect does not benefit the patient.[26] The former quantitative component also is known as "objective" or "strong" futility because of its exactitude. The latter qualitative component also is known as "subjective" or "weak" futility because it involves a value judgment and therefore may be viewed differently by different persons. Both of these components need to be explored further.

The quantitative aspect of futility is based upon the statistically determined confidence interval (CI) for observing success of treatment. As Schneiderman and colleagues have illustrated the concept, assuming that a therapy is at least plausible for a given condition, if there have been no successes in 100 cases of attempted treatment of the condition with the therapy, it can be said with 95% certainty that there will be no more than three successes in applying the same therapy to the same condition in the next 100 cases. In this example, three successes per 100 trials (0.03) is the upper limit of the 95% CI. If there were no successes in 200 trials, the upper limit of the 95% CI would be 0.015. In 1,000 unsuccessful trials, the upper limit of the 95% CI would be 0.003.[27]

However, there are three important limitations when using CI statistical data for determinations of futility. First, many clinical decisions simply lack sufficient data from which to make such precise statistical calculations. Although the emerging field of clinical outcome studies is supplying much needed data for clinical decisions, there remain many areas in which data are inadequate for prognostic purposes.[28] Many outcome studies in neurology contain Class III or IV evidence, such as that from natural history studies, uncontrolled case series, or expert opinion.[29] In the absence of valid outcome studies, clinicians must rely solely on their accumulated experience and that of colleagues. However, recall of accumulated experience is a notoriously inaccurate method of determining therapeutic effect and prognosis because it is susceptible to psychological distortions such as last-case bias.[30] Relying solely on experience also can perpetuate systematic errors that cannot be corrected until a more reliable evidence base is available.

Second, the outcome data must be valid, interpreted correctly, and applied appropriately. Some outcome data are invalid because they have been obtained from faulty studies. Some poorly designed studies create the fallacy of the self-fulfilling prophesy by deriving outcome conclusions without adequately controlling the variable in question (see chapter 8).[31] In other, better designed studies, erroneous conclusions have been drawn from valid data. Basing bedside clinical decisions on outcome data requires rigorous scrutiny of both the validity and interpretation of the data. Even with flawlessly performed and applied studies, prognostic data remain inherently probabilistic and therefore more accurately predict outcomes for groups than for individuals.[32] A recent study of the accuracy of the most commonly accepted prognostic scale for gravely ill ICU patients, the APACHE III, showed a striking error in that it significantly overestimated a hopeless prognosis.[33]

Third, there is no precise and universally agreed upon numerical threshold for the quantitative component of futility. Is a therapy futile if its chances for producing improvement are 0.001, 0.01, or 0.1? There is a continuum of outcome probabilities in clinical medicine. The point on this continuum at which futility occurs is inherently arbitrary and will be delineated differently by different physicians and patients and in various clinical settings.[34]

The qualitative aspects of futility are even more controversial. Who is to determine and by what standards, what should be considered the minimum quality of a patient's life or minimum improvement in a patient's condition to exceed the threshold for futility? Most people agree that a treatment that succeeds only in prolonging the life of a patient in an irreversible vegetative state does not benefit the patient and hence is futile on a qualitative basis. But how should we apply this concept of futility to the religious patient who believes that human life of any quality should be sustained and therefore wishes to continue such treatment? In this instance, a treatment that would be regarded as futile by the large majority of physicians and patients would not be regarded as futile by this patient. (See the case of Helga Wanglie discussed below.)

This conflict highlights the nagging question of who should be authorized to determine, on a qualitative basis, that a particular therapy is futile: the physician, the patient and family, or society? Ordinarily, physicians believe they alone possess the authority to determine the medical benefits of treatments they prescribe. There is consensus that if, in a physician's opinion, a therapy is not beneficial, the physician has no obligation to offer the therapy.[35] For example, neurologists and neurosurgeons—not patients or families—have the knowledge and experience to determine if surgical removal of a large intracerebral hemorrhage is likely to improve a patient's neurological outcome.

While granting physicians the exclusive authority to determine therapeutic benefit usually is justified, does this authority extend to telling the family of a patient in a vegetative state that the treatment maintaining the patient's life is producing no benefit when the family believes it is? In this instance, is futility a medical determination and therefore the appropriate professional domain of the physician, or is it simply a value judgment based upon the physician's perception about the patient's quality of life? If a futility determination in this context is merely a value judgment based upon moral, political, or economic

considerations, it is not at all clear that physicians have any greater professional prerogative or authority to determine it than laymen.[36]

Rationing of health care is another factor in the futility discussion. It is axiomatic that health-care resources are finite and that implicit or explicit allocation and rationing decisions are a necessity. If the costs and finitude of health-care resources were not a factor, it would be more easily defensible to provide care that is futile or, at least, of the most marginal utility. However, the reality is inescapable that health care currently is rationed, especially high-technology care in intensive care units, the most common site of futility debates.[37] Therefore, taking a hard look at the utility of treatment becomes relevant in the discussion of what counts as futile care. Under these circumstances, according to concepts of justice, expensive medical care of zero or the most marginal utility that utilizes scarce resources cannot be justified because doing so also requires withholding care from arguably more meritorious cases.[38]

A coherent concept of futility, however, is not dependent on rationing considerations. Irrespective of financial conditions or resource scarcity, the professional integrity of physicians and nurses is relevant to futility decisions. Professional integrity comes under attack if physicians and nurses are forced to provide inappropriate treatments against their better judgment. Physicians and nurses have argued that they should not be required to compromise their professional integrity and dignity by being forced into purely technical roles that violate their professional prerogatives as a result of unreasonable demands for inappropriate, futile treatment by patients or families.[39]

The incidence of truly futile interventions is lower than many clinicians have assumed. Amir Halevy and colleagues found that only 0.9% of patients treated in ICUs have a predicted mortality greater than 90%.[40] Using a broader definition of "potentially ineffective care," Daniel Cher and Leslie Lenert found that 4.8% of Medicare patients hospitalized in California in 1994 qualified for this designation because they died within 100 days of admission and expended total hospital costs above the 90th percentile.[41] Ramesh Sachdeva and colleagues found that only 2.7% of patient-days in a pediatric ICU met at least one of the definitions of medical futility for some of the days.[42] As noted in the discussion of the SUPPORT study in chapter 8, these types of data on outcomes of critically ill patients must be interpreted in light of clinical reality. The determination that a critically ill patient also is terminally ill often can be made more accurately in retrospect.[43] Keith Berge and colleagues showed that unrealistic family expectations of outcomes of critically ill ICU patients led to increased resource utilization without survival benefits.[44]

ILLUSTRATIVE CASES

To understand the concept of medical futility better it is useful to study examples of how the concept has been employed in neurological practice. I discuss five clinical examples commonly regarded as futile: cardiopulmonary resuscitation (CPR) on patients with terminal illnesses, treating the brain-dead patient, treating the patient with an irreversible vegetative state, providing life-sustaining therapy (LST) for the anencephalic infant, and providing LST for the patient with advanced dementia and multi-organ failure. I illustrate each example with a highly publicized medicolegal case report or a case from my experience.

Futility in Do-Not-Resuscitate Orders: The Case of Catherine Gilgunn

The concept of CPR futility is based upon outcome studies of the success of CPR in hospitalized patients with different diagnoses. As discussed in chapter 8, these studies show that not a single inpatient with metastatic cancer, acute stroke, sepsis, or pneumonia on whom CPR was attempted survived to hospital discharge.[45] Some physicians thereafter advocated the routine use of Do-Not-Resuscitate (DNR) orders based on quantitative futility for such patients. In a decision analysis model, Donald Murphy and David Matchar proposed establishing thresholds for appropriate use of CPR and other life sustaining therapies,

embodying probability of benefit, collective preferences of patients, and the cost of marginal benefits. They argued that life-sustaining therapies such as CPR should not be routinely offered or provided to groups of patients for whom marginal cost-effectiveness is inordinately high because that makes CPR medically or economically inappropriate.[46]

Murphy and Thomas Finucane extended this argument to suggest that hospitals adopt policies permitting physicians not even to offer the option of CPR to patients or their lawful surrogates when the chances of CPR success were very low. In their review of CPR outcome data, they concluded that the following clinical conditions were sufficiently futile to qualify under this policy: metastatic cancer, Child's class C cirrhosis, AIDS with at least two episodes of *Pneumocystis carinii* pneumonia, dementia requiring long-term care, coma lasting longer than 48 hours, multiple organ system failure without improvement after at least three days in the intensive care unit, and unsuccessful out-of-hospital cardiac arrest.[47]

There is a consensus among physicians and the public that physicians are required neither to offer nor to discuss futile therapies with patients. Thus, for example, because outcome data are conclusive that hyperbaric oxygen treatment does not improve multiple sclerosis, a neurologist is not required even to mention the existence of this therapy when discussing therapeutic options with a multiple sclerosis patient. Adopting this doctrine, Murphy and others have argued that when physicians determine that CPR is a futile form of therapy, they are not obligated even to offer it to patients as an option. Physicians therefore should be authorized to write a DNR order without a patient or surrogate's consent and hospital policies should be amended to accommodate this change.[48]

While this is a coherent argument, the problem with adopting such a policy is that, unlike the case of hyperbaric oxygen therapy in MS, the existence of CPR is widely known and assumed by most patients to be provided. I believe that a more reasonable position is for the physician, when possible, to explain to a patient whose underlying disorder is one in which CPR would be futile, that the physician has written a DNR order and why. This dialogue with the patient or surrogate at once acknowledges that the physician has given thoughtful consideration to the use of CPR and has rejected it as a harmful and ineffective therapy in this instance. This dialogue requires tact and compassion, and is most easily conducted when there is an established patient-physician relationship. The overwhelming majority of patients and surrogates will understand the medical-evidence basis for concluding that CPR is futile, agree with the decision for a DNR order, and be grateful for the physician's communication and care.[49]

The practice of patient notification of a DNR order is consistent with the desire which patients, families, and surrogates have expressed in surveys, to participate in decisions involving resuscitation and receiving life-sustaining treatment.[50] If dying patients or their surrogates demand CPR despite the best attempts of the physician to reason with them, there is no moral duty of the physician to order it because it is ineffective therapy. However, the prudent physician should consider the implications of this decision and act accordingly. The public should be educated that CPR is ineffective and inappropriate therapy for most dying patients. To counteract the grossly misleading images commonly conveyed by the media,[51] this education should help to diminish unreasonable demand for CPR and increase understanding and acceptance of the reality of dying from a terminal illness.[52] One study found that few internal medicine residents were using the futility rationale to avoid discussing DNR orders with patients.[53] The United States Department of Veterans Affairs policy mandates discussing DNR orders with patients or surrogates in the setting of futility and provides a procedure to mediate resulting disputes similar to that outlined later in the chapter.[54]

The highly publicized case of Catherine Gilgunn addressed the question whether a determination of medical futility was sufficient grounds for a physician to write a DNR order and remove LST against the wishes of a surrogate. Mrs. Gilgunn was 71 years old when she was admitted to Massachusetts General Hospital for a series of complicated medical problems including hip fractures, diabetes, Parkinson's disease, breast cancer, heart disease, and chronic urinary tract infections. While hospitalized she developed status epilepticus leading to brain damage, coma, and ventilator dependency. Her daughter Joan assumed the role of surrogate by agreement of the family. Mrs. Gilgunn was treated for several weeks without recovery after which her physicians determined that further treatment was futile. Although Joan expressed the continued wish that "everything be done," Mrs. Gilgunn's attending physician wrote a DNR order following a consultation with the Optimum Care Committee chairman Dr. Edwin Cassem.[55] After a protest from Joan, the DNR order was reversed.

At this point, a new attending physician, Dr. William Dec, met with Mrs. Gilgunn to notify her that in his opinion her mother's case was hopeless. Another approval by Dr. Cassem and hospital legal counsel led Dr. Dec to rewrite the DNR order over the persistent protest of Joan. Dr. Dec then ordered the ventilator to be weaned and Mrs. Gilgunn died five days later. Joan met with Dr. Dec only once and did not meet with Dr. Cassem, or any member of the Optimum Care Committee. After Mrs. Gilgunn's death, Joan sued Dr. Dec, Dr. Cassem, and the hospital for withdrawing the ventilator over her objection, claiming that this act caused her mother to die.

After a widely publicized trial, a jury concluded that ventilator therapy and CPR for Mrs. Gilgunn was indeed futile and found in favor of the defendant physicians and hospital. However, the legal precedential value of this case is categorically limited because it was a jury verdict without an appellate court ruling on potentially contestable issues such as jury instructions and objections to the evidence. Therefore, although the jury accepted the theory of futility advanced by the defendants, in the absence of appellate review, *Gilgunn* offers physicians no legal support to invoke futility and probably will have little influence on future cases.[56] However, it was the first case in which laymen accepted a medical futility rationale. *Gilgunn* demonstrated the importance of ongoing communication between physicians and surrogates and also showed the limits of mediation by ethics committees and the necessity to define medical goals collaboratively.

Futility in the Persistent Vegetative State: The Case of Helga Wanglie

The application of the concept of futility to the persistent vegetative state (PVS) was highlighted by the case of Helga Wanglie in Minneapolis in 1991.[57] Mrs. Wanglie was 85 years old when she developed a PVS from hypoxic-ischemic brain damage suffered during a cardiopulmonary arrest. Unlike most PVS patients, she was ventilator-dependent and had failed trials of weaning. After she remained in this state for several months, her examining neurologists stated with a high degree of certainty that she would never regain awareness. Her physicians therefore told her family that they planned to withdraw the ventilator because it was providing her no medical benefit.[58]

However, her husband, daughter, and son disagreed with any suggestion to withdraw treatment and insisted that the ventilator treatment be continued. Although initially they denied that Mrs. Wanglie had previously made known her treatment preferences, later they reported that "she did not want anything done to shorten or prematurely take her life." When asked the reasons for this decision, in light of the dismal prognosis, Mr. Wanglie responded, "That may be true but we hope for the best." Mr. Wanglie indicated that only God can take a life and that the doctors should not play God.[59] The family did, however, consent to a DNR order.

Mrs. Wanglie's husband, an attorney, refused the physician's suggestions that Mrs. Wanglie be transferred to another facility or that the family obtain a court order mandating her continued treatment with the ventilator. Of note, financial incentives or disincentives for either the family or hospital were minimized because her medical bills were being paid fully by insurance. Because of the attending physician's judgment that the medical staff was providing inappropriate care, the hospital decided to go to court to resolve the dispute. They asked the court to appoint an independent conservator to judge whether Mrs. Wanglie

should remain on the ventilator. The husband filed a petition to be named her conservator and the court subsequently agreed in a finding that he could best represent her interests. As expected, he continued to refuse to allow her ventilator to be withdrawn. The hospital continued her ventilator therapy until she died after having lived a year in PVS.[60]

One of Mrs. Wanglie's hospital staff physicians, Steven Miles, later argued that his decision to terminate her ventilator treatment was ethically justified on the grounds that it was providing her no medical benefit because she was in a PVS from which she never could recover awareness.[61] Miles categorized ventilator therapy for Mrs. Wanglie as "inappropriate" because it provided her "no medical benefit." Although Miles later denied that his decision to stop the ventilator was based on a concept of "futility,"[62] his usage of "no medical benefit" is equivalent to the qualitative or subjective concept of futility outlined above and accepted by many scholars using the term.[63]

Recent attention has been directed to the distinction between a patient's request for a therapy and a patient's refusal of a therapy. Physicians are morally and legally obligated to respect the valid, rational treatment refusal of a competent patient or a lawful surrogate but have no correlative duty to honor a patient's request for a therapy that the physician believes to be inappropriate, ineffective or dangerous.[64]

In the Wanglie case, Miles and the other treating physicians believed strongly that continued ventilator treatment was providing her no medical benefit. Accordingly, they wished to discontinue the treatment even though doing so likely would lead directly to her death. Her family offered reasons why they believed that continued treatment was both justified and in accordance with her previously stated wishes. The disagreement centered on differing interpretations of the value to Mrs. Wanglie and others of her continued life in a PVS, and of the authority of physicians alone to make such determinations. It also relied on her physicians' following accepted medical practice standards.

I believe that Mr. Wanglie's decision was rational, although I disagree with it substantively and would not have made that decision for myself or for a member of my family. Indeed, surveys have shown that a large majority of people have indicated that if they were in a PVS without hope for recovery, they would prefer to be allowed to die from nontreatment.[65] However, when a loving family member has made a rational decision to continue ventilator treatment and thereby prolong life, I believe that physicians are ethically obligated to respect it, so long as doing so does not directly harm another patient and it does not violate accepted medical practice standards. If there were a shortage of ventilators and a more viable patient were competing for Mrs. Wanglie's ventilator, I would agree with the position taken by the Society of Critical Care Medicine that a PVS patient should be removed from the ventilator to permit it to be used by another patient who could benefit more from its use.[66]

Using the term "medical benefit" to describe a treatment that sustains a person's life is potentially misleading. True medical benefit, such as, for example, the benefit gained from choosing carbamazepine in a case of complex partial seizures, may be a judgment that is the exclusive domain of physicians, but the decision whether a patient should live or die usually does not occupy that realm. Purely and simply it is a value judgment over which physicians can exert no specialized professional claim. Physicians can counsel families but should not overrule their decisions unless they are irrational or directly harm other patients. I believe that if, after adequate counseling, the family wished to keep her alive on the ventilator, the physicians should have complied.[67]

Only our society can resolve the futility debate. If, through democratic process, we were to enact a national policy saying that we no longer can afford to treat patients in long-standing PVS who have no hope for recovery of awareness because we desperately need that money for more meritorious health-care expenditures, then physicians could unilaterally declare such cases futile (or not medically indicated) and discontinue further life-sustaining treatment. Our society has not yet achieved that level of consensus on this policy. Therefore, I believe that physicians alone

cannot make that decision. Developing such a consensus is an important objective of a national health-care policy.[68] Although courts of law may not be the ideal venue to resolve these conflicts, until a national policy exists, intractable conflicts like these that cannot be settled at the hospital level probably should be referred for judicial review to fairly balance the rights of patients, families, and others.[69]

Futility in Treating the Anencephalic Infant: The Case of Baby K

In 1993 and 1994, an anencephalic infant known as Baby K became the focus of a widely publicized ethical and legal debate in 1993 and 1994 regarding medical futility.[70] Anencephaly was diagnosed prenatally but the mother refused to have the pregnancy terminated as recommended by her physician. The baby, named Stephanie Keene, (but always referred to as Baby K in legal and public documents) was born by caesarian delivery at Fairfax Hospital in Falls Church, Virginia, on October 13, 1992. At her mother's insistence, she was immediately placed on a ventilator because of respiratory distress. Two pediatric neurological evaluations and computed tomography scans disclosed unequivocal anencephaly. The baby's mother refused to permit the hospital staff to write a DNR order or to withdraw the ventilator even though it was obvious that the case was hopeless and further treatment futile. The reason for this decision was later stated by a judge: "Ms. H. has a firm Christian faith that all life should be protected. She believes that God will work a miracle if that is His will. Otherwise, Ms. H. believes God, and not other humans, should decide the moment of her daughter's death."[71]

The physicians caring for the infant wished to discontinue her treatment because that was standard neonatal care for anencephalic infants. Because of the dispute, they consulted their legal counsel who suggested obtaining a court order authorizing them to discontinue treatment. Fearing a lawsuit from the mother, they sought a court order to immunize the hospital and staff against potential liability by seeking judicial affirmation of the appropriate standard of medical care in the management of anencephaly. Ironically, the judge hearing the case not only refused to provide the order they requested but insisted that they continue aggressive treatment of the infant under section 504 of the Rehabilitation Act of 1973 and the American with Disabilities Act of 1990.[72] As a result, the child was treated on a ventilator and survived infancy, unlike all other anencephalic infants.[73] She died on April 5, 1995, at nearly 30 months of age.[74]

The lower court decision was sustained on appeal to the United States Fourth Circuit Court of Appeals in February 1994, on a two-to-one decision. Oddly, the Court cited the Emergency Medical Treatment and Active Labor Act (Emergency Treatment Act or EMTALA) of 1985 in their decision. This law was enacted to prevent discriminatory "dumping" of uninsured patients by hospital emergency rooms and mandated appropriate emergency care irrespective of the ability to pay. The Court ruled only on the narrow issue of whether anencephalic infants represented a justified exception to the treatment requirements of the Emergency Treatment Act. They ruled that an anencephalic infant in respiratory distress was not an exception.[75] The dissenting justice argued that the Emergency Treatment Act was irrelevant in this case because patient dumping was not at issue, and that it was disingenuous to separate the emergency complications of anencephaly from the diagnosis itself because there is "no medical treatment that can improve her condition."[76] A writ of *certiorari* for review by the U.S. Supreme Court was denied.

The question at issue is whether the child's mother had the right to insist upon a treatment regarded by all physicians and by society as futile. Is such a wish rational? A strong argument could be made that it is an irrational wish, particularly given the reasons she holds it. She hoped for a miracle to cure her daughter. Relying on this wish as the only basis for choosing aggressive therapy is irrational. It is similar to the family of the brain dead patient claiming that he will be reanimated by a miracle and thereby demanding continued ventilator treatment. Such a wish is not simply highly improbable, it is impossible. Although the baby's mother may be a sincere believer, religious

faith in miracles alone cannot justify the irrationality of her wish.[77] If the mother's view had been simply, "the longer she lives, the better," it would have been more difficult to call the treatment futile, analogously to the family's reasoning in the Wanglie case.

Society has recognized that anencephalic life is of such limited benefit to the infant that there is no medical mandate to provide LST. For example, although third-trimester elective abortions are otherwise uniformly banned, they are permitted to allow anencephalic infants to die.[78] Anencephalic infants have a uniformly dismal prognosis and anencephaly is classified as a terminal neonatal illness. From data collected by the Medical Task Force on Anencephaly, it appears that Baby K has the dubious distinction of establishing the record for longevity for an anencephalic infant, as well as for receiving aggressive treatment.[79] Is the mother's moral claim valid for this degree of treatment of Baby K?

This conflict could have been prevented. The treating physicians could reasonably have withheld ventilatory treatment from the baby at birth as a standard-of-care issue because anencephalic infants ordinarily do not receive such aggressive treatment. Secondly, the treating physicians could have avoided soliciting advice from legal counsel and simply treated this anencephalic infant like all others, permitting her to die by purposeful non-treatment. It was unnecessary for them to request a court order for immunity from liability. Of course, doing so backfired in this case. The treating physicians were entirely within their authority to permit the infant to die because aggressive treatment in anencephaly is futile and allowing anencephalic infants to die represents the usual standard of care. When asked by the mother about ventilator treatment and other aggressive care for the infant, the physicians could have responded, as was suggested by Father John Paris and colleagues in their discussion of a related case, "I am sorry, but we don't do that here."[80]

There are some analogies between the cases of Baby K and Helga Wanglie. Both had profoundly diminished lives with no hope of recovery. In both cases, the families pushed for aggressive treatment that was considered inappropriate and not indicated by the treating physicians. One difference is that Baby K had no prior life and not the remotest possibility of becoming aware of herself or her surroundings, much less of developing a personality. This tragically malformed infant had no chance of attaining meaningful human development. Mrs. Wanglie had lived a rich life and her final illness was the culmination of this life. Her family's wish to continue her existence a bit longer, which was meaningful to the family, arguably is more rational than Baby K's mother's wish to prolong a hopeless and meaningless anencephalic existence awaiting a miracle.

A second difference between the cases is that the accepted standard of medical practice is clearer for managing anencephaly than for managing patients with ventilator-dependent PVS. Anencephalic infants are not treated or resuscitated but some PVS patients are treated aggressively for prolonged periods depending on surrogate consent or refusal. Therefore a physician cannot rely on an unambiguous medical practice standard to justify unilaterally stopping treatment of a PVS patient as a physician could in withholding treatment in anencephaly.

Courts deciding such cases should rule that neither physicians nor hospitals have the duty to prolong a hopeless, meaningless, and futile anencephalic existence because of an irrational wish of the child's mother. The Court should uphold the authority of physicians to rely on the standard of medical care to govern their decisions in the case of life support for anencephalic infants. Physicians should not be required to prescribe meaningless and wasteful forms of medical treatment merely because some people irrationally wish others to receive them. For their part, physicians should not only establish the standards of medical care but also have the courage to adhere to them without first demanding unconditional legal immunity.[81]

Futility in Treating a Brain-Dead Patient

The family of a 56-year-old brain dead man refused to accept that he was dead and insisted upon further treatment until an agreement could be reached. The patient had suffered an out-of-hospital cardiac arrest and was resuscitated after 25 minutes of ventricular fibrillation and asystole. Thereafter, he never regained any measurable brain functions on serial neurological examinations. Apnea testing was positive for apnea. EEG showed electrocerebral silence. Brain stem auditory evoked potentials were absent. Radionuclide angiogram showed absence of intracranial blood flow. Vasopressor drugs were required to maintain blood pressure. Approximately 16 hours after admission, he was declared dead by brain criteria.[82]

The neurologist spoke to his wife and brother, explaining the concept of brain death and its irreversibility and offering organ donation. Family members were shocked, rejected organ donation, and did not believe that it was possible for a person to be dead and remain warm, have a heartbeat, and make urine. Several detailed conversations carried out over two days explaining the conceptual and legal basis of brain death and the utter futility of further treatment were to no avail. The neurologist considered simply ordering extubation over the protests of the family on the grounds of futility but wished to avoid unnecessarily antagonizing them.

On hospital day 3, the patient's brother announced that his cousin, a physiologist, wanted to review the patient's EEG. This was urgently arranged and after examining the EEG, the cousin declared the case hopeless. As a consequence, the family agreed to extubation which was performed immediately.

This case demonstrated how both the lack of trust in the physician and difficulty conceptualizing brain death interfered with proper medical care. Brain death is a clear case where both the quantitative and qualitative components of futility are met. No treatment can restore the patient's life and continued treatment of a dead body is meaningless. Most instances of disputes with families over the diagnosis of brain death result from the emotional inability of family members to accept the diagnosis of death because of the presence of heartbeat and circulation.[83] The continued presence of heartbeat and circulation provides false encouragement to some families that there may be hope for neurological recovery.

These cases need to be handled sensitively. First, valid religious objections to brain death determination should be inquired about and respected if present.[84] I believe that briefly continuing support of ventilation is a compassionate response until the family accepts the fact of death.[85] The length of such treatment must be determined case by case, but physicians remain on firm ethical and legal grounds to discontinue all treatment immediately, once death has been declared, even over the objection of family members, basing this action on futility and the provisions of state law.[86]

Futility in Life-Sustaining Therapy for the Dying Patient with Advanced Dementia

A patient with advanced dementia and progressive multi-organ failure whose son demanded LST exemplified both quantitative and qualitative futility issues.[87] An 84-year-old woman with advanced Alzheimer's disease was transferred from a nursing home to the ICU for treatment of pneumonia and multi-organ failure. In the nursing home, her dementia had progressed to the point that she was mute, doubly incontinent, and unable to recognize family members. She had contractures of all extremities and moaned when she was moved.

On hospital admission, she was deeply comatose. She received ventilator treatment for respiratory and cardiac failure and intravenous antibiotics for sepsis. She then developed acute renal tubular necrosis. Her physicians counseled her son that the most appropriate treatment for her was palliative care, given the prognosis of her underlying disease and the exceedingly small likelihood of her recovering from multi-organ failure.

Her son, who was also her Durable Power of Health Care, insisted that she be treated aggressively with a ventilator, antibiotics, and hemodialysis. Her attending physician claimed that further life-prolonging therapy in her condition was futile because it could not help her achieve her health-care goals of recovery of cognition. The Ethics Committee was asked to mediate the dispute.

The ethics consultants interviewed her son and other family members at length. Her son said "she was a fighter" and had previously indicated to him her wish to be treated aggressively and that doctors not "give up" on her. He understood her poor prognosis but claimed his actions were in accordance with his understanding of her treatment preferences and he wished to fulfill them.[88] The ethics consultants met with him several times to discuss his decision. They explored with him the meaning of "doing everything" for her. One consultant asked him if he would instruct her physicians to begin looking for a heart and lung organ donor because of her cardiac and respiratory failure. He replied that organ transplantation for her was a ridiculous idea but the consultant made him aware that even he (the son) was not doing everything possible. Nevertheless, he continued to insist on aggressive treatment. The nephrologists, however, refused to dialyze her, claiming that she was not a "qualified candidate" for dialysis because of her advanced dementia. Her son accepted this judgment and she died six days later, still on the ventilator.

This case illustrates a serious treatment dispute over futility and the inability of the ethics consultants to mediate it successfully. It also shows how physicians who possess certain technical skills or maintain control over certain high-technology therapies (e.g., surgery, dialysis) may simply refuse to provide it, claiming that the patient is not an appropriate candidate, and how that claim at times may end the dispute. Many surrogates will accept this pronouncement whereas they may not accept a physician's claim that the patient cannot have a ventilator or medications. The case also pointed out that when patients say they "want everything done," this statement is made in ignorance of all the therapies available and usually means that they wish not to be abandoned and to be actively treated. The ethics consultants doubted that the patient's true preference would be to have aggressive therapy in her present state and believed that the best active treatment was palliative care.[89] They concluded that they were not going to convince her son but anticipated an uphill battle to convince a court to name a new surrogate for her.

Her physicians were prepared simply to stop her ventilator treatment on the grounds of futility but preferred the solution that ensued.

CONCEPTUALIZATIONS OF MEDICAL FUTILITY

Some scholars view the medical futility dispute as fundamentally a power struggle between the patient/surrogate and physician to determine which party prevails.[90] Should respect for patient self-determination empower patients or their surrogates to prevail or should the professional autonomy granted by society to physicians authorize them to decide on behalf of their patients?[91] Should physicians' social duty to responsibly shepherd society's scarce resources and their professional training to decide when specific therapies are appropriate empower them alone to determine when, why, and for whom they will be used? Viewing the futility dispute as a power struggle, Bethany Spielman proposed bargaining strategies for patients and physicians similar to those used in out-of-court dispute resolution.[92]

Other scholars have viewed futility disputes as a breakdown of the patient-physician relationship. John Lantos pointed out that the futility debate can be conceptualized in two distinct ways. One concept asks the question whether a physician has a moral obligation to provide a treatment requested by a patient, simply because the patient wants it, irrespective of benefits, costs, or other factors. The second asks whether physicians may decide, using their own values and without even considering the patient's perceptions or values, that a treatment's benefit is so low that it need not even be offered. He concluded that framing futility in terms of the conflict between patients' rights and physicians' prerogatives is unhelpful. Lantos concluded that futility can be understood better as deficiencies in the physician-patient relationship resulting from four factors: power, money, trust, and hope.[93]

The physician-patient relationship is based upon trust, honesty, fidelity, and good communication. In the setting of secure trust and effective communication, futility problems usually do not arise. Futility issues usually arise in the following circumstances: (1) poor communication; (2) mistrust; (3) ignorance or grossly unrealistic expectations of outcome by family members; (4) confusion among family members resulting from conflicting messages; (5) a dogged determination "to do everything possible" irrespective of probabilities, arising from fierce loyalty or neurosis; or (6) the psychological inability of a family member to abandon hope, give up, and admit failure.[94] Family members showing these last two attitudes must be compassionately counseled until they realize that "letting go" by allowing a hopelessly ill loved one to die should not be construed as abandonment. [95]

PREVENTING AND RESOLVING DISPUTES OVER MEDICAL FUTILITY

Medical futility disputes are easier to prevent than to resolve. Most disputes occur in the ICU and involve decisions to initiate or maintain LST. Critical care decisions often must be made quickly without the benefit of unambiguous data or lengthy explanations to families. Critical care physicians usually have no prior relationship with the patient or family on which to base trust. Family members are anxious, fearful, and emotionally distraught. They may harbor unrealistic expectations because of their overconfidence in the miracles of modern medical technology. It is a compliment to critical care physicians that futility disputes occur relatively rarely in this emotionally charged situation. Most ICU physicians succeed in establishing strong relationships with patients, surrogates, and other family members that permit good decision-making practices and appropriate levels of medical care.

Failure of communication is the cause of many disputes. Excellent communication between physicians and family members can help them understand the patient's illness and make realistic decisions based on up-to-date, accurate information about diagnosis and prognosis, but communication in the ICU is difficult under most circumstances. Commonly, families meet teams of physicians including critical care and other specialists, consultants and house officers, as well as medical students. They frequently rotate services. Therefore, a patient who is in the ICU for several weeks may come under the care of dozens of physicians. Nurses also rotate shifts frequently. Often, there is inadequate space and ambience in the ICU for physicians to sit and have a calm discussion with family members. Family members may visit at irregular times, hear conflicting information, and get mixed messages from different professionals. Family members often ask lengthy questions that require more time to answer than busy physicians may have available. They commonly ask questions about prognosis for which confident answers cannot be given. This circumstance produces anxiety in physicians that may lead them to avoid the family. Moreover, family members commonly harbor fears and anxieties that may alter their perception of the reality of the situation.

Families of critically ill and dying patients have emotional and informational needs that should be addressed by ICU physicians and nurses. It widely believed that adequately satisfying these needs can help prevent futility disputes. The Ethics Committee of the Society of Critical Care Medicine enumerated these needs as listed in Table 10-1.[96] The American College of Critical Care Medicine Task Force recently published practice guidelines for the support of family members of ICU patients.[97] The failure to meet family members' emotional and informational needs can cause a type of post-traumatic stress disorder among family members of ICU patients.[98] Alexandre Lautrette and colleagues showed recently that implementing a proactive communication strategy in the ICU with brochures and increased time for conferences with family members diminished their subsequent bereavement.[99] Randall Curtis and colleagues have described the techniques of holding an ICU family conference and explored its benefits and limitations.[100]

Family members' unrealistic expectations about treatment are an important factor damaging the patient-physician relationship. An unfortunate problem is commonly inherited by ICU physicians but is not of their creation. In an attempt to calm anxious family members, referring physicians may reassure them that once the critically ill patient reaches the

TABLE 10-1   Emotional and Informational Needs of Family Members of Dying Patients

1. To be with the dying patient
2. To be helpful to the dying patient
3. To be informed of the dying patient's changing condition
4. To understand what is being done to the patient and why
5. To be assured of the patient's comfort
6. To be comforted
7. To ventilate emotions
8. To be assured that their decisions were right
9. To find meaning in the dying of their loved one
10. To be fed, hydrated, and rested

Modified from Ethics Committee of the Society of Critical Care Medicine.[96]

academic medical center, the miraculous technology and highly-skilled physicians there surely will be able to help or cure the patient. This message instantly raises the family's expectations of therapy to a level higher than may be appropriate for the patient's condition. Because of the unrealistic expectations communicated by the referring physician, critical care physicians may be thrown on the defensive from their first conversation with family members when they try to explain the poor prognosis and counsel limitation of treatment. One experienced academic physician I know routinely tells referring physicians that he will accept the critically ill patient in transfer only on the condition that the referring physician makes no promises to the family about the successes of ICU treatment.

Another cause of futility disputes is a family's insistence that every possible therapy be used to maintain their loved one's life, irrespective of age, prognosis, or the patient's suffering resulting from the treatment. I have performed ethics consultations in several difficult cases in which family members vigorously expressed this sentiment in their zeal to keep an elderly and infirmed relative alive as long as possible. In some cases, family members expressed their motivation as love for the patient; in others they claimed they were following the patient's wishes. Despite compassionate counseling, family members became angry at physicians and ethics committee members who advocated palliative care because of the patient's poor prognosis and suffering resulting directly from the continued aggressive treatment. In one recent case, a family member accused the hospital of committing "geriatric genocide." These troubling cases illustrate the sometimes unbridgeable chasm between physicians and family members over the appropriate goals of treatment.

Thomas Prendergast outlined a series of strategies for ICU physicians to prevent futility disputes.[101] He argued that declaring a proposed treatment to be futile is a poor strategy for resolving end-of-life disputes because it created an adversarial relationship between the physician and patient/surrogate. As an alternative, Prendergast proposed the series of strategies to minimize conflicts and negotiate treatment limits listed in Table 10-2. Prendergast also explained how to apply the mediation and communication strategies developed by Fisher, Ury, and Patton for the business community to resolving disputes in the ICU. The mediation strategies comprise four elements: (1) identify the problem and separate it from the people involved; (2) focus on interests, not positions; (3) use objective criteria; and (4) invent options for mutual gains.[102] In an educational intervention carried out in over 225 hospitals, Joseph Fins and Mildred

---

TABLE 10-2 Strategies to Minimize Conflicts and Negotiate Treatment Limits in the ICU

1. Keep patients and families informed
2. Identify other staff members to facilitate good patient relations
3. Promote realistic expectations
4. Strive for accuracy in prognosis
5. Maintain continuity of care
6. Be compassionate and flexible
7. Show firmness about limits
8. Beware of making decisions based on economic market forces

Modified from Prendergast[101]

Solomon studied the elements of communication necessary to resolve futility disputes in the ICU. They found that good communication required not only the use of clear and understandable language but also clinicians' self-awareness and recognition of the early stages of impending disputes, psychological insight into the cause of disputes, and an institutional culture that promoted good communication with families.[103]

In the small number of cases in which strategies of mediation and open communication fail to resolve the dispute, ICU physicians can request assistance in dispute resolution from social workers, chaplains, or the hospital ethics committee. A growing number of hospital ethics consultations now are ordered for dispute resolution. Robert Orr and Dennis deLeon explained the techniques of dispute resolution by hospital ethics committees and consultants, including the techniques of negotiation, mediation, and arbitration.[104] Most ethics committees practice mediation, a technique in which the ethics consultants are invited as a neutral party with allegiance only to the patient's interests. They work with both parties through mutual understanding and compromise to facilitate a resolution to the conflict that is in the patient's best interests.[105] A study of the process of ethics consultation has confirmed the success of this approach.[106]

LEGAL AND POLICY SOLUTIONS

Advocates of employing a concept of medical futility to resolve disputes in end-of-life care have proposed institutional and community-wide policies that explain how futility will be determined and stipulate the mechanism to resolve futility disputes.[107] In an influential editorial in 1993 on future management objectives for the American health-care system, then *JAMA* editor George Lundberg urged physicians to define medical futility and suggested that hospitals develop guidelines for resolving futility disputes.[108]

The current legal status for physicians to assert medical futility as grounds for unilaterally withholding or withdrawing therapy remains ambiguous. As noted in the cases of

Helga Wanglie and Baby K, and in the few other futility cases adjudicated, courts have not supported this position. A few state legislatures have enacted laws incorporating the concept of medical futility. In 2000, California enacted the Health Care Decisions Law permitting physicians to refuse to provide futile end-of-life care. Although this law's primary intent was to integrate and simplify advance directives, it contained a provision for physicians and hospitals to refuse to provide requested treatment if it "requires medically ineffective health care or health care contrary to generally accepted health-care standards applicable to the health-care provider or institution."[109] The Texas Advance Directives act of 1999 (see below) contains a similar provision.[110] The existence of such a law might have provided legal support allowing the doctors caring for Baby K and Helga Wanglie to unilaterally discontinue LST.

Several medical societies and scholars have drafted procedural policies to integrate the concept of futility into medical practice. In their consensus statement regarding futile and inadvisable treatments, the Ethics Committee of the Society of Critical Care Medicine recommended that all institutional futility policies have the following characteristics: (1) they are disclosed in the public record; (2) they reflect moral values acceptable to the community; (3) they are not based exclusively on prognostic scoring systems; (4) they articulate appellate mechanisms; and (5) they are recognized by the courts.[111] An additional desirable feature is uniformity: futility policies should use standardized definitions of futility. A review in 2000 of futility policies in 26 hospitals in California showed that the futility definitions used by most hospitals were similar, a finding that adds support to the concept that uniform futility policies can establish a practice standard.[112]

In an influential report, the American Medical Association Council on Ethical and Judicial Affairs recommended a stepwise, algorithmic procedural policy for physicians to follow when faced with futility disputes in end-of-life care. The policy permitted a physician's unilateral cessation of therapy only after all other avenues of negotiation had been tried

and failed. It admonished physicians to conduct the steps listed in Table 10-3 in order.[113] The limits of this process resulting from patients' cultural beliefs were discussed recently.[114]

Given the wide medical practice differences in futility determinations, medical futility remains a plausible concept only if is embraced by a community of physicians and patients. Several groups have produced community-wide futility policies. Others have proposed that a widespread consensus on hospital futility policies may help establish legal standards of practice. Hospital futility policies should not be freestanding but a component of integrated hospital policies governing all decision making for limitation of treatment.[115] Hospital futility policies should be drafted with community input to represent a collective, communal perspective of shared values.[116] National medical societies can aid this process by devising best medical practice guidelines on futility.[117]

A few groups have implemented community-wide futility policies. The Houston City-Wide Task Force on Medical Futility, a consortium of representatives from leading hospitals in Houston, drafted a futility policy that was endorsed by most of the major hospitals in Houston and by the Harris County Texas Medical Society. The policy requires that patients or their surrogates be included in

---

TABLE 10-3 An Algorithm for Physicians Faced with Futility Disputes in the ICU

1. Deliberate values with surrogates and transfer patients to the care of another physician if the values conflict
2. Conduct shared decision making using outcome data and value judgments
3. Involve consultants if disagreements about data arise
4. Involve the hospital ethics committee
5. Transfer the patient to another physician within the institution
6. Transfer the patient to another hospital
7. Only if all these measures fail may physicians unilaterally cease the futile intervention.

Modified from the American Medical Association Council on Ethical and Judicial Affairs[113]

prognosis and treatment discussions from the beginning. It insists that physicians may not act unilaterally. It preserves the right of patients to be transferred to other institutions willing to care for them and avoids patient abandonment by either the physician or the institution. It provides a process for trying to accommodate the patient's or surrogate's wishes. It offers an institutional review mechanism to patients or surrogates to guarantee due process. One advantage of city-wide cooperation was the incorporation of community input into the guidelines.[118] A group of hospitals in northern California made a similar attempt but did not implement the policy because of fear of legal liability.[119]

Even communities of patients and physicians may not comprise sufficiently large groups, however, and state law may be necessary to address futility disputes satisfactorily. In 1999, Texas became the first state to adopt a law regulating end-of-life decision making that included a provision to resolve medical futility disputes. The Texas Advance Directives Act of 1999 provided a series of rules for physicians to follow in futility disputes. These rules require hospital ethics consultation to mediate the dispute. If mediation fails, attempts should be made to transfer the patient to another physician or facility willing to provide the desired care. Only if no such person or facility can be identified can the physician unilaterally withhold the treatment found to be futile. Patients and surrogates can request judicial intervention to postpone the withdrawal of therapy which a judge may order if the court finds that with more time, a physician or institution could be found to provide the requested care. Physicians who follow the rules are granted immunity from civil and criminal liability for unilateral cessation of therapy.[120]

A study of the first two years' experience in settling futility disputes under the Texas Advance Directives Act found that it increased the volume of hospital ethics consultations, markedly reduced the time spent in resolving futility disputes, and improved communication between physicians and surrogates.[121] A later, larger study showed that only a minority of Texas hospitals had ever used the act, that most often when it was invoked, an agreeable

solution was reached before the 10-day waiting period had elapsed, and that there were very few cases in which LST was discontinued against the wishes of surrogates or family members.[122]

The most prominent futility case considered under the Texas Advance Directives Act was that of Emilio Gonzalez, an 18-month-old boy dying of Leigh's disease. He had been in an ICU on ventilator support for five months. His physicians ruled his case hopeless because he had a progressive neurometabolic disease and advocated removing him from the ventilator. However, his parents opposed this action. The hospital ethics committee was consulted who opined that although the LST was maintaining his life, it was providing him no medical benefit because of his prognosis. Under the Texas Advance Directives Act, the hospital offered a judicial appeal and transfer to another facility before stopping LST. With the assistance of advocacy groups, a judge extended the 10-day deadline, but Emilio died before a final judicial decision was reached.[123] The framing of the dispute in the popular press contrasted the cruel hospital and physicians who wanted Emilio to die against his loving parents who wanted him to live. The fact that Emilio was from a lower socioeconomic, disenfranchised minority group also was emphasized.

Haavi Morreim pointed out that a coercive struggle between physicians and patients lies at the root of the futility argument. She emphasized the essential role of community input to resolve the conflict. Physicians through professional authority try to coerce patients and their families into accepting their concept of futility whereas patients and families through threats of legal action try to coerce physicians into accepting their concept of the value of life. The solution to optimally accommodate the conflicting interests is to establish a set of rules for the expenditure of health-care resources that is broadly agreed upon by the public. For example, if the public achieved consensus that anencephalic infants should not be placed on ventilators, then physicians could confidently assert the authority not to order such aggressive treatment even over the objection of patients' families. Similarly, if there were a consensus that other profoundly and permanently brain-damaged patients with dismal prognoses would not receive certain types of aggressive treatment, there would be no basis for a struggle between physicians and patients or families over the desirability of treatment.[124]

Another proposed solution to the futility issue is "informed consent for medical rationing." According to a novel theory of economic informed consent, patients can be offered the opportunity to purchase less expensive health insurance if they provide consent in advance to permit their physicians to withhold treatments of marginal benefit and not to inform them of decisions not to employ certain treatments when futility exists.[125] Whether such a libertarian doctrine would be practical in the clinical setting or even lawful appears dubious, because of its inherent discrimination, but it remains to be tested.

FUTILITY AND RATIONING

A complete analysis of medical futility also should consider concepts of justice and economics. Although futility and rationing are distinct concepts, implicit in the concept of futility is the finitude of health-care resources.[126] Given the presence of a global health-care budget, prescribing inappropriate therapy for one patient automatically requires limiting the resources available to others. An ethically important harm from prescribing a futile therapy is that others may be hurt indirectly by the squandering of resources.[127] Thus we must assess the validity of an individual's desire to maintain futile therapy in the context of the harms that it produces to the rest of society. How much claim should one person have over the finite resources of society when the demand is for futile therapy or for therapy with the most marginal of benefits?

The community of patients that forms our society should collectively decide its health-care goals and how it chooses to spend its finite health-care resources. Consensus can be developed through community meetings and the political process, such as that which occurred

in the development of the diagnosis-related groups (DRG) priority lists for the Oregon Medicaid budget.[128] Only once we, as a community of citizen-patients, agree on the most desirable way to spend our health-care dollars can we begin jointly to resolve these conflicts of medical futility.[129]

If we as a society decide that we can no longer can afford to maintain indefinite supportive treatment for anencephalic infants or patients in irreversible vegetative states because these health-care goals are viewed as less compelling than competing, meritorious goals, these activities will be defined as futile and public financial support for them will be withdrawn.[130] This process exemplifies the necessary task of setting health care limits, which our publicly elected officials and health care professionals must work together to determine.[131] However, the exact cost savings resulting from discontinuing futile treatment may be less than many people assume.[132]

FUTURE DIRECTIONS

Where does the debate over medical futility currently stand? Ideally, disputes about end-of-life care in which physicians assert futility to justify unilateral discontinuation of requested therapy are best prevented. Strategies for ICU physicians to minimize such disputes include optimizing communication with patients and surrogates by being available, approachable, and compassionate; providing accurate and realistic prognoses on an ongoing basis; addressing the emotional needs of surrogates and supporting them through their lonely ordeal; empathically considering the surrogate's perspective; providing excellent palliative care; and, in some cases, offering a trial of therapy to prove its futility.

Despite communicating optimally and providing end-of-life care of high quality, physicians cannot completely avoid treatment disputes. These disputes can be resolved best within the context of a societal consensus encompassing both the process and content elements of appropriate medical care of the critically ill and dying patient. Process consensus involves societal agreement on how disputes can be fairly mediated through procedures that respect the rights of patients, surrogates, and physicians. A fair process includes adequate communication of prognosis and treatment options, reasonable attempts to transfer the patient to a willing physician or institution, involvement of the hospital ethics committee as a mediator, and offering an appeal opportunity for judicial review. Content consensus involves community-wide agreement on what constitutes appropriate medical care at the end of life and, in general, what constitutes appropriate expenditures of scarce communal medical resources.

The recently enacted, bold end-of-life treatment statutes of Texas and California are noteworthy societal attempts to resolve the medical futility debate. Legislative action probably is necessary because courts have been unwilling to grapple with the substantive questions of the medical futility debate.[133] Judicial unwillingness to enter the futility debate is best exemplified by the Baby K case, in which a federal district court ruling completely sidestepped the substantive issues. Absent state law, community-wide multi-institutional futility policies, such as the Houston consortium, can help. Absent community-wide hospital consortia, individual hospitals can craft futility policies following national recommendations.[134] But even reasonably crafted laws like the Texas Advance Directives Act can fail in the court of public opinion as exemplified in publicity surrounding the Emilio Gonzalez case.

Neurologists have an important policy role in the futility debate. They can help design hospital futility policies that, in addition to ensuring a fair process, embrace an ethic of care by espousing the principles of palliative medicine and following national recommendations for end-of-life care.[135] Neurologists can further inform the debate by creating and implementing evidence-based clinical practice guidelines incorporating prognosis and futility considerations.[136]

More work needs to be performed on the concept and determination of medical futility.[137] (1) We should acknowledge that the word "futility" is being used too loosely and urge that it be restricted to a precise definition such as that used here. (2) We should actively support research into properly designed outcome studies that clearly measure the efficacy of our technological treatments, because obtaining and applying these data is a prerequisite to a determination of futility. (3) Physicians need to develop broadly acceptable clinical practice guidelines based on the outcome data. (4) In the context of futility, physicians need to emphasize an ethic of caring for the terminally-ill patient, embracing proper palliative care and adequate attention to the comfort and dignity of the dying patient.[138] (5) Physicians should be taught to practice optimal skills of communication to prevent conflicts, and mediation skills to employ when treatment conflicts arise. (6), Hospitals should draft futility policies that try to accommodate patients' treatment wishes, create fair mechanisms for appeals in situations of irresolvable conflict, and permit overruling patient wishes only as a last resort. (7) As a society, we need to engage in frank discussions about the goals of medical care and the design of social policy governing the spending of our limited financial resources to set limits optimally and fulfill those goals. As politicians design national health care plans, they should incorporate these ethical considerations into health-care public policy.[139] All these steps will help advance the goal shared by physicians and families: to see that critically ill and dying patients receive the most effective and appropriate medical care.

NOTES

1. Jecker NS, Schneiderman LJ. Medical futility: the duty not to treat. *Camb Q Healthc Ethics* 1993;2:151–159 and Miles SH. Medical futility. *Law Med Health Care* 1992;20:310–315.

2. President's Commission for the Study of Ethical Problems in Medicine and Biomedical and Behavioral Research. *Deciding to Forgo Life-Sustaining Treatment: Ethical, Medical and Legal Issues in Treatment Decisions.* Washington, DC: US Government Printing Office, 1983:219.

3. 1984 Amendments to the Child Abuse Prevention and Treatment Act. PL 98–457, 1984. The "Baby Doe" regulations are discussed in detail in chapter 13.

4. American Medical Association Council on Ethical and Judicial Affairs. Guidelines for the appropriate use of do-not-resuscitate orders. *JAMA* 1991;265:1868–1871 and American Heart Association. Part 2: Ethical issues. *Circulation* 2005;112 (Suppl):IV-6-IV-11, also available at http://www.circulation.org.

5. Helft PR, Siegler M, Lantos J. The rise and fall of the futility movement. *N Engl J Med* 2000;343:293–296. Although the term "futility" appeared first in 1987, the concept had been discussed earlier. See the description of its early history in Jonsen AR. Intimations of futility. *Am J Med* 1994;96:107–109.

6. Portions of this chapter were adapted, with permission, from Bernat JL. Medical futility: definition, determination, and disputes in critical care. *Neurocrit Care* 2005;2:198–205. © Humana Press.

7. Youngner SJ. Who defines futility? *JAMA* 1988;260:2094–2095.

8. *Jacobellis v. State of Ohio*, 84 S Ct 1676 (1964) cited in Truog RD, Brett AS, Frader J. The problem with futility. *N Engl J Med* 1992;326:1560–1564.

9. For detailed accounts of the different meaning of "futility" to different physicians, see Solomon MZ. How physicians talk about futility: making words mean too many things. *J Law Med Ethics* 1993;21:231–237.

10. The same rigorous process of identifying the definition and criterion was followed in the analysis of death in chapter 11 and the analysis of persistent vegetative state in chapter 12.

11. Temkin O, Temkin CL (eds). *Ancient Medicine: Selected Papers of Ludwig Edelstein*. Baltimore: Johns Hopkins University Press, 1967:97–98, as cited in Lantos JD, Singer PA, Walker RM, et al. The illusion of futility in medical practice. *Am J Med* 1989;87:81–84.

12. Hippocrates. The art. In Reiser SJ, Dyck AJ, Curran WJ, eds. *Ethics in Medicine: Historical Perspectives and Contemporary Concerns*. Cambridge, MA: MIT Press, 1977:6–7, as cited in Truog RD, Brett AS, Frader J. *N Engl J Med* 1992:1560. For a history of the concept of futility in Hippocratic medicine, Baconian science, and nineteenth century medicine, see Jecker NS. Knowing when to stop: the limits of medicine. *Hastings Cent Rep* 1991;21(3):5–8.

13. Feldman DM, Rosner F (eds). *Compendium on Jewish Medical Ethics: Jewish Moral, Ethical, and Religious Principles in Medical Practice*. 6th ed. New York: Federation of Jewish Philanthropies, 1984:101, as cited in Lantos JD, Singer PA, Walker RM, et al. *Am J Med* 1989:81–82.

14. Kely G. Medico-Moral Problems. St. Louis: Catholic Hospital Association, 1958:135 and Ramsey P. *The Patient as Person: Explorations in Medical Ethics*. New Haven, Yale University Press, 1970:124–144, as cited in Lantos JD, Singer PA, Walker RM, et al. *Am J Med* 1989:82.

15. *Oxford English Dictionary*, 2nd ed. Oxford: Oxford University Press, 2006.

16. This example was used in Schneiderman LJ, Jecker NS, Jonsen AR. Medical futility: its meaning and ethical implications. *Ann Intern Med* 1990;112:949–954. For the story of Danaus and the Danaïds, see Hamilton E. *Mythology: Timeless Tales of Gods and Heroes*. New York: Mentor Books, 1942:281–282.

17. Nakao MA, Axelrod S. Numbers are better than words: verbal specifications of frequency have no place in medicine. *Am J Med* 1983;74:1061–1065. The percentages cited are from Lantos JD, Singer PA, Walker RM, et al. *Am J Med* 1989:82.

18. Frick S, Uehlinger DE, Zuercher Zenklusen RM. Medical futility: predicting outcome in intensive care unit patients by nurses and doctors—a prospective comparative study. *Crit Care Med* 2003;31:456–461.

19. Rodriguez KL, Young AJ. Perceptions of patients on the utility or futility of end-of-life treatment. *J Med Ethics* 2006;32:444–449.

20. Schneiderman LJ, Jecker NS, Jonsen AR. *Ann Intern Med* 1990:950.

21. See Grant ER. Medical futility: legal and ethical aspects. *Law Med Health Care* 1992;20:330–335; Cranford RE, Gostin L. Futility: a concept in search of a definition. *Law Med Health Care* 1992;20:307–309; and Truog RD, Brett AS, Frader J. *N Engl J Med* 1992:1563.

22. For a selection of the key works on futility by Lawrence Schneiderman and colleagues, see Schneiderman LJ, Jecker NS, Jonsen AR. Medical futility: its meaning and ethical implications. *Ann Intern Med* 1990;112:949–954; Schneiderman LJ, Jecker N. Futility in practice. *Arch Intern Med* 1993;153:437–441; Schneiderman LJ. The futility debate: effective versus beneficial intervention. *J Am Geriatr Soc* 1994;42:883–886; Schneiderman LJ, Jecker NS. *Wrong Medicine: Doctors, Patients, and Futile Treatments*. Baltimore: Johns Hopkins University Press, 1995; and Schneiderman LJ, Jecker NS, Jonsen AR. Medical futility: responses to critiques. *Ann Intern Med* 1996;125:669–674.

23. Schneiderman LJ, Jecker NS, Jonsen AR. *Ann Intern Med* 1990:950–951. The possibility of rare success despite the presence of futility was discussed in Wanzer SH, Adelstein SJ, Cranford RE, et al. The physician's

responsibility toward hopelessly ill patients. *N Engl J Med* 1984;310:955–959. They observed: "The rare report of a patient with a similar condition who survived is not an overriding reason to continue aggressive treatment."

24. Schneiderman LJ, Jecker NS, Jonsen AR. *Ann Intern Med* 1990:951.

25. Schneiderman LJ, Jecker NS, Jonsen AR. *Ann Intern Med* 1990:950–952. I disagree with the contention of these authors that there is an important distinction between the mathematical calculation to determine quantitative futility and the analogous calculation in clinical decision analysis.

26. The first part of the criterion was adapted from the definition suggested in Schneiderman LJ, Jecker NS, Jonsen AR. *Ann Intern Med* 1990:951.

27. Schneiderman LJ, Jecker NS, Jonsen AR. *Ann Intern Med* 1990:951–952.

28. Knaus WA, Wagner DP, Lynn J. Short-term mortality predictions for critically ill hospitalized adults: science and ethics. *Science* 1991;254 389–394 and Knaus W. Ethical implications of risk stratification in the acute care setting. *Camb Q Healthc Ethics* 1993;2:147–149.

29. For an example of the benefits and limitations of tabulated outcome studies on critically ill patients following massive cerebral infarction and hemorrhage, see Wijdicks EFM, Rabinstein AA. Absolutely no hope? Some ambiguity of futility of care in devastating acute stroke. *Crit Care Med* 2004;32:2332–2342.

30. See Tversky A, Kahneman D. Judgment under uncertainty: heuristics and biases. *Science* 1974;185:1124–1131 and Poses RM, Bekes C, Copare FJ, et al. The answer to "What are my chances, doctor?" depends on whom (sic) is asked: prognostic disagreement and inaccuracy for critically ill patients. *Crit Care Med* 1989;17:827–833.

31. The problem of invalid data because of the fallacy of the self-fulfilling prophesy in poorly designed studies was discussed in Shewmon DA, De Giorgio CM. Early prognosis in anoxic coma. *Neurol Clin* 1989;7:823–843 and Becker KJ, Baxter AB, Cohen WA, et al. Withdrawal of support in intracerebral hemorrhage may lead to self-fulfilling prophecies. *Neurology* 2001;56:766–772. See the further discussion of the fallacy of the self-fulfilling prophesy in chapter 8.

32. The limitations on determining futility by simply using outcome data without carefully interpreting them was pointed out in Truog RD. Can empirical data establish futility? *J Clin Ethics* 1992;3:315–316.

33. Berge KH, Maiers DR, Schreiner DP, et al. Resource utilization and outcome in gravely ill intensive care unit patients with predicted in-hospital mortality rates of 95% or higher by APACHE III scores: the relationship with physician and family expectations. *Mayo Clin Proc* 2005;80:166–173. This study showed that the APACHE III scores predicted outcomes that were five times more pessimistic than those observed.

34. Prendergast TJ. Futility and the common cold: how requests for antibiotics can illuminate care at the end of life. *Chest* 1996;107:836–844.

35. For a debate on whether physicians alone should determine futility, see Brody H. The physician's role in determining futility. *J Am Geriatr Soc* 1994;42:875–878 and Veatch RM. Why physicians cannot determine if care is futile. *J Am Geriatr Soc* 1994;42:871–874.

36. See Alpers A, Lo B. Futility: not just a medical issue. *Law Med Health Care* 1992;20:327–329 and Loewy EH, Carlson RA. Futility and its wider implications: a concept in need of further examination. *Arch Intern Med* 1993;153:429–431.

37. See McGregor M. Technology and the allocation of resources. *N Engl J Med* 1989;320:118–120; Engelhardt HT Jr, Rie MA. Intensive care units, scarce resources, and conflicting principles of justice. *JAMA* 1986;255:1159–1164; and Kalb PE, Miller DH. Utilization strategies for intensive care units. *JAMA* 1989;261: 2389–2395.

38. Jecker NS, Schneiderman LJ. Futility and rationing. *Am J Med* 1992;92:189–196.

39. In my hospital, many requests for ethics consultation have come from ICU nurses who are angry at being required to provide daily intensive care for patients in futile situations. They believe such care is professionally destructive and demeaning. For a study showing the causal relationship between nurses providing futile treatment and their subsequent emotional exhaustion, see Meltzer LS, Huckabay LM. Critical care nurses' perceptions of futile care and its effect on burnout. *Am J Crit Care* 2004;13:202–208.

40. Halevy A, Neal RC, Brody BA. The low frequency of futility in an adult intensive care unit setting. *Arch Intern Med* 1996;156:100–104.

41. Cher DJ, Lenert LA. Method of Medicare reimbursement and the rate of potentially ineffective care of critically ill patients. *JAMA* 1997;278:1001–1007.

42. Sachdeva RC, Jefferson LS, Coss-Bu J, Brody BA. Resource consumption and the extent of futile care among patients in a pediatric intensive care unit setting. *J Pediatrics* 1996;128:742–747.

43. Swanson JW, McCrary SV. Doing all they can: physicians who deny medical futility. *J Law Med Ethics* 1994;22:318–326.

44. Berge KH, Maiers DR, Schreiner DP, et al. Resource utilization and outcome in gravely ill intensive care unit patients with predicted in-hospital mortality rates of 95% or higher by APACHE III scores: the relationship with physician and family expectations. *Mayo Clin Proc* 2005;80:166–173.

45. Bedell SE, Delbanco TL, Cook EF, et al. Survival after cardiopulmonary resuscitation in the hospital. *N Engl J Med* 1983;309:569–576 and Taffet GE, Teasdale TA, Lucho RJ. In-hospital cardiopulmonary resuscitation. *JAMA* 1988;260:2069–2072; Moss AH. Informing the patient about cardiopulmonary resuscitation: when the risks outweigh the benefits. *J Gen Intern Med* 1989;4:349–355. Predictably, later studies of outcomes of CPR among hospitalized patients reveal higher rates of survival because, with the increase in prevalence of DNR orders, resuscitation is not being attempted on many of the sicker hospitalized patients. See Ballew KA, Philbrick JT, Caven DE, Schorling JB. Predictors of survival following in-hospital cardiopulmonary resuscitation. *Arch Intern Med* 1994;154:2426–2432.

46. Murphy DJ, Matchar DB. Life-sustaining therapy: a model for appropriate use. *JAMA* 1990;264: 2103–2108.

47. Murphy DJ, Finucane TE. New do-not-resuscitate policies: a first step in cost control. *Arch Intern Med* 1993;153:1641–1648.

48. Murphy DJ, Finucane TE. *Arch Intern Med* 1993:1647. Others believe that the only justification for unilateral DNR orders is quantitative futility. See Waisel DB, Truog RD. The cardiopulmonary resuscitation-not-indicated order: futility revisited. *Ann Intern Med* 1995;122:304–308.

49. Others are in agreement with the desirability of notifying patients or their surrogates of patients' DNR status in this setting. See Youngner SJ. Futility in context. *JAMA* 1990;264:1295–1296; Scofield GR. Is consent useful when resuscitation isn't? *Hastings Cent Rep* 1991;21(6):28–36; American Medical Association Council on Ethical and Judicial Affairs. *JAMA* 1991:1871; and Alpers A, Lo B. When is CPR futile? *JAMA* 1995;273: 156–158.

50. Lo B, McLeod GA, Saika G. Patient attitudes to discussing life-sustaining treatment. *Arch Intern Med* 1986;146:1613–1615 and Frankl D, Oye RK, Bellamy PE. Attitudes of hospitalized patients toward life support—a survey of 200 medical inpatients. *Am J Med* 1989;86:645–648.

51. The unrealistically high rate of CPR successes in television medical dramas was quantified in Diem SJ, Lantos JD, Tulsky JA. Cardiopulmonary resuscitation on television: miracles and misinformation. *N Engl J Med* 1996;334:1578–1582.

52. Tomlinson T, Brody H. Futility and the ethics of resuscitation. *JAMA* 1990;264:1276–1280.

53. Curtis JR, Park DR, Krone MR, Pearlman RA. Use of the medical futility rationale in do-not-attempt-resuscitation orders. *JAMA* 1995;273:124–128.

54. Cantor MD, Braddock CH III, Derse AR, et al. Do-not-resuscitate orders and medical futility. *Arch Intern Med* 2003;163:2689–2694.

55. See the discussion in chapter 5 of the Massachusetts General Hospital Optimum Care Committee and how it differs from most other hospital ethics committees.

56. *Gilgunn v. Massachusetts General Hospital et al.* Super Ct Civ Action no 92–4820, Suffolk Co, Mass, *verdict*, (April 21, 1995.) I have relied on the following analysis for the facts and interpretation of this case: Capron AM. Abandoning a waning life. *Hastings Cent Rep* 1995;25(4):24–26. I also spoke with Dr. Edwin Cassem about this case on April 13, 1997.

57. For a discussion of the medical aspects of the persistent vegetative state and issues involved in termination of medical treatment, see chapters 7 and 12.

58. I abstracted the facts of the Wanglie case from Miles SH. Informed demand for "non-beneficial" medical treatment. *N Engl J Med* 1991;325:512–515.

59. The quoted statements are from Cranford RE. Helga Wanglie's ventilator. *Hastings Cent Rep* 1991;12(4):23–24.

60. *In re Helga Wanglie*, Fourth Judicial District (Dist Ct, Probate Ct Div) PX-91–283, Minnesota, Hennepin County.

61. Miles SH. *N Engl J Med* 1991; Miles SH. Legal procedures in *Wanglie*: a two-step, not a sidestep. *J Clin Ethics* 1991;2:285–286 and Miles SH. Interpersonal issues in the Wanglie case. *Kennedy Inst Ethics J* 1992;2:61–72.

62. Miles SH. Letter to the editor. *Hastings Cent Rep* 1994;24(1):46.

63. The Dartmouth-Hitchcock Medical Center policy uses the term "medically ineffective care" rather than "futility" because of the controversial and emotional issues raised by the term "futility."

64. See Gert B, Bernat JL, Mogielnicki RP. The moral distinction between patient refusals and requests. *Hastings Cent Rep* 1994;24(4):13–15 and the further discussion of this subject in chapter 8.

65. Frankl D, Oye RK, Bellamy PE. *Am J Med* 1989:645–648.

66. Society for Critical Care Medicine. Consensus report on the ethics of forgoing life-sustaining treatments in the critically ill. *Crit Care Med* 1990;18:1435–1439.

67. Others are in agreement with this position. See Angell M. A new kind of "right-to-die" case. *N Engl J Med* 1991;325:511–512; Ackerman F. The significance of a wish. *Hastings Cent Rep* 1991;21(4):27–29; Callahan D. Medical futility, medical necessity: the-problem-without-a-name. *Hastings Cent Rep* 1991;21(4):30–35; Veatch RM, Spicer CM. Medically futile care: the role of the physician in setting limits. *Am J Law Med* 1992;18:15–36; and Klepper H, Truog RD. Treating the patient to benefit others. *Camb Q Healthc Ethics* 1997;6:306–311.

68. Societal consensus as a prerequisite to implementing decisions to terminate treatment based on futility is discussed in Johnson DH. Helga Wanglie revisited: medical futility and the limits of autonomy. *Camb Q Healthc Ethics* 1993;2:161–170 and in Rie MA. The limits of a wish. *Hastings Cent Rep* 1991;21(4):24–27.

69. The merit of referral to court of cases such as Wanglie was debated in Mishkin DB. The next *Wanglie* case: the problems of litigating medical ethics. *J Clin Ethics* 1991;2:282–286 and in Capron AM. In re Helga Wanglie. *Hastings Cent Rep* 1991;21(5):26–28.

70. Other ethical issues in managing infants with anencephaly are discussed in chapters 11 and 13.

71. The facts about the case of Baby K were abstracted from McCarthy M. Anencephalic baby's right to life? *Lancet* 1993;342:919; Annas GJ. Asking the courts to set the standards of emergency care—the case of Baby K. *N Engl J Med* 1994;330:1542–1545; and from a conversation with Robert S. Chabon, M.D., J.D., Medical Director, Fairfax Hospital, Falls Church, Virginia, August 19, 1993.

72. *In the matter of Baby K*, 832 F. Supp 1022 (E.D. Va 1993). The Baby Doe regulations initially arising from section 504 of the Rehabilitation Act of 1973 which mandate certain types of treatment to critically ill neonates, specifically excluded anencephalic infants. The Baby Doe regulations have been reissued as discussed in chapter 13.

73. The medical facts about anencephaly, including diagnosis, treatment, and survival, are discussed in chapter 11. For a discussion of medical futility issues in neonates with other disorders, particularly extreme prematurity with many medical problems, see Fine RL, Whitfield JM, Carr BL, Mayo TW. Medical futility in the neonatal intensive care unit: hope for a resolution. *Pediatrics* 2005;116:1219–1222.

74. Facts about Baby K, including the date of her death and her name, were reported in Glover JJ, Rushton CH. Introduction: from Baby Doe to Baby K: evolving challenges in pediatric ethics. *J Law Med Ethics* 1995;23:5–6.

75. *In the matter of Baby K*, 16 F. 3d 590 (4th—Cir 1994). This ruling was discussed in Annas GJ. Asking the courts to set the standard of emergency care—the case of Baby K. *N Engl J Med* 1994;330:1542–1545. The legal arguments in support of the mother of Baby K have been described by her attorney in Flannery EJ. One advocate's viewpoint: conflicts and tensions in the baby K case. *J Law Med Ethics* 1995;23:7–12.

76. As reported in Annas GJ. Asking the courts to set the standards of emergency care—the case of Baby K. *N Engl J Med* 1994;330:1542–1545.

77. The reasons for the generally negative public and scholarly responses to the religious grounds for her decision stated by Baby K's mother are discussed in Post SG. Baby K: medical futility and the free exercise of religion. *J Law Med Ethics* 1995;23:20–26.

78. Chervenak FA, Farley MA, Walters L, et al. When is termination of pregnancy in the third trimester morally justifiable? *N Engl J Med* 1984;310:501–504 and Walsh JL, McQueen MM. The morality of induced delivery of the anencephalic fetus prior to viability. *Kennedy Inst Ethics J* 1993;3:357–369.

79. The Medical Task Force on Anencephaly. The infant with anencephaly. *N Engl J Med* 1990;322:669–674.

80. Paris JJ, Schreiber MD, Statter M, et al. Beyond autonomy—physicians' refusal to use life-prolonging extracorporeal membrane oxygenation. *N Engl J Med* 1993;329:354–357.

81. Annas GJ. Asking the courts to set the standards of emergency care–the case of Baby K. *N Engl J Med* 1994;330:1542–1545. This point was made specifically in the context of medical futility. See Johnson SH, Gibbons VP, Goldner JA, Wiener RL, Eton D. Legal and institutional policy responses to medical futility. *J Health Hosp Law* 1997;30:21–36.

82. For a review of tests for determining brain death, see Wijdicks EFM. The diagnosis of brain death. *N Engl J Med* 2001;344:1215–1221 and the discussion in chapter 11.

83. Hardwig J. Treating the brain dead for the benefit of the family. *J Clin Ethics* 1991;2:53–56.

84. For a discussion of New Jersey's law providing an exclusion on brain death determination on religious grounds, see Olick RS. Brain death, religious freedom, and public policy: New Jersey's landmark legislative

initiative. *Kennedy Inst Ethics J* 1991;4:275–288. For religious claims by families for other inappropriate treatment, see Orr RD, Genesen LB. Requests for inappropriate treatment based on religious beliefs. *J Med Ethics* 1997;23:142–147.

85. Cranford RE. Discontinuation of ventilation after brain death. Policy should be balanced with concern for the family. *BMJ* 1999;318:1754–1755.

86. See the discussion in chapter 11 on the legal issues in the care of the brain dead patient.

87. See chapter 15 for a discussion of the ethical issues in withholding or withdrawing treatment for patients with advanced dementia.

88. For a thoughtful discussion of a similar case, see Fried TR, Gillick MR. The limits of proxy decision making: overtreatment. *Camb Q Healthc Ethics* 1995;4:524–529.

89. The American Academy of Neurology published guidelines for neurologists helping families define appropriate therapy for patients with advanced dementia. See American Academy of Neurology Ethics and Humanities Subcommittee. Ethical issues in the management of the demented patient. *Neurology* 1996;46:1180–1183. See also Luchins DJ, Hanrahan P. What is appropriate health care for end-stage dementia? *J Am Geriatr Soc* 1993;41:25–30.

90. For example, see Morreim EH. Profoundly diminished life: the casualties of coercion. *Hastings Cent Rep* 1994;24(1):33–42 and Daar JF. Medical futility and implications for physician autonomy. *Am J Law Med* 1995;21:221–240. The legal precedents for using futility arguments are reviewed in Menikoff J. Demanded medical care. *Ariz St Law J* 1998;30:1091–1126.

91. Edmund Pellegrino pointed out that the futility debate "underscores a growing ethical conflict between the autonomy of the physician and of the patient." Pellegrino ED. Ethics. *JAMA* 1993;270:202–203.

92. Spielman B. Bargaining about futility. *J Law Med Ethics* 1995;23:136–142 and Spielman B. Futility and bargaining power. *J Clin Ethics* 1995;6:44–52.

93. Lantos JD. Futility assessments and the doctor-patient relationship. *J Am Geriatr Soc* 1994;42:868–870.

94. Youngner SJ. Applying futility: saying no is not enough. *J Am Geriatr Soc* 1994;42:887–889.

95. Hardwig J. Families and futility: forestalling demands for futile treatment. *J Clin Ethics* 2005;16:335–344.

96. Ethics Committee of the Society of Critical Care Medicine. Recommendations for end-of-life care in the intensive care unit: the Ethics Committee of the Society of Critical Care Medicine. *Crit Care Med* 2001;29:2332–2348.

97. Davidson JE, Powers K, Hedayat KM, et al. Clinical practice guidelines for support of the family in the patient-centered intensive care unit: American College of Critical Medicine Task Force 2004–2005. *Crit Care Med* 2007;35:605–622.

98. Azoulay E, Pouchard F, Kentish-Barnes N, et al. Risk of post-traumatic stress symptoms in family members of intensive care unit patients. *Am J Respir Crit Care Med* 2005;171:987–994.

99. Lautrette A, Darmon M, Megarbane B, et al. A communication strategy and brochure for relatives of patients dying in the ICU. *N Engl J Med* 2007;356:469–478.

100. Curtis JR, Patrick DL, Shannon SE, Treece PD, Engelberg RA, Rubenfeld GD. The family conference as a focus to improve communication about end-of-life care in the intensive care unit: opportunities for improvement. *Crit Care Med* 2001;29(2 Suppl):N26–N33 and Curtis JR, Engelberg RA, Wenrich MD, Shannon SE, Treece PD, Rubenfeld GD. Missed opportunities during family conferences about end-of-life care in the intensive care unit. *Am J Respir Crit Care Med* 2005;171:844–849.

101. Prendergast TJ. Resolving conflicts in end-of-life care. *New Horiz* 1997;5:62–71.

102. Fisher R, Ury W, Patton B. *Getting to Yes: Negotiating Agreement Without Giving In*, 2nd revised edition. New York, Viking Penguin Books, 1991.

103. Fins JJ, Solomon MZ. Communication in intensive care settings: the challenge of futility disputes. *Crit Care Med* 2001;29 Suppl:N10–N15.

104. Orr RD, deLeon D. The role of the clinical ethicist in conflict resolution. *J Clin Ethics* 2000;11:21–30.

105. West MB, Gibson JM. Facilitating medical ethics case review: what ethics committees can learn from mediation and facilitation techniques. *Camb Q Healthc Ethics* 1992;1:63–74.

106. Jurchak M. Report of a study to examine the process of ethics case consultation. *J Clin Ethics* 2000;11:49–55.

107. Tomlinson T, Czlonka D. Futility and hospital policy. *Hastings Cent Rep* 1995;25(3):28–35.

108. Lundberg GD. American health care system management objectives. The aura of inevitability becomes incarnate. *JAMA* 1993;269:2554–2555.

109. Foubister V. California law facilitates advance directives. *Am Med News*, August 14, 2000:10–12.

110. Texas Advance Directives Act of 1999. *Texas Health and Safety Code* ch. 166 (Vernon Supp. 1999).

111. Society of Critical Care Medicine Ethics Committee. Consensus statement of the Society of Critical Care Medicine's Ethics Committee regarding futile and other possibly inadvisable treatments. *Crit Care Med* 1997;25:887–891.

112. Schneiderman LJ, Capron AM. How can hospital futility policies contribute to establishing standards of practice? *Camb Q Healthc Ethics* 2000;9:524–531.

113. American Medical Association Council on Ethical and Judicial Affairs. Medical futility in end-of-life care: report of the Council on Ethical and Judicial Affairs. *JAMA* 1999;281:937–941.

114. Wojtasiewicz ME. Damage compounded: disparities, distrust, and disparate impact in end-of-life conflict resolution policies. *Am J Bioethics* 2006;6:8–12.

115. Tomlinson T, Czlonka D. Futility and hospital policy. *Hastings Cent Rep* 1995;25(3):28–35.

116. Spielman B. Collective decisions about medical futility. *J Law Med Ethics* 1994;22:152–160.

117. White LJ. Clinical uncertainty, medical futility and practice guidelines. *J Am Geriatr Soc* 1994;42:899–901.

118. Halevy A, Brody BA. A multi-institution collaborative policy on medical futility. *JAMA* 1996;276:571–574.

119. Bay Area Network of Ethics Committees (BANEC) Nonbeneficial Treatment Working Group. Nonbeneficial or futile medical treatment: conflict resolution guidelines for the San Francisco Bay Area. *West J Med* 1999;170:287–290.

120. Fine RL. The Texas Advance Directives Act of 1999: politics and reality. *HEC Forum* 2001;13:59–81.

121. Fine RL, Mayo TW. Resolution of futility by due process: early experience with the Texas Advance Directives Act. *Ann Intern Med* 2003;138:743–746. The same authors later showed how futility disputes over life-sustaining treatment of critically ill neonates could be resolved under the Act. See Fine RL, Whitfield JM, Carr BL, Mayo TW. Medical futility in the intensive care unit: hope for a resolution. *Pediatrics* 2005;116:1219–1222.

122. Smith ML, Gremillion G, Slomka J, Warneke CL. Texas hospitals' experience with the Texas Advance Directives Act. *Crit Care Med* 2007;35:1271–1276.

123. Truog RD. Tackling medical futility in Texas. *N Engl J Med* 2007;357:1–3.

124. Morreim EH. Profoundly diminished life: the casualties of coercion. *Hastings Cent Rep* 1994;24(1):33–42.

125. Hall MA. Informed consent to rationing decisions. *Milbank Q* 1993;71:669–676.

126. Jecker NS, Schneiderman LJ. *Am J Med* 1992:192–194.

127. See Danis M, Churchill LR. Autonomy and the common weal. *Hastings Cent Rep* 1991;21(1):25–31 and Callahan D. Symbols, rationality, and justice: rationing health care. *Am J Law Med* 1992;18:1–13. Also see the discussion on rationing and justice in chapter 3.

128. Hadom DC. Setting health care priorities in Oregon: cost-effectiveness meets the rule of rescue. *JAMA* 1991;265:2218–2225 and Daniels N. Is the Oregon rationing plan fair? *JAMA* 1991;265:2232–2235.

129. Jecker NS, Schneiderman LJ. *Am J Med* 1992:195. This position is similar to the communitarian philosophy of medical ethics advocated in Emanuel EJ. *The Ends of Human Life: Medical Ethics in a Liberal Polity.* Cambridge, MA: Harvard University Press, 1991.

130. Payne SK, Taylor RM. The persistent vegetative state and anencephaly: problematic paradigms for discussing futility and rationing. *Semin Neurol* 1997;17:257–263. Payne and Taylor argued that futility was not a good paradigm for discussing the problems of decision making for the patient in a persistent vegetative state. This issue is discussed further in chapter 12. For a discussion of the necessity to develop ethically sound social policies, see Jecker NS. Integrating medical ethics with normative theory: patient advocacy and social responsibility. *Theor Med* 1990;11:125–139.

131. Murphy DJ, Povar GJ, Pawlson LG. Setting limits in clinical medicine. *Arch Intern Med* 1994;154:505–512.

132. For a study quantifying the modest savings resulting from reducing ICU care at the end of life, see Luce JM, Rubenfeld GD. Can health care costs be reduced by limiting intensive care at the end of life? *Am J Respir Crit Care Med* 2002;165:750–754.

133. For a review of court rulings on medical futility cases, see Menikoff J. Demanded medical care. *Ariz St Law J* 1998;30:1091–1126.

134. For ideal policies, see American Medical Association Council on Ethical and Judicial Affairs. Medical futility in end-of-life care: report of the Council on Ethical and Judicial Affairs. *JAMA* 1999;281:937–941 and

Society of Critical Care Medicine Ethics Committee. Consensus statement of the Society of Critical Care Medicine's Ethics Committee regarding futile and other possibly inadvisable treatments. *Crit Care Med* 1997;25:887–891.

135. Ethics Committee of the Society of Critical Care Medicine. Recommendations for end-of-life care in the intensive care unit: the Ethics Committee of the Society of Critical Care Medicine. *Crit Care Med* 2001;29:2332–2348.

136. Schneiderman LJ, Capron AM. How can hospital futility policies contribute to establishing standards of practice? *Camb Q Healthc Ethics* 2000;9:524–531.

137. These objectives were adapted from Schneiderman LJ, Jecker N. *Arch Intern Med* 1993:440.

138. Schneiderman LJ, Faber-Langendoen K, Jecker NS. Beyond futility to an ethic of care. *Am J Med* 1994;96:110–114.

139. See Dougherty CJ. Ethical values at stake in health care reform. *JAMA* 1992;268:2409–2412 and Wolf SM. Health care reform and the future of physician ethics. *Hastings Cent Rep* 1994;24(2):28–41.

ETHICAL ISSUES IN NEUROLOGICAL SYNDROMES

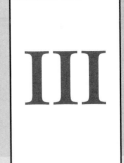

Brain Death

11

"Brain death" is a colloquial term for human death determined by brain criteria. It is used when observable functions of the brain have ceased irreversibly even though other organs continue to function through technological support. Major areas of agreement about brain death have been achieved over the past four decades—a consensus that has permitted all states in the United States, all Canadian provinces, and many other countries to enact brain death statutes and regulations. However, a few stubborn areas of philosophical controversy centering on the definition and criterion of human death remain. There also remain several unresolved ethical issues surrounding the determination of brain death and the use of the brain dead patient for organ transplantation, research, and teaching.

Although the term "brain death" is hallowed by four decades of consensual usage, it is an unfortunate and misleading term because it implies erroneously that there are two types of death: brain death and ordinary death. In fact, death remains a unitary phenomenon but it may be determined in two ways: (1) by showing the irreversible cessation of breathing and circulation; or (2) by showing the irreversible cessation of clinical brain functions when breathing and circulation are mechanically supported. The latter determination is called "brain death."

HISTORY

Although brain death is a phenomenon of only the last half-century, philosophical and practical issues concerning the definition and determination of human death have been discussed since antiquity. The ancients addressed an important question: what organ of the body represents the essence of life, because, without its function the body is dead? Greek physicians held that the heart was "the seat of life; the first organ to live and the last to die."[1] Because the heart was the essence of life and created the vital spirits, the absence of heartbeat was regarded as the principal sign of death. Greek and Roman medical experts believed that neither respiration nor brain function was essential to life, although both Hippocrates and Galen held that the brain was the source of reason, sensation, and motion.

The 12th century rabbi and physician-scholar Moses Maimonides can be regarded as the father of brain death because he first argued that a decapitated person was immediately dead, despite the presence of movements of some muscles. For the preceding millennium, ancient Hebrew law (Halachah) had provided that breathing, not heartbeat, was the essence of life and accordingly, cessation of respiration was the defining aspect of death. Maimonides took a step further toward the concept of brain death when he asserted that the "spasmodic jerking" of the decapitated body did not represent evidence of life because the muscle movements were not indicative of a central control.[2] Thus, Maimonides believed that the central controlling mechanism of locomotion was as essential to life as was breathing. Today, these profound insights remain essential to the concept of brain death.

Throughout the 18th and 19th centuries, the general public expressed fear of incorrect death determination and resultant inappropriate burial of the living. These fears were the subject of several short stories by Edgar Allen Poe[3] and resulted in the marketing and sale, by the Russian Count Karnice-Karnicki and others, of above-ground bell-ringing and flag-waving devices attached to caskets to detect breathing that could alert people to exhume a recently buried person who was erroneously declared dead and buried. The omnipresence of the fear of premature burial has continued to impel physicians to design tests of death that have zero false-positive determinations.

The implementation of the positive-pressure mechanical ventilator in the 1950s ushered in the contemporary era of brain death. For the first time, patients who had suffered irreparable damage to the brain that had rendered them permanently apneic could have their heartbeat and circulation sustained temporarily by positive-pressure support of their respiration. The depth of unresponsiveness associated with this profound degree of brain damage had not been observed before because, previously, all such patients had died immediately from apnea.

The first careful descriptions of patients on ventilators who had undergone functional destruction of the brain were reported by French neurologists, neurosurgeons, and neurophysiologists. Mollaret and Goulon coined the term le coma dépassé (a state beyond coma, irretrievable coma) to acknowledge that the constellation of utter unresponsiveness, deep tendon areflexia, cranial nerve areflexia, apnea, and absent electroencephalographic activity was unprecedented in the annals of coma observation. Although initially they did not conclusively assert that such patients were dead, they did believe that le coma dépassé was qualitatively unlike any form of coma previously reported.[4]

A number of isolated case reports and commentaries were published over the next decade that further consolidated the clinical features of the state that came to be called brain death. Most patients reached this tragic state because they were resuscitated and ventilated following severe head trauma, hypoxic-ischemic brain damage from cardiac arrest or asphyxia, or massive stroke. With aggressive ventilatory and other intensive support, physicians could sustain cardiac activity for several days or, more rarely, weeks. But were such patients alive or dead?

In a landmark paper published in 1968, an ad hoc committee of Harvard Medical School faculty, including ten physicians, a theologian, a lawyer, and a historian of science, first formulated criteria to assert that patients with irreversible apnea, areflexia, and complete unresponsiveness from devastating brain damage were legally dead.[5] Analyses of the writings of the committee chairman, Henry K. Beecher, suggest that the committee was motivated by a desire to permit withdrawal of treatment in hopeless cases and to facilitate organ transplantation. Despite the misleading title of their report, the committee stated that their "primary purpose [was] to define irreversible coma as a new criterion of death."[6]

Over the succeeding two decades, numerous investigators and commentators added refinements to the concepts and tests proposed by the Harvard Ad Hoc Committee, which further consolidated the clinical findings in brain death and the philosophical basis for regarding brain dead patients as dead.[7] The attraction of the brain death concept was so strong that only two years after the Harvard report, the state of Kansas enacted the first statute of death incorporating the new concept of brain death, even before it received a rigorous biophilosophical justification.[8] In 1981, the President's Commission for the Study of Ethical Problems in Medicine and Biomedical and Behavioral Research chose Defining Death as the topic of their first book. The President's Commission strongly endorsed both the concept of brain death and the desirability of adopting uniform statutes of death among jurisdictions.[9] They cited the analysis of death authored by my Dartmouth colleagues, Bernard Gert and Charles Culver, and me [10] as the rigorous philosophical justification that brain death was the equivalent of human death.[11] A contemporaneous report by the Law Reform Commission of Canada also reached the conclusions that brain death was a valid concept and should be uniformly incorporated into law.[12]

By the turn of the 21st century, the practice of declaring brain death had become so well-accepted throughout the developed world and much of the developing world that only a minority of scholars continued to regard it as a philosophical or ethical controversy. The worldwide acceptance of brain death continues to grow: it is practiced in over 80 countries at present, and even countries such as Denmark, Japan, and Saudi Arabia that previously had questioned or rejected brain death now accept it.[13]

PHILOSOPHICAL BASIS FOR REGARDING BRAIN DEATH AS DEATH

Until the past generation, philosophical discussions of death concerned metaphysical rather than biological considerations. Prior to the advent of positive-pressure ventilators, death was a biologically unitary phenomenon: when one organ system critical to life failed irreversibly, other organ system failures followed rapidly and unequivocal death occurred within minutes. Patients who stopped breathing quickly lost heartbeat and blood pressure. Hypoxic-ischemic destruction of the brain and other organs followed with subsequent rigor mortis, putrefaction, and dissolution of the organism. A similar chain of events could be triggered by loss of heartbeat. One did not have to consider whether an organism that had lost certain vital functions while retaining others was alive or dead because such an occurrence was technically impossible.

With the development of the positive-pressure mechanical ventilator and characterization of *le coma dépassé*, the life status of the "brain-dead" patient became ambiguous. Brain-dead patients possess certain characteristics previously associated with life: they are warm, have spontaneous heartbeat and systemic circulation, produce urine, and absorb and metabolize administered food. Yet they also possess certain characteristics previously associated with death: they are utterly unresponsive to even the most noxious stimuli, are apneic, make no spontaneous movements, and have few internal mechanisms of physiologic homeostasis. Are such patients alive or dead?

The new ambiguity in death determination was a technological artifact. Technology had produced an example showing us that our previous understanding of death was ambiguous and incomplete. Now that it was possible for a patient to have lost one set of vital functions (brain functions) while retaining others (circulation, albeit mechanically supported), physicians alone could no longer determine death. Physicians could not develop and apply clinical tests and examination procedures to diagnose death at the bedside because it was unclear what the tests were intended to measure. A concept or definition of death had to be agreed upon before the tests to measure it could be formulated and used.

A rigorous philosophical analysis of death should be conducted in four sequential phases that proceed from the conceptual and intangible to the measurable and tangible.[14] First, scholars must formulate the *paradigm* of death by agreeing on the nature and boundaries of the topic to be discussed. Second, philosophers must propose a concept or *definition* of death. The task is to analyze our intuitions, attitudes, and practices of death determination, and from these, distill the essence of the ordinary meaning of the word "death" that has been rendered ambiguous by technology. In short, this is the philosophical task of making explicit the traditional implicit concept of death that we all hold. The third task is the philosophical and medical task of identifying the *criterion* of death. The criterion of death is the general, measurable standard of death that shows the definition has been fulfilled by being both a necessary and sufficient condition for death. The criterion can be used in a statutory or operational definition of death. Finally, physicians have the medical task of developing and validating a battery of *bedside tests, operations, and procedures* to show conclusively that the criterion has been satisfied.[15] With a few exceptions, most scholars in this area have accepted our method of analysis, if not our conclusions.[16]

The Paradigm of Death

A prerequisite for any rigorous analysis of death is to agree on the paradigm of death: a set of assumptions and conditions about the nature of death that frame the argument by making explicit the nature and boundaries of the topic to be discussed and the class of phenomena to which it belongs.[17] Although not all scholars share these assumptions, it is difficult to imagine achieving consensus on a philosophical analysis of death unless they are accepted because the assumptions in the paradigm frame the argument. Much of the published disagreement on the analysis of death stems from failure to accept the paradigm. For example, the failure to agree with the assumption that death is fundamentally a biological phenomenon creates a paradigm noncongruence that precludes choosing a definition of death. Similarly, the failure to agree that all organisms must be either alive or dead makes it impossible to choose a unitary criterion of death.[18] The paradigm of death has seven assumptions:

1. "Death" is a non-technical word that we use familiarly. The goal of any analysis is to make explicit the implicit consensually accepted meaning of the word "death" that we all understand and use accurately. The goal is not to formulate a new definition of death, to contrive a redefinition of death to further a social, political, philosophical, or medical agenda, or to overanalyze the concept of death to an abstract metaphysical level that is clinically irrelevant.[19]

2. Death, like life, is fundamentally a biological phenomenon. It is a term that we all use correctly to refer to the cessation of the life of a formerly living organism. We all know that the practices surrounding dying, death determination, burial, and mourning have rich and profound social, cultural, anthropological, legal, religious, and historical aspects. I disagree with scholars who hold that death is fundamentally a social determination that can be contrived.[20] As a biological phenomenon, death is not arbitrarily determined by society but is an independent and immutable physical point terminating the life of an organism. The paradigm thus considers the ontology of death, not its normative aspects.

3. The concept of death is univocal among higher animal species. We refer to the same concept when we say our dog died as we do when we say our grandfather died. A concept of death should not be delineated uniquely to *Homo sapiens*. Further, in this context, we restrict our purview to the death of the human organism, not the death of a human cell, tissue, or organ. Determining the death of organ subsystems is a valid biophilosophical task but is not the task at hand here.

4. "Death" is a term that can be applied directly and categorically only to living organisms. All living organisms must die and only living organisms can die. When we say "a person died," we refer to the death of the formerly living organism that embodied the person. In this sense, it is more accurate to say "a human being died." Personhood can cease but cannot die except metaphorically as in the phrase "the death of a culture." All metaphorical, non-biological uses of "death" mean cessation.

5. Death is irreversible. It is impossible to return from being dead. Irreversibility is not merely a limitation of current technology; it is an intrinsic and inescapable element of the definition of death. The term "clinically dead" simply shows the limited contribution that observation can make to the diagnosis. Patients recovering after resuscitation from cardiac arrest have recovered from dying, not from death. Similarly, patients later describing so-called "near-death" experiences may have returned from incipient dying but not from being dead.[21]

6. Death is an event and not a process. Alive or dead are the only two possible underlying states of a higher organism. The two states can be mapped as mutually exclusive (non-overlapping) and jointly exhaustive (no other) sets.[22] All higher organisms must be either alive or dead; they cannot be neither or both. Conversely, dying and bodily disintegration are processes that happen to organisms: dying while the organism is alive, and disintegration after the organism is dead. Death is best viewed as

the event that separates the processes of dying and disintegration. Death must be an event: the transition from the bodily state of alive to that of dead is inherently discontinuous and sudden because there is no intervening state.[23] The timing of the event of death may not be determinable at an exact moment or may be known only in retrospect.

7. Physicians should be able to determine death with a high degree of reproducibility and accuracy, at least in retrospect, using relatively simple bedside tests. The tests for death should be delineated and validated to eliminate the possibility of false-positive determinations.

Unacceptable Definitions of Death

The definition and criterion of death have been the subject of religious and secular debate for centuries. In certain religious writings, death is singularly characterized by the departure of the soul from the body. This definition is unsatisfactory for medical purposes because it does not generate a measurable criterion. Moreover, secularists and religious persons agree that although the loss of the soul represents a belief about what happens at the time of death, losing the soul is not the implicit meaning of the concept of death and is not what we mean to communicate by the word "death."

Some conservative secular clinicians, in times past, have advocated a definition of death as the physical dissolution of the body. They argued that only by awaiting the irreversible changes of rigor mortis or putrefaction could physicians be certain that death had occurred. The social undesirability and utter impracticality of a criterion based on this definition are obvious.[24]

A more plausible but still conservative definition of death is the irreversible loss of all functions of bodily cells. However, because it is generally accepted that hair and nails continue to grow for several days following the customary determination of death, a criterion from this definition would produce too many false-negative declarations of death to be useful clinically.

The Whole Brain Definition and Criterion

The whole brain formulation of death was advocated by the Harvard Ad Hoc Committee, the President's Commission, the Law Reform Commission of Canada, Julius Korein, and in a series of papers, by me and my colleagues Charles Culver and Bernard Gert.[25] It is the legal formulation accepted throughout the United States, all Canadian provinces, and in most countries accepting brain death. The tests for brain death determination throughout the world are based on the whole brain formulation.

We defined death as the permanent cessation of the critical functions of the organism as a whole. In this formulation, by "organism as a whole" we refer not to the whole organism (the sum of the parts of the organism) but rather to the set of functions of integration, control, and behavior that provide the unity of the organism and are greater than the sum of the organism's parts. Critical functions of the organism as a whole subsume the coordination and integration of organ subsystems, the generation of vital functions, and the set of physiologic homeostatic mechanisms that permit the organism to survive and thrive in a dangerous environment, by responding to internal and external stimuli in such a way as to favor its continued health.[26]

The concept of the organism as a whole was formulated in 1916 by the biologist Jacques Loeb.[27] Loeb pointed out that organisms possess hierarchies of functions that integrate bodily subsystems and that through their interrelatedness create the unity of the organism. Modern biophilosophers use the term emergent functions to capture this phenomenon with greater conceptual clarity. An emergent function is a property of a whole that is not possessed by any of its component parts and cannot be reduced to one or more of its component parts.[28] The organism's emergent functions, such as human consciousness, arise from the interrelatedness of the components but cannot be found in any single component.

More specifically, critical functions of the organism as a whole include: (1) vital functions of spontaneous breathing and the autonomic control of circulation; (2) integrating functions that assure the homeostasis of the organism, such as appropriate physiologic responses to baroreceptors and chemoreceptors, neuroendocrine feedback loops, and temperature control; and (3) consciousness which is required for the organism to respond to its needs for hydration, nutrition, and protection, among others.

The organism as a whole may continue to function despite loss of some parts of the organism, such as a limb or a kidney, and despite replacement of some parts or functions, such as by hemodialysis or the insertion of a prosthetic joint. But once the organism as a whole is lost permanently, the organism is dead because its unity is gone forever, despite the continued functioning of some of its subsystems. In this instance, the mechanically supported, independent, uncoordinated, and directionless continued functioning of certain organ subsystems is meaningless because the organism as a whole no longer is present. This state is conceptually analogous to the continued growth of a person's cultured epithelial cells in a flask after the person has died.[29]

The criterion of death showing that the organism-as-a-whole definition is fulfilled is the permanent cessation of clinical functioning of the whole brain. The "whole brain" refers to the cerebral hemispheres, diencephalon, cerebellum, and brain stem. All regions of the brain are required to serve the critical functions of the organism as a whole. The cerebral hemispheres are necessary for awareness, food-seeking, memory, planning, and avoiding danger. The diencephalon is necessary for regulation of temperature, fluid and electrolytes; neuroendocrine and autonomic function; processing of all sensory input; and memory. The brain stem is necessary for wakefulness, breathing, blood pressure control, all motor output, and nearly all sensory input.

"Clinical functions" are those functions that clinicians can assess by bedside physical examination. Clinical functions do not include instrumentally measured functions of nests of neurons that may have survived the illness or injury producing brain death. After brain death, some residual hemispheric neuronal activity can be measured by electroencephalography, some

hypothalamic neuroendocrine activity of cells producing antidiuretic hormone can be assayed, and a small amount of cortical neuronal metabolism can be measured by positron emission tomography.[30] In these instances, isolated nests of neurons have survived the global insult and continue to function independently. But because the neurological examination reveals an absence of clinical functions, these small, independent, multifocal areas of functioning cells do not contribute materially to the organism's clinical functions and thus do not count as evidence of functioning of the organism as a whole.

The whole brain formulation contains a fail-safe mechanism not present in other brain formulations. Following the primary insult producing brain death (traumatic brain injury, intracranial hemorrhage, hypoxic-ischemic neuronal damage during cardiac arrest or anoxia are the most common causes),[31] diffuse brain swelling produces markedly elevated intracranial pressure (ICP). When ICP exceeds mean arterial blood pressure, no intracranial blood flow can occur and the neurons not killed by the primary insult are destroyed secondarily by ischemic infarction.

The whole brain formulation is not a new definition of death but simply makes explicit the implicit traditional definition of death. The clinical examination for death throughout history has required searching for evidence of responsiveness, pupillary reaction to light, breathing, and heartbeat. The first three tests, taken together, directly measure whole brain functioning. Only the detection of heartbeat is not a direct sign. But since heartbeat stops within minutes of cessation of respiration, and since respiration is generated by the brain, all traditional clinical bedside tests for death have assessed whole brain functioning.

The Higher Brain Formulation

The higher brain formulation[32] has provided a popular alternative definition and criterion of death since its introduction in 1975 by Robert Veatch and its later conceptual consolidation by Michael Green and Daniel Wikler, Stuart Youngner and Edward Bartlett, and others.[33] The higher brain formulation holds that death is best defined as the permanent loss of that which is essential to the nature of man. This definition produces the "neocortical death" criterion, in which only the functions of the neocortex must be permanently lost for death because their loss eliminates the "experiential and social integrating function [that] is the essential element in the nature of man, the loss of which is to be called death."[34] Veatch rejected the idea that death is related to an organism's "loss of the capacity to integrate bodily function" claiming that "man is, after all, more than a sophisticated computer."[35] By a strict application of this criterion, anencephalic infants and patients in a persistent vegetative state, both tragic clinical disorders featuring continued functioning of the brain stem but severely depressed or absent functioning of the cortex, would be classified as dead.

The conceptual basis of the higher brain formulation rests on the premise that consciousness and cognition are the essential characteristics of the life of the human organism, and their permanent absence is death. According to this account, it is the cerebral cortex, not the brain stem or other lower centers, that serves awareness, thinking, ability to experience, memory, and personal identity. The brain stem centers serve only integrative and coordinating functions that conceivably could be replaced with a machine.[36] Thus, according to the higher brain formulation, the continued functioning of the brain stem and diencephalon are irrelevant to the determination of death.

The higher brain formulation has intuitive and practical attractions. From a practical perspective, it instantly solves the vexing problem of the disposition of patients in a persistent vegetative state (PVS); they are dead. It also instantly solves the dilemma of whether anencephalic infants can be used as multi-organ donors (discussed below); they can. The intuitive attraction is that almost nobody would wish to continue living in a PVS. Because of the tragic, meaningless, unconscious existence of patients in a PVS, some people consider them "as good as dead." Indeed there are compelling reasons to allow PVS patients to die by withdrawing life-sustaining treatment, if

that was their treatment preference, as discussed in chapter 12.

However, there are serious and inescapable conceptual and practical flaws in accepting the higher brain formulation as a definition and criterion of death. First, unlike the whole brain formulation that attempts to make explicit the implicit traditional definition of death, the higher brain formulation represents a clear example of redefining death. At no point in history and in no society or culture have spontaneously breathing persons been declared dead. Severely brain-damaged or otherwise moribund persons may have been allowed to die in many cultures, but in none were they diagnosed as dead while still breathing.

The non-univocality of death is another definitional problem. Because death is a purely biological phenomenon and not an arbitrarily defined conceptual entity, it should be univocal across species of higher animals and should not be delineated idiosyncratically for *Homo sapiens*.

The neocortical criterion of death has a slippery slope problem: what is the necessary number of cortical neurons that must cease to function permanently for brain death? Patients in PVS comprise a broad spectrum featuring varying degrees of brain damage, ranging from focal states of cortical laminar or pseudolaminar necrosis to global "neocortical death" with absent EEG activity.[37] In all cases, consciousness and cognition are absent. Are all such patients dead? What about those nearly vegetative patients with advanced dementia who have lost their personality, memory, language, and continence? Surely they too have lost "that which is significant to the nature of man."

Veatch observed that a similar slippery slope problem exists for whole brain death.[38] The critical difference is that for whole brain death, the slippery slope problem produces no practical complications because it does not alter the bedside determination of death. The opposite is the case for the slippery slope problem produced by the higher brain formulation. Prognosticating with confidence that the PVS patient will not recover awareness usually cannot be accomplished on the basis of a few examinations. Prognostication for the patient in PVS following an hypoxic-ischemic injury often requires several weeks of careful observation and examination.[39] It is counterintuitive to the concept of death to argue that a physician must examine a patient for several weeks to determine if he is dead.

A practical problem arises in burial of the vegetative patient. Such patients have spontaneous respiration, heartbeat, and airway protective reflexes, such as gag and cough. Should they be buried or cremated with these functions intact or should they be given a lethal injection to abolish them? In the latter situation, why should such an injection be necessary if they are really dead? Our revulsion toward burying breathing, heart beating PVS patients results from the fact that, at an intuitive level, despite their profound neurological impairment and our belief that, in some ways, they may be "as good as dead," we recognize that they are alive.

Some supporters of the higher brain formulation have suggested that because the brain stem functions primarily to regulate the body's physiologic systems, it could be replaced with a machine. This argument was intended to demote the importance of the brain stem in cognitive processing.[40] These authors, however, have misunderstood the critical importance of the brain stem in generating consciousness. The brain stem ascending reticular activating system that projects to the cerebral hemispheres is an indispensable anatomic substrate for wakefulness, which is a prerequisite for awareness, cognition, and memory. This system, therefore, could not be replaced mechanically without invoking the same advanced science fiction required to imagine that the cerebral cortex could be replaced by a computer.[41]

The rightful use of the higher brain formulation is to determine the loss of personhood, not death. Personhood is a psychosocial, spiritual, and legal concept characterized by uniquely human characteristics and capacities,[42] in contrast to life, which is a biological phenomenon. Living organisms can die but personhood cannot die, except metaphorically. Personhood can be lost, which is what happens to the higher brain patient. Loss of personhood may be adequate grounds for individuals to refuse further life-sustaining treatment, a subject discussed further in chapter 12, but claiming that loss of personhood is death represents a radical redefinition of death. It has been accepted nowhere outside the academy.

The Brain Stem Formulation

Brain death, as determined in the United Kingdom, requires the permanent cessation of only brain stem functioning, a formulation referred to as "brain stem death."[43] This conceptualization and its acceptance in the United Kingdom were largely the result of the work of Christopher Pallis.[44] Pallis accepted that death was defined as the cessation of functioning of the organism as a whole. He believed the best criterion for this definition was irreversible cessation of brain stem functioning. He observed correctly that most of the bedside tests for brain death, such as pupillary light/dark reflexes, other cranial nerve reflexes, and tests for apnea, directly measured functions of the brain stem. This is true primarily because the clinical functions served by many areas of the brain, including the frontal, parietal, temporal, and occipital lobes, thalamus, hypothalamus, and basal ganglia cannot be tested accurately in a comatose subject. The crux of Pallis's argument was that the brain stem contains and controls the *capacities* for consciousness and respiration, and acts as a through-station for all motor output from the hemispheres and all sensory input to the hemispheres except vision and olfaction.

The brain stem formulation is attractive but contains one serious conceptual flaw and one practical shortcoming. By not requiring cessation of hemispheric cortical function, there exists the possibility of a state in which a patient remains conscious despite having lost all clinical evidence for other brain stem functioning. Such a completely locked-in syndrome could be diagnosed only by EEG or cortical metabolic rate measurements. Despite its great improbability, even the theoretical possibility of such a state favors use of the whole brain formulation. The brain stem formulation also has a practical problem. In those instances in which confirmatory tests for brain death are desirable, using EEG or measurements of intracranial blood flow or cortical neuronal metabolic rates, these tests would show hemispheric activity and thus be useless to confirm "brain stem death."

In a whimsical moment, Pallis also considered the possibility of such a case. He wrote the following limerick that he remarked could have been penned by one of the *tricoteuses* (knitters) who sat by the guillotine in Paris in 1793 during the French Revolution, as memorably exemplified by Charles Dickens's Madame Defarge in *The Tale of Two Cities*:

> *We knit on, too blasées to ask it:*
> *"Could the tetraparesis just mask it?*
> *When the brain stem is dead*
> *Can the cortex be said*
> *To tick on, in the head, in the basket?"*[45]

Brain stem death is quite similar to whole brain death in that both share the same definition but differ somewhat in their criterion. In the future, the criterion of whole brain death will likely move more in the direction of brain stem death. Future technologic advances in the laboratory assessment of focal neuronal functioning, using such techniques as positron emission tomography (PET), single photon emission computed tomography (SPECT), functional magnetic resonance imaging (fMRI), quantitative electroencephalography (QEEG), and magnetoencephalography (MEG) will permit the identification and location of those brain neurons that are critical to the functioning of the organism as a whole. It will be only this set of neurons and their connections whose function must irreversibly cease for brain death to be determined. Laboratory criteria, no matter how sophisticated, can only complement clinical criteria and not replace them.

The Circulation Formulation

The traditional tests for death assess the permanent absence of breathing and circulation. These tests continue to be useful to diagnose death in the large majority of deaths uncomplicated by mechanical ventilation because apnea and circulatory arrest quickly produce destruction of the brain. One group of theorists rejects the concept of brain death entirely and holds that death is the permanent cessation of systemic blood circulation. Patients declared brain dead by the accepted tests are not dead according to the circulation formulation, because they have persistent heartbeat and circulation. At present, this formulation has gained acceptance among some conservative Catholic scholars and a few physicians and philosophers.[46] Over the past decade, the circulation formulation has achieved greater popularity as a result of the publications of Alan Shewmon, its most rigorous and eloquent advocate (see below).[47]

TESTS FOR BRAIN DEATH

The next task is for physicians to devise sets of tests and procedures to show that the criterion of death has been satisfied. Most patients who die are not mechanically ventilated prior to death. In such instances, "cardiopulmonary" tests that show the permanent absence of breathing and circulation are sufficient. Brain death tests are necessary only for the patient receiving mechanical ventilation.

Numerous sets of brain death tests have been studied since the 1968 Harvard Ad Hoc Committee Report, but those proposed by the 1981 President's Commission medical consultants have achieved the widest acceptance.[48] In 1995, these tests were subjected to an evidence-based analysis by Eelco Wijdicks, which culminated in a practice guideline published that year by the American Academy of Neurology.[49] The tests were delineated in such a way as to eliminate the possibility of false-positive determinations, even though doing so generated the probability of some false-negative determinations. The tests have been validated thoroughly. There has never been an established case in which a patient fulfilled properly performed and interpreted tests for brain death and recovered at all. This validation is in ironic contrast to the occasional instance in which a physician incorrectly diagnoses death using cardiopulmonary tests.

The test batteries in use today are essentially identical, requiring a demonstration that all clinical brain functions are absent and that the loss of functions results from an irreversible structural lesion, and not from a potentially reversible metabolic or toxic condition.[50] In practice, these goals are accomplished by performing a bedside examination showing utter unresponsiveness to noxious and all other stimuli, true apnea (tested correctly), and the absence of all reflexes served by the brain stem and cranial nerves, such as pupillary, corneal, gag, cough, and vestibulo-ocular reflexes. Deep tendon reflexes and other reflexes mediated by the spinal cord may persist. Any possible contribution to absent brain functions resulting from metabolic and toxic disorders must be excluded, such as depressant drug intoxication, the use of a neuromuscular junction blocking agent, hypothermia, and shock.

The absence of clinical brain functions must persist for a predetermined time, after which a second examination is performed to demonstrate the continued absence of clinical brain functions. It is presumed that clinical brain functions were absent throughout the interval between examinations. The necessary duration of the interval between serial examinations varies as a function of the age of the patient, the disorder producing brain death, and the use of confirmatory laboratory tests. In general, the interval is longer in younger patients and in those whose disorders were produced by hypoxic-ischemic damage. The specific methods and procedures of the bedside tests and of the laboratory confirmatory tests for brain death are beyond the scope of this chapter, but are available in standard texts.[51]

The moment of death is the time at which the patient fulfills the second set of brain death tests. Until that time, the patient is considered incipiently brain dead. Although such a practice at first appears arbitrary, declaring death at that time is consistent with the practice of determining death using cardiopulmonary tests. A physician called to the bedside of a hospitalized patient who has been found dead in bed will declare the time of death to be the time he examined the patient and ascertained a prolonged absence of breathing and heartbeat. The patient may have died several hours earlier. The somewhat

arbitrarily delineated moment of death shows that brain death can be determined only in retrospect.[52]

Electrophysiologic and neuroimaging tests for brain death can be performed to expedite and confirm the clinical determination. These tests are useful in several circumstances: (1) to facilitate timely organ procurement; (2) to make the diagnosis when a complete clinical examination cannot be performed; and (3) to assist less experienced examiners in making the diagnosis. An adequate electrophysiologic determination includes EEG, brain stem auditory evoked potentials, and somatosensory evoked potentials, all of which must be absent. It is preferable to perform a study showing the absence of intracranial blood flow because this finding proves the irreversibility of the process.[53] Imaging studies to prove absent intracranial blood flow include radionuclide angiography, transcranial Doppler ultrasonography (TCD), magnetic resonance angiography or perfusion scanning, computed tomographic angiography, and SPECT.[54] Most physicians declaring brain death rely on a confirmatory study. Radionuclide angiography is ordered most commonly but younger physicians prefer TCD.[55] There is evidence that neurosurgeons and critical care physicians conducting brain death determinations rely more on intracranial blood flow tests and neurologists rely more on clinical tests.[56]

BRAIN DEATH IN CHILDREN AND NEONATES

The determination of brain death in young children and neonates differs from that in adults in one critical respect: how thoroughly the bedside tests for brain death have been validated in this age group.[57] The Medical Consultants for the Diagnosis of Death of the President's Commission cautioned that the tests for brain death had not been validated sufficiently in children under five years of age.[58] Subsequently, the Task Force for the Determination of Brain Death in Children was impaneled from representatives of the American Academy of Neurology, the American Neurological Association, and the American

Academy of Pediatrics to study the available data on brain death in children and neonates and make recommendations for physicians.

Their 1987 report *Guidelines for the Determination of Brain Death in Children* permitted brain death declaration in any full-term infant over the age of one week. Children over the age of one year were treated exactly the same as adults. Children from two months to one year must have a confirmatory test such as electroencephalogram or radionuclide intracranial blood flow study in addition to fulfilling the clinical tests showing absence of all clinical brain functions for an interval of 24 hours. Infants from one week to two months must fulfill the same clinical and confirmatory test criteria over an interval of 48 hours.[59]

The *Guidelines* generally were accepted by neurologists and pediatricians, except for those that pertained to determining brain death in infants under the age of two months. Joseph Volpe pointed out the practical limitations of attempting to determine brain death in neonates. Most neonates with this degree of brain damage have suffered perinatal injuries, especially diffuse hypoxic-ischemic insults. Often, there is not sufficiently accurate historical information about the duration and severity of this insult to confidently predict irreversibility. Second, the role of hypotension cannot be fully appreciated. Third, brain imaging techniques cannot accurately quantify the extent of brain damage. Thus, the essential criteria of irreversibility and totality of functional loss often cannot be met.[60]

Alan Shewmon pointed out that the false-positive error rate in neonatal brain death determination is no less than 0.02. He showed that even with more recorded experience, this error rate will not fall significantly. This problem, he argued, results from reliance for the declaration of brain death on tests of brain function rather than on tests of brain structure. Shewmon believes that neonatologists should rely only on unequivocal evidence of structural, irreversible brain damage, such as completed rostrocaudal, transtentorial brain herniation.[61]

From a practical perspective, the principal indication for formal brain death determination in a neonate or young infant is to permit the brain-dead infant to serve as an organ donor. The determination of brain death never has been a prerequisite for termination of medical treatment in the setting of hopeless brain damage. (See discussions on withholding and withdrawing life-sustaining treatment in chapters 8, 12, and 13.) Reports of the experience of conducting brain death determination in pediatric and neonatal intensive care units show results similar to those in adult ICUs,[62] unfortunately, including the same disappointingly high degree of noncompliance by physicians in using established test batteries.[63] Recent experiences have been published describing the challenging medical and ethical issues involved in pronouncing brain death in children.[64]

THE STATUTORY DEFINITION OF DEATH

The final task is to draft a statute of death recognizing the irreversible cessation of brain functioning as the legal criterion of death. Statutory recognition of brain death is desirable because it both acknowledges biological reality and provides physicians the authority to determine death when patients are receiving ventilatory support. Since 1970, when Kansas became the first state to incorporate brain death in a statutory definition of death, all other states in the United States have enacted statutes of death incorporating brain death, except New York, which issued an administrative regulation legalizing brain death.[65] By the turn of the 21st century, nearly all Western and developed countries had enacted brain death laws and many other countries also had done so.[66]

An ideal statute of death should accurately recapitulate the whole brain concept of death and offer practical guidance to physicians regarding when the brain death tests should be employed and when the cardiopulmonary tests are sufficient. An ideal statute first should state the criterion of death as the permanent cessation of the clinical functions of the brain. Then it should make clear that death can be determined in one of two ways: in the patient without mechanical ventilation, by showing the permanent cessation of respiration and circulation; and in the patient with mechanical ventilation, by the permanent absence of clinical functions of the brain.

In 1972, Alexander Capron and Leon Kass designed a model death statute incorporating brain death, which they revised in 1978.[67] This statute created two equal criteria of death instead of explaining that death had a single criterion but could be determined in two ways. In 1975, the American Bar Association created another model death statute with a correct single brain criterion that failed to clarify that most determinations of death rely on permanent cessation of respiration and circulation.[68]

By far, the most influential American model death statute was published in 1981 by the President's Commission in their work *Defining Death*. Their model statute, the Uniform Determination of Death Act (UDDA), was proposed for adoption by all American jurisdictions. With the assistance of the National Conference of Commissioners of Uniform State Laws, the UDDA eventually was adopted by about half of states in the United States as their statute of death and most of the others adopted a variation of it. The UDDA provides:

> An individual who has sustained either (1) irreversible cessation of circulatory and respiratory functions, or (2) irreversible cessation of all functions of the entire brain, including the brain stem, is dead.
> A determination of death must be made in accordance with accepted medical standards.[69]

In 1981, Charles Culver, Bernard Gert, and I drafted a model statute clarifying the criterion and tests of death, which we modified in 1982 to incorporate language compatible with the UDDA.[70] We criticized the UDDA as incorrectly elevating the tests of death into criteria of death rather than maintaining a single whole brain criterion with two tests. Our model statute provides:

> An individual who has sustained irreversible cessation of all functions of the entire brain, including the brain stem, is dead. In the absence of artificial means of cardiopulmonary support, death may be determined by the prolonged absence of spontaneous circulatory and respiratory functions. In the presence of artificial means of cardiopulmonary support, death must be determined by tests of brain function. In both situations, the determination of death must be made in accordance with accepted medical standards.

Our statute has the advantage of conceptual clarity and practical utility. It clarifies that irreversible cessation of brain functioning is the sole criterion of death, but that the criterion can be determined by two separate tests, depending upon the clinical circumstances. Although this statute represents an improvement over the UDDA, states choosing a brain death statute in the future probably should select the UDDA. At this point, the UDDA's practical advantage of obtaining uniformity in statutory language among states probably outweighs our statute's abstract advantage of greater conceptual clarity.

OPPOSITION TO BRAIN DEATH

A group of scholars has opposed the concept of brain death since it was first introduced in the 1960s.[71] I discussed the opposition to the whole brain criterion by the advocates of the higher brain formulation. Despite Robert Veatch's exaggerated claims that the concept of whole brain death is in "impending collapse" or is "dead" itself,[72] after over three decades of writings, the higher brain theorists have failed to convince any medical societies in the world to change their criterion of death or any jurisdictions to convert their brain death laws from the whole brain to the higher brain formulation.

During the 1990s, a new group of opponents emerged to refute not simply the whole brain criterion but the entire concept of brain death. The current opponents argue three positions: (1) brain death is philosophically incoherent as a concept of human death; (2) brain death is a legal fiction that once may have been justified but now no longer serves a useful social purpose; and (3) brain death is incompatible with the belief systems of Christianity and Judaism.

Conceptual Confusion and Legal Fiction

Several scholars have pointed out inconsistencies in the whole brain formulation. Robert Veatch argued that the principal claim made by whole brain advocates was false, namely that *all* functions of the entire brain were absent, because some brain dead patients retained rudimentary EEG activity and secretion of antidiuretic hormone.[73] This theme was echoed by Baruch Brody and Amir Halevy in a similar critique.[74] These scholars cited the UDDA, the model death statute proposed by the President's Commission codifying the whole brain formulation, which states in part: "an individual who has sustained ... irreversible cessation of all functions of the entire brain, including the brain stem, is dead."[75]

Notwithstanding the sweeping language of the UDDA, the discussion in the President's Commission report providing the context for the proposed statute made it clear that the term "functions" applied only to clinical functions, as I have defined them, not to laboratory-measured cellular physiologic activities. Thus, the whole brain formulation stipulated in the UDDA remains compatible with any degree of preserved neuronal activity that does not contribute to a clinical function.

Robert Truog argued that brain death is an anachronism that should be abandoned.[76] He pointed out that when the brain death concept was formulated in the 1960s, there was no acceptable professional standard permitting the discontinuation of ventilators and other forms of life-sustaining therapy on hopelessly ill patients with massive brain damage. By declaring these patients dead, physicians could legally discontinue life-sustaining measures. But now that legal standards permit withholding and withdrawing life-sustaining therapy, we no longer need to rely on determining brain death. The only remaining use of brain death is to permit unpaired vital organ donation. Truog then suggested that vital organ donation could be accomplished through means other than by declaring the donor dead, such as by relying on patient or family consent in a hopelessly ill, dying patient who is "beyond harm."

In a similar vein, Robert Taylor argued that brain death represents a "legal fiction" that is no longer necessary in contemporary society.[77] He pointed out that the concept of brain death is analogous to the legal fiction of "legal blindness." We all know that many patients determined to be legally blind in fact retain some vision. But their visual loss is so severe that for legal purposes it is functionally equivalent to blindness. The concept of legal blindness is a useful fiction created by law that permits these patients to receive the same societal benefits that had been reserved for the utterly blind. Similarly, he argued, we all know that brain dead patients are not truly dead but only hopelessly and incipiently dying. We simply employ the convenient legal fiction of "brain death" to permit uncontested termination of life-sustaining treatment and to facilitate multi-organ procurement.

It is certainly true that brain death no longer is a necessary condition for discontinuing life-sustaining treatment and that its major utilitarian benefit is to permit unpaired vital organ transplantation and uncontested termination of life-sustaining treatment. However, the fact that it may be useful today in these ways does not necessarily alter the coherence of whole brain death as a concept of death. In contrast to these criticisms, Alan Shewmon's claim that brain death is conceptually incoherent represents a more serious challenge.

Spinal Integration and Chronic Cases

In a series of articles over the past decade, Alan Shewmon waged a penetrating attack on the brain death concept.[78] These articles are particularly fascinating because, prior to 1994, Shewmon was one of the strongest proponents of brain death.[79] Like Robert Taylor and the philosopher Josef Siefert,[80] Shewmon now holds that the human is not dead until circulation ceases irreversibly. In the circulation formulation that he proposes, the brain is simply one organ among many and enjoys no special significance in death determination.

Shewmon cites two lines of data to support his contention. First, he criticizes the whole brain concept's reliance on the brain's unique capacity to integrate, regulate, and maintain homeostasis. He points out that other structures in the body, especially the spinal cord, perform integrating functions, and that therefore it is arbitrary to impart a unique value to those particular integrating and regulating functions performed by the brain.[81] Thus, even accepting death as the permanent cessation of the critical functions of the organism as a whole, he argues that loss of whole brain function does not necessarily achieve this standard.

Shewmon's second line of argument features cases he termed "chronic brain death." He reported a series of patients who were declared brain dead but who had respiration and other functions supported technologically for prolonged periods: several months in a number of cases and, in one extraordinary case, for 16 years.[82] A few of these patients were pregnant women who were physiologically maintained for several months to permit live birth of viable neonates by Cesarean delivery. Shewmon argued that it is counterintuitive to the concept of death to consider that dead people could do what those patients have done: gestate infants, grow and experience puberty (as in the case of the child maintained for 16 years), or have circulation and other organ functions maintained for prolonged periods. Jeffrey Spike and Jane Greenlaw similarly discussed a brain dead patient maintained for many months in a state they called "persistent brain death."[83]

In response to the integration-regulation criticism, Eelco Wijdicks and I pointed out that these capacities of the brain are not the sole evidence of functions of the organism as a whole: the vital functions of respiration and circulation as well as consciousness are critical functions. In response to the chronic cases, we first respectfully question whether all the patients Shewmon cited were unequivocally brain dead. Some of the cases were not reported in sufficient detail to be certain that they had undergone proper tests for apnea, for example. Granted, however, that at least some of these patients were unequivocally brain dead, we view the existence of the "chronic" cases as rare outliers. They show evidence that our intensive care technology now occasionally succeeds in producing instances of physiological support of heroic proportions.

But we do not conclude that the existence of these cases necessarily must change our concept of death.[84]

I concede that the doctrine of whole brain death remains imperfect and that my attempts and those of others to respond to its shortcomings noted by critics remain inadequate. Yet, its conceptual soundness, intuitive appeal, universal acceptance by medical societies and lawmakers, and widespread societal acceptance mean that it is coherent biologically and has succeeded as public policy.[85]

RELIGIOUS ATTITUDES ABOUT BRAIN DEATH

The major Western religions generally have accepted the concept of brain death.[86] Even in the early writings on brain death, most Protestant, Roman Catholic, and Jewish commentators pronounced that the declaration of brain death was compatible with the tenets and ancient texts of their religions.[87] However, some conservative Roman Catholic and Orthodox Jewish scholars hold that the contemporary determination of brain death violates their religious doctrines, as they interpret them.

Acceptance by Christianity

Religious scholars and other authorities in Christianity have stated that brain death is entirely consistent with Christian religious beliefs and traditions. Among Protestants, this acceptance is essentially universal, even among fundamentalist groups.[88] Among Roman Catholics, the acceptance is general but not universal. Over the past two decades, four Vatican Pontifical Councils and Academies charged with studying this issue opined that brain death was consistent with Roman Catholic beliefs and teachings.[89] The Catholic church magisterium first took an official position in August, 2000, when, in an address to the International Congress of the Transplantation Society meeting in Rome, Pope John Paul II formally endorsed brain death as fully consistent with Roman Catholic teachings.[90] In 2007, the Pontifical Academy of Sciences affirmed this position.[91]

There have been a few opponents of brain death who have asserted that the concept of brain death is inconsistent with Roman Catholic, and even Christian, belief systems. Most vocal in this area over the past 30 years has been Paul Byrne.[92] Yet, even before the Pope's pronouncement, it was clear that his opinion was marginalized within Roman Catholic circles. The conservative Roman Catholic bioethics institute, the National Catholic Bioethics Center (formerly called the Pope John Center), held that Byrne was incorrect and that brain death was fully consistent with the teachings of Roman Catholicism.[93] More recently, they concluded that Pope John Paul's endorsement of brain death should quell the disagreement by Byrne and other skeptics on Roman Catholic religious grounds.[94]

As a matter of practice, there is almost never a religious issue raised among any Christians regarding brain death determination. Brain death is determined in Roman Catholic hospitals throughout the world and organ donation is permitted without exception. It seems unlikely that the Vatican will reverse its position permitting brain death determination in the near future.

Acceptance by Judaism

Judaism lacks the Roman Catholic structure of doctrinal authoritarianism: there are no "top-down" rulings on issues of religious doctrine. Rather, individual learned rabbis and other scholars apply traditional Jewish law (Halachah) to contemporary questions, analyzing and discussing biblical and Talmudic writings and ancient rabbinic teachings to formulate positions of Jewish law. The approach of this area of scholarship is somewhat analogous to that of American constitutional law, in which contemporary scholars attempt to divine the intent of the constitutional framers on novel issues. Understandably, this scholarly discourse produces disagreement. There remains an unresolved rabbinic debate on whether brain death is human death according to Jewish law.[95]

Some Orthodox rabbis, such as the rabbi-scientist Moshe Tendler believe that brain death is compatible with Halachic law because it is the physiological equivalent of decapitation. In the 12th century, Maimonides wrote that a decapitated body was immediately dead and that transient muscle twitches observed in the decapitated body were not signs of life. Tendler and the physician-talmudist Fred Rosner cite the Talmudic tract, discussed by Rashi, in which it is stated that breathing, not heartbeat, is the primary sign of life. Using these two citations, Tendler and Rosner conclude that brain death is consistent with Jewish law.[96]

The opposite conclusion was reached by the prominent Orthodox rabbis and Talmudic scholars David Bleich and Ahron Soloveichik.[97] They pointed out that there is a difference between a sign of death and death itself. They explained that ancient rabbis considered the cessation of respiration as the cardinal sign of death because it implied a prior cessation of heartbeat. They concluded that physicians cannot determine death according to Jewish law in the presence of spontaneous heartbeat.

In practice, brain death is accepted by essentially all Reform and Conservative Jews. Orthodox Jews are split between those endorsing the Tendler-Rosner position and those endorsing the Bleich-Soloveichik position. In general, only the strictest Orthodox sects, such as the Chasidim, consistently embrace the latter position. This group represents only a small minority of practicing Jews in Western countries.

Acceptance by Islam

Initially, Islam had not supported the equivalency of brain death and human death. However, the good accruing from organ transplantation generated a reconsideration of this question by Islamic scholars and authorities. The Council of Islamic Jurisprudence Academy resolved, in its third session in Amman, Jordan in 1986, to support the concept of brain death in the kingdom of Saudi Arabia and in other Islamic countries. Consequently, following a fatwah approving brain death determination, the Ullamah Council in Saudi Arabia confirmed the practice of brain death and permitted it in the kingdom of Saudi Arabia.[98] The Saudi tests to determine brain death are essentially identical to those proposed by the

American Academy of Neurology and practiced worldwide. The Sixth International Conference of Islamic Jurists, held in Jeddah, addressed the many of the issues of organ transplantation from brain dead patients.[99]

Acceptance by Other Religions

The question of Hindu acceptance of brain death has been the topic of conferences held in Bombay and Madras. A bill was passed by the Indian legislature in 1993 called the Transplantation of Human Organs Act that contains provisions for determining brain death.[100] There have not been specific pronouncements on brain death, of which I am aware, from Confucianism and other Eastern religions.

The situation in Japan is unique and worthy of note. Over the past generation, the Japanese traditional Shinto and Buddhist concepts of death requiring cessation of heartbeat and breathing have collided with technological attempts to westernize Japanese medicine including the introduction of brain death and organ transplantation.[101] Scholarly works, medical and scientific society advocacy, and public debates over the past two decades have led Japanese society to gradually accept the practices of brain death and multi-organ procurement. The anthropologist Margaret Lock has conducted the most detailed study of the social and cultural processes in Japan leading to the conditional acceptance of brain death and organ donation.[102]

American Death Laws with Religious Provisions

Since Kansas's pioneering brain death statute in 1970, all states have enacted either statutory recognition of brain death or administrative regulations permitting brain death determination. This legal recognition introduced a problem. What if the determination of brain death violated a patient's religious beliefs? Would or should physicians be permitted to determine a patient's death in this way despite this conflict?

In 1991, New Jersey became the first state to include an explicit religious exemption for declaring brain death. Subsequently, the New York state legislature passed administrative regulations containing a similar provision. The relevant part of the New Jersey statute provides: "The death of an individual shall not be declared upon the basis of neurological criteria . . . when such a declaration would violate the personal religious beliefs or moral convictions of that individual and when that fact has been communicated to, or should . . . reasonably be known by, the licensed physician authorized to declare death."[103] Although this law was sponsored by members of the Orthodox Jewish community who rejected brain death as human death, the law applies to any citizen who can show the stipulated criterion. By comparison, the New York administrative regulation requires physicians to "mandate notification of an individual's next of kin" and allow for a "reasonable accommodation to an individual's religious or moral objections to the use of neurologic criteria to diagnose death."[104]

To implement the New Jersey religious exemption, members of the patient's family must approach the responsible physician with evidence of "reason to believe" that the brain death declaration would violate the patient's religious beliefs. The duty falls on family members to assert this right and requires that they have clear knowledge of the patient's religious beliefs. Oral statements are sufficient.[105]

The physician of a brain-dead patient who is faced with a family's religious opposition to brain death determination has a dilemma. Because brain death determination is lawful in most jurisdictions, the physician probably has no legal requirement not to declare brain death. However, should he choose to determine brain death, he has an ethical duty not to act on this determination when it is likely that the family's opposition is based on coherent, valid, and well-established religious grounds, and is not simply an emotional or psychological inability to accept a dire diagnosis and prognosis.[106] Physicians probably should continue to ventilate such patients rather than extubating them despite the fact that they fulfill brain-death tests. But because such patients have a "zero prognosis" for recovery, physicians have no compelling ethical duty to treat them aggressively. Some physicians would maintain ventilation, but reduce vasopressor medication and other support, and await the inevitable asystole in a few hours to days. Other physicians would continue all aggressive treatment out of respect for the family's religious beliefs.

The question of how much diversity in death statute policy a society can tolerate has been the subject of several essays.[107] A few libertarian scholars believe that patients should be given the choice to decide which of several different criteria of death applies to them when their own death is determined.[108] For example, if a person subscribed to the higher brain formulation of death, she would be declared dead if she were in a persistent vegetative state. I believe that if such a free choice-driven concept were legislated it would create legal and medical chaos. It seems more coherent to design death statutes that stipulate justified exceptions.

FAMILY OPPOSITION TO BRAIN DEATH

The emotional or psychological inability to accept the hopeless diagnosis and prognosis of the brain dead patient is a more common reason than a religious conviction for families to request continuation of ventilator treatment. For some families, it is counterintuitive to accept that their loved one is dead given the patients' obvious signs of life, such as heartbeat, warm skin, and urine production. Family members' desperate hope for recovery often is a barrier to their acceptance of the finality of the diagnosis. Physicians and nurses may compound the problem by conveying internally contradictory messages to families by referring to the ventilator as a "life-support system" or to endotracheal extubation as "allowing them to die." In these instances a conflict may arise between the physician and family about the necessity to continue ventilatory and other means of aggressive physiologic support.[109]

If one accepts that brain death is human death determined by an alternative method, one could make a strong argument that families have no more right to interfere in the physician's bedside determination of death by brain tests than by circulatory tests. By this account, physicians declaring brain death have no duty to seek permission from families or even to inform them of the plan to extubate the patient after brain death declaration. Two state courts held that physicians were permitted to ignore a family's desire to maintain their loved one on a ventilator once brain death was determined.[110]

Physicians have several ethical responsibilities in this situation. First, they have a duty to communicate effectively with the patient's family. They should carefully explain the concept, practice, and legality of brain death determination, stressing particularly that the patient is not simply in coma, but that the patient is biologically and legally dead and *cannot* recover. Both physicians and nurses should carefully avoid using internally contradictory phrases, such as referring to the ventilator as "life support," that convey mixed messages to families and add confusion to the family's grief.[111] In particular, physicians should explain that were it not for the ventilator, the issue of brain death determination would not have arisen, because the patient would have died immediately from cessation of respiration and heartbeat. Physicians should also state their certainty of the diagnosis and explain that no patient fulfilling brain death tests has ever recovered irrespective of treatment.

Inaccurate knowledge of brain death by both medical professionals and the public is a barrier to effective communication. The public remains seriously confused on this topic. A telephone survey study of Ohio residents revealed that although 98% had heard of the term "brain death," only one-third believed that someone who was brain dead was legally dead.[112] One reason for this confusion is that media depictions of brain death frequently are inaccurate. A recent study of the use of the term "brain death" in *The New York Times* disclosed that in 62% of the articles in which it was mentioned, it was discussed incorrectly or in a confusing manner that would lead readers to believe that a brain dead patient was alive.[113] Even experienced intensive care physicians and nurses have conceptual and terminological confusion about brain death and frequently use the term incorrectly.[114] A more recent study of fourth year medical students' concepts of death revealed a clearer understanding of brain death.[115]

The majority of families will accept the explanation of brain death and not oppose extubation. A minority will reject this explanation and demand continued treatment, either because they do not understand or accept the concept of brain death or they think the physician's diagnosis may be in error. These cases need compassionate and diplomatic management. The physician has the choice between extubating the patient over the opposition of the family or continuing to ventilate the patient. In the latter instance, physicians are not obligated to maintain other forms of aggressive support, such as vasopressor drugs that are usually necessary to maintain an adequate blood pressure. In these instances, it may be easier for families to tolerate the patient's circulatory death with the ventilator maintained. Such a death appears more natural and will cause them less anxiety from uncertainty. Physicians have an ethical duty to help relieve a family's anxiety when possible, but this duty must be balanced carefully against their responsibility to conserve scarce medical resources and their duty not to prescribe futile therapies.[116]

The issue of continued hospitalization insurance coverage after brain death declaration is another factor. Some insurance carriers may refuse to pay for hospitalization expenses once it is clear that the patient is brain dead. Physicians have the duty to explain this possibility to families, for whom it may be a relevant factor in their position.

It is desirable for hospitals to provide procedural policies that prescribe the optimal management of the brain-dead patient and the fair resolution of disputes. The brain death practice guidelines from the California Medical Association and Canadian Medical Association are exemplary.[117] There is evidence that brain death determination is practiced differently by physicians in different hospitals[118] and that medical record documentation of brain death determinations in some institutions is not optimal.[119]

DEATH BRAIN AND ORGAN TRANSPLANTATION

Although the concept of brain death arose before the advent of multi-organ transplantation, the demand for multi-organ donors has been the principal force promoting the popularization and legalization of brain death. The practices of multi-organ procurement and brain death determination are thus inextricably linked. Brain dead patients serve as the only proper donor for hearts, and continue to represent the major donor for lungs, livers, pancreases, small intestines, and kidneys. Additionally, expanding programs in organ donation after cardiac death (formerly called non-heart-beating organ donation) provide additional kidneys and livers.[120] Living whole organ donation provides kidneys, and living partial donation provides partial livers and lungs.[121] Several ethical issues of organ transplantation are relevant to the cadaveric brain dead donor.[122]

Since the earliest days of organ transplantation, physicians have known of a potential conflict of interest: the organs of a brain-dead donor are retrieved for another person's benefit. Thus the donor is used as the means to the end of organ donation. To protect the donor from being incorrectly diagnosed as brain dead simply to permit organ procurement, it is axiomatic that the organ donor must be dead (the "dead-donor rule"[123]) and that no member of the transplantation team may participate in the donor's brain death determination. This strict separation of roles is especially important in the organ donor after cardiac death, given the necessary preceding decision to discontinue life-sustaining therapy. Neither should the physician declaring brain death participate in the procurement procedure.[124] There is evidence that "uncoupling" the brain death determination from the organ procurement process in the family's mind also improves the donation consent rate.[125]

The ethical foundation for organ donation is the concept of beneficence. The potentially transplantable organs are no longer of value to the dead patient, but can save or prolong the life or improve the health of the recipient. This fact creates an ethical duty for the physician caring for a brain-dead patient. The physician has the ethical duty of rescue: to offer the family the possibility of organ donation and to encourage its performance by explaining the goods that could result both to the recipient and to the family. If the family is interested, the physician can contact the organ donation coordinator to answer the family's technical questions, obtain consent, and proceed with the procurement. There is evidence that the rates for donation consent are higher when the consent process is conducted by trained organ donor personnel who can clearly explain brain death to families and answer logistic questions authoritatively and compassionately.[126] Donation rates also increase with the use of standardized protocols that remove the treating physician from conducting the donation discussion.[127] Families who have previously discussed organ donation topics are more likely to consent.[128]

Families consenting to organ donation often derive significant benefits. They are comforted to realize that because of the organ gift from their loved one, another person's life can be saved or function restored. This knowledge often creates transcendent meaning and good from an otherwise meaningless death, particularly in the common instance of massive head trauma in young patients. Families are further comforted to think that the life spirit of their loved one "lives on" in another person.[129]

The rule of veracity must be followed when speaking to families about organ transplantation. The limitations and possible failures should be discussed as well as the success rates.[130] Coercion should never be employed, either covertly by exaggerating transplant success rates and thereby manipulating the family to provide consent, or overtly by insisting that they agree to transplantation as a condition of further care.[131]

Many patients previously will have completed Uniform Donor Cards or will have indicated on their driver's license that they wish to be organ donors in the event of their death, according to the provisions of the Uniform Anatomical Gift Act.[132] In both cases as a matter of practice, the families usually also are asked to provide consent. Gaining their consent is

usually easier in these instances because it can be framed accurately as simply following the patient's expressly stated wishes, as in following the terms of a will.[133] In some settings, out of respect for the family's wishes, organ donation is not performed if the next-of-kin refuses, even if the patient previously had completed a Uniform Donor Card.

Some scholars have advocated that current practices be changed to require only the patient's prior consent and to eliminate the requirement for the family's consent.[134] Other ideas that have been explored to increase donation rates include: (1) mandated choice, a system requiring an organ donation decision each time a driver's license is renewed; (2) presumed consent, a policy that would automatically permit organ donation in the absence of clear advance refusal;[135] and (3) financial compensation for the family of the organ donor.[136] A working group impaneled by the Ethics Committee of the American Society of Transplant Surgeons concluded that any financial compensation was troublesome because it blurred the distinction between the organs as gifts and as commodities. They felt that trials of partial reimbursement for funeral expenses could be studied in a pilot project.[137]

In contemporary American practice, organ procurement organizations (OPOs), the regional networks of organ sharing, practice widely varying policies of consent for organ donation. In one survey of OPOs, 31% followed the wishes of the deceased only, 31% followed the next of kin's wishes only, 21% procured organs if neither party objected, 13% procured organs if either party consented or neither objected, and 3% followed none of these practices.[138] The need for a more uniform national policy is obvious.[139]

There are legal requirements in the United States to seek families' consent for organ and tissue donation in the setting of circulatory death and brain death. Over 90% of states in the United States have enacted statutes requiring physicians to inquire from families about consent for organ and tissue donation. All hospitals receiving Medicare or Medicaid funds must have policies in place for "required request." Perhaps because of physicians' negative reactions resulting from the mandatory nature of these regulations, these laws have not had the desired impact of significantly increasing rates of organ donation.[140] Regulations from the U.S. Department of Health and Human Services Center for Medicare and Medicaid Services further require hospitals to monitor incipiently brain dead patients and report them to local OPOs before they are removed from ventilators, and to designate and train hospital staff to request organ donation.[141]

If the family provides consent for organ donation, following the second set of brain death tests, the patient is declared dead and mechanical ventilation and other aggressive physiologic treatment is continued through the moment of procurement. If organ donation is refused or if the patient is not a suitable candidate for procurement, the patient is extubated once brain death has been determined by the second set of tests.[142]

One major unresolved ethical issue involving transplantation from brain-dead donors is the extent to which treatment protocols can be prescribed that are in the best interest of the organ recipient but may not be in the best interest of the organ donor. Certain donor treatment protocols may be intended to assure healthy procured organs but may interfere with the ordinary management or the brain death determination of the donor. The related concept of "elective ventilation" remains controversial. By this protocol, "unsalvageable" patients with massive brain injury are admitted solely to determine brain death and permit organ procurement, rather than being extubated and allowed to die in emergency rooms. The practice of elective ventilation has been defended on the grounds of beneficence given the good that accrues from the procured organs.[143]

The patient who has satisfied his first brain death test battery but is in the interval before the second examination has been completed can be considered to be incipiently brain dead. Such patients may suffer hypotension, diabetes insipidus, cardiac arrhythmia, and hypoxemia. Should these potentially lethal complications be treated to permit organ donation or should the incipiently brain-dead, hopelessly-ill patient be permitted to die from them? What if it will take many hours to ready

the operating room for procurement? How long is it reasonable to maintain aggressive physiologic support to permit organ procurement that otherwise would be omitted?

Because of the good that accrues to the organ recipients and to the family of the donor, I believe that a small degree of harm to the donor's dignity and the donor's family's emotional state is justified. The harms produced by delaying the diagnosis of brain death or by physiologically supporting the brain-dead patient include indignity from a prolonged intensive care unit admission of no benefit to the patient, delay of burial and life-closure, emotional trauma to the family, and financial expense to the family and to society. I believe that a reasonable compromise that balances both sets of interests is to permit a delay of up to 24 hours before completing the second test battery and declaring brain death in those patients from whom organ procurement is planned. During this time the incipiently brain-dead donor can be aggressively supported awaiting the completion of logistical details, thereby permitting successful multi-organ procurement.[144]

ANENCEPHALIC NEONATES AS MULTI-ORGAN DONORS

The decade-long history of the use of anencephalic infants as multi-organ donors is a fascinating story combining science, ethics, and public policy. In the mid-1980s, the first accounts were published of using living anencephalic neonates as multi-organ donors. Proponents of this practice justified it using a variety of claims, including: (1) anencephalic neonates are brain-dead because they are born essentially without a brain;[145] (2) anencephalic neonates are not brain-dead at birth but will become brain-dead within a short time;[146] (3) anencephalic neonates are not dead but it is justifiable to kill them to retrieve their organs because they will inevitably die within a very short time, irrespective of treatment;[147] (4) anencephalic neonates are not persons and therefore may be sacrificed for their organs;[148] (5) anencephalic neonates are neither dead nor alive, but occupy a "special category" between the two states;[149] or (6) anencephalic neonates are alive, but either the dead-donor rule or the brain-death statute should be amended legally to permit organ retrieval from them.[150] Do these justifications make sense? Does the net benefit to society exceed the net harm from this practice?

Anencephaly is the congenital absence of the skull, scalp, and forebrain caused by a failure of cranial neurulation in the first month of fetal gestation. The cerebral hemispheres are absent and the brain stem is affected variably. The diagnosis is usually obvious by inspection but related conditions can confuse the inexperienced observer. The prevalence in the United States is 0.29 to 6.7 per 1,000 births, the lower values corresponding to areas where prenatal screening programs are in effect. Today, most cases of anencephaly are diagnosed prenatally and fetuses are therapeutically aborted.[151] Half of anencephalic infants carried to term are still-born. Of those surviving birth, half die within the first 24 hours, and only 5% remain alive at one week, with death usually resulting from purposeful nontreatment. Anencephaly is a terminal illness.[152]

Most observers, aside from neonatologists, are unaware that the neurological functioning of the anencephalic infant appears remarkably similar to that of a normal neonate. The ability of the neonate to cry, suck, swallow, cough, breathe, sneeze, and have sleep-wake cycles is mediated by the brain stem, which remains largely intact in anencephaly, at least temporarily.[153] It is generally believed that anencephalic neonates have a diminished or absent capacity for suffering because of the absence of the cerebral cortex, but such an assertion is difficult to prove merely on the basis of observing the differences between their behavior and that of normal neonates.

It is clear that anencephalic infants are not brain-dead. Moreover, studies on the natural history of anencephaly reveal that the infants die from respiratory failure, cardiac arrhythmia, or sepsis and usually do not progress to brain death. Of those few who do progress to brain death, in the majority of cases, their organs will have been rendered unsuitable for transplantation because of hypoxic-ischemic damage or infection. Thus, awaiting brain death to procure their organs is not a feasible strategy.[154]

Amending the whole brain definition of death or the legal criterion of death to permit declaring anencephalic neonates dead is not desirable. To assert that obviously living infants are dead is to ignore biological reality and to commit the fallacy of using the higher brain formulation as a definition of death, as discussed previously. To destroy the serviceable and accepted concept of whole brain death simply to solve this particular problem is unwise on utilitarian grounds because it produces more harm than the good it creates.[155] Additionally, to argue that anencephalic infants are not persons, and therefore surgeons should be permitted to kill them to procure their organs violates the dead-donor rule, the ethical axiom of organ transplantation.

To argue that anencephalic infants are in a unique life-state between death and life is also conceptually troubling. What reasons can be given that are adequate to justify the rejection of one of the most basic dichotomies in biology, the distinction between life and death? Are anencephalics so unique? What about the life status of infants with other related congenital malformations?

The American Medical Association and the American Academy of Pediatrics have policies respecting the dead-donor rule that require anencephalic infants to be dead before their organs can be procured.[156] By the mid-1990s, most neonatologists, philosophers, ethicists, and legal scholars reached a consensus that the use of living anencephalic neonates as multi-organ donors is not desirable or feasible and that such programs should be abandoned.[157] Such infants are not brain-dead, do not become brain-dead, and should not be reclassified to permit killing them for their organs. Beneficial and coherent concepts and laws of brain death should not be changed to accommodate this practice because the net harm to society outweighs the net benefit.[158]

At the time this consensus was reached, the American Medical Association Council on Ethical and Judicial Affairs (CEJA) unexpectedly recommended that the AMA's previous policy should be reversed to permit anencephalic infants to be used as multi-organ donors.[159] Both the substance and timing of this recommendation surprised observers. There was substantial opposition to this position by physicians, ethicists, and medical societies throughout the country, including the American Academy of Neurology. They pointed out that a broad consensus had been reached that this practice constituted both bad medicine and bad public policy. As a result of these protests and the unresolved scientific question of residual consciousness in anencephalic neonates, the AMA suspended the CEJA recommendation and reasserted their previous policy banning this activity.[160]

MATERNAL BRAIN DEATH AND LIVE BIRTH

Over the past few decades, a dozen or so cases have been published describing in detail the lengthy physiologic support of brain-dead pregnant women until their fetuses were sufficiently mature for delivery.[161] In three of the most carefully described cases, one brain-dead mother was supported for seven days, one for nine weeks, and one for over 15 weeks.[162] These cases are remarkable on several counts: (1) for the physicians' technologic prowess in successful, long-term management of the brain-dead mother's circulatory failure, respiratory failure, endocrine failure, and nutrition, as well as successful treatment of the complications of infection, hypothermia, disseminated intravascular coagulation, and diabetes insipidus;[163] (2) for maintaining the health of the fetus to permit it to grow to maturity; and (3) for the profound ethical and social questions they raise.

The fundamental ethical issue is the same conflict of interest issue raised in the cases discussed previously of patients whose brain death declaration was purposely delayed to permit them to serve as organ donors. To what extent is it ethically justified to create harms to one person to help another? More specifically, how much harm can be done to the brain-dead mother and her family to permit the birth of the child? The justice question is whether society should make a disproportionate expenditure to rescue a single life when that money could be used by many others for preventive health or other health goals.

Analysis of this ethical dilemma begins with a statement of the physician's duty to the patient. In obstetrics, the physician has the ethical duty to promote the best medical interest of two patients: the mother and the prospective infant.[164] Ordinarily the interests of both parties are compatible, in that what is good for the mother is good for the fetus. In those instances in which interests conflict, generally the interests of the mother should take precedence. This priority is the ethical basis of permitting abortion in those instances in which the mother's health is in jeopardy. In the present case, however, the mother has no further medical interests because she is dead. The obstetrician's principal ethical duty then shifts to the fetus. The obstetrician is obligated to try to rescue the fetus if possible.[165]

What is the balance of harms and goods? The harms produced by continued physiologic support of the brain-dead mother include: (1) the indignity to the mother of a prolonged intensive care unit admission which cannot benefit her health and for which her body is used as an incubator; (2) the delay of maternal death determination, burial, and life-closure; (3) the emotional trauma on the family; and (4) the financial expense to the family and to society.[166] The benefit is the potential rescue of a young life that otherwise would have been lost.

The actual chance of successful fetal salvage must be made clear before a rational decision can be made to support the brain-dead mother. In most cases of profound fetal immaturity, it will be impossible to maintain maternal health long enough to permit a healthy child to be born. In general, the closer the fetus is to term, the greater the probability of achieving a live, healthy birth.

How much is this benefit worth and who should make the decision? Of course, a human life is of inestimable value. If the father of the prospective child had a loving relationship with the brain-dead mother, he probably is best poised to weigh the relevant factors and to decide. He must consider the harms enumerated above, the chances for fetal abnormality, and his own emotional state and willingness to be a single parent. Generally, the physician should be supportive and try to encourage salvage of the fetus. The duty to encourage the husband to permit fetal salvage grows with increasing fetal age, because of the increasing chance of success in producing a live, healthy birth and the decreasing duration of required maternal physiologic support.[167]

Jay Kantor and Iffath Hoskins argued that the most useful model for analyzing the conflicting ethical issues in such cases is that the brain-dead prospective mother is analogous to a cadaver organ donor. If the prospective mother had stated her wishes in advance, they should be followed, even if doing so led to the death of a fetus at a relatively advanced gestational age. If her wishes were not known, the surrogate decision maker should decide using a standard of substituted judgment.[168] In a comprehensive legal review of the subject, Daniel Sperling suggested that if the prospective mother left clear instructions of her wishes for treatment these should be followed. Because that situation is unlikely, balancing burdens against benefits, treatment should be conducted only if the following three criteria are met: (1) the fetus is in the third trimester; (2) there is at least a 75% probability of successful fetal outcome; and (3) the medical treatment will last less than 14 days or until it is clear that fetal success exceeds 85%.[169]

RESEARCH AND TEACHING USING BRAIN DEAD PATIENTS

The brain-dead patient represents a valuable resource for research and clinical teaching because he retains many normally functioning physiologic subsystems when ventilatory and circulatory support is maintained. The brain-dead patient is an ideal research subject for potentially lethal experiments that could not be performed on live patients, because he cannot possibly be harmed physically, regardless of the danger of the research protocol. Similarly, brain-dead and circulatory dead patients may offer opportunities for trainees to practice certain life-saving skills, such as endotracheal intubation, that arguably cannot be learned any other way.

The potential research and teaching value of the brain-dead patient raises several ethical issues. Under what conditions is it ethically acceptable to conduct research using brain-dead subjects that cannot possibly help the patient? How should consent be obtained or is consent unnecessary because the patient is dead? When can brain-dead patients serve as teaching subjects? Should consent be requested, and by whom, and how? [170]

A utilitarian ethical analysis compares the benefits and burdens resulting from using the brain-dead as a research or teaching subject. There is no essential ethical distinction that turns on whether the patient has been declared dead by brain or circulatory tests. The potential benefits are the generation of scientific information that may help future patients and that cannot be obtained in any other way. Physician trainees can perfect procedural skills that could be applied to save lives of other patients. The burdens result from the failure to respect dead bodies and treat them with dignity, the evils produced by deception if consent is omitted, and the pain caused to families by asking for consent to perform procedures on their dead loved one.

Several commentators have formulated sets of criteria designed to maximize the benefits of research on the brain dead while minimizing the harms. There is consensus on the following guidelines: (1) at no time should the research team participate in the brain death determination; (2) all protocols should be reviewed and approved by the Institutional Review Board (IRB) to assure scientific validity and patient protection; and (3) exclusion criteria should be present to permit organ transplantation and not to preclude or interfere with autopsy.[171] Mechanisms for effective research oversight must be established and followed.[172]

John La Puma formulated additional guidelines to assure that the benefits gained by conducting research on brain-dead subjects exceed the burdens borne to make the research ethically acceptable: (1) the dignity and humanity of the body should never be violated, even in the pursuit of the most valuable scientific knowledge; (2) the experiment should be precisely designed and limited to a few minutes or hours instead of days or weeks; (3) the diagnosis of brain death must be unequivocal, made in accordance with the standard of care and by the patient's clinicians; (4) the fully voluntary, knowledgeable consent of the next-of-kin is necessary; if possible, the next-of-kin should act as the patient would; (5) the experiment's medical importance must be clear and vital to clinicians; that is, the results should be likely to yield valuable information, such as safe, efficacious, innovative treatment for a lethal or severely disabling disease; (6) prospective review and approval of the research protocol by an IRB, with its community and ministry members in attendance, is necessary; and (7) any charges for the time or resources spent on "life-support" systems after the declaration of death should be paid for by the investigators, not by the patient or the patient's family or their insurance carrier.[173]

Using newly dead patients (including the brain-dead) as subjects for physician trainees to practice procedural skills, such as endotracheal intubation, has been conducted clandestinely in the past. Only in the last few decades has this practice been discussed and analyzed ethically. Almost without exception, practicing on the newly dead has taken place without consent from the family.

Defenders of the practice justify it by claiming that no harm is caused to the dead patient and much benefit is gained as the result of physicians learning a life-saving skill that could help future patients. They claim that skills such as endotracheal intubation cannot be learned except by human practice and it is dangerous to practice on live patients. Some defenders have made the claim that the dead have no interests and that therefore they cannot be harmed.[174] Critics of the practice assert that harms are produced by unauthorized manipulation of dead bodies, that it is wrong in principle to conduct teaching exercises requiring this degree of invasion of the human body without first obtaining consent, and that using sophisticated anatomical models has rendered this unethical practice unnecessary. Defenders counter that asking for consent is hurtful to the family and that it would be better for all involved if the family remained unaware.[175]

First, it is unclear whether any procedures require the sole use of dead patients for practice.[176] Second, explicit, and not merely presumed, consent is required for any invasive procedures on a dead body,[177] which is why explicit consents are necessary for routine autopsies. Presumed consent is a fall-back position, used in emergencies and, even then, only when it is impossible to obtain consent from a patient or surrogate. No emergency exists when a patient dies. On balance, practicing on the newly dead without consent is unethical because the benefits do not justify the harms. The suggestion that physicians can practice on the newly dead because of presumed consent, implicit permission granted on admission unless families or patients had previously denied consent, is disingenuous and coercive, because patients and families are unaware of this rule.[178] The concept of presumed consent would be acceptable only if it were part of a clearly stipulated hospital policy known to families in advance.[179]

NOTES

1. The early history of determining death was discussed in Pernick MS. Back from the grave: recurring controversies over defining and diagnosing death in history. In Zaner RM (ed). *Death: Beyond Whole brain Criteria*. Dordrecht, the Netherlands: Kluwer Academic Publishers, 1988:17–74. For an account of twentieth century events in brain death, see Pallis C. Brainstem death. In Braakman R (ed). Head Injury. In Vinken PJ, Bruyn GW, Klawans HL (eds). *Handbook of Clinical Neurology*. vol 57 (revised series, vol 13), Amsterdam: Elsevier Science Publishers, 1990:441–496.

2. Soloveichik A. The Halakhic definition of death. In Rosner F, Bleich JD. *Jewish Bioethics*. New York: Sanhedrin Press, 1979:296–302.

3. See, especially, The Fall of the House of Usher and The Premature Burial. In Poe EA. *The Complete Edgar Allen Poe Tales*. New York: Avenel Books, 1981:199–212, 432–441.

4. Mollaret P, Goulon M. Le coma dépassé (mémoire préliminaire). *Rev Neurol* 1959;101:3–15. See also Jouvet M. Diagnostic électro-souscorticographique de la morte du système nerveux central au cours de

certaine comas. *Electroencephalogr Clin Neurophysiol* 1959;2:805–808; and Wertheimer P, Jouvet M, Descotes J. A propos du diagnostic de la morte du système nerveux dans les comas avec arrêt respiratoire traités par respiration artificielle. *Presse Méd* 1959;67:87–88. The historical importance of these papers was discussed in Wijdicks EFM. The landmark Le coma dépassé. In Wijdicks EFM (ed) *Brain Death.* Philadelphia: Lippincott Williams & Wilkins, 2001:1–4.

5. A definition of irreversible coma. Report of the Ad Hoc Committee of the Harvard Medical School to Examine the Definition of Brain Death. *JAMA* 1968;205:337–340.

6. For the history of the landmark Harvard report, see Giacomini M. A change of heart and a change of mind? Technology and the redefinition of death in 1968. *Soc Sci Med* 1997;44:1465–1482; Pernick MS. Brain death in a cultural context: the reconstruction of death 1967–1981. In Youngner SJ, Arnold RM, Schapiro R (eds). *The Definition of Death: Contemporary Controversies.* Baltimore: Johns Hopkins University Press, 1999:3–33; Belkin GS. Brain death and the historical understanding of bioethics. *J Hist Med Allied Sci* 2003;58:325–361; Wijdicks EFM. The neurologist and Harvard criteria for brain death. Neurology 2003;61:970–976; and Diringer MN, Wijdicks EFM. Brain death in historical perspective. In Wijdicks EFM (ed) *Brain Death.* Philadelphia: Lippincott Williams & Wilkins, 2001:5–27.

7. Notable original observations, studies, commentaries, and syntheses in the mid-history of brain death include the following: Mohandas A, Chou SN. Brain death: a clinical and pathologic study. *J Neurosurg* 1971;35:211–218; Task Force on Death and Dying of the Institute of Society, Ethics, and the Life Sciences. Refinements in the criteria for the determination of death: a reappraisal. *JAMA* 1972;221:48–53; Jørgenson PB, Jørgenson EO, Rosenklint A. Brain death: pathogenesis and diagnosis. *Acta Neurol Scand* 1973;49:355–367; van Till HAH. Diagnosis of death of comatose patients under resuscitation treatment: a critical review of the Harvard report. *Am J Law Med* 1976;2:1–40; Veatch RM. *Death, Dying, and the Biological Revolution: Our Last Quest for Responsibility.* New Haven: Yale University Press, 1976; Conference of Royal Conferences and Faculties of the United Kingdom. Diagnosis of brain death. *Lancet* 1976;2:1069–1070; Veith FJ, Fein JM, Tendler MD, et al. Brain death I. A status report of medical and ethical considerations. *JAMA* 1977;238:1651–1655; Veith FJ, Fein JM, Tendler MD, et al. Brain death II. A status report of legal considerations. *JAMA* 1977;238:1744–1748; Collaborative Study of Cerebral Survival. An appraisal of the criteria of cerebral death. *JAMA* 1977;237:982–986; American Neurological Association. Revised statement regarding methods for determining that the brain is dead. *Trans Am Neurol Assoc* 1977;102:192–193; Korein J (ed). Brain Death: Interrelated Medical and Social Issues. *Ann NY Acad Sci* 1978;315:1–454; Black PM. Brain death. Parts I and II. *N Engl J Med* 1978;299:338–344, 393–401; Pallis C. *ABC of Brainstem Death.* London: British Medical Journal Publishers, 1983; and Walker AE. *Cerebral Death,* 3rd ed. Baltimore: Urban & Schwarzenberg, 1985.

8. Curran WJ. Legal and medical death—Kansas takes the first step. *N Engl J Med* 1971;284:260–261. The pioneering bill to make brain death determination lawful in Kansas was co-authored and lobbied by Dr. Creighton Hardin, an influential Professor of Surgery at the University of Kansas Medical Center. http://www.kumed.com/bodyside.cfm?id=2036 (Accessed February 13, 2007).

9. President's Commission for the Study of Ethical Problems in Medicine and Biomedical and Behavioral Research. *Defining Death. Medical, Ethical, and Legal Issues in the Determination of Death.* Washington, DC: US Government Printing Office, 1981.

10. Bernat JL, Culver CM, Gert B. On the definition and criterion of death. *Ann Intern Med* 1981;94: 389–394.

11. President's Commission, 1981:35–36.

12. Law Reform Commission of Canada. *Criteria for the Determination of Death.* Ottawa: Law Reform Commission of Canada, 1981.

13. Wijdicks EFM. Brain death worldwide: accepted fact but no global consensus on diagnostic criteria. *Neurology* 2002;58:20–25. For several essays reflecting recent thinking about the philosophical, legal, and public policy issues in brain death, see Youngner SJ, Arnold RM, Schapiro R (eds). *The Definition of Death: Contemporary Controversies.* Baltimore: Johns Hopkins University Press, 1999.

14. Most of the following analysis was developed in Bernat JL, Culver CM, Gert B. On the definition and criterion of death. *Ann Intern Med* 1981;94:389–394; Bernat JL, Culver CM, Gert B. Defining death in theory and practice. *Hastings Cent Rep* 1982;12(1):5–9; Bernat JL. The definition, criterion, and statute of death. *Semin Neurol* 1984;4:45–51; Bernat JL. How much of the brain must die in brain death? *J Clin Ethics* 1992;3:21–26; Bernat JL. A defense of the whole brain concept of death. *Hastings Cent Rep* 1998;28(2):14–23; and Bernat JL. The biophilosophical basis of whole brain death. *Social Philosophy & Policy* 2002;19:324–342.

15. An analysis using sequential levels also was conducted in Capron AM, Kass LR. A statutory definition of the standards for determining human death: an appraisal and a proposal. *Univ Penn Law Rev* 1972;121:87–118. Capron and Kass used four levels: concepts, standards, criteria, and tests/procedures.

16. Exceptions include Shewmon DA, Shewmon ES. The semiotics of death and its medical implications. *Adv Exper Med Biol 2004*;550:89–114 and Chiong W. Brain death without definitions. *Hastings Cent Rep* 2005; 35(6):20–30.

17. This section was based on the analyses of the paradigm of death in Bernat JL. Philosophical and ethical aspects of brain death. In Wijdicks EFM (ed). *Brain Death*. Philadelphia: Lippincott Williams & Wilkins, 2001:171–187; Bernat JL. The biophilosophical basis of whole brain death. *Social Philosophy & Policy* 2002;19:324–342; and Bernat JL. The whole brain concept of death remains optimum public policy. *J Law Med Ethics* 2006;34:35–43.

18. I have responded to critiques of each of these assumptions in Bernat JL. A defense of the whole brain concept of death. *Hastings Cent Rep* 1998;28(2):14–23 and Bernat JL. The whole brain concept of death remains optimum public policy. *J Law Med Ethics* 2006;34:35–43.

19. For example, Linda Emanuel analyzed the concept of death in such abstract metaphysical depth, she rendered it devoid of its ordinary meaning. She wrote "there is no state of death … to say 'she is dead' is meaningless because 'she is' is not compatible with 'dead.'" Emanuel LL. Reexamining death: the asymptotic model and a bounded zone definition. *Hastings Cent Rep* 1995;25(3):27–35.

20. For an example of a scholar who holds that death determination is social and contrived, see Veatch RM. The conscience clause: how much individual choice in defining death can our society tolerate? In, Youngner SJ, Arnold RM, Schapiro R (eds). *The Definition of Death: Contemporary Controversies*. Baltimore: John Hopkins University Press, 1999:137–160.

21. For example, see the descriptions in Parnia S, Waller DG, Yeates R, Fenwick P. A qualitative and quantitative study of the incidence, features, and etiology of near death experiences in cardiac arrest survivors. *Resuscitation* 2001;48:149–156.

22. This terminology, based on "fuzzy set" theory applied to the analysis of death, is described in Halevy A, Brody B. Brain death: reconciling definitions, criteria, and tests. *Ann Intern Med* 1993;119:519–525. The authors, disagreeing with the paradigm, argued that alive and dead were best conceptualized as fuzzy sets, a concept that the world does not divide itself neatly into sets and their complements. They concluded that attempting to identify a definition and criterion of death was a futile exercise.

23. The question whether death is an event or process was the subject of classic debate thirty years ago. Morison RS. Death: process or event? *Science* 1971;173:694–698 and Kass LR. Death as an event: a commentary on Robert Morison. *Science* 1971;173:698–702. Alan and Elisabeth Shewmon argued that this debate was linguistically based and had become tiresome because, according to mathematical analysis by the nonlinear dynamic theory of discontinuous events, death obviously was an event. Shewmon DA, Shewmon ES. The semiotics of death and its medical implications. *Adv Exper Med Biol* 2004;550:89–114.

24. Pallis C. *Handbook of Clinical Neurology*, 1988 quotes an unnamed author of a 1740 paper entitled "The uncertainty of the signs of death and the danger of precipitate interments" who asserted that putrefaction was the only totally reliable sign of death.

25. President's Commission, *Defining Death* 1981; Law Reform Commission of Canada. *Criteria for the Determination of Death*. Ottawa: Law Reform Commission of Canada, 1981. Korein J. *Ann NY Acad Sci* 1978; Korein J. Brain states: death, vegetation, and life. In Cottrell JE, Turndorf H (eds). *Anesthesia and Neurosurgery* 2nd ed. St. Louis: CV Mosby, 1986; Bernat JL, Culver CM, Gert B. *Ann Intern Med* 1981; Bernat JL, Culver CM, Gert B. *Hastings Cent Rep* 1982; and Bernat JL. *J Clin Ethics* 1992.

26. The original definition of death I proposed with Charles Culver and Bernard Gert omitted the adjective "critical." I explain the reason for this modification in Bernat JL. A defense of the whole brain concept of death. *Hastings Cent Rep* 1998;28(2):14–23.

27. Loeb J. *The Organism as a Whole*. New York: G.P. Putnam's Sons, 1916.

28. Mahner M, Bunge M. *Foundations of Biophilosophy*. Berlin: Springer-Verlag, 1997:29–30.

29. I offer a rigorous biophilosophical account of the organism as a whole based on the concept of emergent functions in Bernat JL. The biophilosophical basis of whole brain death. *Social Philosophy & Policy* 2002; 19:324–342.

30. A number of investigators have studied cellular neuronal functioning after brain death. For continued neuroendocrine functioning after brain death, see Outwater KM, Rockoff MA. Diabetes insipidus accompanying brain death in children. *Neurology* 1984;34:1243–1246 and Fiser DH, Jiminez JF, Wrape V, et al. Diabetes insipidus in children with brain death. *Crit Care Med* 1987;15:551–553. For continued EEG

activity after brain death, see Grigg MM, Kelly MA, Celesia GG, et al. Electroencephalographic activity after brain death. *Arch Neurol* 1987;44:948–954 and Darby J, Yonas H, Brenner RP. Brain stem death with persistent EEG activity: evaluation by xenon-enhanced computed tomography. *Crit Care Med* 1987;15:519–521. For continued neuronal metabolism after brain death, see Darby JM, Yonas H, Gur D, et al. Xenon-enhanced computed tomography in brain death. *Arch Neurol* 1987;44:551–554; and Ashwal S, Schneider S, Thompson J. Xenon computed tomography measuring cerebral blood flow in the determination of brain death in children. *Ann Neurol* 1989;25:539–546. Additional similar studies are reviewed in Truog RD, Fackler JC. Rethinking brain death. *Crit Care Med* 1992;20:1705–1713.

31. Staworn D, Lewison L, Marks J, Turner G, Levin D. Brain death in pediatric intensive care unit patients: incidence, primary diagnosis, and the clinical occurrence of Turner's triad. *Crit Care Med* 1994;22:1301–1305.

32. This section was adapted from Bernat JL. How much of the brain must die in brain death? *J Clin Ethics* 1992;3:21–26.

33. Veatch RM. The whole brain oriented concept of death: an outmoded philosophical formulation. *J Thanatol* 1975;3:13–30; Green MB, Wikler D. Brain death and personal identity. *Philosophy Public Aff* 1980;9:105–133; Youngner SJ, Bartlett ET. Human death and high technology: the failure of the whole brain formulations. *Ann Intern Med* 1983;99:252–258. See also Gervais K. *Redefining Death*. New Haven: Yale University Press, 1987; Devettere RJ. Neocortical death and human death. *Law Med Health Care* 1990;18:96–104; and Veatch RM. *Death, Dying, and the Biological Revolution. Our Last Quest for Responsibility,* 2nd ed. New Haven: Yale University Press, 1989:15–44.

34. Veatch RM. *J Thanatol* 1975:18.

35. Veatch RM. *J Thanatol* 1975:23.

36. Green MB, Wikler D. *Philosophy Publ Aff* 1980:112–114.

37. On the persistent vegetative state, see Bernat JL. Chronic disorders of consciousness. *Lancet* 2006;367:1181–1192 and the discussion in chapter 12. For the most severe examples, see Brierley JB, Adams JH, Graham DI, Simpsom JA. Neocortical death after cardiac arrest: a clinical, neurophysiological and neuropathological report of two cases. *Lancet* 1971;2:560–565.

38. Veatch RM. Brain death and slippery slopes. *J Clin Ethics* 1992;3:181–187.

39. For a tightly argued and evidence-based defense of this position, see Shewmon DA, de Giorgio CM. Early prognosis in anoxic coma: reliability and rationale. *Neurol Clin* 1989;7:823–844.

40. Green MB, Wikler D. *Philosophy Publ Aff* 1980:113–114 and Youngner SJ, Bartlett EB. *Ann Intern Med* 1983:257–258.

41. This point was argued carefully in Lamb D. *Death, Brain Death, and Ethics*. Albany, NY: State University of New York Press, 1985.

42. For one philosopher's critique of concepts of personhood, see Beauchamp TL. The failure of theories of personhood. *Kennedy Inst Ethics J* 1999;9:309–324.

43. Conference of Medical Royal Colleges and their Faculties in the United Kingdom. Diagnosis of brain death. *BMJ* 1976;2:1187–1188 and Conference of Medical Royal Colleges and their Faculties in the United Kingdom. Memorandum on the diagnosis of death. *BMJ* 1979;1:322.

44. Christopher Pallis wrote a series of six articles in the early 1980s published in the *British Medical Journal* that were collected and published later as the book: Pallis C. *ABC of Brainstem Death*. London: British Medical Journal Publishers, 1983.

45. Pallis C. *ABC of Brainstem Death*: 32.

46. For an ultra-conservative Roman Catholic perspective, see Byrne PA, O'Reilly S, Quay PM. Brain death—an opposing viewpoint. *JAMA* 1979;242:1985–1990; Evers JC, Byrne PA. Brain death: still a controversy. *Pharos* 1990;53(4):10–12; and Seifert J. Is brain death actually death? A critique of redefinition of man's death in terms of 'brain death.' *The Monist* 1993;76:175–202. For a unique variation on this theme in which the authors argue that it is acceptable to harvest organs from the brain dead, but that death occurs only at asystole, see Halevy A, Brody B. Brain death: reconciling definitions, criteria, and tests. *Ann Intern Med* 1993;119:519–525.

47. Shewmon DA. Chronic "brain death:" meta-analysis and conceptual consequences. *Neurology* 1998;51:1538–1545 and Shewmon DA. The brain and somatic integration: insights into the standard biological rationale for equating "brain death" with death. *J Med Philosophy* 2001;26:457–478.

48. The test battery recommended by the President's Commission was reprinted in several medical journals. See Report of the Medical Consultants on the Diagnosis of Death to the President's Commission for the Study of Ethical Problems in Medicine and Biomedical and Behavioral Research. Guidelines for the determination of death. *JAMA* 1981;246:2184–2186.

49. Wijdicks EF. Determining brain death in adults. *Neurology* 1995;45:1003–1011 and Quality Standards Subcommittee of the American Academy of Neurology. Practice parameters for determining brain death in adults [summary statement]. *Neurology* 1995;45:1012–1014.

50. For current summaries of accepted brain death tests, see Wijdicks EFM. The diagnosis of brain death. *N Engl J Med* 2001;344:1215–1221; Canadian Neurocritical Care Group. Guidelines for the diagnosis of brain death. *Can J Neurol Sci* 1999;26:64–66; and Haupt WF, Rudolf J. European brain death codes: a comparison of national guidelines. *J Neurol* 1999;246:432–437.

51. See, for example, Wijdicks EFM. The diagnosis of brain death. *N Engl J Med* 2001;344:1215–1221 and Bernat JL. Brain death. In Laureys S, Tononi G (eds). *The Neurology of Consciousness: Cognitive Neuroscience and Neuropathology.* Amsterdam: Elsevier, 2008 (in press).

52. This practice is consistent with the "T4" time of death offered by Joanne Lynn and Ronald Cranford in Lynn J, Cranford RE. The persisting perplexities in the determination of death. In, Youngner SJ, Arnold RM, Schapiro R (eds). *The Definition of Death: Contemporary Controversies.* Baltimore: Johns Hopkins University Press, 1999:101–114.

53. For my argument that confirmatory testing should be performed more routinely, see Bernat JL. On irreversibility as a prerequisite for brain death determination. *Adv Exper Med Biol* 2004;550:161–168.

54. For reviews of these technologies, see Young B, Lee D. A critique of ancillary tests of brain death. *Neurocritical Care* 2004;1:499–508 and Shemie SD, Pollack MM, Morioka M, Bonner S. Diagnosis of brain death in children. *Lancet Neurology* 2007;6:87–92.

55. Boissy AR, Provencio JJ, Smith CA, Diringer MN. Neurointensivists' opinions about death by neurological criteria and organ donation. *Neurocrit Care* 2005;3:115–121.

56. Nanda A, Schmidley J. Diagnosing brain death—is it still clinical? (Abstract P03.114) *Neurology* 2007;68 (Suppl 1):A137.

57. For reviews on determining brain death in infancy and childhood, see Ashwal S. Brain death in the newborn. Current perspectives. *Clin Perinatol* 1997;24:859–882 and Shemie SD, Pollack MM, Morioka M, Bonner S. Diagnosis of brain death in children. *Lancet Neurology* 2007;6:87–92.

58. Report of the Medical Consultants on the Diagnosis of Death to the President's Commission for the Study of Ethical Problems in Medicine and Biomedical and Behavioral Research. Guidelines for the determination of death. *JAMA* 1981;246:2184–2186.

59. Task Force for the Determination of Brain Death in Children. Guidelines for the determination of brain death in children. *Arch Neurol* 1987;44:587–588.

60. Volpe JJ. Brain death determination in the newborn. *Pediatrics* 1987;80:293–297. See also Freeman JM, Ferry PC. New brain death guidelines in children: further confusion. *Pediatrics* 1988;81:301–303.

61. Shewmon DA. Caution in the definition and diagnosis of infant brain death. In Monagle JF, Thomasma DC (eds). *Medical Ethics: A Guide for Health Professionals.* Rockville, MD: Aspen Publishers, 1988:39 and Shewmon DA. Commentary on Guidelines for the Determination of Brain Death in Children. *Ann Neurol* 1988;24:789–791.

62. Staworn D, Lewison L, Marks J, Turner G, Levin D. Brain death in pediatric intensive care unit patients: incidence, primary diagnosis, and the clinical occurrence of Turner's triad. *Crit Care Med* 1994;22:1301–1305 and Parker BL, Frewen TC, Levin SD, et al. Declaring brain death: current practice in a Canadian pediatric critical care unit. *CMAJ* 1995;153:909–916.

63. Mejia RE, Pollack MM. Variability in brain death determination practices in children. *JAMA* 1995; 274:550–3.

64. Ashwal S. Brain death in the newborn. Current perspectives. *Clin Perinatol* 1997;24:859–82; Banasiak KJ, Lister G. Brain death in children. *Curr Opin Pediatr* 2003;15:288–93 and Shemie SD, Pollack MM, Morioka M, Bonner S. Diagnosis of brain death in children. *Lancet Neurology* 2007;6:87–92.

65. Beresford HR. Brain death. *Neurol Clin* 1999;17:295–306.

66. Wijdicks EFM. Brain death worldwide: accepted fact but no global consensus on diagnostic criteria. *Neurology* 2002;58:20–25.

67. Capron AM, Kass LR. A statutory definition of the standards for determining human death: an appraisal and a proposal. *Univ Penn Law Rev* 1972;121:87–118; Capron AM. Legal definition of death. *Ann NY Acad Sci* 1978;315:349–362.

68. House of Delegates redefines death, urges redefinition of rape, and undoes the Houston Amendments. *Am Bar Assoc J* 1975;61:463–464.

69. President's Commission. *Defining Death.* 1981:160.

70. Bernat JL, Culver CM, Gert B. *Ann Intern Med* 1981:393 and Bernat JL, Culver CM, Gert B. *Hastings Cent Rep* 1982:8.

71. This section was modified from Bernat JL. Philosophical and ethical aspects of brain death. In Wijdicks EFM (ed) *Brain Death*. Philadelphia: Lippincott Williams & Wilkins, 2001:171–187.

72. Veatch RM. The impending collapse of the whole brain definition of death. *Hastings Cent Rep* 1993;23(4):18–24 and Veatch RM. The death of whole brain death: the plague of the disaggregators, somaticists, and mentalists. *J Med Philosophy* 2005;30:353–378.

73. Veatch RM. *Hastings Cent Rep* 1993:19.

74. Halevy A, Brody B. Brain death: reconciling definitions, criteria, and tests. *Ann Intern Med* 1993;119: 519–525.

75. President's Commission. *Defining Death*. 1981:160.

76. Truog RD. Is it time to abandon brain death? *Hastings Cent Rep* 1997;27(1):29–37.

77. Taylor RM. Reexamining the definition and criterion of death. *Semin Neurol* 1997;17:265–270.

78. Shewmon DA. "Brainstem death," "brain death" and death: a critical re-evaluation of the purported equivalence. *Issues Law Med* 1998;14:125–145; Shewmon DA. Spinal shock and "brain death": somatic pathophysiological equivalence and implications for the integrative-unity rationale. *Spinal Cord* 1999;37:313–324; Shewmon DA. Chronic "brain death:" meta-analysis and conceptual consequences. *Neurology* 1998;51:1538–1545; Shewmon DA. The brain and somatic integration: insights into the standard biological rationale for equating "brain death" with death. *J Med Philosophy* 2001;26:457–478; and Shewmon DA, Shewmon ES. The semiotics of death and its medical implications. *Adv Exper Med Biol* 2004;550:89–114.

79. For the compelling account of how and why Alan Shewmon changed his mind about the validity of brain death, from being one of its strongest supporters to one of its most vocal critics, see Shewmon DA. Recovery from 'brain death:' a neurologist's apologia. *Linacre Q* 1997;64(1):30–96.

80. Seifert J. Is brain death actually death? A critique of redefinition of man's death in terms of 'brain death.' *The Monist* 1993;76:175–202.

81. Shewmon DA. Spinal shock and "brain death": somatic pathophysiological equivalence and implications for the integrative-unity rationale. *Spinal Cord* 1999;37:313–324.

82. Shewmon DA. Chronic "brain death:" meta-analysis and conceptual consequences. *Neurology* 1998;51:1538–1545. An autopsy on the extraordinary patient (mentioned in this article) who was declared brain dead at age four and thereafter was physiologically maintained for 16 years confirmed that he was brain dead by showing no evidence of brain neurons. See Repertinger S, Fitzgibbons WP, Omojola MF, Brumback RA. Long survival following bacterial meningitis-associated brain destruction. *J Child Neurol* 2006; 21:591–595.

83. Spike J, Greenlaw J. Ethics consultation: persistent brain death and religion: must a person believe in death to die? *J Law Med Ethics* 1995;23:291–294.

84. Wijdicks EFM, Bernat JL. Chronic "brain death:" meta-analysis and conceptual consequences. (letter) *Neurology* 1999;53:1639–1640.

85. This conclusion also was reached by Alexander Capron, the distinguished legal scholar and former Executive Director of the President's Commission for the Study of Ethical Problems in Medicine and Biomedical and Behavioral Research. See Capron AM. Brain death—well settled yet still unresolved. *N Engl J Med* 2001;344:1244–1246. A similar conclusion was reached by the bioethicist Dan Wickler. See Wickler D. Brain death: a durable consensus. *Bioethics* 1999;7:239–241. Most recently, this conclusion also was reached by the United States President's Council on Bioethics in their report: Controversies in the Determination of Death: White Paper of the President's Council on Bioethics. Draft of September 2007. Personal communication, Edmund D. Pellegrino, Chairman, September 27, 2007. Their full report will be accessible at www.bioethics.gov.

86. This section was modified from Bernat JL. Religious issues in brain death. Presented at the 52nd Annual Meeting of the American Academy of Neurology, San Diego, CA, April 30, 2000. (©American Academy of Neurology.)

87. See review by Veith FJ, Fein JM, Tendler MD, et al. Brain death I. A status report of medical and ethical considerations. *JAMA* 1977;238:1651–1655 and Veith FJ, Fein JM, Tendler MD, et al. Brain death II. A status report of legal considerations. *JAMA* 1977;238:1744–1748.

88. Campbell CS. Fundamentals of life and death: Christian fundamentalism and medical science. In, Youngner SJ, Arnold RM, Schapiro R (eds). *The Definition of Death: Contemporary Controversies*. Baltimore: John Hopkins University Press, 1999:194–209.

89. White RJ, Angstwurm H, Carrasco de Paula I (eds). *Working Group on the Determination of Brain Death and its Relationship to Human Death.* Scripta Varia 83. Vatican City: Pontifical Academy of Sciences, 1992; Pontifical Council for Pastoral Assistance. *Charter for Health Care Workers.* Boston: St. Paul Books and Media, 1994; Pontifical Academy of Life, Vatican City. (Msgr. Elio Sgreccia, Vice-President of the Pontifical Academy for Life, personal communication, September 14, 2000); and Pontifical Academy of Sciences. *The Signs of Death.* Scripta Varia 110. Vatican City: Pontifical Academy of Sciences, 2007.

90. Pope John Paul II. Address of the Holy Father John Paul II to the 18th International Congress of the Transplantation Society, August 29, 2000, Rome. http://www.vatican.va/holy_father/john_paul_ii/speeches/2000/jul-sep/documents/hf_jp-ii_spe_20000829_transplants_en.html (Accessed July 7, 2007).

91. Personal correspondence from Bishop Marcelo Sánchez Sorondo, Chancellor of the Vatican Pontifical Academy of Sciences, January 15, 2007. See Pontifical Academy of Sciences. *The Signs of Death.* Scripta Varia 110. Vatican City: Pontifical Academy of Sciences, 2007.

92. Byrne PA, O'Reilly S, Quay PM. Brain death—an opposing viewpoint. JAMA 1979;242:1985–1990 and Evers JC, Byrne PA. *Pharos* 1990:10–12.

93. Furton EJ. Reflections on the status of brain death. *Ethics and Medics* 1999;24(10):2–4.

94. Furton EJ. Brain death, the soul, and organic life. *The National Catholic Bioethics Quarterly* 2002;2:455–470.

95. The current rabbinic debate on the Jewish definition of death is explained in Rosner, F. The definition of death in Jewish law. In Youngner SJ, Arnold RM, Schapiro R (eds). *The Definition of Death: Contemporary Controversies.* Baltimore: John Hopkins University Press, 1999:210–221.

96. Tendler MD. Cessation of brain function: ethical implications in terminal care and organ transplants. *Ann NY Acad Sci* 1978;315:394–407 and Rosner F, Tendler MD. Definition of death in Judaism. *Journal of Halacha and Contemporary Society* 1989;17:14–31.

97. Bleich JD. Establishing criteria of death. In Rosner F, Bleich JD (eds). *Jewish Bioethics.* New York: Sanhedrin Press, 1979:277–295; Bleich JD. Of cerebral, respiratory and cardiac death. *Tradition* 1989;24(3):44–66; and Soloveichik A. The Halakhic definition of death. In Rosner F, Bleich JD (eds). *Jewish Bioethics.* New York: Sanhedrin Press, 1979:296–302.

98. Yaqub BA, Al-Deeb SM. Brain death: current status in Saudi Arabia. *Saudi Med J* 1996;17:5–10.

99. Abomelha MS, Al Kawi MZ. Brain death. *Saudi Kidney Dis Transplant Bull* 1992;3:177–179. See also Albar MA. Organ transplantation—an Islamic perspective. *Saudi Med J* 1991;12:280–284. I am grateful to Dr. Saeed Bohlega and Dr. Edward Cupler of the Neurology Department of the King Faisal Specialist Hospital and Research Centre in Riyadh, Saudi Arabia for providing this information.

100. Jain S, Maheshawari MC. Brain death—the Indian perspective. In, Machado C (ed). *Brain Death.* Amsterdam: Elsevier, 1995:261–263.

101. See Lock M. Contesting the natural in Japan: moral dilemmas and technologies of dying. *Culture, Medicine and Psychiatry* 1995;19:1–38; Kimura R. Japan's dilemma with the definition of death. *Kennedy Inst Ethics J* 1991;1:123–131; and Akabayashi A. Finally done—Japan's decision on organ transplantation. *Hastings Center Rep* 1997;27(5):47.

102. Lock M. *Twice Dead: Organ Transplants and the Reinvention of Death.* Berkeley, CA: University of California Press, 2002.

103. New Jersey Declaration of Death Act. NJSA 26, Ch 6, A1–8, 1991.

104. NY Comp Codes, Rules & Regs, Title 10, § 400.16(d), (e)(3), 1992.

105. Olick RS: Brain death, religious freedom, and public policy: New Jersey's landmark legislative initiative. *Kennedy Inst Ethics J* 1991;4:275–288.

106. Orr RD, Genesen LB. Requests for inappropriate treatment based on religious beliefs. *J Med Ethics* 1997;23:142–147. See also Spike J, Greenlaw J. Ethics consultation: persistent brain death and religion: must a person believe in death to die? *J Law Med Ethics* 1995;23:291–294.

107. Miles S. Death in a technologic and pluralistic culture. In Youngner SJ, Arnold RM, Schapiro R (eds). *The Definition of Death: Contemporary Controversies.* Baltimore: John Hopkins University Press, 1999:311–318.

108. Veatch RM. The conscience clause: how much individual choice in defining death can our society tolerate? In Youngner SJ, Arnold RM, Schapiro R (eds). *The Definition of Death: Contemporary Controversies.* Baltimore: John Hopkins University Press, 1999:137–160 and Brock DW. The role of the public in public policy on the definition of death. In Youngner SJ, Arnold RM, Schapiro R (eds). *The Definition of Death: Contemporary Controversies.* Baltimore: John Hopkins University Press, 1999:293–307.

109. For example, see Miedema F. Medical treatment after brain death: a case report and ethical analysis. *J Clin Ethics* 1991;2:50–52 and Hardwig J. Treating the brain dead for the benefit of the family. *J Clin Ethics* 1991;2:53–56.

110. *In Re Bowman,* 617 P2d 731 (WN Sup Ct 1980) and *Matter of Haymer,* 450 NE 2d 940 (Ill App 1983).

111. Molinari GF. Brain death, irreversible coma, and words doctors use. *Neurology* 1982;32:400–402.

112. Siminoff LA, Burant C, Youngner SJ. Death and organ procurement: public beliefs and attitudes. *Kennedy Inst Ethics J* 2004;14:217–234.

113. Laskowski KR, Ackerman AL, Friedman AL. Opportunity to improve clarity about brain death: analysis of 95,221 articles in the 2005 NY Times. Abstract #1098 Presented at the World Transplant Congress, Boston, July 24, 2006.

114. Youngner SJ, Landefeld S, Coulton CJ, et al. "Brain death" and organ retrieval: a cross-sectional survey of knowledge and concepts among health professionals. *JAMA* 1989;261:2205–2210.

115. Frank JI. Perceptions of death and brain death among fourth-year medical students: defining our challenge as neurologists (abstract). *Neurology* 2001;56(suppl 3):A429.

116. Cranford RE. Discontinuation of ventilation after brain death. Policy should be balanced with concern for the family. *BMJ* 1999;318:1754–1755. See the discussion in chapter 10 on futility in brain death.

117. For examples of optimal policies for conducting brain death in practice, see Shaner DM, Orr RD, Drought T, Miller RB, Siegel M. Really, most SINCERELY dead: policy and procedure in the diagnosis of death by neurologic criteria. *Neurology* 2004;62:1683–1686 and Shemie SD, Doig C, Dickens B, et al. Severe brain injury to neurological determination of death: Canadian forum recommendations. *CMAJ* 2006;174:S1–S13.

118. Powner DJ, Hernandez M, Rives TE. Variability among hospital policies for determining brain death in adults. *Crit Care Med* 2004;32:1284–1288; Mejia RE, Pollack MM. Variability in brain death determination practices in children. *JAMA* 1995;274:550–553; and Hornby K, Shemie SD, Teitelbaum J, Doig C. Variability in hospital-based brain death guidelines in Canada. *Can J Anaesth* 2006;53:613–619.

119. Wang MY, Wallace P, Gruen JP. Brain death documentation: analysis and issues. *Neurosurgery* 2002;51: 731–736.

120. For data on non-heart-beating organ donation, see Bernat JL, D'Allesandro AM, Port FK, et al. Report of a national conference on donation after cardiac death. *Am J Transplantation* 2006:6:281–291. For a more general review, see Institute of Medicine. *Non-Heart-Beating Organ Transplantation: Practice and Protocols.* Washington, DC: National Academy Press, 2000.

121. See, for example, Marcos A, Fisher RA, Ham JM, et al. Selection and outcome of living donors for adult to adult right lobe transplantation. *Transplantation* 2000;69:2410–2415 and Starnes VA, Woo MS, MacLaughlin EF, et al. Comparison of outcomes between living donor and cadaveric lung transplantation in children. *Ann Thorac Surg* 1999;68:2279–2283. For a discussion of the ethical issues in living donor partial organ transplants, see Singer PA, Siegler M, Wittington PF, et al. Ethics of liver transplantation with living donors. *N Engl J Med* 1989;321:620–622.

122. For a review of the ethical issues in organ procurement from cadaveric donors, see Arnold R, Siminoff L, Frader J. Ethical issues in organ procurement: a review for intensivists. *Crit Care Clin N Am* 1996;12:29–48.

123. Robertson JA. The dead donor rule. *Hastings Cent Rep* 1999;29(6):6–14.

124. American Medical Association Judicial Council. Ethical guidelines for organ transplantation. *JAMA* 1968;205:341–342 and Merrill JP. Statement of the Committee on Morals and Ethics of the Transplantation Society. *Ann Intern Med* 1971;75:631–633.

125. Hauptman PJ, O'Connor KJ. Procurement and allocation of solid organs for transplantation. *N Engl J Med* 1997;336:363–372.

126. Franz HS, DeJong W, Solfe SM, et al. Explaining brain death: a critical feature of the donation process. *J Transplant Coord* 1997;7:13–21 and Gortmaker SL, Beasley CL, Sheehy L, et al. Improving the request process to increase family consent for organ donation. *J Transplant Coord* 1998;8:210–217.

127. Helms AK, Torbey MT, Hacein-Bey L, Chyba C, Varelas PN. Standardized protocols increase organ and tissue donation rates in the neurocritical care unit. *Neurology* 2004;63:1955–1957.

128. Siminoff LA, Gordon N, Hewlett J, Arnold RA. Factors influencing families' consent for donation of solid organs for transplantation. *JAMA* 2001;286:71–77.

129. Douglass GE, Daly M. Donor families' experience of organ donation. *Anaesth Intensive Care* 1995;23: 96–98.

130. The elements of informed consent for organ donation have been formulated most completely for living organ donation but many of them also apply to surrogate consent for cadaveric organ donation after brain death or cardiac death. See Steiner RW, Gert B. Ethical selection of living kidney donors. *Am J Kidney Dis* 2000;36:677–686.

131. For a discussion of the *Strachan* case in which a family of a brain-dead patient was wrongly coerced by the treating physicians into consenting for organ donation, see Annas GJ. Brain death and organ donation: you can have one without the other. *Hastings Cent Rep* 1988;18(3):28–30.

132. The Uniform Anatomical Gift Act, 8A ULA § 15 (1987).

133. This outcome was found by Siminoff LA, Burant C, Youngner SJ. Death and organ procurement: public beliefs and attitudes. *Kennedy Inst Ethics J* 2004;14:217–234.

134. Kluge EH. Decisions about organ donation should rest with potential donors, not next of kin. *CMAJ* 1997;157:160–161. See also May T, Aulisio MP, DeVita MA. Patients, families, and organ donation: who should decide? *Milbank Q* 2000;78:336.

135. American Medical Association Council on Ethical and Judicial Affairs. Presumed consent and mandated choice for organs from deceased donors. In, *Code of Medical Ethics of the American Medical Association: Current Opinions with Annotations*, 2006–2007 edition. Chicago: American Medical Association, 2006:62–63 and Spital A. Mandated choice for organ donation: time to give it a try. *Ann Intern Med* 1996;125:66–69.

136. American Medical Association Council on Ethical and Judicial Affairs. Financial incentives for organ procurement: ethical aspects of future contracts for cadaveric donors. *Arch Intern Med* 1995;155:581–689.

137. Arnold R, Bartlett S, Bernat J, et al. Financial incentives for cadaver organ donation: an ethical reappraisal. *Transplantation* 2002;73:1361–1367.

138. Wendler D, Dickert N. The consent process for cadaveric organ procurement. How does it work? How can it be improved? *JAMA* 2001;285:329–333.

139. Capron AM. Reexamining organ transplantation. *JAMA* 2001;285:3334–3335.

140. Evans RW, Orians CE, Ascher NL. The potential supply of organ donors: an assessment of the efficiency of organ procurement efforts in the United States. *JAMA* 1992;267:239–246.

141. U.S. Department of Health and Human Services Center for Medicare and Medicaid Services. Requirements for Approval and Reapproval of Transplant Centers to Perform Organ Transplants; Final Rule. (42 CFR 405, 482, 488, and 498) *Federal Register* 2007;72:15198–15280. (March 30, 2007.) http://www.cms.hhs.gov/CertificationandComplianc/downloads/Transplantfinal.pdf (Accessed July 7, 2007).

142. For the criteria to be an organ donor and the principles of management of potential organ donors, see Wood KE, Becker BN, McCartney JG, D'Allesandro AM, Coursin DB. Care of the potential organ donor. *N Engl J Med* 2004;351:2730–2739.

143. Browne A, Gillett G, Tweeddale M. The ethics of elective (non-therapeutic) ventilation. *Bioethics* 2000; 14:42–57.

144. I have defended this practice in Bernat JL. Ethical issues in brain death and organ transplantation. *Neurol Clin* 1989;7:715–728.

145. Harrison MR. The anencephalic as organ donor. *Hastings Cent Rep* 1986;16(2):21–22 and Holzgreve W, Beller FK, Buchholz B, et al. Kidney transplantation from anencephalic donors. *N Engl J Med* 1987;316: 1069–1070.

146. There are technical difficulties in the determination of brain death in the anencephalic neonate. See Walters JW, Ashwal S. Organ prolongation in anencephalic infants: ethical and medical issues. *Hastings Cent Rep* 1988;18(5):19–27.

147. Zaner RM. Anencephalics as organ donors. *J Med Philosophy* 1989;14:61–78.

148. Cefalo RC, Engelhardt HT Jr. The use of fetal and anencephalic tissue for transplantation. *J Med Philosophy* 1989;14:25–44. For a critique of this position, see Willke JC, Andrusko D. Personhood redux. *Hastings Cent Rep* 1988;18(5):30–33.

149. Cranford RE, Roberts JC. Use of anencephalic infants as organ donors: crossing a threshold. In: Kaufman HH (ed). *Pediatric Brain Death and Organ Retrieval.* New York: Plenum Press, 1989 and Ethics and Social Impact Committee. Anencephalic infants as sources of transplantable organs. *Hastings Cent Rep* 1988;18(5):28–30.

150. Truog RD, Fletcher JC. Anencephalic newborns. Can organs be transplanted before brain death? *N Engl J Med* 1989;321:388–390; Walters JW. Yes—the law on anencephalic infants as organ sources should be changed. *J Pediatr* 1989;115:824–828; Sass HM. Brain life and brain death: a proposal for a normative agreement. *J Med Philosophy* 1989;14:45–60; and Diaz JH. The anencephalic organ donor: a challenge to existing moral and statutory laws. *Crit Care Med* 1993;21:1781–1786.

151. See Walsh JL, McQueen MM. The morality of induced delivery of the anencephalic fetus prior to viability. *Kennedy Inst Ethics J* 1993;3:357–369.

152. Medical Task Force on Anencephaly. The infant with anencephaly. *N Engl J Med* 1990;322:669–674; Shewmon DA. Anencephaly: selected medical aspects. *Hastings Cent Rep* 1988;18(5):11–18; and Shinnar S, Arras J. Ethical issues in the use of anencephalic infants as organ donors. *Neurol Clin* 1989;7:729–743.

153. Shewmon DA. *Hastings Center Rep* 1988:13–14.

154. Physicians at Loma Linda University have amassed the greatest experience with anencephalic organ donors. In their protocol, the infants were treated aggressively in intensive care units pending their development of brain death. Because so few anencephalic neonates were eventually suitable organ donors, they suspended their program. See Peabody JL, Emery JR, Ashwal S. Experience with anencephalic infants as prospective organ donors. *N Engl J Med* 1989;321:344–350. Others have called for a general moratorium on this practice. See Fost N. Organs from anencephalic infants: an idea whose time has not yet come. *Hastings Cent Rep* 1988;18(5):5–10.

155. Hanger LE. The legal, ethical, and medical objections to procuring organs from anencephalic infants. *Health Matrix* 1995;5:347–368.

156. American Medical Association Council on Ethical and Judicial Affairs. Report 14: *Anencephalic infants as organ donors.* Chicago, December, 1988; American Academy of Pediatrics Committee on Bioethics. Infants with anencephaly as organ sources: ethical considerations. *Pediatrics* 1992;89:1116–1119.

157. See Shewmon DA, Capron AM, Peacock WJ et al. The use of anencephalic infants as organ sources: a critique. *JAMA* 1989;261:1773–1781; Arras JD, Shinnar S. Anencephalic newborns as organ donors: a critique. *JAMA* 1988;259:2284–2285; Medearis DN, Holmes LB. On the use of anencephalic infants as organ donors. *N Engl J Med* 1989;321:391–393; Capron AM. Anencephalic donors: separate the dead from the dying. *Hastings Cent Rep* 1987;17(2):5–9; Fost N. *Hastings Cent Rep* 1988:5–10; and Steinberg A, Katz E, Sprung CL. Use of anencephalic infants as organ donors. *Crit Care Med* 1993;21:1787–1790.

158. Bard JS. The diagnosis is anencephaly and the parents ask about organ donation: now what? A guide for hospital counsel and ethics committees. *West New Engl Law Rev* 1999;21:49–95.

159. American Medical Association Council on Ethical and Judicial Affairs. The use of anencephalic neonates as organ donors. *JAMA* 1995;273:1614–1618.

160. Plows CW. Reconsideration of AMA opinion on anencephalic neonates as organ donors. *JAMA* 1996;275:443–444. For the history of this fascinating episode of medical-ethical-legal politics, see Walters J, Ashwal S, Masek T. Anencephaly: where do we now stand? *Semin Neurol* 1997;17:249–255.

161. For a useful review and analysis of the published cases of maternal brain death, see Farragher RA, Laffey JG. Maternal brain death and somatic support. *Neurocrit Care* 2005;3:99–106.

162. Dillon WP, Lee RV, Tronolone MJ. Life support and maternal brain death during pregnancy. *JAMA* 1982;248:1089–1091; Field DR, Gates EA, Creasey RK, et al. Maternal brain death during pregnancy: medical and ethical issues. *JAMA* 1988;260:816–820; and Bernstein IM, Watson M, Simmons GM, et al. Maternal brain death and prolonged fetal survival. *Obstet Gynecol* 1989;74:434–437.

163. For details on the medical and nutritional management of the brain dead mother, see Nuutinen, LS, Alahuta SM, Heikkinen JE. Nutrition during ten-week life support with successful fetal outcome in a case with fatal maternal brain damage. *J Parent Ent Nutrition* 1989;13:432–435 and Catanzarite VA, Willms DC, Holdy KE, Gardner SE, Ludwig DM, Cousins LM. Brain death during pregnancy: tocolytic therapy and aggressive maternal support on behalf of the fetus. *Am J Perinatol* 1997;14:431–434.

164. Mattingly SS. The maternal-fetal dyad: exploring the two-patient obstetrical model. *Hastings Cent Rep* 1992;22(1):13–18.

165. See Siegler M, Wikler D. Brain death and live birth. *JAMA* 1982;248:1101–1102 and Veatch RM. Maternal brain death: an ethicist's thoughts. *JAMA* 1982;248:1102–1103.

166. In one report, the cost to society for a successful fetal rescue in this setting was estimated at $2.4 to 3.0 million. Spike J. Brain death, pregnancy, and posthumous motherhood. *J Clin Ethics* 1999;10:57–65.

167. Loewy EH. The pregnant brain dead and the fetus: must we always try to wrest life from death? *Am J Obstet Gynecol* 1987;157:1097–1101.

168. Kantor JE, Hoskins IA. Brain death in pregnant women. *J Clin Ethics* 1993;4:308–314. For a rebuttal of this position, see Glover JJ. Incubators and organ donors. *J Clin Ethics* 1993;4:342–346.

169. Sperling D. Maternal brain death. *Am J Law Med* 2004;30:453–500.

170. Wicclair MR. Informed consent and research involving the newly dead. *Kennedy Inst Ethics J.* 2002;12:351–372.

171. Coller BS, Scudder LE, Berger HJ, et al. Inhibition of human platelet function in vivo with a monoclonal antibody: with observations on the newly dead as experimental subjects. *Ann Intern Med* 1988;109:635–638. See also Martyn RM. Using the brain dead for medical research. *Utah Law Rev* 1986;1:1–28 and Fost N. Research on the brain dead. *J Pediatr* 1980;96:54–56.

172. Wicclair MR, DeVita M. Oversight of research involving the dead. *Kennedy Inst Ethics J.* 2004;14:143–164.

173. La Puma J. Discovery and disquiet: research on the brain dead. *Ann Intern Med* 1989;109:606–608.

174. Nelkin D, Andrews L. Do the dead have interests? Policy issues for research after life. *Am J Law Med* 1998;24:261–291.

175. Orlowski JP, Kanoti GA, Mehlman MJ. The ethics of using newly dead patients for teaching and practicing intubation techniques. *N Engl J Med* 1988;319:439–441; Orlowski JP, Kanoti GA, Mehlman MJ. The ethical dilemma of permitting the teaching and perfecting of resuscitation techniques on recently expired patients. *J Clin Ethics* 1990;1:201–205; and Benfield DG, Flaksman RJ, Lin TH, et al. Teaching intubation skills using newly deceased infants. *JAMA* 1991;265:2360–2363.

176. Burns JP, Reardon FE, Truog RD. Using newly deceased patients to teach resuscitation procedures. *N Engl J Med* 1994;331:1652–1655.

177. American Medical Association Council on Ethical and Judicial Affairs. Performing procedures on the newly deceased patient for training purposes. In *Code of Medical Ethics of the American Medical Association: Current Opinions with Annotations*, 2006–2007 edition. Chicago: American Medical Association, 2006:262–263.

178. This possibility is mentioned as an option but is not necessarily advocated by Orlowski JP, Kanoti GA, Mehlman MJ. *N Engl J Med* 1988:440 and Orlowski JP, Kanoti GA, Mehlman MJ. *J Clin Ethics* 1990:204.

179. Perkins HS, Gordon AM. Should hospital policy require consent for practicing invasive procedures on cadavers? The arguments, conclusions, and lessons from one ethics committee's deliberations. *J Clin Ethics* 1994;5:204–210 and Hayes GJ. Issues of consent: the use of the recently dead for endotracheal intubation training. *J Clin Ethics* 1994;5:211–216.

Disorders of Consciousness

12

Managing patients with disorders of consciousness presents challenging ethical issues for neurologists and neurosurgeons and raises vexing questions. How can physicians be certain that the patient is unconscious and unable to experience pain and suffering? How confidently can physicians prognosticate the probability and quality of the patient's recovery? What duration of aggressive treatment is necessary before physicians can predict outcome with reasonable certainty? What is the appropriate level of treatment for the patient at each stage of illness? How should physicians counsel family members? Who makes treatment decisions for the incapacitated patient and by what criteria? How do physicians resolve conflicts among family members over medical treatment?

Disorders of consciousness comprise a continuum of severity from the deepest coma to the mildest confusional state and a spectrum of prognosis from the reversible to the permanent. Most physicians aggressively treat patients with coma hoping for improvement (excluding those who are brain dead), at least until their prognosis becomes clear. Irrespective of its cause, true eyes-closed coma usually is a temporary state lasting from between a few hours to a few weeks. Thereafter, most comatose patients achieve one of three outcomes: they die, they enter a vegetative state (VS), or they recover consciousness to a varying degree from a minimally conscious state (MCS) to normality.[1] The VS and MCS may be transient stages during recovery after an acute brain injury or illness or may be chronic stable states that persist for months or years without improvement. Patients remaining in chronic VS and MCS account for the most difficult ethical issues encountered in the treatment of unconscious patients.

THE VEGETATIVE STATE AND THE MINIMALLY CONSCIOUS STATE

The vegetative state (VS) is a disorder of consciousness that ironically combines wakefulness and lack of awareness. When it occurs as a chronic stable disorder, it is commonly called the "persistent vegetative state" (PVS). Patients reach a VS after suffering a pathological process that has produced widespread dysfunction of cerebral cortical neurons, thalamic neurons, or the white matter connections between the cortex and thalamus, but that largely spares brain stem and hypothalamic neurons. The most common causes of VS are head trauma, stroke, and neuronal hypoxia and ischemia suffered during cardiopulmonary arrest.[2]

The VS is an artifact of modern technology because, formerly, most patients with brain injuries sufficient to cause this disorder would have died. Technologically advanced methods of restoring such patients to relatively normal health through cardiopulmonary resuscitation and other treatment often succeed. When these attempts fail to restore normal neurological function, surviving patients may be left in VS, a condition that some physicians have termed "a state worse than death."[3] The tragedy and meaninglessness of a chronically non-cognitive existence create difficult ethical problems in the management of VS patients. In the United States in March 2005, many of these problems were brought to intense public scrutiny during the sensationalized dying of Theresa Schiavo.

History

In 1972, Bryan Jennett and Fred Plum coined the name "persistent vegetative state" and defined its essential clinical features, although others earlier had recognized and provided brief descriptions of similar states.[4] Jennett and Plum observed that many patients rendered comatose from head trauma and other brain injuries progressed after several weeks from a typical eyes-closed, comatose state to an eyes-open unresponsive and unaware state. Although sleep-wake cycles returned and they were awake, these patients appeared to be utterly unaware of themselves and their environment. To the fullest extent that could be determined, they were incapable of thinking, remembering, feeling, or experiencing. With adequate medical and nursing care, young patients could remain in this state for many months or years.

Jennett and Plum chose the term "vegetative" to capture the essential characteristic of these patients. As they pointed out, vegetative is defined in the Oxford English Dictionary as "a merely physical life, devoid of intellectual activity or social intercourse . . . an organic body capable of growth and development but devoid of sensation and thought." In retrospect, the term "vegetative" was an unfortunate choice because of its unintended similarity to the pejorative term "vegetable," a term sometimes callously applied to non-cognitive patients. Jennett and Plum chose the adjective "persistent" to indicate that these patients had remained in this noncognitive state for a long time. The authors purposely avoided the term "permanent," connoting a definite prognosis, because they recognized that often it is impossible to make such a prognosis with a high degree of certainty. Subsequently, other commentators have tried to equate the term "persistent" with the term "permanent" but, because some VS patients ultimately recover awareness, persistence is not

synonymous with permanence. Stated another way, persistent vegetative state denotes a diagnosis whereas permanent vegetative state denotes a prognosis.

Over the past few decades, a number of case reports, a small series of patients, and several reviews have highlighted the clinical features and natural history of VS.[5] Further, VS has been the subject of much writing in clinical ethics[6] and the focus of several landmark high court rulings in the United States involving termination of life-sustaining treatment, most notably the cases of Karen Ann Quinlan, Paul Brophy, Nancy Beth Cruzan, and Theresa Schiavo.[7] Despite the quantity of such writings, nagging areas persist in which lack of consensus has confounded discussion, especially surrounding the diagnostic criteria and prognosis of the VS.

In an attempt to address the medical and ethical problems in the management of VS patients, several medical societies have formulated diagnostic criteria and propounded prognostic assessments for VS.[8] Although these efforts have been welcomed, they have not been accepted universally. Critics point out that statements of medical societies are learned assertions that do not necessarily result from an evidence-based review of the scientific literature.

The Multi-Society Task Force on PVS was impaneled in 1991 to try to achieve an evidence-based consensus on the medical aspects of VS. The Task Force was composed of experts representing the American Academy of Neurology, the American Neurological Association, the American Association of Neurological Surgeons, the American Academy of Pediatrics, and the Child Neurology Society. In formulating their report, the Task Force members reviewed the world literature on VS and studied relevant databases such as the National Institute of Neurological Disorders and Stroke Traumatic Coma Data Bank. Drafts of the report were circulated widely among other experts in the field of consciousness disorders to assure that the Task Force findings and conclusions represented the mainstream of current thought. The 1994 Task Force report was the most authoritative summary of medical facts on VS at that time.[9] In the

United Kingdom, the Royal College of Physicians Working Group [on "Permanent Vegetative State"] published their findings in 1996 with a clarification in 2003 that reached many of the same conclusions as the Task Force.[10]

Although the Task Force report generally was regarded as authoritative,[11] it was criticized in some circles for failing to include representatives from rehabilitation medicine (who provide care for most VS patients), for overstating the confidence with which it asserted that VS patients were noncognitive,[12] and for using circular reasoning about awareness in the definition of VS.[13] The Quality Standards Subcommittee of the American Academy of Neurology subsequently derived practice parameters for the management of patients in VS from the Task Force report.[14] The American Academy of Neurology is revisiting the subject of VS and is expected to publish an updated report in 2008 or 2009.

The terminology of the vegetative state has been plagued with confusion since it was coined. The modifiers "persistent" and "permanent" cause ambiguity. I agree with Bryan Jennett that it is best to use the term "VS" as a diagnosis without a preceding modifier such as "persistent" or "permanent."[15] The prognosis for a VS patient's recovery of awareness is a critically important issue but it should be addressed separately, not by incorporating it into the name of the syndrome. In this chapter, I use "VS" to describe the syndrome and "PVS" only when necessary for historical accuracy.

Definition, Criteria, and Clinical Features of the Vegetative State

The Multi-Society Task Force on PVS operationally defined the VS as "a condition of complete unawareness of the self and the environment accompanied by sleep-wake cycles with either complete or partial preservation of brain stem and hypothalamic autonomic functions." A VS may be a transient stage in the recovery from a diffuse brain insult or may be a chronic condition. The Task Force followed the 1972 usage of Jennett and Plum by defining PVS as a VS lasting longer than one month.[16]

The Task Force developed clinical diagnostic criteria for VS as listed in Table 12-1. The possible behavioral repertoire of VS patients is listed in Table 12-2. Patients in VS thus demonstrate intact sleep-wake cycles and can blink,

---

TABLE 12-1 Criteria for Diagnosing the Vegetative State

- Unaware of self and environment
- No of interaction with others
- No sustained, reproducible, or purposeful voluntary behavioral response to visual, auditory, tactile, or noxious stimuli
- No language comprehension or expression
- No blink to visual threat
- Present sleep-wake cycles
- Preserved autonomic and hypothalamic function to survive for long intervals with medical/nursing care
- Preserved cranial nerve reflexes
- Bowel and bladder incontinence

Modified from Bernat JL. *Lancet* 2006;367:1181–1192.

TABLE 12-2 Potential Behavioral Repertoire of Patients in a Vegetative State

- Sleep-wake cycles with eyes closed, then open
- Spontaneous breathing
- Spontaneous blinking and roving eye movements
- Nystagmus
- Vocalization of sounds but no words
- Brief, unsustained visual pursuit
- Grimacing to pain, changing facial expressions
- Yawning; chewing jaw movements
- Swallowing of saliva
- Nonpurposeful limb movements; arching of back; decorticate limb posturing
- Flexion withdrawal from noxious stimuli
- Brief movements of head or eyes toward sound or movement
- Auditory startle
- Startle myoclonus
- Sleep-related erections

Modified from Bernat JL. *Lancet* 2006;367:1181–1192.

move their eyes, swallow, vocalize sounds, breathe, grimace, and move their limbs. They may exhibit unsustained visual pursuit for a few seconds as well. Stereotyped movements resulting from intact subcortical motor reflexes may be present. Despite their repertoire of motor activities, VS patients execute none in response to command nor do they execute movements in a purposeful way that would suggest the presence of an aware, experiencing, responsive intellect.[17]

The intact subcortical motor functions, brain stem reflexes, breathing, and generally preserved autonomic functions in VS patients result because brain stem and hypothalamic neurons are largely spared by the pathological process that destroyed or disconnected cerebral cortical and thalamic neurons. The VS patient retains wakefulness and alertness because the ascending reticular activating system of the brain stem is spared. Because the cerebral cortex or thalami are diffusely damaged or disconnected, awareness of self and environment is abolished and all cognition is absent despite wakefulness.

Patients in VS commonly are classified as unconscious, but the use of the term "consciousness" in this context is ambiguous. In their famous monograph, Fred Plum and Jerome Posner pointed out that normal consciousness has two necessary components: (1) wakefulness or alertness, served by the ascending reticular activating system of the brain stem and its thalamic and hemispheric projections; and (2) awareness of self and environment served by the cerebral cortex and its connections with itself, the thalami, and other subcortical structures.[18]

Patients in a typical eyes-closed coma are classified as unconscious because they lack both the wakefulness and awareness components of consciousness. Patients in VS possess wakefulness but lack awareness; thus they possess only one component of consciousness. Because both components are necessary for normal consciousness, and the absence of awareness is the most relevant characteristic of unconsciousness,[19] VS patients reasonably may be classified as unconscious. That the VS patient possesses a relatively intact alerting mechanism is of no functional value in the absence of the capacity for awareness and cognitive experience.

The VS is distinct from other states of unconsciousness or severe paralysis. Brain death (chapter 11) requires the irreversible loss of all clinical functions of the brain, including those of the hypothalamus and brain stem. Coma is a pathological state of eyes-closed unconsciousness without sleep-wake cycles, which results from impairment of the ascending reticular activating system in the brain stem. The apallic syndrome is a particularly severe form of PVS.[20] Akinetic mutism is a state of severe abulia with preserved awareness following bilateral orbitofrontal or bilateral cingulate gyrus lesions.[21] The locked-in syndrome (chapter 14) is a state of pseudo-coma featuring profound paralysis but preserved awareness; it usually caused by an acute, large lesion of the pons, usually of vascular origin, though similar states of profound paralysis with intact awareness can result from advanced states of neuromuscular diseases. In a clever turn of phrase, Hannah Kinney and Martin Samuels called the VS a "locked out" syndrome because the cerebral cortex is disconnected from the external world, in contrast to the "locked in" syndrome in which the patient has preserved awareness but profound paralysis.[22] Because the criteria of VS have become accepted it is desirable to abandon using the overlapping terms apallic syndrome and akinetic mutism.

Definition, Criteria, and Clinical Features of the Minimally Conscious State

Just as patients evolve from coma to VS several weeks following a diffuse brain insult, some patients may recover from VS weeks or months later to enter a state of unresponsiveness in which awareness is present, at least to some extent, and at some times. This state recently has been called the minimally conscious state (MCS).

Although patients in this condition have been described for years, classifying them as MCS, primarily by experts in traumatic brain injury rehabilitation, is a product only of the past decade.[23] The Aspen Neurobehavioral

Conference impaneled a task force to study the available literature and seek consensus-based recommendations regarding the diagnosis, prognosis, and management of MCS. The report of the Aspen Neurobehavioral Conference defines the MCS as "a condition of severely altered consciousness in which minimal but definite behavioral evidence of self or environmental awareness is demonstrated." They require that patients in MCS show "limited but clearly discernable self or environmental awareness on a reproducible or sustained basis" by demonstrating one or more behaviors, including following simple commands, gesturing yes/no answers to questions, intelligible verbalizations, purposeful behavior, appropriate smiling or crying, reaching for and touching objects, and pursuit eye movements.[24] The criteria for MCS are listed in Table 12-3 and the potential behavioral repertoire of a patient with MCS is listed in Table 12-4. The differential characteristics of VS, MCS, coma, brain death, and locked-in syndrome are displayed in Table 12-5.

Like the VS, the MCS may occur as a transient stage in the recovery after severe head injury or other brain insult, or it may be a chronic, stable condition. With continued recovery, some patients emerge from MCS to a higher state of awareness. Evidence for this improvement is present if the patient can

TABLE 12-3 Criteria for Diagnosing the Minimally Conscious State

- Globally impaired responsiveness
- Limited but discernable evidence of awareness of self and environment as demonstrated by the presence of one or more of the following behaviors
- Following simple commands
- Gestural or verbal responses to yes/no questions
- Intelligible verbalization
- Purposeful behavior: movements or affective behaviors that occur in contingent relation to relevant environmental stimuli and are not simply reflexive movements (see Table 12-4)

Modified from Bernat JL. *Lancet* 2006;367:1181–1192.

TABLE 12-4 Potential Behavioral Repertoire of Patients in a Minimally Conscious State

- Follow simple commands
- Gesture yes/no answers
- Verbalize intelligently
- Vocalize or gesture in direct response to a question's linguistic content
- Reach for objects demonstrating a clear relationship between object location and direction of reach
- Touch and hold objects in a manner that accommodates the size and shape of the object
- Sustain visual pursuit of moving stimuli
- Smile or cry appropriately to linguistic or visual content of emotional but not of affectively neutral topics or stimuli

Modified from Bernat JL. *Lancet* 2006;367:1181–1192.

engage in functional interactive communication or use two different objects functionally. It is essential for clinicians to distinguish VS from MCS.

Critics of the term "MCS" point out that the mere fact that these patients were poorly responsive did not necessarily imply that their consciousness was deficient. I believe that the term "minimally responsive state" more accurately describes their behavior.[25] This term was used for these patients in the neuro-rehabilitation literature before "MCS" was coined.[26] It is unclear why the more descriptive term "minimally responsive state" was abandoned in favor of "MCS." Other critics worry that the category called MCS was created from within the continuum of brain-injured patients to accelerate the devaluation of their lives and to permit a more casual decision to discontinue their treatment.[27]

Patients with impaired consciousness, in whom the diagnosis of VS or MCS is being considered, need to be examined carefully and systematically to assess their level of awareness. Several clinical assessment scales that target responses of conscious awareness have been developed, tested, and validated in brain-injured patients.[28] Physicians should examine patients in a distraction-free environment

TABLE 12-5 A Comparison of Vegetative State, Minimally Conscious State, and Related Disorders*

	Awareness	Wakefulness	Brain Stem/ Respiratory	Motor	EEG	Evoked Potentials	PET/fMRI	Comment
Brain Death	Absent	Absent	Absent	Absent	ECS	Absent	Absent cortical metabolism	Legally dead in most jurisdictions
Coma	Absent	Absent	Depressed, variable	Reflex or posturing	Polymorphic delta, burst-suppression	BAER variable; cortical ERPs often absent	Resting <50%	Prognosis variable
Vegetative State	Absent	Present, intact sleep-wake cycles	Intact	Reflex, non-purposeful	Delta, theta, or ECS	BAER preserved; cortical ERPs variable	Resting <50%; primary areas stimulatable	Prognosis variable
Minimally Conscious State	Intact but poorly responsive	Intact	Intact	Variable with purposeful movements	Nonspecific slowing	BAER preserved; cortical ERPs often preserved	Reduced; secondary areas also stimulatable	Prognosis variable
Locked-In Syndrome	Intact but communication difficult	Intact	Intact breathing; often brain stem signs	Quadriplegia, pseudobulbar palsy	Usually normal	BAER variable; cortical ERPs normal	Normal or nearly normal	Not a disorder of consciousness

*ECS: electrocerebral silence; BAER: brain stem auditory evoked responses; ERP: event-related potentials
The table lists typical findings that are not necessarily present in all patients.
Modified from Bernat JL. *Lancet* 2006;367:1181–1192.

after tapering sedative medications to maximize the patients' alertness.[29] Commands to follow tasks should attempt to elicit responses that lie within patients' capacities. Visual, auditory, tactile, noxious, and olfactory stimuli should be administered. Raising patients upright to 85 degrees on a tilt table can improve their responsiveness.[30] Nurses and caregivers should be interviewed to determine if they have witnessed patient behaviors suggesting awareness. If so, they should be asked to elicit them for the examiner.

Limits of Diagnostic Certainty: The Role of Functional Neuroimaging Studies

By definition, VS patients are unaware. But how can physicians be certain that they are utterly unaware and incapable of thinking, suffering, or having any cognitive experience? Is it possible that VS patients are aware but we simply lack the means to detect evidence of their cognitive life and thus erroneously deny its presence?[31] Do the motor responses of VS patients to noxious stimuli, such as limb withdrawal or facial grimace, indicate that they can consciously perceive pain and thus suffer?[32] Of course, if the patient is found to be aware, the correct diagnosis must change from VS to MCS.

There is a fundamental and irreducible biological limitation in knowing for certain whether any other person possesses a conscious life. No person can directly experience the consciousness of another. We can ascertain another person's quality and quantity of consciousness solely by inference. We interact with others and infer in them a particular level of conscious life on the grounds of their behavior and, in particular, the quality and quantity of their responses to our stimuli. If patients' responses to our stimuli are markedly deficient or absent, we may reasonably infer a reduction in the quality and quantity of their consciousness.

Thus, it remains possible that VS patients are actually aware, and neurologists erroneously make an incorrect diagnosis by asserting that their awareness and cognitive life is absent when it is actually present.[33] This type

of diagnostic error has been made in the past, most commonly by the careless examiner of a patient with locked-in syndrome who, because of lack of response and pinpoint pupils, is erroneously labeled as unconscious (see chapter 14). Two studies of patients diagnosed as VS who then were carefully examined by experienced clinicians showed that 37% and 43% of the patients actually were aware and therefore in a MCS, not in a VS.[34] It is probable these patients initially were in a VS but that they had improved over time to MCS and evidence for their awareness was not detected until they were re-examined.

Family members commonly assert that VS patients respond to them even when physicians cannot detect evidence of it.[35] It is essential for neurologists to carefully examine patients with impaired responsiveness searching for any evidence of awareness. Routinely, I ask family members or nurses who have detected awareness behaviors to demonstrate them to me. Only if awareness is unequivocally absent should physicians diagnose VS.

In the previous edition of this book, I concluded that, despite an irreducible limitation of proof, we could justifiably conclude that properly diagnosed VS patients were incapable of any conscious experience, including the experience of pain or suffering. Now, in light of several recent provocative functional neuroimaging reports discussed below, I am no longer so certain. Previously, I cited three lines of empirical evidence that VS patients were unaware.[36] First, the motor responses exhibited by VS patients to verbal, visual, auditory, somasthetic, or noxious stimuli achieve a level of complexity no greater than primitive involuntary subcortical reflexes seen in unequivocally comatose patients. VS patients respond to verbal and auditory stimuli by opening or randomly moving their eyes. They follow no commands. Their eyes and head can follow a visual stimulus briefly, but they show no signs of purpose, attention, planning, recognition, or sustained optical tracking or visual fixation. In response to noxious or other somatosensory stimuli, they assume stereotyped motor postures and have increased autonomic activity. The repertoire of VS patients' motor responses to stimuli, thus, while not excluding the presence of cognitive life, shows no convincing evidence of it.

Second, pathological studies of VS reveal diffuse cortical laminar or pseudolaminar necrosis or widespread bilateral thalamic necrosis in the majority of nontraumatic cases of VS and diffuse axonal injury in those cases in which VS was caused by head trauma.[37] Based on our understanding of the anatomical structures necessary for awareness, we would expect the extent and severity of these lesions to produce a disorder so profound that VS patients could not retain any degree of awareness.[38] There is obvious circularity in this reasoning, however, because our knowledge of the anatomy of consciousness is based on clinical-anatomic correlation.

Third, early functional neuroimaging studies revealed that VS patients had markedly diminished resting rates of cortical glucose consumption suggesting severe diffuse impairment of cortical function. Regional cerebral metabolic rates of glucose consumption (rCMRglc) measured by positron emission tomography (PET) scanning, a reliable indicator of cerebral cortical metabolism, are depressed to levels less than one-half normal values, a range seen in comatose patients and in normal individuals in the deepest planes of general anesthesia.[39] The cerebral cortical functioning in VS patients thus is similar to that of normal patients in deep general anesthesia, who, as everyone agrees, are insensate and utterly incapable of experience.

More recent functional neuroimaging studies using PET and functional MRI (fMRI) to assess cortical responses to stimulation have further clarified the physiology of consciousness. That resting cerebral neuronal metabolism is abnormally depressed in VS patients does not necessarily mean that it might not be appropriately increased in response to stimulation. In a study of auditory processing in VS, Steven Laureys and colleagues used PET scanning to test for increases in regional cerebral blood flow and cerebral metabolism in response to auditory stimulation. They found that auditory click stimuli activated auditory cortex bilaterally but did not activate the contralateral auditory association cortex, the posterior parietal association area, the anterior

cingulate cortex, or the hippocampus of patients in VS. They concluded that the activation of auditory cortices in isolation, without the multimodal and limbic areas, could not lead to the integrative processes believed to be necessary for awareness.[40] In a subsequent study, they showed evidence for the return of normal thalamocortical conductivity after recovery from VS.[41]

Reviews of over a decade of functional neuroimaging studies in VS with PET and fMRI by Steven Laureys and colleagues and by Nicholas Schiff and colleagues have reached common conclusions.[42] In VS patients, auditory, visual, and somatosensory stimuli can activate primary sensory areas but generally fail to activate secondary cortical areas and distributed cortical networks believed to be necessary for awareness. The absence of activation of higher order multimodal association cortices that provide the brain's integrated, distributed neuronal networks is evidence that VS patients lack awareness.

Functional neuroimaging studies in MCS patients show very different results. Cortical activation to spoken voice studies in MCS patients show generally intact distributed language networks.[43] In my recent review of these studies, I concluded "These preliminary functional imaging data suggest that some MCS patients retain sufficient cortical connectivity to support cognitive and linguistic processes, and may not be as 'minimally conscious' as their impaired responsiveness suggests."[44]

Two recent provocative functional neuroimaging reports raise fascinating and disturbing questions about the sensitivity of the neurological examination to detect awareness. Adrian Owen and colleagues studied a 23-year-old woman in VS five months after a traumatic brain injury. When she was told to imagine playing tennis and think about the ball being hit back and forth across the net, her supplementary motor area was activated. When she was asked to imagine visiting each room in her house, activity was recorded in her parahippocampal gyrus, posterior parietal lobe, and lateral premotor cortex. Both findings were similar to the cortical activations recorded in normal controls with the same stimuli. The investigators concluded that "beyond any doubt [the patient] was consciously aware of herself and her surroundings." Six months later, she began to show clinical evidence of awareness.[45] In retrospect, given this evidence that she was aware, it is reasonable to conclude that she was in a MCS despite her clinical diagnosis of VS made by competent examiners.

H.B. Di and colleagues reported two patients clinically diagnosed as VS who showed cortical activation of perisylvian language cortex, similar to findings recorded in MCS patients, evoked by hearing their names spoken by a familiar voice. The small subgroup of VS patients who showed evoked cortical activation later developed clinical evidence for awareness whereas the larger subgroup of VS patients showing no activation did not.[46] In an accompanying editorial, David Rottenberg and I opined that, although it is difficult to draw important conclusions from a few isolated reports, these cases suggested that the neurological examination, at times, may be insensitive to determine awareness. We predicted that once fMRI stimulation techniques become standardized and validated as a result of carefully studying many more patients, they will become an important ancillary test to the neurological examination in determining the diagnosis and prognosis of patients with VS and MCS.[47]

Pathogenesis, Pathology, and Epidemiology

Patients may reach a VS or MCS following diffuse brain injury or illness. The most common and poignant cases are young, previously healthy patients who have suffered massive head trauma. The second most common etiology is a nontraumatic event such as hypoxic-ischemic neuronal damage resulting from cardiopulmonary arrest. Infants born with anencephaly are in VS but poorly responsive infants born with hydranencephaly or other severe congenital malformations typically show fragments of awareness behavior and thus usually are in MCS.[48]

Formerly, VS was believed to be the common endpoint of chronic neurodegenerative diseases, such as Alzheimer's, Parkinson's, Creutzfeldt-Jakob, or Huntington's disease.[49] Although most experienced neurologists have

seen cases of neurodegenerative diseases so far advanced that the patient was unresponsive, a study examining the frequency of such instances found that cases of true VS are rare. Ladislav Volicer and colleagues carefully examined 88 patients with the most advanced Alzheimer's disease in an Alzheimer's chronic care facility. Of three independent examiners, two diagnosed VS in two patients and one examiner diagnosed VS in five patients. The examinations were repeated two months later after they had better standardized their examination procedures. In the second examination, VS was diagnosed by one examiner in six patients and not at all by the other two.[50] Thus, MCS is a more common diagnosis than VS in patients with endstage neurodegenerative diseases.

The Multi-Society Task Force based its estimates of the prevalence of VS in the United States on reported cases, data bank entries such as the NINDS Traumatic Coma Data Bank, and assumptions that VS resulted from endstage neurodegenerative diseases. The Task Force estimated the prevalence of VS in the United States as 10,000 to 25,000 adults and 4,000 to 10,000 children.[51] Given the rarity sof VS in endstage neurodegenerative diseases of adults and children, these are overestimates. More exact point prevalence studies which show a prevalence of 19 cases per million, yield an estimated total prevalence in the United States of about 6,000 patients.[52]

A review of the pathology of VS by Hannah Kinney and Martin Samuels found that VS has three patterns: (1) diffuse, widespread cortical damage such as that resulting from hypoxic-ischemic encephalopathy suffered during cardiopulmonary arrest; (2) diffuse, widespread damage to the subcortical hemispheric white matter, such as that resulting from diffuse axonal injury in traumatic brain injury; and (3) profound damage to both thalami resulting from stroke, hypoxia-ischemia, or other injuries. Each of these distributions results in a disconnection of the cerebral cortex from the external world. The destruction or isolation of the cortex is responsible for the absence of awareness in VS patients.[53] A neuropathological study of 49 patients in VS by J.H. Adams and colleagues confirmed these three patterns.[54] In hypoxic-ischemic neuronal damage from cardiac arrest, ischemia produces greater neuronal necrosis than hypoxia.[55]

In the same issue of the *New England Journal of Medicine* in which part 1 of the Task Force report was published, Hannah Kinney and colleagues reported the neuropathology of the celebrated VS case of Karen Ann Quinlan. Contrary to expectations, Quinlan's thalami were more severely damaged than her cerebral cortex, although she did have bilateral cortical damage particularly in the occipital poles and the parasagittal parieto-occipital regions. As expected, her brain stem remained largely intact. Her profound VS was attributed to the disconnection of her cortex from the external world resulting from her profound bilateral thalamic damage.[56]

Vegetative and Minimally Conscious State in Childhood

Vegetative and minimally conscious states are particularly tragic in children. Children may sustain the same traumatic, cerebrovascular, and hypoxic-ischemic acute brain insults as adults.[57] Additionally, MCS in childhood may result from severe cases of developmental and degenerative disorders.[58] Most children with severe neurodevelopmental defects are not in a VS. Alan Shewmon and colleagues reported four children with severe congenital brain malformations involving the absence or near-absence of the cerebral cortex, all of whom showed evidence of discriminate awareness, possibly reflecting the development of higher processing by the hypothalamus or brain stem made possible by neural plasticity.[59] As is true in adults, the importance of conducting a careful neurological examination searching for signs of awareness is obvious. These findings also point out the capacity of young children with developmental defects to evolve alternative neural pathways.

The Child Neurology Society Ethics Committee commissioned a survey of pediatric neurologists to record their personal experience with PVS. Of the 26% of the members completing the survey, 93% believed that PVS could be diagnosed in children over two years,

70% believed it could be diagnosed in children between two months and two years, and only 16% believed that it could be diagnosed in infants younger than two months. Fully 86% believed that the younger the patient, the longer he or she should be observed before being diagnosed with PVS. As is also true for the determination of brain death in infants, pediatric neurologists believe that a period of observation longer than that used for adults is necessary before PVS can be diagnosed reliably, particularly in infants younger than two months. PVS in children older than two years has the same essential characteristics as PVS in adults. Seventy-eight percent of the respondents in the study believed that PVS could be diagnosed in children with severe developmental disorders.[60]

Limits of Prognostic Certainty

The prognosis for improvement in VS and MCS depends on its etiology and duration.[61] Adults or children with neurodegenerative diseases or children with developmental disorders who develop MCS have no hope for recovery because these disorders are progressive and irreversible. An exception is the patient with neuronal damage not severe enough to produce VS who intercurrently develops infection, fever, electrolyte imbalance, dehydration, drug toxicity, or another cause of metabolic or toxic encephalopathy. Such patients may cycle between VS and MCS, the former when the superimposed metabolic or toxic disorder is present and the latter once the metabolic or toxic disorder is resolved.

Whether a patient rendered vegetative after head trauma or cardiopulmonary arrest is likely to recover awareness is a critical question that the physician must address before devising a treatment plan that is in accordance with the patient's and family's wishes and within the standards of good medical care. Any discussion of the ethical and legal issues surrounding decisions to either continue or stop life-sustaining treatment in the PVS patient must be preceded by the physician's clear statement of the patient's probability of recovering awareness.[62]

The Multi-Society Task Force on PVS studied the existing data on the probability of recovering awareness in acute VS. The task force was able to formulate three general rules governing prognosis of VS patients: (1) the probability for recovery of awareness is greater for patients who develop VS following head trauma than for those who develop VS following stroke or hypoxic-ischemic brain damage; (2) children recover better than adults after suffering equivalent brain injuries; (3) early prognostic signs are unreliable predictors of recovery of awareness.[63]

Reliable probabilities for recovery of awareness are difficult to discern from published studies. Most studies are biased because of their retrospective rather than prospective design. Most studies failed to provide confidence limits for predictive values, thus limiting the positive predictive value of an alleged prognostic sign when the number of patients studied was small. Outcome measures were unclear in many of the studies because VS was not distinguished from severe disability or nonsurvival.[64]

Most importantly, many patients were provided less than maximal medical treatment when their physicians judged that they had a poor prognosis. Although such decisions may have been correct medically and ethically, they make poor science because the patients' actual pattern of recovery with full treatment cannot be known. Publishing outcome data that incorporate the prognosis of these patients contributes to the fallacy of the self-fulfilling prophecy.[65] One study showed that clinical prediction algorithms in patients with severe head injuries clearly influenced the intensity of the treatment they received: patients with a better prognosis were treated more aggressively, whereas those with a poorer prognosis were treated less aggressively.[66]

These facts must be considered when interpreting the Task Force data that VS carried a 70% mortality at three years and a 84% mortality at five years.[67] These data do not necessarily reflect the natural history of maximally-treated VS but rather the experiential history of VS, including the reality that life-sustaining treatment was eventually withheld from many patients.

Despite these limitations, the Multi-Society Task Force made three general prognostic conclusions: (1) Recovery of awareness from traumatic VS is rare after one year. (2) Recovery of awareness after nontraumatic (cardiopulmonary arrest, stroke) VS is rare after three months and exceedingly rare after one year. (3) Although functional recovery in children is better than in adults with comparable injuries, the majority of VS patients recovering awareness after six months in traumatic VS or after three months in nontraumatic VS still show sustained severe disability with quadriparesis, pseudobulbar palsy, and dementia.[68] The Task Force acknowledged several well-documented late recoveries of awareness after nontraumatic events, the longest of which occurred after 22 months.[69] They investigated numerous popular accounts of late recovery from coma and VS and found none that fell outside the parameters of their conclusions.[70]

Investigators have attempted to refine prognostic indicators further in the years since the Task Force report was published. Christian Madl and colleagues found that the bilateral absence of the cortical evoked potential N20 peak was associated with 100% mortality in a group of 86 patients in nontraumatic coma or VS.[71] A meta-analysis of studies of early predictors of poor outcome in hypoxic-ischemic coma or PVS found that the bilateral absence of cortical somatosensory evoked potentials within the first week was most highly predictive of not recovering awareness.[72] In a series of 80 adult patients with traumatic VS from diffuse axonal injury who were studied by MRI, Andreas Kampfl and colleagues found that patients with hemorrhagic lesions in the corpus callosum and dorsolateral brain stem were less likely to recover awareness.[73]

There are few reliable data on prognosis in MCS. The longer MCS persists, the lower the probability of recovery. In the subgroup of patients initially in MCS from acute traumatic brain injury, 40% regain full consciousness within 12 weeks of injury and 50% regain independent function at one year.[74] Among the subgroup of severely injured patients in prolonged MCS, one study showed a heterogeneity of outcome without reliable early predictors.[75]

One recent case of a very late unexpected recovery from MCS was reported widely in the press and studied carefully by investigators. Terry Wallis sustained a traumatic brain injury at age 19 (presumed to have been diffuse axonal injury) and progressed from coma to VS to MCS over several months. He remained in a stable MCS for 19 years—his only communication ability was nodding and grunting—after which he spontaneously began speaking in coherent full sentences. Diffusion tensor imaging study of his white matter, in comparison to that of another patient with diffuse axonal injury who was in MCS for six years and who did not recover, showed increased axonal activity that they interpreted as axonal regrowth in large regions of the posterior bilateral hemispheric white matter. The investigators postulated that late regrowth of severed axons accounted for his remarkably improved language function, but accepted that his was an extraordinary and probably an unprecedented case.[76]

DETERMINING THE APPROPRIATE LEVEL OF MEDICAL TREATMENT

Physicians determining the appropriate level of medical treatment for a VS or MCS patient need to consider: (1) medical issues—reaching the correct diagnosis and prognosis; (2) ethical issues—determining the treatment preferences of the patient and identifying the surrogate decision maker; and (3) legal issues—understanding the laws governing decision making for incompetent patients. The ethical, legal, and procedural issues of continuing or discontinuing life-sustaining treatment (LST), including artificial hydration and nutrition (AHN), are discussed in chapter 8.

Treatment of a VS patient requires the same comprehensive medical and nursing care as in a comatose patient. Nutrition and hydration must be provided by feeding gastrostomy tube, with nutritional requirements calibrated according to metabolic demands.[77] Most VS patients are not ventilator-dependent, but most require tracheostomy tubes for airway protection. Nursing care must be vigilant with excellent skin care and frequent turning to prevent decubitus ulcers and frequent passive range of motion exercises to prevent contractures.

Pulmonary toilet is necessary to prevent pneumonia. Many patients develop recurrent pulmonary and urinary tract infections that require courses of antibiotics. For most medically stable VS patients, however, the only ongoing LST they receive is AHN by gastrostomy tube. Early treatment in a neurorehabilitation unit specializing in brain injury[78] is preferable because of evidence that early intensive neurorehabilitation improves outcome.[79] Spasticity often requires aggressive treatment.[80] MCS patients may require individualized communication systems developed by speech-language pathologists.

Attempts to improve responsiveness of VS patients by using sensory, electrical, or pharmacological stimulation have been disappointing but most studies represent class III evidence making conclusions ambiguous. Sensory stimulation programs providing music, voices, visual images, smells, and touching have strong intuitive appeal but systematic reviews have not shown efficacy in improving awareness.[81] Deep brain electrical stimulation of the thalamus or mesencephalic reticular formation induces no unequivocal benefit in VS.[82] Treatment with drugs including levodopa, amphetamines, tricyclic antidepressants, amantadine, bromocriptine, and anticonvulsants has had mixed results.[83] Levodopa and amantadine appear to be most useful when parkinsonian features are present, but they benefit patients in MCS more than those in VS.[84] A preliminary report of one patient in a chronic stable MCS showed improved responsiveness and arousal resulting from deep-brain stimulation of the intralaminar nuclei.[85] Another recent report showed that zolpidem produced clinical and PET scan evidence of improvement in a patient in MCS following an anoxic injury.[86] Clinicians should carefully consider the benefits and risks of initiating trials of stimulant medications or other treatments in MCS patients.

Ethical Considerations

Despite the fact that the VS patient is unconscious, continued respect for the patient's autonomy remains an important goal. Surrogate decision makers should identify and try to follow the patient's previously expressed wishes for treatment. If a patient's expressed wishes are unknown, the surrogate decision maker should be asked to try to recreate the decision that the patient would have made, were he able to decide (the standard of substituted judgment). This decision may not necessarily represent the decision that the surrogate would personally choose if he or she were in the patient's predicament.[87]

Written advance directives such as living wills (see chapter 4) provide reliable but usually only general evidence of patients' treatment preferences. Verbal conversations with family members, friends, or physicians may also represent evidence of preferences. Courts generally place a higher premium on written directives than on oral directives because the former are presumed to reflect careful consideration of the issues, whereas the latter may have been uttered casually without thoughtful deliberation.

The surrogate decision maker who lacks clear evidence of the patient's prior wishes can neither fulfill a desire to respect the patient's autonomy nor exercise substituted judgment. The surrogate then must rely on the ethical concepts of nonmaleficence and beneficence in trying to reach a decision that avoids harms and promotes good. The surrogate should balance the burdens resulting from continued treatment against the benefits accrued by continued treatment, and follow a best interest standard. (See chapters 4 and 8.)

The ethical concept of justice also becomes relevant to the patient in an irreversible VS. Whether large sums of money and dedicated technological support should be devoted to maintaining the life of a permanently noncognitive patient is a relevant issue for family members and society. Some commentators have offered arguments based on a model of medical futility, claiming that, in the ethical hierarchy, concepts of justice should trump the claims of autonomy.[88] (See chapter 10.)

One unanswered ethical question for the surrogate to consider is the probability threshold for recovery of awareness that mandates continued treatment. This question must be answered individually because it is based on personal values. Some patients would not wish aggressive or burdensome medical treatment if their chance for recovery of awareness were below 0.1. Others might draw the line at 0.01 or 0.001. There is no consensus on the precise probability threshold that satisfies the standard of "ethical acceptability." This issue is considered further in the discussion of medical futility in chapter 10.

Some patients will have executed specific advance directives anticipating the possibility of a vegetative existence. (See chapter 4.) In the most common of these directives, patients have indicated in writing that they wish treatment to be withheld if they enter a vegetative state without reasonable hope for recovery of awareness, because they want to be allowed to die. Under these circumstances, the attending physician should follow the patient's directive and withdraw LST once the prognosis is reasonably clear.

More commonly, family members may relate informal statements previously uttered by a patient. For example, the patient may have told a family member that he never wanted to be "kept alive as a vegetable" and insisted on being allowed to die rather than to maintain a hopeless and meaningless existence "on a machine." Physicians and surrogate decision makers should explore the exact circumstances of these discussions to determine if this information is reliable and relevant to the current medical situation.

Some families, such as the Wanglie family discussed in chapter 10, demand continued treatment despite the futility of an irreversible VS because they believe it is in accordance with the patient's wishes or religious beliefs. In these cases, the continued treatment may appear to benefit the family more than the VS patient.[89] I believe that physicians should continue to provide LST if the decision to continue treatment validly reflects the wishes of the patient as expressed by the surrogate and there are no countervailing considerations. (See discussion in chapter 10.)

In the situation in which no information exists about the patient's previous wishes, the surrogate decision maker must perform a benefit-burden analysis of continued treatment to identify the decision that is in the patient's best interest. The benefit of continued treatment is extending the patient's life. The burdens of treatment in VS are a matter of debate. Some scholars have argued that VS patients can have no burdens caused by continued treatment because they are permanently noncognitive and therefore incapable of experiencing anything.[90] Although it is true that VS patients have no awareness of their plight, their continued vegetative life represents an emotional and financial burden on their family and loved ones. The burden of their dependency is precisely what most chronically ill patients strive to avoid. Because most patients wish to avoid being a burden to their loved ones, particularly without the benefits of conscious experience, I believe that VS patients do incur a burden of treatment.

In my opinion, a physician who must rely on a best-interest standard for his or her decision has no compelling ethical duty to prescribe aggressive treatment to preserve the life of a patient in an irreversible VS, unless there is an explicit directive to treat.[91] There are limitations and risks, however, in employing a best interest standard to choose the level of treatment of a VS patient.[92] When a healthy surrogate makes a quality-of-life assessment of a severely disabled patient, there is frequently a bias toward under-treatment. Surrogates may undervalue continuing a vegetative existence that, for religious or other personal reasons, some patients may believe to be beneficial. Physicians should proceed with caution whenever surrogates employ a best interest standard.

One report poignantly described the legal and social complications that parents and physicians faced in attempting to withdraw hydration and nutrition from a 17-month-old infant in a VS following a hypoxic-ischemic brain injury suffered during status epilepticus. The parents insisted that the child should be allowed to die by withdrawal of hydration and nutrition and the physicians concurred. The case was reviewed by the infant care review committee. State agencies and courts became involved after an anonymous call was placed to the National Child Abuse Hotline in Washington, DC. The parents retained legal counsel to insist that their preferences be followed. After lengthy litigation, the parents' wishes were respected and the child died peacefully from dehydration.[93]

Survey Data

Surveys of patients have shown the expected result that most people would not want to continue living if they were in an irreversible VS. David Frankl and coworkers at UCLA found that 90% of the hospitalized inpatients they surveyed would want to receive life support if, as a result, they could be returned to their previous level of health. Conversely, only 30% wished to receive life support if, as a result, they would be unable to care for themselves after hospital discharge. Approximately 16% requested life support even if their case was hopeless, and only 6% wanted to be treated if they were in a PVS.[94]

These data are instructive in light of the *a priori* assumption held by many judges and legislators (especially in states such as Missouri that require the "clear and convincing" evidentiary standard) that, in the absence of compelling evidence to the contrary, irreversible VS patients should receive full medical support. This assumption is based on the state's interest in protecting incompetent citizens. Perhaps it should be re-examined in light of the health goals that citizens really wish for themselves, rather than guided by a paternalistic legal principle. People generally wish to receive aggressive medical treatment when it can help them achieve their health goals of restoring their capacity to function, at least to a minimal level.

In the absence of evidence to the contrary, I believe that a more reasonable default position for our society would be to provide citizens aggressive medical treatment if doing so can help them to achieve their health goals. According to this principle, once the diagnosis of irreversible VS has been reached with a high level of certainty, patients would not receive LST unless they had indicated this wish in an advance directive or it represents the treatment decision of their surrogate.

Two surveys of physicians assessed their opinions about the nature of PVS and its appropriate treatment. Kirk Payne and colleagues surveyed neurologists and nursing home directors in the United States. They found that 13% believed that PVS patients have awareness; 30% said PVS patients could feel pain. Fewer than

9% believed that medical complications should be treated in PVS and 89% said it was ethical to withdraw AHN. Slightly fewer than half believed that PVS patients should be declared dead and 20% said it would be ethical to hasten PVS patients' deaths by lethal injection.[95] In an accompanying editorial, Eric Cassell pointed out that these discouraging data show the depth of confusion about PVS, even among neurologists, and the obvious need for improved education.[96]

Andrew Grubb and colleagues conducted a similar survey of British neurologists, neurosurgeons, orthopedic surgeons, and physiatrists about treatment of VS patients. Over 90% of physicians reported that it would be appropriate not to treat infections or other life-threatening conditions and 65% approved of the withdrawal of AHN. Surprisingly, fewer than half the physicians thought that an advance directive should have a decisive influence in determining treatment-limiting decisions.[97] The survey revealed a discrepancy between ethical requirements and clinical practices because so many physicians would not provide the treatment that the patient wished.

Families of VS patients also have been surveyed. In a study of 33 family members of 62 VS patients in four Milwaukee nursing homes, the majority wished continuation of therapeutic interventions for the patients. The mean age of the patients was 73 years; the majority had become vegetative from progressive dementia. Interestingly, 90% of the family members believed that the patients retained some degree of awareness.[98] They probably were correct. Ladislaw Volicer and colleagues showed that physicians erroneously diagnose VS in elderly demented nursing home residents.[99] It is likely that family members refused to accept the diagnosis of VS, perhaps for valid reasons, and that this sentiment influenced their otherwise surprising preference for aggressive treatment.

Legal Issues in the Vegetative State: The Quinlan, Cruzan, and Schiavo Cases

Legal factors in decision making for VS patients, including withdrawing or withholding LST and AHN, were discussed in chapter 8 where I reviewed the important judicial rulings in *Quinlan, Brophy, Barber,* and *Cruzan.* To summarize that discussion, every United States citizen has a constitutionally protected right to accept or refuse LST, including AHN. This right is not extinguished by incapacity but is transferred to a legally authorized surrogate decision maker to exercise on behalf of the incompetent patient. States retain statutory authority to determine the standards of evidence of patients' previously stated wishes and the extent to which surrogates are permitted to refuse AHN on behalf of patients. As explained in chapter 8, physicians who discontinue LST of patients who have validly refused therapy or whose lawful surrogates have validly refused therapy are not liable for criminal homicide if the patient dies as a result. Nor should such an act be called passive euthanasia because the patient died of the underlying disease, which was terminal in the absence of LST.[100]

Quinlan was a landmark ruling because it first clarified that surrogates were permitted refuse LST on behalf of incompetent patients. The *Quinlan* ruling initiated a change in medical practice by permitting physicians to withdraw LST from a PVS patient once it had been refused by the lawful surrogate even if the patient died as a result.[101] *Cruzan* was an important ruling because the U.S. Supreme Court found a constitutional basis for all citizens to refuse unconditionally LST or any other therapy they did not want, including AHN. The Court confirmed that a surrogate was permitted to exercise that right on behalf of the incompetent patient.[102]

In March 2005, the poignant case of the vegetative state patient Theresa Schiavo was a staple of daily headlines throughout print and broadcast media in the United States, in which the vicious dispute within her family over whether to continue or stop her AHN was highlighted. She had been in a VS for 15 years as a result of suffering profound hypoxic-ischemic neuronal damage suffered during an at-home cardiac arrest in 1990 at age 26. Throughout her illness, several neurologists confirmed she was in a VS without hope for recovery of awareness. Her EEG showed electrocerebral silence and her brain CT scan showed profound cortical atrophy. A trial of thalamic deep-brain stimulation early in her course failed to improve her condition.[103]

At issue were two questions: (1) Was she in an irreversible VS from which no recovery was possible? (2) Was her husband correct that it was her true wish not to continue living in a permanently noncognitive state thus justifying his decision to remove her gastrostomy feeding tube? There was a highly publicized and intractable dispute among her family over her wishes. Her husband (her lawful surrogate in Florida) claimed she would want the feeding tube removed to permit her to die but her parents insisted she would not want it removed and wished to live. Mrs. Schiavo had completed no advance directives that might have clarified the issue.

After an extensive legal process involving evidentiary hearings during which the testimonies of friends, relatives, and medical experts were heard and assessed, Pinellas County Court judge George Greer ruled that expert opinion had established she was in a PVS from which no recovery was possible. He further ruled that removing her feeding tube was in accordance with her wishes, given her diagnosis and prognosis, and ordered it to be removed. Judge Greer concluded that the evidence that removing her feeding tube represented her true wishes was "reliable," "credible," and "clear and convincing." After a lengthy legal process during which his ruling was sustained repeatedly by state and federal appellate courts, and after unprecedented[104] and unpopular[105] legislative involvement by both the Florida legislature and the United States Congress to reverse the ruling, her feeding tube was removed and she died.

Each of the courts hearing *Schiavo* cited the legal precedent in the analogous U.S. Supreme Court ruling in *Cruzan*, also involving a young woman in a prolonged, post-cardiac-arrest VS in which the question of removing her feeding tube was litigated. *Cruzan* differed from *Schiavo* in that there was no dispute among her family members, all of whom wanted her feeding tube removed because they concurred that it was in accordance with her prior wishes. But the other facts about the two cases were so similar that *Cruzan* was the obvious precedent. In

fact, the ruling in *Cruzan* was so relevant that there were no novel legal issues raised in *Schiavo* prior to legislative interference. The unique features of *Schiavo* were the intense publicity, particularly the sensationalized family dispute that flagrantly violated her privacy and that of her family, the polarizing involvement of political action groups advocating on each side of the dispute, and the unconstitutional intrusion by the legislatures of Florida and the United States which enacted laws solely to influence her case.[106]

Schiavo produced an increased public awareness of the vexing problems inherent in making clinical decisions for patients with disorders of consciousness. Most medical centers thereafter recorded a spike in public interest in completing advance directives, presumably to prevent similar disputes over treatment. A less beneficial consequence of *Schiavo* has been a continuing multi-state effort to rewrite statutes governing decision making for incompetent patients as they pertain to withholding AHN. Several states recently have tightened the criteria by which lawful surrogates are empowered to withhold or withdraw dying patients' AHN by requiring explicit written consent of the patient in an advance directive.[107] Representing the American Academy of Neurology, Dana Bacon and colleagues expressed concern that some of these laws may perversely harm neurological patients by unwisely restricting the authority of lawful surrogates to make decisions patients would have wanted, particularly those lacking the foresight to have put their treatment preferences into writing.[108]

In the United Kingdom, the principal legal precedent in withholding AHN from a PVS patient was *Airedale N.H.S. Trust v. Bland*. In this decision, the House of Lords ruled that it was lawful for a physician to cease tube feedings for a PVS patient even though this act would lead invariably to the patient's death and (most remarkably) that the physician's intent in doing so was to kill the patient. As *Schiavo* did later, *Bland* created a firestorm of controversy.[109]

As a procedural matter, it is desirable to ask for an oversight consultation by the hospital ethics committee in cases in which the physician is considering ordering a level of treatment that will predictably shorten the life of a patient who is not terminally ill. The hospital ethics committee should ascertain that: (1) physicians have reached a clear diagnosis and prognosis; (2) advance directives, if available, are followed; and (3) the previous wishes of the patient and the present wishes of the family or surrogate are followed. These actions that protect the patient and secondarily the physician are discussed further in chapter 8.

The ethics consultant called to assist in making decisions concerning VS patients should restrict advice to providing procedural oversight. In one opinion survey, ethics consultants were asked to provide advice based on hypothetical vignettes involving treatment decisions on VS patients. The content of their answers revealed a striking discordance. Of seven paradigmatic vignettes, the ethics consultants agreed only on the "easy" one in which the VS patient's advance directive and family both refused further LST.[110] Because of inconsistency in substantive advice, ethics consultants should focus on process issues by assuring that the diagnosis and prognosis have been established and that an appropriate decision-making process has been followed by the attending physician. The structure and function of hospital ethics committees and the role of ethics consultants are discussed further in chapter 5.

Physicians can minimize medical malpractice liability if they practice according to prevailing medical standards. (See chapter 4.) In the setting of care of the VS patient, those standards include making and communicating a correct diagnosis and prognosis; attempting to follow the previously expressed treatment wishes of the patient using written or verbal advance directives or, if they are unavailable, following the current treatment decision of the lawful surrogate; ordering a treatment plan consistent with these wishes; and maintaining the patient's dignity and comfort.

Medical Society Positions

Several medical societies have published statements reflecting best medical practices in the care of VS patients. The American Academy of Neurology position statements of 1989 and 1995 are undergoing revision.[111] Additional position papers have been published by the American Neurological Association,[112] the British Medical Association,[113] the Royal College of Physicians,[114] and the Italian Neurological Society.[115] For physicians practicing in the United States, the American Medical Association Council on Ethical and Judicial Affairs (CEJA) published the most influential policy statement. The CEJA statement summarizes a physician's duties in decisions to withhold or withdraw LST on VS patients and epitomizes many points I discussed in this chapter.

Withholding or Withdrawing Life-Prolonging Medical Treatment. The social commitment of the physician is to sustain life and relieve suffering. Where the performance of one duty conflicts with the other, the preferences of the patient should prevail. If the patient is incompetent to act in his own behalf and did not previously indicate his preferences, the family or other surrogate decision maker in concert with the physician, must act in the best interest of the patient.

For humane reasons, with informed consent, a physician may do what is medically necessary to alleviate severe pain, or cease or omit treatment to permit a terminally ill patient to die when death is imminent. However, the physician should not intentionally cause death. In deciding whether the administration of potentially life-prolonging medical treatment is in the best interest of the patient who is incompetent to act in his own behalf, the surrogate decision maker and physician should consider several factors, including: the possibility for extending life under humane and comfortable conditions; the patient's values about life and the way it should be lived; and the patient's attitudes toward sickness, suffering, medical procedures, and death.

Even if death is not imminent but a patient is beyond doubt permanently unconscious, and there are adequate safeguards to confirm the accuracy of the diagnosis, it is not unethical to discontinue all means of life prolonging medical treatment.

Life-prolonging medical treatment includes medication and artificially or technologically supplied respiration, nutrition or hydration. In treating a terminally ill permanently unconscious patient, the dignity of the patient should be maintained at all times.[116]

Withholding or Withdrawing Life-Prolonging Medical Treatment–Patients' Preferences. A competent, adult patient may, in advance, formulate and provide a valid consent to the withholding or withdrawal of life-support systems in the event that injury or illness renders that individual incompetent to make such a decision. The preference of the individual should prevail when determining whether extraordinary life-prolonging measures should be undertaken in the event of terminal illness. Unless it is clearly established that the patient is terminally ill or permanently unconscious, a physician should not be deterred from appropriately aggressive treatment of a patient.[117]

The Roman Catholic Position

In an allocution in 2004, Pope John Paul II stated that artificial feeding tubes for hydration and nutrition for patients in vegetative states were "not a medical act" and that their use "always represents a natural means of preserving life" that is an element of "normal care." Therefore, as a moral matter, their use is ordinary and obligatory and their removal is "euthanasia by omission." This statement was met with consternation by American Roman Catholic scholars and leaders because it appeared to depart from several decades of consistent Church teaching that such treatment was "extraordinary" and, therefore, was not obligatory.[118]

Exactly how United States Catholic hospitals would respond to this allocution was unclear and was the subject of much conjecture. In July 2005, the United States Conference of Catholic Bishops requested that the Vatican clarify their position. In the interim, some knowledgeable American commentators doubted that the allocution would have much effect on American end-of-life treatment practices, particularly in light of the decisions Pope John Paul II made about his own dying.[119]

In September 2007, Pope Benedict XVI approved the response of the Congregation for the Doctrine of the Faith to the question of the United States Catholic Bishops to clarify Pope John Paul II's allocution. The Congregation for the Doctrine of the Faith stated that patients in vegetative states, with few exceptions, have a moral right to artificial food and hydration. Artificial food and hydration are not obligatory only when they are "excessively burdensome" or because the patient cannot assimilate food and liquids, "their provision becomes altogether useless."[120] It remains to be seen what effect this clarification has on medical practices in Catholic hospitals in the United States.

Legal Issues in the Minimally Conscious State

The importance of distinguishing the MCS from the VS was illustrated in the tragic case of Nancy Jobes. While pregnant, Mrs. Jobes suffered pelvic fractures in an automobile accident. Her four-month-gestation fetus died *in utero*. During surgery to remove the dead fetus she suffered a cardiopulmonary arrest and consequent diffuse hypoxic-ischemic brain damage. Thereafter, she was diagnosed as in a PVS. After she had survived for five years in PVS, her husband asked her physicians to remove her feeding tube to permit her to die, an act he claimed was in accordance with her prior stated wishes.

In the ensuing litigation, she was examined by four prominent neurologists with internationally recognized expertise in disorders of consciousness to determine if she was in a true PVS. Two of the expert neurologists concluded that she was in a PVS and the other two that she was in a MCS (although they did not use that term because it had not been coined yet). Ironically, to resolve the conflicting opinion, the judge examined Mrs. Jobes himself and pronounced her to be in a PVS and approved the petition to remove her feeding tube.[121]

I criticized several aspects of this case.[122] The Jobes case underscored the clinical difficulty in performing and interpreting neurological examinations in severely brain damaged patients and the ambiguity arising when even a skilled examiner tries to perceive minimal evidence of awareness in a severely brain-damaged patient.

The judge concluded that the two neurologists who found Mrs. Jobes to be aware had lost their objectivity in the matter because of their strong moral beliefs that it was wrong for such patients to have feeding tubes removed, a factor he said caused them to see evidence of awareness where none existed. However, I believe a more plausible explanation is that the examiners were correct because she was in a MCS on good days and in a VS on bad days. Such a so-called "remitting" vegetative state[123] may constitute a baseline MCS with minimal awareness that, when complicated by metabolic or toxic factors such as the effect of medications, fever, infection, or electrolyte imbalance, descends temporarily to a VS.

A nationally publicized feeding tube removal case demonstrated that a MCS patient's retained consciousness restricted the authority of a lawful surrogate to refuse AHN on the patient's behalf. A middle-aged man, Robert Wendland, was in a chronic MCS resulting from head trauma he suffered during a motor vehicle accident seven years earlier. He had completed no advance directives. In a premonition of *Schaivo*, his wife and his mother hotly disputed the level of treatment he should receive. His wife claimed that he would want his gastrostomy feeding tube removed to allow him to die, because of her belief that he wished never to live in a state of severe disability. Wendland's mother wished to maintain his gastrostomy tube feedings to keep him alive, claiming that he would want to continue to live under these circumstances.

As a consequence of national publicity, *Wendland*, like *Schiavo*, became politicized. "Right-to-die" advocates, including some medical ethicists and the American Civil Liberties Union, supported his wife's position while disability-rights advocates, and other medical ethicists, supported his mother's position. In 2001, the California Supreme Court ruled that his conservator could not order removal of his feeding tube. The court argued that because Wendland remained conscious, a higher standard of evidence was required than would have been necessary in an unconscious (VS) patient for discontinuing AHN, an act that would lead to his death. The court required clear and convincing evidence that Wendland "wished to refuse life-sustaining treatment or that to withhold such treatment would have been in his best interest."[124] The court ruled that neither of these criteria was met. As in *Schiavo*, the dispute most likely could have been prevented if Wendland had executed an advance directive.[125]

It is unclear to me why the court ruled that the presence or absence of a patient's awareness changed the evidentiary standard for a surrogate's decision making. One could plausibly argue the opposite position that, because of retained awareness, a patient's suffering in an MCS exceeds that of in a PVS, there is an even higher duty to follow a patient's preferences for treatment. The *Wendland* decision made the more general point that courts have been slow to assimilate new neuroscience information about states of impaired consciousness.

NOTES

1. Posner JB, Saper CB, Schiff ND, Plum F. *Plum and Posner's Diagnosis of Stupor and Coma*, 4th ed. New York: Oxford University Press, 2007:357.

2. I have recently reviewed the medical aspects of VS and MCS in Bernat JL. Chronic disorders of consciousness. *Lancet* 2006;367:1181–1192.

3. Feinberg WM, Ferry PC. A fate worse than death: the persistent vegetative state in childhood. *Am J Dis Child* 1984;138:128–131.

4. Jennett B, Plum F. Persistent vegetative state after brain damage: a syndrome in search of a name. *Lancet* 1972;1:734–737.

5. For recent reviews, see Jennett B. *The Vegetative State: Medical Facts, Ethical and Legal Dilemmas*. Cambridge: Cambridge University Press, 2002; Laureys S, Owen AM, Schiff ND. Brain function in coma, vegetative state, and related disorders. *Lancet Neurology* 2004;3:537–546; the symposium on VS and MCS in *NeuroRehabilitation* 2004; 19(2); Giacino J, Whyte J. The vegetative and minimally conscious states: current knowledge and

remaining questions. *J Head Trauma Rehabil* 2005;20:30–50; Wijdicks EFM, Cranford RE. Clinical diagnosis of prolonged states of impaired consciousness in adults. *Mayo Clin Proc* 2005;80:1037–1046; and Bernat JL. Chronic disorders of consciousness. *Lancet* 2006;367:1181–1192.

6. See, for example, Cranford RE. Termination of treatment in the persistent vegetative state. *Semin Neurol* 1984;4:36–44; Bernat JL. The boundaries of the persistent vegetative state. *J Clin Ethics* 1992;3:176–180; Brody B. Special ethical issues in the management of PVS patients. *Law Med Health Care* 1992;20:104–115; and Celesia GG. Persistent vegetative state: clinical and ethical issues. *Theor Med* 1997;18:221–236.

7. For reviews, see Emanuel EJ. A review of the ethical and legal aspects of terminating medical care. *Am J Med* 1988;84:291–301; Beresford HR. Legal aspects of termination of treatment decisions. *Neurol Clin* 1989;7:775–788; and Weir RF, Gostin L. Decisions to abate life-sustaining treatment for nonautonomous patients: ethical standards and legal liability for physicians after Cruzan. *JAMA* 1990;264:1846–1853.

8. The most notable examples are: American Academy of Neurology. Position of the American Academy of Neurology on certain aspects of the care and management of the persistent vegetative state patient. *Neurology* 1989;39:125–126; American Medical Association Council on Scientific Affairs and Council on Ethical and Judicial Affairs. Persistent vegetative state and the decision to withdraw or withhold life support. *JAMA* 1990;263:426–430; Institute of Medical Ethics Working Party on the Ethics of Prolonging Life and Assisting Death. Withdrawal of life-support from patients in a persistent vegetative state. *Lancet* 1991;337:96–98; American Neurological Association Committee on Ethical Affairs. Persistent vegetative state: report of the American Neurological Association Committee on Ethical Affairs. *Ann Neurol* 1993;33:386–391; and British Medical Association. *BMA Guidelines on Treatment Decisions for Patients in Persistent Vegetative States.* London: British Medical Association, 1996.

9. Multi-Society Task Force on PVS. Medical aspects of the persistent vegetative state. Parts I and II. *N Engl J Med* 1994;330:1499–1508, 1572–1579. The members of the Task Force were Stephen Ashwal and Ronald Cranford (co-chairmen), James Bernat, Gastone Celesia, David Coulter, Howard Eisenberg, Edwin Myer, Fred Plum, Marion Walker, Clark Watts, and Teresa Rogstad. The American Neurological Association representatives published a separate report containing many of the same findings as the Task Force. See American Neurological Association Committee on Ethical Affairs. Persistent vegetative state: report of the American Neurological Association Committee on Ethical Affairs. *Ann Neurol* 1993;33:386–391.

10. Royal College of Physicians Working Group. The permanent vegetative state. *J Roy Coll Phys Lond* 1966;30:119–121 and Royal College of Physicians. The vegetative state: guidance on diagnosis and management: a report of the working party of the Royal College of Physicians. *Clin Med* 2003;3:249–54.

11. For example, the British review by Adam Zeman accepted the authority of the Task Force statements. See Zeman A. Persistent vegetative state. *Lancet* 1997;350:795–799. The work of the Task Force also was commended in an editorial in the *British Medical Journal.* Howard RS, Miller DH. The persistent vegetative state: information on prognosis allows decisions to be made on management. *BMJ* 1995;310:341–342.

12. Howsepian AA. The 1994 Multi-Society Task Force consensus statement on the persistent vegetative state: a critical analysis. *Issues Law Med* 1996;12:3–29. This article criticized the Multi-Society Task Force for its sloppy use of English in, for example, conflating the meanings of "permanent" and "irreversible."

13. Shewmon DA. A critical analysis of conceptual domains of the vegetative state: sorting fact from fancy. *NeuroRehabilitation* 2004;19:343–7.

14. American Academy of Neurology Quality Standards Subcommittee. Practice parameters: assessment and management of patients in the persistent vegetative state (summary statement). *Neurology* 1995;45:1015–1018.

15. Jennett B. *The Vegetative State: Medical Facts, Ethical and Legal Dilemmas.* Cambridge University Press, Cambridge, 2002:4. For a similar recommendation, see American Congress of Rehabilitation Medicine. Recommendations for use of uniform nomenclature pertinent to patients with severe alterations of consciousness. *Arch Phys Med Rehabil* 1995;76:205–209.

16. Multi-Society Task Force on PVS. *N Engl J Med* 1994:1500.

17. Multi-Society Task Force on PVS. *N Engl J Med* 1994:1500.

18. For the discussion in the long-awaited 4th edition, see Posner JB, Saper CB, Schiff ND, Plum F. *Plum and Posner's Diagnosis of Stupor and Coma,* 4th ed. New York: Oxford University Press, 2007:5–6.

19. Zeman A. Consciousness. *Brain* 2001;124:1263–1289. See also the fascinating anthology of papers addressing the problem of consciousness from a variety of disciplines: Block N, Flanagan O, Güzeldere G (eds). *The Nature of Consciousness: Philosophical Debates.* Cambridge, MA: MIT Press, 1997.

20. Ore GD, Gerstenbrand F, Lucking CH. *The Apallic Syndrome.* Berlin: Springer-Verlag, 1977.

21. Mega MS, Cohenour RC. Akinetic mutism: disconnection of frontal-subcortical circuits. *Neuropsychiat Neuropsychol Behav Neurol* 1997;10:254–259.

22. Kinney HC, Samuels MA. Neuropathology of the persistent vegetative state: a review. *J Neuropathol Exp Neurol* 1994;53:548–558. Ethical issues in patients in the locked-in syndrome are discussed in chapter 14.

23. For example, see Giacino JT, Kalmar K. The vegetative and minimally conscious states: a comparison of clinical features and functional outcomes. *J Head Trauma Rehabil* 1997;12:36–51 and Childs NL, Cranford RE. Termination of nutrition and hydration in the minimally conscious state: contrasting clinical views. *J Head Trauma Rehabil* 1997;12:70–78.

24. Giacino JT, Ashwal S, Childs N, et al. The minimally conscious state: definition and diagnostic criteria. The Aspen Neurobehavioral Conference Consensus Statement. *Neurology* 2002;58:349–353.

25. Bernat JL. Questions remaining about the minimally conscious state. *Neurology* 2002;58:337–338.

26. For example, see Whyte J, DiPasquale MC. Assessment of vision and visual attention in minimally responsive brain injury patients. *Arch Phys Med Rehabil* 1995;76:804–810 and Wilson FC, Harpur J, Watson T, Morrow JI. Vegetative state and minimally responsive patients—regional survey, long-term case outcomes and service recommendations. *NeuroRehabilitation* 2002;17:231–236.

27. Coleman D. The minimally conscious state: definition and diagnostic criteria (letter). *Neurology* 2002;58:506 and Shewmon DA. The minimally conscious state: definition and diagnostic criteria (letter). *Neurology* 2002;58:506.

28. I reviewed these assessment scales in Bernat JL. Chronic disorders of consciousness. *Lancet* 2006;367:1181–1192.

29. Strens LHA, Mazibrada G, Duncan JS, Greenwood R. Misdiagnosing the vegetative state after severe brain injury: the influence of medication. *Brain Inj* 2004;18:213–218.

30. Elliott L, Coleman M, Shiel A, et al. Effect of posture on levels of arousal and awareness in vegetative and minimally conscious state patients: a preliminary investigation. *J Neurol Neurosurg Psychiatry* 2005;76:298–299.

31. A.A. Howsepian excoriated the Task Force members for failing to exercise a "measured degree of agnosticism about the structure of PVS patients' mental lives" and for making glib assertions that PVS patients are unequivocally noncognitive and nonsentient. See Howsepian AA. The 1994 Multi-Society Task Force consensus statement on the persistent vegetative state: a critical analysis. *Issues Law Med* 1996:3–29.

32. Some experienced clinicians believe that VS patients can feel pain and suffer. For example see McQuillen MP. Can people who are unconscious or who are in the persistent vegetative state feel pain? *Issues Law Med* 1991;6:373–383.

33. Bernat JL. The boundaries of the persistent vegetative state. *J Clin Ethics* 1992;3:176–180. The uncertainty about whether VS patients remain utterly unaware has led some physicians to recommend the humane practice of talking routinely to apparently unresponsive patients on the chance that, in fact, they are aware. See La Puma J, Schiedermayer DL, Gulyas AE, Siegler M. Talking to comatose patients. *Arch Neurol* 1988;45:20–22.

34. Childs NL, Mercer WN, Childs HW. Accuracy of diagnosis of persistent vegetative state. *Neurology* 1993;43:1465–1467 and Andrews K, Murphy L, Munday C, Littlewood C. Misdiagnosis of the vegetative state: retrospective study in a rehabilitation unit. *BMJ* 1996;313:13–16.

35. One scholar made the provocative but unverifiable claim that family members can possess subconscious, non-rational, and non-quantifiable "tacit knowledge and intuition" that allows them to communicate with loved ones who are unconscious VS patients. See White MT. Diagnosing PVS and minimally conscious states: the role of tacit knowledge and intuition. *J Clin Ethics* 2006;17:62–71.

36. This argument was developed in Bernat JL. *J Clin Ethics* 1992;3:179–180; Multi-Society Task Force on PVS. *N Engl J Med* 1994;330:1501–1502; American Academy of Neurology. *Neurology* 1989;39:125–126; and American Medical Association Council on Scientific Affairs and Council on Ethical and Judicial Affairs. *JAMA* 1990;263:427. The data supporting the conclusion that pain is perceived only during consciousness were summarized in Pitts GC. An evolutionary approach to pain. *Perspect Biol Med* 1994;37:275–284.

37. These data are reviewed in Multi-Society Task Force on PVS. *N Engl J Med* 1994:1504–1505.

38. Kinney HC, Samuels MA. Neuropathology of the persistent vegetative state: a review. *J Neuropathol Exp Neurol* 1994;53:548–558.

39. Levy DE, Sidtis JJ, Rottenberg DA, et al. Difference in cerebral blood flow and glucose utilization in vegetative versus locked-in patients. *Ann Neurol* 1987:22:673–682.

40. Laureys S, Faymonville ME, Degueldre C, et al. Auditory processing in the vegetative state. *Brain* 2000;123:1589–1601.

41. Laureys S, Faymonville ME, Luxen A, Lamy M, Franck G, Maquet P. Restoration of thalamocortical conductivity after recovery from persistent vegetative state. *Lancet* 2000;355:1790–1791.

42. These studies are summarized in Kobylarz EJ, Schiff ND. Functional imaging of severely brain-injured patients. *Arch Neurol* 2004;61:1357–1360; Laureys S, Owen AM, Schiff ND. Brain function in coma, vegetative state, and related disorders. *Lancet Neurology* 2004;3:537–546; and Bernat JL. Chronic disorders of consciousness. *Lancet* 2006;367:1181–1192.

43. Schiff ND, Rodriguez-Moreno D, Kamal A, et al. fMRI reveals large-scale network activation in minimally conscious patients. *Neurology* 2005;64:514–523 and Laureys S, Perrin F, Faymonville ME, et al. Cerebral processing in the minimally conscious state. *Neurology* 2004;63:916–918.

44. Bernat JL. Chronic disorders of consciousness. Laureys S 2006;367:1181–1192.

45. Owen AM, Coleman MR, Boly M, Davis MH, Laureys S, Pickard JD. Detecting awareness in the vegetative state. *Science* 2006;313:1402.

46. Di HB, Yu SM, Weng XZ, et al. Cerebral response to patients' own name in the vegetative and minimally conscious states. *Neurology* 2007;68:895–899.

47. Bernat JL, Rottenberg DA. Conscious awareness in PVS an MCS: the borderlands of neurology. *Neurology* 2007;68:885–886. A similar point was made in Giacino JT, Hirsch J, Schiff N, Laureys S. Functional neuroimaging applications for assessment and rehabilitation planning in patients with disorders of consciousness. *Arch Phys Med Rehabil* 2006;87(12 Suppl 2):S67–S76. For a discussion of these cases and their implications, see Owen AM, Coleman MR, Boly M, Davis MH, Laureys S, Pickard JD. Using functional magnetic resonance imaging to detect covert awareness in the vegetative state. *Arch Neurol* 2007;64:1098–1102.

48. Shewmon DA, Holmes GL, Byrne PA. Consciousness in congenitally decorticate children: developmental vegetative state as self-fulfilling prophecy. *Dev Med Child Neurol* 1999;41:364–374.

49. Walshe TM, Leonard C. Persistent vegetative state: extension of the syndrome to include chronic disorders. *Arch Neurol* 1985;42:1045–1047.

50. Volicer L, Berman SA, Cipolloni PB, Mandell A. Persistent vegetative state in Alzheimer disease: does it exist? *Arch Neurol* 1997;54:1382–1384.

51. Multi-Society Task Force on PVS. *N Engl J Med* 1994:1503.

52. Stephan C, Haidinger G, Binder H. Prevalence of persistent vegetative state/apallic syndrome in Vienna. *Eur J Neurol* 2004;11:461–466. A study of VS prevalence in the Netherlands found only 2 cases/million but this study did not record patients living at home. See Lavrijsen JC, van den Bosch JS, Koopmans RT, van Weel C. Prevalence and characteristics of patients in a vegetative state in Dutch nursing homes. *J Neurol Neurosurg Psychiatry* 2005;76:1420–424.

53. Kinney HC, Samuels MA. Neuropathology of the persistent vegetative state: a review. *J Neuropathol Exp Neurol* 1994;53:548–558.

54. Adams JH, Graham DI, Jennett B. The neuropathology of the vegetative state after an acute brain insult. *Brain* 2000;123:1327–1338.

55. Simon RP. Hypoxia versus ischemia. *Neurology* 1999;52:7–8 and Miyamoto O, Auer RN. Hypoxia, hyperoxia, ischemia, and brain necrosis. *Neurology* 2000;54:362–371.

56. Kinney HC, Korein J, Panigrahy A, Dikkes P, Goode R. Neuropathological findings in the brain of Karen Ann Quinlan. The role of the thalamus in the persistent vegetative state. *N Engl J Med* 1994;330:1469–1475.

57. Ashwal S. Pediatric vegetative state: epidemiological and clinical issues. *NeuroRehabilitation* 2004;19:349–360.

58. Ashwal S. Medical aspects of the minimally conscious state in children. *Brain Develop* 2003;25:535–545.

59. Shewmon DA, Holmes GL, Byrne PA. Consciousness in congenitally decorticate children: developmental vegetative state as self-fulfilling prophecy. *Dev Med Child Neurol* 1999;41:364–374.

60. Ashwal S, Bale JF Jr, Coulter DL, et al. The persistent vegetative state in children: Report of the Child Neurology Society Ethics Committee. *Ann Neurol* 1992;32:570–576.

61. Multi-Society Task Force on PVS. *N Engl J Med* 1994:1572.

62. Howard RS, Miller DH. The persistent vegetative state: information on prognosis allows decisions to be made on management. *BMJ* 1995;310:341–342. For a broader discussion on ethical issues in prognosis, see Bernat JL. Ethical aspects of determining and communicating prognosis in critical care. *Neurocrit Care* 2004;1:107–118.

63. Multi-Society Task Force on PVS. *N Engl J Med* 1994:1572–1575.

64. An important exception is the careful study of Levy DE, Caronna JJ, Singer BH, et al. Predicting outcome from hypoxic-ischemic coma. *JAMA* 1985;253:1420–1426. These investigators used confidence intervals and clearly distinguished outcomes.

65. Shewmon DA, De Giorgio CM. Early prognosis in anoxic coma. *Neurol Clin* 1989;7:823–843. The same point of the fallacy of the self-fulfilling prophecy was made more recently in Becker KJ, Baxter AB, Cohen WA, et al. Withdrawal of support in intracerebral hemorrhage may lead to self-fulfilling prophecies. *Neurology* 2001; 56:766–772.

66. Murray LS, Teasdale GM, Murray GD, et al. Does prediction of outcome alter patient management? *Lancet* 1993;341:1487–1491.

67. The original Task Force Report erroneously calculated the mortality rate for PVS at 82% for three years and 95% at five years. These data were recalculated and a correction published with the correct figures in Ashwal S, Cranford R. Medical aspects of the persistent vegetative state—a correction. *N Engl J Med* 1995;332:130.

68. Multi-Society Task Force on PVS. *N Engl J Med* 1994:1575–1576. Several of the recovered cases are detailed in Andrews K. Recovery of patients after four months or more in the persistent vegetative state. *BMJ* 1993;300:1597–1600.

69. Snyder BD, Cranford RE, Rubens AB, Bundlie S, Rockswold GE. Delayed recovery from postanoxic persistent vegetative state. *Ann Neurol* 1983;14:152. I reviewed the other reported cases of delayed recovery in Bernat JL. Chronic disorders of consciousness. *Lancet* 2006;367:1181–1192.

70. The public is fascinated with the idea of delayed recovery from coma. To some extent, the public may be misled by inaccurately reported newspaper stories. See Wijdicks EFM, Wijdicks MF. Coverage of coma in headlines of US newspapers from 2001 through 2005. *Mayo Clin Proc* 2006;81:1332–1336.

71. Madl C, Kramer L, Yeganehfar W, et al. Detection of nontraumatic comatose patients with no benefit of intensive care treatment by recording of sensory evoked potentials. *Arch Neurol* 1996;53:512–516.

72. Zandbergen EGJ, de Haan RJ, Stoutenbeek CP, Koelman JHTM, Hijdra A. Systematic review of early prediction of poor outcome in anoxic-ischaemic coma. *Lancet* 1998;352:1808–1812.

73. Kampfl A, Schmutzhard E, Franz G, et al. Prediction of recovery from post-traumatic vegetative state with cerebral magnetic-resonance imaging. *Lancet* 1998;351:1763–1767.

74. Giacino JT. The vegetative and minimally conscious states: consensus-based criteria for establishing diagnosis and prognosis. *NeuroRehabilitation* 2004;19:293–298.

75. Lammi MH, Smith VH, Tate RL, Taylor CM. The minimally conscious state and recovery potential: a follow-up study two to five years after traumatic brain injury. *Arch Phys Med Rehabil* 2005;86:746–754.

76. Voss HU, Uluğ AM, Dyke JP, et al. Possible axonal regrowth in late recovery from the minimally conscious state. *J Clin Invest* 2006;116:2005–2111. For commentaries on this study, see Laureys S, Boly M, Maquet P. Tracking the recovery of consciousness from coma. *J Clin Invest* 2006;116:1823–1825 and Fins JJ, Schiff ND, Foley KM. Late recovery from the minimally conscious state: ethical and policy implications. *Neurology* 2007;68:304–307.

77. For details, see American Dietetic Association. Position of the American Dietetic Association: legal and ethical issues in feeding permanently unconscious patients. *J Am Diet Assoc* 1995;95:231–234.

78. Andrews K. Managing the persistent vegetative state: early skilled treatment offers the best hope for optimal recovery. *BMJ* 1992;305:486–487.

79. Eilander HJ, Wijnen VJ, Scheirs JG, de Kort PL, Prevo AJ. Children and young adults in a prolonged unconscious state due to severe brain injury: outcome after an early intensive neurorehabilitation programme. *Brain Inj* 2005;19:425–436.

80. Montané E, Vallano A, Laporte JR. Oral antispastic drugs in nonprogressive neurologic diseases: a systematic review. *Neurology* 2004;63:1357–1363.

81. Lombardi F, Taricco M, De Tanti A, Telaro E, Liberati A. Sensory stimulation of brain-injured individuals in coma or vegetative state: results of a Cochrane systematic review. *Clin Rehabil* 2002;16:464–472.

82. Yamamoto T, Kobayashi K, Kasai M, Oshima H, Fukaya C. Katayama Y. DBS therapy for the vegetative state and minimally conscious state. *Acta Neurochir Suppl* 2005;93:101–104.

83. I reviewed these studies in Bernat JL. Chronic disorders of consciousness. *Lancet* 2006;367:1181–1192.

84. Whyte J, Katz D, Long D, et al. Predictors of outcome in prolonged posttraumatic disorders of consciousness and assessment of medication effects: a multicenter study. *Arch Phys Med Rehabil* 2005;86:453–462.

85. Schiff ND, Giacino JT, Kalmar K, et al. Behavioural improvements with thalamic stimulation after severe traumatic brain injury. Nature 2007;448:600–603.

86. Brefel-Courbon C, Payoux P, Ory F, et al. Clinical and imaging evidence of zolpidem effect in hypoxic encephalopathy. *Ann Neurol* 2007;62:102–105. During 2007, I was contacted by several families of MCS patients to report similar improvement following zolpidem treatment.

87. Wade DT. Ethical issues in diagnosis and management of patients in the permanent vegetative state. *BMJ* 2001;322:352–354. See the discussion in President's Commission for the Study of Ethical Problems in

Medicine and Biomedical and Behavioral Research. *Making Health Care Decisions: The Ethical and Legal Implications of Informed Consent in the Patient-Practitioner Relationship*. Washington, DC: US Government Printing Office; 1982:178–179.

88. Kirk Payne and Robert Taylor argued that PVS patients do not comprise good paradigmatic cases for discussing medical futility. See Payne SK, Taylor RM. The persistent vegetative state and futility: problematic paradigms for discussing futility and rationing. *Semin Neurol* 1997;17:257–263.

89. Klepper H, Truog RD. Treating the patient to benefit others. *Camb Q Healthc Ethics* 1997;6:306–313.

90. Beresford HR. Legal aspects of termination of treatment decisions. *Neurol Clin* 1989;7:775–788.

91. Other commentators have reached this conclusion. See President's Commission for the Study of Ethical Problems in Medicine and Biomedical and Behavioral Research. *Deciding to Forego Life-Sustaining Treatment: Ethical, Medical, and Legal Issues in Treatment Decisions*. Washington, DC: US Government Printing Office; 1983:171–196; Hastings Center. *Guidelines on the Termination of Life-Sustaining Treatment and the Care of the Dying*. Briarcliff Manor, NY: Hastings Center, 1987:29; and Weir RF. *Abating Treatment with Critically Ill Patients: Ethical and Legal Limits to the Medical Prolongation of Life*. New York: Oxford University Press; 1989:322–367.

92. Dresser RS, Robertson JA. Quality of life and non-treatment decisions for incompetent patients: a critique of the orthodox approach. *Law Med Health Care* 1989;17:234–244.

93. Leicher CR, DiMario FJ Jr. Termination of nutrition and hydration in a child with vegetative state. *Arch Pediatr Adolesc Med* 1994;148:87–92.

94. Frankl D, Oye RK, Bellamy PE. Attitudes of hospitalized patients toward life support: A survey of 200 medical inpatients, *Am J Med* 1989;86:645–648. For more detailed descriptions of the reasons given for refusing life-sustaining medical treatment in VS and related states, see Pearlman RA, Cain KC, Patrick DL, et al. Insights pertaining to patient assessments of states worse than death. *J Clin Ethics* 1993;4:33–40.

95. Payne K, Taylor RM, Stocking C, Sachs GA. Physicians' attitudes about the care of patients in the persistent vegetative state: a national survey. *Ann Intern Med* 1996;125:104–110.

96. Cassell E. Clinical incoherence about persons: the problem of the persistent vegetative state. *Ann Intern Med* 1996;125:146–147.

97. Grubb A, Walsh P, Lambe N, Murrells T, Robinson S. Survey of British clinicians' views on management of patients in persistent vegetative state. *Lancet* 1996;348:35–40. Physicians in Japan generally have a more tolerant attitude to long-term treatment of VS patients. See Asai A, Maekawa M, Akiguchi I, et al. Survey of Japanese physicians' attitudes toward the care of adult patients in persistent vegetative state. *J Med Ethics* 1999;25:302–308.

98. Tresch DD, Sims FH, Duthie EH Jr, et al. Patients in a persistent vegetative state: attitudes and reactions of family members. *J Am Geriatr Soc* 1991;39:17–21.

99. Volicer L, Berman SA, Cipolloni PB, Mandell A. Persistent vegetative state in Alzheimer disease: does it exist? *Arch Neurol* 1997;54:1382–1384.

100. For a review of legal issues in VS, see Beresford HR. The persistent vegetative state: a view across the legal divide. *Ann N Y Acad Sci* 1997;835:386–394. For a discussion and citations of the cases of Quinlan and Cruzan, among others, see chapter 8.

101. For a commentary on *Quinlan*, see Beresford HR. The Quinlan decision: problems and legislative alternatives. *Ann Neurol* 1977;2:74–81. See the further discussion in chapter 8.

102. For commentaries on Cruzan, see Meisel A. A retrospective on *Cruzan*. *Law Med Health Care* 1992;20:340–353; Capron AM (ed). Medical decision-making and the "right to die" after *Cruzan*. *Law Med Health Care* 1991;19:1–104; and White BD, Siegler M, Singer PA, et al. What does *Cruzan* mean to the practicing physician? *Arch Intern Med* 1991;151:925–928. See the further discussion in chapter 8.

103. The medical and legal facts of the Schaivo case were abstracted from Hook CC, Mueller PS. The Terri Schiavo saga: the making of a tragedy and lessons learned. *Mayo Clin Proc* 2005;80:1149–1160; Cranford RE. Facts, lies, and videotapes: the permanent vegetative state and the sad case of Terri Schiavo. *J Law Med Ethics* 2005;33:363–371; and Wolfson J. Erring on the side of Theresa Schiavo: reflections of the special *guardian ad litem*. *Hastings Cent Rep* 2005;35(3):16–19.

104. For the political and constitutional issues raised, see Annas GJ. "Culture of life" politics at the bedside—the case of Terri Schiavo. *N Engl J Med* 2005;352:1710–1715 and Gostin LO. Ethics, the constitution, and the dying process: the case of Theresa Marie Schiavo. *JAMA* 2005;293:2403–2407.

105. Twelve national opinion surveys, conducted in March and April 2005, showed that the efforts of elected politicians to intervene in the Schiavo case were opposed by the majority of Americans. See Blendon RJ, Benson JM, Herrmann MJ. The American public and the Terri Schiavo case. *Arch Intern Med* 2005;165:2580–2584.

106. There is a voluminous literature on the significance of the Schiavo case. See, for example, Quill TE. Terri Schiavo—a tragedy compounded. *N Engl J Med* 2005;352:1710–1715; Perry JE, Churchill LR, Kirshner HS. The Terri Schiavo case: legal, ethical, and medical perspectives. *Ann Intern Med* 2005;143:744–748; and Caplan AL, McCartney JJ, Sisti DJ (eds). *The Case of Terri Schiavo: Ethics at the End of Life.* Amherst, NY: Prometheus Books, 2006.

107. For a review of state laws governing physicians' orders to withhold or withdraw artificial hydration and nutrition in permanently unconscious patients, see Larriviere D, Bonnie RJ. Terminating artificial nutrition and hydration in persistent vegetative state patients: current and proposed state laws. *Neurology* 2006:66:1624–1628.

108. Bacon D, Williams MA, Gordon J. Position statement on laws and regulations concerning life-sustaining treatment, including artificial nutrition and hydration, for patients lacking decision-making capacity. *Neurology* 2007;68:1097–1100.

109. Keown J. Restoring moral and intellectual shape to the law after *Bland. Law Quart Rev* 1997;113:481–503.

110. Fox E, Stocking C. Ethics consultants' recommendations for life-prolonging treatment of patients in a persistent vegetative state. *JAMA* 1993;270:2578–2582.

111. American Academy of Neurology. Position of the American Academy of Neurology on certain aspects of the care and management of the persistent vegetative state patient. *Neurology* 1989;39:125–126 and American Academy of Neurology Quality Standards Subcommittee. Practice parameters: assessment and management of patients in the persistent vegetative state (summary statement). *Neurology* 1995;45:1015–1018. Committees of the American Academy of Neurology are currently writing new position papers on VS and PCS which are expected to be published in 2009.

112. American Neurological Association Committee on Ethical Affairs. Persistent vegetative state: report of the American Neurological Association Committee on Ethical Affairs. *Ann Neurol* 1993;33:386–391.

113. British Medical Association. *BMA Guidelines on Treatment Decisions for Patients in Persistent Vegetative States.* London: British Medical Association, 1996.

114. Royal College of Physicians. The vegetative state: guidance on diagnosis and management: a report of the working party of the Royal College of Physicians. *Clin Med* 2003;3:249–54.

115. Bonito V, Primavera A, Borghi L, Mori M, Defanti CA. The discontinuation of life support measures in patients in a permanent vegetative state. *Neurol Sci* 2002;23:131–139.

116. American Medical Association Council on Scientific Affairs and Council on Ethical and Judicial Affairs. Persistent vegetative state and the decision to withdraw or withhold life support. *JAMA* 1990;263:429 (©1990, American Medical Association; reprinted with permission).

117. American Medical Association Council on Scientific Affairs and Council on Ethical and Judicial Affairs. *JAMA* 1990:429–430 (©1990, American Medical Association; reprinted with permission).

118. Shanon TA, Walter JJ. Implications of the papal allocution on feeding tubes. *Hastings Cent Rep* 2004;34(4):18–20. See also Hamel RP, Walter JJ (eds). *Artificial Nutrition and Hydration and the Permanently Unconscious Patient: The Catholic Debate.* Washington, DC: Georgetown University Press, 2007.

119. Sulmasy DP. Terri Schiavo and the Roman Catholic tradition of forgoing extraordinary means of care. *J Law Med Ethics* 2005;33:359–362.

120. William Cardinal Levada. Prefect, Congregation for the Doctrine of the Faith. Responses to certain questions of the United States Conference of Catholic Bishops concerning artificial nutrition and hydration. August 1, 2007. http://www.vatican.va/roman_curia/congregations/cfaith/documents/rc_con_cfaith_doc_20.html (Accessed October 1, 2007).

121. *In re Jobes,* 108 NJ 394, 529 A2d 424 (1987).

122. Bernat JL. The boundaries of the persistent vegetative state. *J Clin Ethics* 1992;3:176–180.

123. Thomasma DC, Brumlik J. Ethical issues in the treatment of patients with a remitting vegetative state. *Am J Med* 1984;77:373–377.

124. Lo B, Dornbrand L, Wolf LE, Groman M. The Wendland case – withdrawing life support from incompetent patients who are not terminally ill. *N Engl J Med* 2002;346:1489–1493. For an additional commentary on the Wendland case, see Dresser R. The conscious incompetent patient. *Hastings Cent Rep* 2002;32(3):9–10.

125. For a description of this case from an expert witness neurologist who supports the patient's wife's position, see Nelson LJ. Cranford RE. Michael Martin and Robert Wendland: beyond the vegetative state. *J Contemp Health Law Policy* 1999;15:427–453.

Severe Neurological Disorders in Neonates

13

Over the past three decades, the neonatal intensive care unit (NICU), also called the intensive care nursery (ICN), has been the site of a continuing controversy over to what extent to treat critically ill neonates with profound congenital neurological abnormalities. Advances in resuscitative and life-support technology have made it possible to rescue many neonates who would have died despite maximal treatment only a short time ago. Because many of these infants remain profoundly disabled and some may never develop the capacity to experience meaningful, cognitive lives, most neonatologists have practiced "selective treatment" of at least some of them. The concept of selective treatment refers to a practice in which some neurologically damaged neonates are chosen to receive life-sustaining therapy (LST) and others, because of their dismal neurological prognosis, are permitted to die of their underlying abnormalities by withholding life-sustaining therapy.

Selective treatment raises vexing ethical questions. Should all critically ill neonates with profound congenital anomalies be treated or what severity of congenital anomaly justifies withholding or withdrawing LST? Who should decide which neonates should receive LST and which should be allowed to die? By what criteria should such decisions be made? What standards of decision making should be employed? How should disputes over the decision to treat be resolved? How should the law regulate this decision-making process? What relevance should cost factors play in decision making? How should society balance its duty to provide expensive, high-technology care for a few profoundly disabled citizens with its competing duty to provide medical care for the remainder of the population?

Public and scholarly debates on these questions over the past three decades have resulted in the convening of numerous conferences, the writing of a number of books and journal articles,[1] and the drafting of laws in the United States to regulate the practice of selective treatment of disabled infants. Over the past two decades, neonatology practices have evolved to become more uniform, suggesting an emerging consensus. However, this consensus has not become sufficiently widespread to permit the drafting of universally acceptable clinical practice guidelines for selective treatment.

A major stumbling block in developing a consensus is the irreducible medical uncertainty in determining the prognosis of neonates with congenital neurological abnormalities. Unless neonatologists can state with a high degree of certainly that the prognosis for survival or cognitive functioning of these neonates is exceedingly poor, many scholars and physicians believe that the medical profession has an overwhelming ethical duty to treat them. Most neonatologists have simply adopted the policy of "treat, wait, and see" that sidesteps the question of early selective treatment. Although this policy of treatment appears reasonable in the face of an uncertain prognosis, adopting it may create additional suffering for patients and family, produce tremendous expense to society, and delay the difficult decision to withdraw treatment until the infant is older.[2]

In this chapter, I review the history and current practices of neonatologists in selective treatment of severely neurologically impaired neonates. I discuss the principal ethical and legal issues involved and highlight the roles and conflicts of the principal decision makers, including parents, neonatologists, infant care review committees, and the courts. I discuss the results of opinion surveys and practice data regarding selective treatment. I conclude with a series of recommended clinical practice guidelines incorporating relevant ethical and medical considerations.

HISTORY

Infanticide has a long and infamous history in many cultures but it has been practiced for social, cultural, economic, and criminal reasons more than for medical ones.[3] There is an important distinction between infanticide and withholding medical treatment to allow a seriously ill infant to die. Infanticide is the purposeful killing or abandoning of an infant, usually with malicious intent, in which the neonate's state of health is irrelevant because the act alone is sufficient to produce death. By contrast, when LST is withdrawn or withheld from a severely ill neonate, the underlying medical condition alone is sufficient to cause death. Rather than being killed, infants are permitted to die of their underlying congenital disorders, which are terminal illnesses in the absence of LST. This accepted medical practice is not classified as infanticide or active euthanasia.[4]

In contemporary neonatology, the practice of selective treatment of neurologically damaged and other severely malformed neonates was highlighted in the early 1970s by the provocative reports of John Lorber in England and Raymond Duff and A.G.M. Campbell in the United States. Selective treatment was practiced earlier but not explicitly reported.[5] In a 1971 article on treatment efficacy in infants with meningomyelocele, Lorber recommended that physicians select the most severely affected babies and allow them to die by purposely not treating them.[6] In 1973, Duff and Campbell reported a consecutive series of 299 neonatal deaths in the nursery at the Yale-New Haven Medical Center in which 14% (43 infants) died because they were purposefully not treated.[7] They explained that the treatment decisions were made by physicians and parents because the baby's prognosis "for meaningful life was extremely poor or hopeless." The diagnoses of the 43 infants who were purposely permitted to die, in order of frequency, were: multiple anomalies, trisomy, cardiopulmonary disease, meningomyelocele, other central nervous system (CNS) disorders, and short bowel syndrome. The following year, the Jesuit theologian Richard McCormick published an influential article in *JAMA* identifying and analyzing the moral issues in these cases and emphasizing the need to establish treatment guidelines.[8]

By the 1980s, the percentages of neonates in NICUs who died as a result of selective treatment were even higher. A figure of 30% was quoted at Hammersmith Hospital in London[9] and a figure of 21% was reported from Aberdeen Maternity Hospital in Scotland.[10] In a NICU study from the University of California at San Francisco during 1989–1992, 73% of the 165 infant deaths resulted from withholding or withdrawal of LST based on a poor prognosis. Diagnoses of the neonates were: intracerebral hemorrhage (39%), necrotizing enterocolitis (29%), extremely low birth weight (28%), congenital abnormalities (24%), and respiratory failure (17%).[11]

Over the past 20 years, there has been a striking evolution of neonatology practices away from selective treatment.[12] In the 1970s, neonates with Down syndrome commonly did not receive standard medical and surgical treatments for curable complications.[13] In 1983, surgery for meningomyelocele was withheld from half of affected infants routinely.[14] But by the 1990s, as a result of federal laws in the United States, such as the "Baby Doe" regulations which mandated treatment and the use of infant care review committees, normative practices had evolved to aggressively treat all but the most severely neurologically damaged, exceedingly premature, and incipiently dying neonates. In summarizing this remarkable practice transformation, Norman Fost observed "A prolonged history of what is now perceived as serious undertreatment of infants with reasonable prospects for living a meaningful life was replaced by an era of serious overtreatment. One form of child abuse, neglect, was replaced by a form of medical battering. In both cases, the interests of the patient seemed to be a casualty."[15]

The resuscitation and aggressive treatment of neonates born with extreme prematurity has created an additional and growing ethical controversy in contemporary American neonatology. It is now commonplace for infants born at 23 to 25 weeks of gestation—and even some at 22 weeks—to receive aggressive support in NICUs, often at the insistence of their parents. Media publicity of cases highlighting the successful treatment of some of these babies (often without also noting the frequent treatment failures and subsequent disabilities) has led to high expectations from parents and to disputes over treatment with neonatologists.[16] There are also poignant cases in which parents refuse resuscitation and aggressive treatment that has been advocated by neonatologists.[17] These disputes between neonatologists and parents over the advisability of neonatal resuscitation have been called the tension between "medical authority and parental autonomy."[18]

Neonatal resuscitation and intensive treatment have advanced technically, but the appropriate application of these advances remains to be determined because of the statistical uncertainty about prognosis. Ethical questions arising in the care of extremely premature neonates now are a more common problem that those arising in the care of congenitally malformed neonates. The American Academy of Pediatrics (AAP) Committee on Fetus and Newborn recently published guidelines for neonatologists. The AAP acknowledges the important role of parents in decision making but states that "the physician's first responsibility is to the patient." They further advise that "The physician is not obligated to provide inappropriate treatment or to withhold beneficial treatment at the request of the parents. Treatment that is harmful, of no benefit, or futile and merely prolonging dying should be considered inappropriate. The physician must ensure that the chosen treatment

. . . is consistent with the best interest of the infant."[19]

Premature babies commonly are classified into three groups: (1) low-birth-weight (LBW) neonates weighing less than 2,500 grams; (2) very-low-birth-weight (VLBW) neonates weighing less than 1,500 grams; and (3) extremely-low-birth-weight (ELBW) neonates weighing less than 750 grams.[20] Advances in NICU technology producing successful outcomes have led neonatologists to treat LBW and VLBW babies routinely. The most vexing ethical issue is whether to treat infants in the ELBW category aggressively or allow them to die.

There is a growing evidence base recording the neurological and developmental outcomes of infants after extremely preterm births. In one study, approximately half of children born at 25 or fewer weeks of gestation have disabilities when tested at 30 months of age, and approximately half of those disabilities are severe.[21] A study of the outcomes at age 6 of extremely preterm births showed that survivors had a 86% rate of moderate-to-severe disability.[22] Another study showed an 86% mortality rate of infants weighing under 600 grams and a 44% mortality rate of infants weighing 600 to 750 grams. Over two-thirds of surviving infants tested at 30 months had impaired mental development.[23] In a study of over 4,000 ELBW infants of birth weight 401 to 500 grams, only 17% survived to discharge and most had serious comorbidities.[24] These data should be shared and discussed with parents when they consider consenting for neonatal resuscitation and other aggressive treatment for ELBW babies.[25] Jonathan Muraskas and colleagues produced an algorithm for decision making in ELBW patients, considering gestational age, birth weight, and parental decision.[26]

DIAGNOSIS AND PROGNOSIS ARE PREREQUISITES TO DECISION MAKING

As is true with clinical decision making in older patients, a clear diagnosis and prognosis are prerequisites for treatment decisions in neonates. Robert Weir and James Bale believe that neonates born with severe neurological and other profound congenital anomalies can be grouped into three general diagnostic and prognostic categories on the basis of the severity of their anomalies and their prognoses. This categorization by diagnosis and prognosis permits an ethical analysis of similar cases within each group and establishes a procedure for decision making in novel cases.[27]

The first category consists of those neonates with lethal anomalies so profound that it is beyond the best efforts of physicians and current technology to sustain their lives. Neonates in the second category have profound anomalies, but some may survive with aggressive treatment. Infants whose disorders are serious but not profound and whose lives generally can be saved with treatment comprise the third category.[28]

In a recent article, Tracy Koogler and colleagues raised an important caveat: the commonly used prognostic term "lethal anomalies" is misleading. Many obstetricians, neonatologists, and geneticists use the term "lethal anomalies" to describe infants with profound neurological compromise, structural abnormalities, or functional disabilities (such as anencephaly, trisomy 13, and trisomy 18), that, if untreated, cause death within a few months, The authors pointed out that what makes these conditions lethal is a medical decision not to treat them aggressively in light of their poor neurological prognosis.[29] This caveat should be kept in mind in the following analysis by Robert Weir and James Bale.

According to the Weir and Bale argument, clinicians have no ethical duty to attempt to treat infants in the first group because they cannot be helped by any therapy. For example, anencephalics do not survive beyond infancy, irrespective of treatment.[30] The current debate about selective treatment principally involves the second group. The survival data on infants in group two are more ambiguous than that for those in group one, but, generally, group two infants have a poor prognosis for survival or cognitive life. Nearly all neonatologists believe that infants in group three should be treated aggressively because their prognosis for survival is good and their prognosis for developing the capacity for intellectual life is at least fair.

The diagnoses in infants in group one (disorders so profound that prolonged survival is impossible or highly improbable) include anencephaly, multiple severe congenital anomalies requiring repetitive efforts to resuscitate, and profound prematurity under 22 weeks of gestation. Even the most conservative, "pro-treatment" neonatologists generally do not advocate treatment of profoundly malformed or extremely premature neonates because treatment attempts are doomed to failure.[31]

The second group of neonatal neurological disorders that many believe justifies selective nontreatment includes hydranencephaly, schizencephaly, holoprosencephaly, trisomy 13, trisomy 18, other severe chromosomal disorders (such as triploidy syndrome and 4p-syndrome), infantile Werdnig-Hoffman disease, X-linked myotubular myopathy, severe perinatal trauma, high myelomeningocele coupled with other major congenital abnormalities, severe high-cervical spinal cord injury with ventilator dependency, and large vein of Galen malformation associated with neonatal congestive heart failure. Also in the second group are disorders that present in infancy but not in the neonatal period: Canavan's disease, Alexander's disease, metabolic-storage diseases (such as Lesch-Nyan syndrome, Tay-Sachs disease, Menkes' disease, and Krabbe's disease), and infantile ceroid lipofuscinosis. The neurological conditions classified in the second group account for less than 1% of all births.[32] Premature babies of 22 to 25 weeks gestation may be added to this list because some can survive with aggressive treatment.[33]

The third group for whom aggressive treatment routinely should be ordered represents the majority of neurologically imperfect newborns. These neonates usually survive in a state of partial disability. Disorders in this group include prematurity (but greater than 25 weeks of gestation), hydrocephalus, most cases of meningomyelocele, most cases of neonatal intraventricular hemorrhage, trisomy 21, many metabolic conditions, such as phenylketonuria, maple syrup urine disease, organic acidemias, and congenital hypothyroidism, and other major congenital central nervous system malformations, such as porencephaly, agenesis of the corpus callosum, and neuronal migration disorders.[34]

Neonatologists first should make the correct diagnosis and assign neurologically impaired infants to the correct group. Usually, this task can be accomplished successfully. Generally, making the diagnosis is easier than making the prognosis with an equivalent level of certainty. Clinical inspection and neuroimaging procedures can diagnose anencephaly and major cranial and spinal malformations with a high degree of certainty. Many genetic disorders can be diagnosed confidently with chromosomal or DNA analysis. Many metabolic disorders can be diagnosed with a high level of certainly by chemical tests.

Clinicians can confidently state the outcome for survival and neurological functioning only for the first group of disorders. In the second and third groups, an inescapable degree of uncertainty exists because of the probabilistic nature of studies on the outcomes of infants with these disorders who were treated and those who were not. A statistical prognosis can be based on clinical findings, such as diagnosis, severity of illness, and presence of comorbid medical problems. This prognosis will be accurate when the outcomes of sizable numbers of similarly affected infants are averaged. However, because an individual case may fall anywhere within the statistical range, only a probabilistic statement can be issued concerning the prognosis in an individual case.[35] Wise neonatologists have adopted the position of "prognostic humility."

Neonatologists have responded to this irreducible uncertainty by adopting one of three general decision-making strategies. The first strategy is a "statistical" approach: generate practice criteria purely from statistics on outcome data that are applied to every subsequent case. For example, a statistical approach would rule that no infant born before 22 weeks gestation would be treated, because outcome data show that treatment is futile in this group.[36] The second strategy is a "wait until near certainty" approach in which all severely ill neonates in categories two and three are treated aggressively until the prognosis becomes certain. This practice is becoming increasingly common in the United States. The third strat-

egy is an "individualized approach" to initiate treatment on every infant in categories two and three and then to permit the parents the option to terminate treatment before the prognosis has become definite. This approach is more common in Great Britain.[37]

Knotty problems result from each approach. The statistical approach assumes that the outcome data on which it is based are sufficiently robust to justify the application of binding treatment rules. Although some outcome data achieve this level of clarity, other data show significant rates of false-negative and false-positive errors. With false-positive errors, viable neonates will be permitted to die unjustifiably. With false-negative errors, nonviable neonates will be treated aggressively, causing unjustified suffering to the patient and family.

One logistical problem limiting the usefulness of outcome studies is that to achieve statistical validity, outcome studies generally require that infants in each class receive uniform treatment. While such a study would comprise good science, it is unrealistic in practice because uniform treatment may be inappropriate in many cases. For example, measuring the outcomes of infants with selected fetal defects solely by seeing how long they live assumes that each infant is treated with uniform aggressiveness. Often, this assumption is erroneous because parents and physicians may feel that aggressive medical treatment is contraindicated in a particular case. Systematically incorporating these outcome data into studies as if they represented the natural history of the treated disease may be misleading and may produce the fallacy of the self-fulfilling prophecy. (See chapter 10.)

Irreducible uncertainty is another limitation of outcome studies. Alan Shewmon has demonstrated the mathematical limits to the certainty of a prognosis of "irreversible" brain damage based on experimental data from outcome studies. The irreducible degree of uncertainty results from the relatively small number of patients available for recruitment into studies from even large institutions or into interinstitutional cooperative outcome studies. When these studies are published, the investigators should also report the statistical confidence intervals to acknowledge the degree of uncertainty resulting from a small sample size.[38]

For example, John Lantos and colleagues studied the outcome of cardiopulmonary resuscitation (CPR) performed on VLBW babies (below 1,500 grams). They found that none of the babies who underwent CPR in the first three days of life survived, and only 36% of the babies who underwent CPR thereafter survived, of whom three-fourths had residual neurological deficits. They concluded that CPR was futile therapy in this group.[39] However, the number of patients they were able to study was necessarily small because of the rarity of performing CPR on VLBW babies. In fact, the reported "75% of patients" with residual neurological deficits actually represented three infants of the four infants studied. The confidence intervals were therefore necessarily very low given the small number. Anyone who attempts to develop practice guidelines from these data must take into account the statistical uncertainty resulting from the necessarily small numbers of patients studied.

The clinician who adopts the wait-until-near-certainty approach inevitably will treat some neonates who should have been permitted to die earlier. Treatment of these nonviable neonates causes them and their families to suffer, places an expensive burden on society, and postpones but does not obviate the need to terminate treatment. In some cases, this approach simply represents unwillingness by the physician or parents to make a psychologically difficult decision to terminate treatment in a timely manner.

The individualized approach permits frequent reassessments and allows the parents to see that the baby will not survive or develop the capacity for any more than a minimally cognitive existence. With this approach, both overtreatment and undertreatment errors can result, but both these errors are less likely to result than errors resulting from the first two approaches.[40] The American Medical Association Council on Ethical and Judicial Affairs opined: "It is not necessary to attain absolute or near-absolute certainty before life-sustaining treatment is withdrawn, since this goal is often unattainable and risks unnecessarily prolonging the infant's suffering."[41]

Cultural factors mold attitudes and influence behaviors of neonatologists when they decide which infants should be treated. In the EURONIC Study Group (European Project on Parents' Information and Ethical Decision Making in Neonatal Intensive Care Units), neonatologists from 10 European countries were surveyed about their attitudes and self-reported practices. Neonatologists' attitudes and practices varied by nationality, especially when comparing the question of preservation of life at any cost versus concerns about the infants' quality of life. Self-reported practices of aggressively treating versus allowing to die followed the reported attitudes.[42] In other published reports from this study, neonatologists' practices correlated positively to the laws of their countries of origin,[43] the extent of participation of parents in the decision making,[44] and the religious and moral beliefs of physicians in different countries.[45]

ETHICAL ISSUES IN TERMINATING LIFE-SUSTAINING TREATMENT

The principal ethical issues involved in withholding or withdrawing LST of neurologically ill neonates may be formulated as three questions: (1) What is the right decision? (2) Who should make the decision? and (3) By what standards should the decision be made?

The Decision to Terminate Treatment: What and How?

The substantive issue of what is the morally correct decision remains the major debatable point in this controversy. Some scholars have oversimplified the debate to the tension between addressing "quality of life" and "sanctity of life."[46] The sanctity of life argument in its purest form states that physicians and parents have the moral duty to rescue the lives of all infants unless it is technologically impossible to do so.[47] The quality of life of the rescued infant is not relevant; the overriding moral duty is to save the life.[48] The only infants who would remain purposely untreated in this scheme are those dying irreversibly and those classified in the first diagnostic group (e.g., anencephalic infants). All infants in the second and third diagnostic group should be treated.

Advocates of the primacy of the infant's quality of life in decision making must prove one critical point: some lives are so miserable and meaningless that they would be better unlived. On first inspection, it is counterintuitive to think that any infant's death would be preferable to her life. We all can imagine deriving some joy of life from even a profoundly disabled existence that would clearly justify supporting life over death. However, consider a child who survives rescue treatment in infancy to end up with severe mental retardation, quadriplegia, blindness, and seizures; who lacks the capacity to think, communicate, or give and receive love; who experiences daily suffering; and who is consigned to a wretched and painful institutional existence requiring custodial care. It is a hopeless existence of unmitigated suffering that those advocating selective treatment strive to prevent by allowing an infant to die.

There may be systematic differences in attitudes between health-care professionals and parents about the harms of a severely disabled life and therefore what is the best course of action for the severely neurologically impaired child. One survey showed that a greater percentage of neonatologists and neonatal nurses than of adolescents and their parents viewed a childhood of profound neurological impairment as a fate worse than death.[49]

Weir and Bale identified five distinct moral positions that different philosophers have advocated in the sanctity of life vs. quality of life debate. These positions range on a continuum from "conservative," in which sanctity of life is the highest ethic, to "liberal," in which quality of life is the highest ethic.[50] The most conservative moral stand dictates treatment for any infant who can be kept alive by technological support. Those irreversibly dying are the only exception in this case. Clinicians and philosophers who take the most liberal stand believe that treatment of any infant may be terminated on the basis of an arcane personhood argument. Because no infant, normal or abnormal, is yet a person, the infant lacks the same rights as a self-aware, rational person; therefore, any infant can be allowed to die.[51]

There are three more intuitively reasonable positions between these two extremes. One focuses on who would make the difficult decision instead of what constitutes the grounds for the decision. This stand gives moral authority to the decision maker's judgment. Although I consider this important question later in the chapter, the procedural issue of who should make the decision should not totally obscure the grounds for that decision. Another position, based purely on a determination of the quality of life, holds that it is morally justified to terminate treatment if the prognosis points to a serious neurological abnormality that would render the quality of life poor for the patient and her family.[52]

The final, and I believe most reasonable, position is based on a careful assessment of the infant's best interests. A best interest judgment incorporates quality-of-life considerations and potential personhood predictions. By taking this stand, a clinician attempts to balance the benefits of the salvaged life against the burdens of that life. When it can be determined that the burdens of the projected life outweigh the benefits, it becomes morally justified to allow the neonate to die by selective treatment. Such a best interest standard has been supported as the most relevant ethical analysis by the majority of physicians, philosophers, and commissions studying this controversy.[53]

The best interest judgment has several advantages. It is a substantive standard, not simply a procedural one. It is a common sense, moderate position that places a high value on neonatal life but recognizes that tragic circumstances can transform the ordinary good of existence into a meaningless life of perpetual suffering.[54] It acknowledges that we are not morally obligated to do everything possible technologically, but that we have the responsibility of stewardship; that is, we should use our technology judiciously for the good of each person and for humankind.

The best interest standard also has limitations, most importantly the innate slippery slope aspect of the quality-of-life issue. How wretched must an infant's quality of life become in the future before it is no longer in her best interest to continue to live? The British pediatrician John Lorber, an early advocate of selective treatment, wrote that a criterion for adequate quality of life should be "the ability to work or marry."[55] Clearly, he aimed far too high. On the other end of the spectrum is the standard articulated in the 1984 United States Child Abuse Amendments (see discussion below), which permitted non-treatment only if an infant was in a permanent coma or incipiently dying.[56] Closer to the mark is the standard proposed by Richard McCormick of "the potential of human relationships associated with the infant's condition."[57]

John Robertson has written eloquently that no one except a handicapped person ever can know the value of a markedly limited quality of life.[58] Although active, healthy adults performing a best interest judgment may choose death over a life of dementia, paraplegia, incontinence, and social isolation, such a judgment is not necessarily relevant to a severely handicapped person. Because the severely handicapped person never may have known the joys of intellectual activity, ambulation, continence, or social interaction, the permanent absence of these capacities would not be as disagreeable to her as their loss would be to a normal person.

The coherence of Robertson's analysis places a strict duty on everyone who employs a quality-of-life determination in a best interest judgment. They have the duty to show convincingly that early death is a preferable alternative to living because life offers only meaningless suffering without the countervailing benefits of self-awareness and social interactions. Clinicians bound by this ethical duty completely reject Lorber's criteria for quality of life and disqualify for selective treatment all patients categorized in diagnostic group three. For example, patients with uncomplicated Down syndrome should be aggressively treated as infants because, despite their multiple disabilities, they often live happy lives.[59]

One of the most difficult issues surrounds the decision to withdraw artificial hydration and nutrition (AHN) from these infants. Although also true in older patients, it is especially true that in neonates the provision of food and fluids is strongly embued with symbolic meaning regarding loving, nurturing,

and parenting.[60] Yet, decisions to withhold or withdraw treatment usually encompass cessation of AHN. In NICU ethics consultations I have performed, and in serving on my hospital infant care review committee, we often suggest offering and assisting oral hydration and nutrition when the baby can suck and swallow, but permit cessation of AHN if the infant satisfies the Baby Doe regulations discussed below.

The American Academy of Pediatrics issued a policy statement emphasizing the primacy of the physician's ordinary duty to treat:

> It is ethically and legally justified to withhold medical or surgical procedures which are clearly futile and will only prolong the act of dying. However, supportive care should be provided, including sustenance as medically indicated and relief of pain and suffering. The needs of the dying person should be respected. The family also should be supported in its grieving.
>
> In cases where it is uncertain whether medical treatment will be beneficial, a person's disability must not be the basis for a decision to withhold treatment. At all times during the process when decisions are being made about the benefit or futility of medical treatment, the person should be cared for in the medically most appropriate ways. When doubt exists at any time about whether to treat, a presumption always should be in favor of treatment.[61]

Another element in the decision to treat is the resource allocation issue: is it reasonable to treat infants with a grim neurological prognosis when the money could be used elsewhere with greater benefit? Tracy Koogler and colleagues rejected this argument, citing data showing that if all profoundly neurologically impaired neonates in NICUs were not treated the cost savings would be inconsequential.[62] However, if costs from the NICU care of ELBW babies were added, it no longer would be inconsequential.[63] Moreover, the costs attendant to rescuing a severely malformed or ill infant do not end with NICU care. These patients frequently are admitted to pediatric ICUs as they get older [64] and require impressive expenditures to cover home or institutional care.

Dana Johnson and colleagues composed six ethical propositions that provide an adequate summary of the relevant ethical issues in balancing the ordinary duty to treat with the best interest doctrine.

1. Each infant born possesses an intrinsic dignity and worth that entitles the infant (within constraints of equity and availability) to all medical and special care that is reasonably thought to be conducive to the infant's well-being.

2. The parent(s) bear the principal moral responsibility for the well-being of their infant and should be the surrogates for their infant, unless disqualified for one of the following reasons: decision-making incapacity, unresolvable disagreements between parents, or choosing a course of action that is clearly against the infant's best interest.

3. The primary role of the attending physician is to be the advocate for his/her patient, the infant. The attending physician must take all reasonable medical measures conductive to the well-being of the infant.

4. When the burden of treatment lacks compensating benefit or treatment is futile, the parent(s) and attending physician need not continue or pursue it.

5. Therapies lack compensating benefit when: (a) they serve merely to prolong the dying process; (b) the infant suffers from intolerable, intractable pain which cannot be alleviated by medical treatment; (c) the infant will be unable to participate even minimally in human experience.

6. In the care of an infant from whom life-sustaining support or curative efforts are withheld, certain provisions are necessary to continue to respect the intrinsic dignity and worth of that infant. These include: (a) warmth and physical and social comforting; (b) enteric feeding and hydration, if compatible with the above ethical proportions; (c) freedom from pain, even if administration of analgesia may inadvertently hasten death.[65]

Who Should Decide?

The next controversy surrounds who should decide whether the severely ill neonate will be treated. Potential decision makers include the parents, the neonatal intensive care unit physicians or nurses, the infant care review committee, the court, or a combination of these parties.

Parents. There is a strong tradition in the Western world, particularly in the United States, that parents should be granted the ultimate authority to make important decisions for their children. The presumption of parental authority grounds the duty of physicians treating children to obtain informed consent from the parents. Our society holds that parents know better than anyone else what is in the best interest of their children, and will actively seek out what is best for their children. The presumption of parental authority over the welfare of their children is so strong that anyone advocating an alternative decision maker has the burden of proof to show that the proposed surrogate is better than the parents.[66] Concurring, the American Medical Association Council on Ethical and Judicial Affairs stated: "In desperate situations involving newborns, the advice and judgment of the physician should be readily available, but the decision whether to exert maximal efforts to sustain life should be the choice of the parents."[67]

Parental authority, however strong, is not unlimited. The presumption of the superiority of the decision making of parents regarding their children can be overruled if there is evidence that the parents' decision is not in the best interest of their child. Some parents, for example, may wish to withhold or withdraw treatment from a slightly disabled child because they lack the desire or means to raise a child with special needs. Parents with particular religious beliefs, such as Christian Scientists or Jehovah's Witnesses, may refuse to permit their child to receive certain treatments that objectively are in the best interest of maintaining the child's health because the treatments in question are contrary to the teachings of their religion. In these instances, the basis for the presumption of parental authority is fallacious because the parents' decision generally is regarded as unfavorable to the child's best interest.[68]

Parents who are Jehovah's Witnesses or Christian Scientists would likely base their refusal of treatment in their child's best interest on their religious beliefs. However, more objective bodies such as courts nearly always rule that, although adults are permitted to die or suffer harm by refusing medical treatment on religious grounds, it is not in the best interest of children to withhold life-saving treatments from them solely on the basis of their parents' religions beliefs. Our society rejects the presumption that children would concur with their parents' ranking of medical treatment as a greater evil than death. Therefore children are presumed to prefer to receive life-saving treatment even though doing so violates their parents' religious beliefs.[69]

There is a powerful tradition in neonatology to follow the parents' wishes regarding neonatal resuscitation and treatment. J.M. Peerzada and colleagues conducted a survey of New England neonatologists regarding their practices when infants were born at the threshold of viability. They found that 93% of neonatologists regarded treating infants born at 23 weeks or earlier to be futile. Yet 33% said they would continue to provide this futile treatment at the parents' request. When neonatologists considered treatment to be of uncertain benefit, all reported that they would resuscitate when the parents requested it, 98% reported that they would resuscitate when parents were unsure, and 76% reported that they would follow parental requests to withhold resuscitation.[70]

Health-Care Professionals. Because neonatologists and neonatal intensive care unit nurses have the greatest experience in caring for severely ill neonates, some have advocated that they should be granted the authority to make the difficult decisions. However, healthcare professionals often have divergent views regarding what is in the best interest of a neonate. Some NICU staff members may believe that it is their professional duty to keep the infant alive as long as possible and at all costs, using whatever technology is necessary to accomplish this task. Others may see it as their duty to facilitate the death of the infant, ending its suffering and the consequent burden on the family, as quickly as possible.[71] The "moral distress" experienced by NICU nurses

over such decision making has been recorded in several surveys and qualitative studies.[72]

Rather than serving as primary or independent decision makers, NICU physicians and nurses should function in a shared decision-making capacity with the parents (see chapters 2 and 4). Health-care professionals have the duty to explain to parents in as great detail as necessary the medical facts about diagnosis, prognosis, and treatment options, because parents need to know these facts in order to make a rational decision. NICU physicians and nurses should recommend a specific course of treatment and work with parents to reach a shared decision.

A contemporary trend in American neonatology is family-centered neonatal care. This practice refers to the inclusion of the parents and grandparents in the day-to-day medical decision making about the severely ill neonate.[73] The concept of holding back no relevant information from parents also has been termed "transparency" in neonatal care.[74] Transparency enhances parents' trust in physicians and enables parents to understand more clearly the meaning on their child's illness. Parents are included as an integral part of the treatment team and participate in daily decision making. On some neonatology services, parents participate in daily work rounds with the treatment medical and nursing teams. Both the American Academy of Pediatrics[75] and the Canadian Paediatric Society[76] have issued official statements supporting the primacy of parents in neonatal medical decision making, especially for severely ill infants and those at the threshold of viability. One parent of an affected patient poignantly described her experience and how being given all relevant medical information was invaluable in boosting her confidence that she made the right decision.[77]

It is equally important for physicians and nurses to provide emotional support for grieving parents. Usually, parents arrive at the hospital in joyful expectation of bringing home a healthy baby. When they learn that they have a severely disabled baby, they face a lifetime of emotional and financial burdens. As a result, they often experience anger, fear, frustration, and grief in dealing with this burden. Careful attention to the parents' psychological needs is imperative as they struggle to reach a treatment decision and thereafter.[78]

The Infant Care Review Committee. The infant care review committee (ICRC) was mandated by the "Baby Doe" regulations (see below) to protect the interests of the neonate. If there is a disagreement between the physicians and the family regarding termination or continuation of medical treatment for a severely ill infant, the ICRC can help resolve the conflict. As discussed in chapter 5, a similar committee called the infant bioethics committee was recommended by the President's Commission for the Study of Ethical Problems in Medicine and Biomedical and Behavioral Research and by the American Academy of Pediatrics. Most institutions have only one committee that serves both functions. The American Academy of Pediatrics Committee on Bioethics recommended that freestanding ICRCs be dissolved and their functions be restructured under the institutional ethics committee.[79]

The ICRC or similar body is not ideally poised to be the decision maker because it is composed of members who, working at a distance from the clinical arena, should not be authorized to make clinical decisions. Further, parents are not permitted to participate in the meetings of many such committees; therefore, their critical input is presented only indirectly. In practice, ICRCs are most useful in obtaining necessary medical facts, resolving disputes, and fostering a fair decision-making process.

I believe that the ICRC ideally should serve two functions. First, it should provide a forum that brings together medical and nursing staffs, parents, and other relevant professionals to jointly discuss the infant's diagnosis, prognosis, and treatment options. The free exchange of information and opinion thus facilitated encourages optimal decision making and conflict resolution.[80] Second, the ICRC should provide procedural oversight of the decision-making process to assure that the infant's best interests are protected.[81]

Surveys of hospitals with neonatology services found that only 52% have functioning ICRCs.[82] In a questionnaire survey of neonatologists, most respondents indicated that they made difficult ethical decisions for neonates by discussing the case with parents and by presenting it to an interdisciplinary clinical care conference. They did not use ICRCs because they were unavailable or they found them neither necessary nor useful.[83]

The Courts. Most people believe that courts provide the greatest objectivity in deliberation, diligence in uncovering the relevant facts about a complex situation, and strictness in protecting the rights of patients to receive due process in decision making. In these ways, formal judicial review potentially can improve the decision-making process concerning critically ill infants.

Judicial process, however, is time-consuming and inefficient. Inevitable delays add further burdens to the overly stressed family and physician. Moreover, judicial process may be confrontational, intimidating, and expensive. Further, there is no *prima facie* reason to believe that a judge has any more expertise or wisdom to decide the right course of action than local decision makers. Judicial review should be reserved for those cases in which: (1) a child's life is in immediate danger because medical treatment has been terminated despite the availability of effective treatment sufficient to return the child to reasonably normal health; or (2) there is an intractable disagreement about appropriate treatment among primary decision makers.[84]

Weir argued that the ideal decision maker should possess four qualities: knowledge of relevant information, impartiality, emotional stability, and consistency.[85] Parents may lack impartiality, emotional stability, and consistency. Physicians, similarly, may lack complete impartiality and consistency. Courts and ICRCs are too distant and bureaucratic to make timely and relevant decisions. Because of these limitations, no decision maker alone should be granted complete authority for medical decisions concerning the severely ill infant.

Weir advocated a sequential decision-making model that incorporates each potential surrogate and provides a system of checks and balances against the limitations of each. The optimal sequence of decision making should proceed from parents to physician to ICRC to court.[86] In Weir's system, the parents are the primary decision makers. The parents' decision can be overridden by the attending physician only with clear evidence that they do not have the best interest of the infant in mind. The physician cannot overrule the parents merely because the two parties disagree. There must be evidence that the parents are inadequate decision makers and thus have failed in their ethical duty as the infant's surrogate: they may be unable to comprehend the relevant medical facts, be emotionally unstable, or appear to put their own interests before those of the neonate.

In decisions to limit or stop LST of infants who are not terminally ill, the ICRC should be asked to provide procedural oversight to assure protection of the infant's best interests. The ICRC can override the physician's decision if there is evidence that the physician is pursuing interests other than those of the seriously ill neonate. For example, he may appear to be in too great a hurry to stop LST before the prognosis is clear, or, conversely, may advocate inappropriately aggressive treatment for an unsalvageable infant. The ICRC decision can be overridden by the court in that rare instance in which the committee, too, fails to function as an adequate surrogate in protecting the infant's best interests.

Palliative Care

Any infant for whom the decision has been made to withdraw or withhold LST needs to be provided with ideal palliative care as described in chapter 7. Palliative care protocols tailored for neonates have been developed that address the needs of patients, families, and staff, and that are designed to provide a pain-free, dignified, family- and staff-supported death for neonates who cannot benefit from LST.[87] Adequate treatment of pain in neonates should be accorded a high priority and has been studied in depth.[88] The emotional needs of the staff and families in the high-stress NICU environment require vigilant attention and thoughtful management.[89] Families need ongoing information to be able to make the right decision for their neonate. The education that family members receive from neonatologists and

neonatal nurses can be supplemented with specially designed brochures and videos.[90] A growing number of hospices have developed perinatal hospice programs to provide palliative care to dying infants.

LEGAL ISSUES

The law constrains decisions to withhold or withdraw medical treatment from seriously ill neonates through several mechanisms: homicide laws, administrative regulations governing child abuse and neglect laws, and medical malpractice law.[91]

Criminal Law

Most physicians do not seriously consider liability for homicide when, following the parents' refusal of LST, they allow a neurologically impaired infant to die. John Robertson has warned, however, that physicians or parents could be held liable if they failed to treat all infants whose demise was easily preventable. According to his legal analysis, at least theoretically, physicians and parents conducting such activity could be liable for criminal offenses ranging from neglect to conspiracy to murder.[92] As a practical matter, however, this warning is probably overstated because criminal law is applied to these decisions extremely rarely.[93]

Nevertheless, Robert Weir believes that existing homicide statutes should be amended to provide immunity for parents and physicians who follow proper decision-making standards in permitting severely ill infants to die. Parents and physicians should apply a best interest standard to the neonate, which permits the termination of LST only in carefully defined and strictly justified medical conditions. The statutory amendment should contain procedural safeguards to bar the application of this practice to neonates who are less severely ill, who fail to achieve a quality of life that reflects someone's arbitrary standard other than that of best interest, or who simply are unwanted by their parents. Using the sequential decision-making model, the statute should stipulate when the ICRC and court will be called to provide oversight.[94]

I believe that as long as physicians and parents making these decisions are not being subjected to criminal prosecution, there is no pressing need to revise criminal homicide statutes to provide them immunity. Existing criminal and common law appears adequate to provide proper legal protection of the infant without unnecessarily complicating the decision-making process further.

Civil Law

Professional liability in neonatal decision making has been alleged in two related claims: actions for "wrongful birth" and actions for "wrongful life." A parent of a seriously ill child can bring an allegation of wrongful birth against a physician, claiming that the physician's negligence resulted in the birth of a defective child. Such allegations may include the physician's failure to offer genetic counseling, genetic testing, or elective abortion to prevent the child's birth, in the face of a high probability of anticipated hereditary or acquired fetal defects.[95] Suits for wrongful life may be brought later by the affected patient for the same set of allegations. Most courts have had difficulty conceptualizing the latter claim and therefore have rejected it.[96]

The most widely analyzed medical malpractice case, *Miller v. HCA*, balanced parental and physician authority to resolve a dispute over the decision to resuscitate an extremely preterm infant.[97] Karla Miller went into labor at 23 weeks gestation at which time her fetus (a girl later named Sidney) weighed an estimated 629 grams. When an amniotic infection ensued, her obstetrician and neonatologist informed her that urgent delivery was necessary despite the fact that a baby born so prematurely probably would not survive or would have profound neurological and other deficits if it did. Karla Miller and her husband then refused resuscitation and other aggressive measures and declined to permit a neonatologist in the delivery room. However, the hospital policy required resuscitation of any baby with a birth weight exceeding 500 grams. A hospital administrator requested that Mr. Miller sign a consent form for neonatal resuscitation but he refused. The neonatologist attending the birth decided that he would determine whether to perform resuscitation only after the baby was born and he could assess her condition. Sidney was born weighing 615 grams. She breathed, cried, and had Apgar scores of three at one minute and six at five minutes. The neonatologist therefore performed resuscitation and ordered mechanical ventilation. Sidney sustained a large intracranial hemorrhage a few days later producing devastating and permanent neurological impairment.

The Millers sued the hospital and its parent company HCA for battery and negligence because they required Sidney's resuscitation which the attending physicians were willing to withhold. A trial court found HCA and the hospital grossly negligent and awarded the Millers over $60 million in total damages. The Texas Court of Appeals overturned the jury verdict in ruling that, under the Texas Natural Death Act, parents could not withhold a child's life-sustaining treatment unless the child's medical condition was declared "terminal." Upon appeal, the Texas Supreme Court sustained the appeals court verdict but cited a different justification. The Court supported the neonatologist's contention that an informed decision about resuscitation could be made only after examining the infant at birth and rejected the validity of the parents' treatment refusal. A concurring judge wrote, "We hold that a physician, who is confronted with emergent circumstances and provides life-sustaining treatment to a minor child, is not liable for first obtaining consent from the parents." The ruling clarified that the refusal of resuscitation by the child's parents was irrelevant. The court decided that the physicians' authority to treat was based not on the doctrine of implied consent but simply on their duty to save the patient's life during an emergency.[98]

Administrative Law

In the Unites States, the most binding legal constraints affecting the medical treatment of seriously ill neonates are the highly publicized "Baby Doe regulations." Baby Doe was born in Bloomington, Indiana, in 1982 with Down syndrome, esophageal atresia, and tracheoesophageal fistula. His physician presented treatment options to the parents, who chose not to consent to surgical repair of the tracheoesophageal fistula and esophageal atresia because of the overall poor prognosis of the infant. Because his condition was inevitably fatal without surgery, the baby was not fed intravenously. The parents' decision was approved by a circuit judge and later upheld by the Indiana Supreme Court. The baby died during an appeal to the U.S. Supreme Court.[99]

Because of the publicity resulting from this case and from the contemporaneous case of nontreatment of a spina bifida patient from Lawrenceville, Illinois, President Reagan instructed the United States Department of Health and Human Services (DHHS) in 1983 to apply and enforce section 504 of the Rehabilitation Act of 1973 to mandate treatment of these infants. Section 504 "forbids recipients of federal funds from withholding from handicapped citizens, simply because they are handicapped, any benefit or services that would ordinarily be provided to persons without handicaps."[100] President Reagan ordered that this law be enforced to prevent future instances of withdrawing or withholding of medical treatment from seriously ill neonates.

Subsequently, the Secretary of DHHS ordered the original "Baby Doe regulations" ("Baby Doe I") to clarify how failure to treat seriously ill neonates was unlawful practice under section 504 of the Rehabilitation Act of 1973. The 1983 Baby Doe I regulations, stated: "it is unlawful . . . to withhold from a handicapped infant nutritional sustenance or medical or surgical treatment required to correct a life-threatening condition, if: (1) the withholding is based on the fact that the infant is handicapped; and (2) the handicap does not render the treatment or nutritional sustenance medically contraindicated."[101]

Baby Doe I was notorious not only for its broad inclusiveness but also for its onerous enforcement mechanisms. The telephone numbers of a toll-free hotline to the federal Office for Civil Rights and to the state child protective services agency were required to be displayed prominently so that anyone observing or suspecting noncompliance with these regulations could easily report the alleged violation to the authorities. Both the Office for Civil Rights and state child protective agencies were required to perform on-site investigations of alleged abuses.[102]

The negative response to these regulations from medical organizations and other groups was immediate and vehement. Medical journal editorials and other opinion pieces explained in detail how these regulations were unjustifiably intrusive, created an environment of fear and intimidation in the NICU, and ultimately would contribute to the worsening, not the betterment, of medical care for infants.[103] When the original regulations later were invalidated by a federal court, DHHS amended them ("Baby Doe I-R") to eliminate the onerous enforcement mechanisms, to list exceptions to the ban on terminating treatment, and to recommend that hospitals form ICRCs to oversee these decisions.[104]

In June 1984, a federal court struck down Baby Doe I-R in ruling that section 504 of the Rehabilitation Act of 1973 was intended to protect handicapped citizens and did not apply to treatment decisions for seriously ill neonates. The lower court opinion was upheld on appeal to the U.S. Supreme Court in 1986.[105]

Despite the invalidation of the original and modified Baby Doe regulations, the United States Congress moved to replace them under the newly enacted Child Abuse Amendment Act of 1984 (PL 98–457), itself a revised version of the Child Abuse and Neglect Prevention and Treatment Act. DHHS then reissued the newest Baby Doe regulations ("Baby Doe II") under the Child Abuse Amendment Act of 1984. Congress thus reclassified selective treatment of neonates as child abuse or neglect. The currently effective Baby Doe II regulations in their entirety provide:

> The term "withholding of medically indicated treatment" means the failure to respond to the infant's life-threatening conditions by providing treatment (including appropriate nutrition, hydration, and medication) which, in the treating physician's (or physicians') reasonable medical judgment, will be most likely to be effective in ameliorating or correcting all such conditions, except that the term does not include the failure to provide treatment (other than appropriate nutrition, hydration, or medication) to an infant when, in the treating physician's (or

physicians') reasonable medical judgment any of the following circumstances apply:

(i) The infant is chronically and irreversibly comatose;
(ii) The provision of such treatment would merely prolong dying, not be effective in ameliorating or correcting all of the infant's life-threatening conditions, or otherwise be futile in terms of the survival of the infant; or
(iii) The provision of such treatment would be virtually futile in terms of the survival of the infant and the treatment itself under such circumstances would be inhumane.[106]

The current Baby Doe regulations remain a source of concern in the neonatology community. In an effort to determine the impact of the Baby Doe regulations on the practices of neonatologists, Loretta Kopelman and colleagues performed a questionnaire survey of 494 practicing neonatologists. They found that 76% of neonatologists believed that the regulations were unnecessary to protect the rights of the infants, 66% believed that the regulations interfered with the parents' right to determine the treatment course that was in their infant's best interests, 60% believed that the regulations did not take into proper account the degree of infants' suffering, and 32% believed that the maximal life-prolonging therapy mandated by the regulations was not in the infants' best interests.[107]

Not only do pediatricians believe that the Baby Doe regulations are unnecessary, many of them fail to understand their provisions. In a 1987 survey of pediatricians in Massachusetts, David Todres and coworkers found that 27% of the respondents incorrectly interpreted the Baby Doe regulations to require maximal life-prolonging therapy even for anencephalic infants.[108] Todres and colleagues repeated the survey in 1999 and found stability of their earlier findings, except that a greater percentage of responders rejected infant review committees as mediators.[109]

In my experience performing ethics consultations on severely ill infants and serving on our hospital ICRC, I find that the Baby Doe regulations are considered seriously in every case of a neonate for whom withholding or withdrawing

LST is considered. There is an inescapable problem in their interpretation, however. Despite their legalistic syntax, the current Baby Doe regulations are inherently ambiguous. For example, the regulations contain the phrase "appropriate nutrition, hydration, or medication." Who is to define what therapy counts as appropriate? Could the attending neonatologist simply assert that AHN for the medical condition of a particular seriously ill neonate is not appropriate? Our hospital attorneys opined that the designers of the regulations inserted the phrase "appropriate" to increase physicians' latitude in determining what treatments should be given, but this important question remains unclear. Similarly, the clause permitting cessation of treatment, "the provision of such treatment would merely prolong dying, not be effective in ameliorating or correcting all of the infant's life-threatening conditions," plausibly could be interpreted as encompassing LST for an irreversible severe congenital neurological disorder.

The American Academy of Pediatrics (AAP) Committee on Bioethics believes that these inherent ambiguities in the Baby Doe regulations provide sufficient elasticity of interpretation that physicians can successfully conduct individualized decision making for infants employing a best interest standard.[110] In a recent article, Loretta Kopelman disagreed strongly with the AAP interpretation and argued that they reached an erroneous conclusion because they misunderstood the Baby Doe regulations and because they removed several of the regulations' key words from their intended context, such as "futile," "inhumane," "appropriate," and "reasonable medical judgment."[111]

The latest controversy over the Baby Doe regulations concerns their applicability to extremely preterm newborns of extreme low birth weight (ELBW). The Baby Doe regulations were not written to address treatment decisions for ELBW patients but have been interpreted by some legal scholars to encompass decisions about their treatment.[112] In ruling in *Miller v. HCA*, as discussed above, the Texas Supreme Court considered the applicability of the Baby Doe regulations to a hospital policy mandating neonatal resuscitation. The ambiguity of whether or how the Baby Doe regulations mandate treatment of ELBW infants has led some commentators to wonder if they should be modified.[113]

There is a tragic irony to the Baby Doe regulations. Although they mandate aggressive medical treatment for the seriously ill infant, no regulations provide for the continuing care of the infant if it survives to return home. The emotional and financial burden on families caring for these infants is enormous. Some families find caring for a severely disabled infant to be an ennobling experience, but others are destroyed by it.[114] A coherent public policy to protect these infants would not ignore their plight and that of their family once their lives had been rescued. Our society has at least as much moral responsibility to provide for the continuing care of these profoundly disabled citizens as it does to guarantee their neonatal care.

In a critique of the Baby Doe regulations, David Stevenson and colleagues predicted that the intrusion of the federal government into medical decision making in the NICU would worsen the quality of neonatal care. As an alternative to the regulations, they suggested:

> "In the true spirit of the Baby Doe legacy, a federal proclamation would probably have sufficed, indicating (1) that the 'best interest' of the child should always come first, with the accommodation of the interests of other participants insofar as they are compatible with those of the child; (2) that decision making should be fair (just) and consistent with the Constitution and its laws, and flexible enough to handle unforeseeable situations; and (3) that any guidelines for decision making should not undermine widely held moral values of our society: the sanctity of life, the equal right of all citizens to life and medical treatment, and the duty of society to protect the weak and the helpless."[115]

GUIDELINES FOR TREATMENT DECISIONS FOR SERIOUSLY ILL NEONATES

The preceding medical, ethical, and legal considerations can be summarized in a set of procedural guidelines that outline when and how LST could be limited or stopped for a seriously ill neonate.[116] Cases should be carefully individualized when clinicians apply these guidelines.

1. *Maintain active communication with the parents at every stage of the infant's care, and encourage their substantive participation in all decision making.*

2. *Establish the diagnosis or diagnoses.* The infant's precise diagnosis or diagnoses should be established confidently by appropriate examinations, tests, and consultations.

3. *Establish the prognosis with and without treatment.* The prognosis for survival and future neurological functioning with and without various types of treatment should be established as confidently as possible. If prognosis cannot be established with a high level of confidence, the probability of confidence should be communicated to the parents and used in subsequent decision making. To the greatest extent possible, the quality of life that the infant will have in the future, should she survive, should be predicted along with an assessment of its benefits and burdens.

4. *Identify and explain available treatment options.* The options for medical, surgical, and rehabilitative treatment should be explained carefully to parents. The process of explanation and question answering is time consuming and can be assisted by other staff, brochures, and videos. It often requires repeated conversations as families assimilate and discuss information.

5. *Provide emotional support and counseling for the family.* Family members require ongoing compassionate emotional support during the difficult decision-making stage.

6. *Assess if parents are adequate decision makers.* The physician should test the rationality of the parents' decision by exploring the reasons for their decision. Simply agreeing with the physician is not a satisfactory test of the adequacy of a decision. If the parents' decision-making capacity is deemed adequate, they are permitted to be the infant's surrogate decision maker. If it is not, the physician has the difficult task of identifying

an alternative surrogate. Physicians should follow parental treatment decisions unless there is evidence they are not deciding in the infant's best interests.

7. *Recommend the level of appropriate treatment.* The physician should discuss the appropriate level of treatment with the parents or other surrogate and should communicate the medical reasons behind the recommendation. The recommendation may be for aggressive treatment, for limited treatment, or for withholding or withdrawing treatment, depending on the physician's assessment of the infant's diagnosis and prognosis and on other factors. Parents need not follow the physician's recommendation.

8. *Assess compliance with the Baby Doe regulations* (United States only). Only permanent coma, incipient death, or permanent and profound impairment of cognitive functioning should be used as a diagnostic or prognostic factor favoring nontreatment.

9. *Provide optimal palliative care to the infant.* A palliative care consultation should be requested if available and if the clinician is unsure how to provide optimal palliative care.

10. *Request that the infant care review committee oversee the case.* Review by the ICRC, the hospital ethics committee, or another neonatologist is generally desirable in cases in which treatment will be limited or terminated because the ICRC can oversee the decision-making process to insure that it protects the infant's interests. This review is particularly important in those instances in which the physician and the parents or other surrogate disagree or the surrogate has made a decision for reasons that are not altruistic.

11. *Refer the case to court for judicial review* (exceptional circumstances only). The court should designate a formal surrogate if there is an intractable disagreement between the physicians and surrogate, if the parents are deemed inadequate surrogates, or if the hospital attorney urges this course of action for valid legal reasons.

NOTES

1. The most carefully argued book on the subject is Weir RF. *Selective Nontreatment of Handicapped Newborns: Moral Dilemmas in Neonatal Medicine.* New York: Oxford University Press, 1984. See also Kuhse H. Singer P. *Should the Baby Live? The Problem of Handicapped Infants.* New York: Oxford University Press, 1985; Murray TH, Caplan AL, eds. *Which Babies Shall Live? Humanistic Dimensions of the Care of Imperiled Newborns.* Clifton, NJ: Humana Press, 1985; Shelp EE. *Born to Die? Deciding the Fate of Critically Ill Newborns.* New York: Free Press, 1986; Anspach RR. *Deciding Who Lives: Fateful Choices in the Intensive Care Nursery.* Berkeley: University of California Press, 1992; and, most recently, Lantos JD, Meadow WL. *Neonatal Bioethics: The Moral Challenges of Medical Innovation.* Baltimore: Johns Hopkins University Press, 2006.

2. Caplan A, Cohen CB, eds. Imperiled newborns. *Hastings Cent Rep* 1987:17(6):5–32.

3. For reviews of infanticide, see Hausfater G, Hardy SB (eds). *Infanticide: Comparative and Evolutionary Perspectives.* New York: Aldine, 1984 and Wissow LS. Infanticide. *N Engl J Med* 1998;339:1239–1241.

4. As discussed in chapter 9, euthanasia remains illegal in nearly all jurisdictions throughout the world. The euthanasia of hopelessly ill newborns is practiced in the Netherlands under the controversial "Groningen Protocol." See Verhagen E, Sauer PJJ. The Groningen Protocol—euthanasia in severely ill newborns. *N Engl J Med* 2005;352:959–962. However, euthanasia is practiced currently in the Netherlands in only 1% of neonatal end-of-life decisions. See Vrakking AG, van der Heide A, Onwuteaka-Philipsen BD, Keij-Deerenberg IM, van der Maas PJ, van der Wal G. Medical end-of-life decisions made for neonates and infants in the Netherlands. *Lancet* 2005;365:1329–1331. For a thoughtful essay arguing that the Groningen Protocol is unethical and unjustified, see Chervenak FA, McCullough LB, Arabin B. Why the Groningen Protocol should be rejected. *Hastings Cent Rep* 2006;36(5):30–33.

5. For a history of selective treatment, see Paris JJ, Ferranti J, Reardon F. From the Johns Hopkins baby to Baby Miller: what have we learned from four decades of reflection on neonatal cases? *J Clin Ethics* 2001;12:207–214.

6. Lorber J. Results of treatment of myelomeningocele: an analysis of 524 unselected cases, with special reference to possible selection for treatment. *Dev Med Child Neurol* 1971:13:279–303.

7. Duff RS, Campbell AGM. Moral and ethical dilemmas in the special care nursery. *N Engl J Med* 1973:289:890–894.

8. McCormick RA. To save or let die: the dilemma of modern medicine. *JAMA* 1974;229:172–176.

9. Whitelaw A. Death as an option in neonatal intensive care. *Lancet* 1986;2:328–331.

10. Campbell AGM. Which infants should not receive intensive care? *Arch Dis Child* 1982;57:569–571.

11. Wall SN, Partridge JC. Death in the intensive care nursery: physician practice of withdrawing and withholding life support. *Pediatrics* 1997;99:64–70. This series included patients with acquired as well as congenital conditions and can be compared to similar data reported from adult ICUs. See Prendergast TJ, Claessens MT, Luce JM. A national survey of end-of-life care for critically ill patients. *Am J Respir Crit Care Med* 1998;158:1163–1167.

12. Fost N. Decisions regarding treatment of seriously ill newborns. *JAMA* 1999;281:2041–2043.

13. Todres ID, Krane D, Howell MC, Shannon DC. Pediatricians' attitudes affecting decision-making in defective newborns. *Pediatrics* 1977;60:197–201 and Shaw A, Randolph JG, Manard B. Ethical issues in pediatric surgery: a nationwide survey of pediatricians and pediatric surgeons. *Pediatrics* 1977;60:588–599.

14. Gross RH, Cox A, Tetyrek R, et al. Early management and decision making for the treatment of myelomeningocele. *Pediatrics* 1983;72:450–458. In the first edition of this book (1994), I discussed the published criteria pediatric surgeons developed for determining which neonates with myelomeningocele should receive surgical closure. The major criterion for treatment was the infant's capacity for intellectual functioning but other criteria also were used. By comparison, today, no cognitively intact neonates are selectively not treated irrespective of their degree of paralysis. For a sample of the older literature and guidelines, see Gross RH. Newborns with myelodysplasia: the rest of the story. *N Engl Med* 1985;312:1632–1634; Charney EB, Weller SC, Sutton LN, et al. Management of the newborn with myelomeningocele: time for a decision making process. *Pediatrics* 1985;75:58–64; Evans RC, Tew B, Thomas MD, et al. Selective surgical management of neural tube malformations. *Arch Dis Child* 1985;60:415–419; Tew B. Evans R. Thomas M, et al. The results of a selective surgical policy on the cognitive abilities of children with spina bifida. *Dev Med Child Neurol* 1985;27:606–614; Freeman JM. Early management and decision making for the treatment of myelomeningocele: a critique. *Pediatrics* 1984;73:564–566; Freeman JM, McDonnell K. Termination of care in newborn infants. *Semin Neurol* 1984;4:30–35; Fost N. Counseling families who have a child with a severe congenital anomaly. *Pediatrics* 1981;67:321–324; and McLaughlin JF, Shurtleff DB, Lamers JY, Stuntz JT, Hayden PW, Kropp RJ. Influence of prognosis on decisions regarding the care of newborn with myelodysplasia. *N Engl J Med* 1985;312:1589–1594.

15. Fost N. Decisions regarding treatment of seriously ill newborns. *JAMA* 1999;281: 2041–2043. For a moving essay written by an experienced pediatric neurologist showing the evolution of his thinking over three decades of practice, and explaining how he became aware of his biases, see Freeman JM. On learning humility: a thirty-year journey. *Hastings Cent Rep* 2004;34(3):13–16.

16. Fine RL, Whitfield JM, Carr BL, Mayo TW. Medical futility in the intensive care unit: hope for a resolution. *Pediatrics* 2005;116:1219–1222.

17. Pinkerton J, Finnerty JJ, Lombardo PA, Rorty MV, Chapple H, Boyle RJ. Parental rights at the birth of a near-viable infant: conflicting perspectives. *Am J Obstet Gynecol* 1997;177:283–290. For the most heartrending account of neonatal overtreatment, see Stinson R, Stinson P. *The Long Dying of Baby Andrew*. Boston: Little, Brown, 1983.

18. McHaffie HE, Laing IA, Parker M, McMillan J. Deciding for imperiled newborns: medical authority or parental autonomy? *J Med Ethics* 2001;27:104–109.

19. American Academy of Pediatrics Committee on fetus and Newborn. Noninitiation or withdrawal of intensive care for high-risk newborns. *Pediatrics* 2007;119:401–403.

20. Carter BS, Stahlman M. Reflections on neonatal intensive care in the US: limited success or success with limits? *J Clin Ethics* 2001;12:215–222.

21. Wood NS, Marlow N, Costeloe K, Gibson AT, Wilkinosn AR. Neurologic and developmental disability after extremely preterm birth. *N Engl J Med* 2000;343:378–384.

22. Marlow N, Wolke D, Bracewell MA, Samara M; Epicure Study Group. Neurologic and developmental disability at six years of age after extremely preterm birth. *N Engl J Med* 2005;352:9–19.

23. Agustines LA, Lin YG, Rumney PJ, et al. Outcomes of extremely low-birth-weight infants between 600 and 750 g. *Am J Obstet Gynecol* 2000;182:1113–1116.

24. Lucey JF, Rowan CA, Shiono P, et al. Fetal infants: the fate of 4172 infants with birth weights of 401 to 500 grams—the Vermont Oxford Network experience (1996–2000). *Pediatrics* 2005;113:1559–1565.

25. Cole FS. Extremely preterm birth—defining the limits of hope. *N Engl J Med* 2000;343:429–430. There is evidence that parental counseling may be inadequate in some practices. See Janvier A, Barrington KJ. The ethics of neonatal resuscitation at the margins of viability: informed consent and outcomes. *J Pediatr* 2005; 147:579–585.

26. Muraskas J, Marshall PA, Tomich P, Myers TF, Gianopoulos JG, Thomasma DC. Neonatal viability in the 1990s: held hostage by technology. *Camb Q Healthc Ethics* 1999;8:160–172.

27. Weir RF, Bale JF Jr. Selective nontreatment of neurologically impaired neonates. *Neurol Clin* 1989;7: 807–821.

28. Weir RF, Bale JF Jr. *Neurol Clin* 1989:808.

29. Koogler TK, Wilford BS, Ross LF. Lethal language, lethal decisions. *Hastings Cent Rep* 2003;33(2):37–41.

30. For the prognosis of anencephaly see Medical Task Force on Anencephaly. The infant with anencephaly. *N Engl J Med* 1990;322:669–674. However, the anecephalic infant Baby K discussed in chapter 10 survived over 2 years with aggressive treatment. Extraordinary cases like Baby K show that "lethal anomalies" are lethal because of a decision not to treat. See note 29.

31. The categories and lists of neurological diagnoses are taken from Weir RF, Bale JF Jr. *Neurol Clin* 1989:808. The data showing the fultility of treatment attempts on babies of less than 22 weeks of gestation are from Allen MC. Donohue PK, Dusman AE. The limit of viability—neonatal outcome of infants born at 22 to 25 weeks' gestation. *N Engl J Med* 1993,329:1597–1601.

32. Weir RF. Bale JF Jr. *Neurol Clin* 1989:808. Personal communication. Dr. Stephen Ashwal. February 4, 1994.

33. Allen MC, Donohue PK, Dusman AE. *N Engl J Med* 1993:1597–1601.

34. Weir RF Bale JF Jr. *Neurol Clin* 1989:808 and Allen MC, Donohue PK, Dusman AE. *N Engl J Med* 1993:1597–1601. Personal communication, Dr. Stephen Ashwal. February 4, 1994.

35. For articles discussing the problem of uncertainty in neonatology, see Coulter DL. Neurologic uncertainty in newborn intensive care. *N Engl J Med* 1987;316:840–844; Fischer AF, Stevenson DK. The consequences of uncertainty: an empirical approach to medical decision making in neonatal intensive care. *JAMA* 1987;258:1929–1931; Beresford EB. Uncertainty and the shaping of medical decisions. *Hastings Cent Rep* 1991;21(4):6–11; and Rhoden NK. Treating Baby Doe: the ethics of uncertainty. *Hastings Cent Rep* 1986;16(4):34–42.

36. Allen MC, Donohue PK, Dusman AE. *N Engl J Med* 1993:1597–1601.

37. Caplan A, Cohen CB, eds. *Hastings Cent Rep* 1987:11–12. General practice guidelines for British pediatricians have been published. The Royal College of Paediatrics and Child Health outlined five situations in which withholding or withdrawing curative medical treatment might be considered: (1) brain death; (2) the permanent vegetative state; (3) the "no chance" situation in which LST merely delays death; (4) the "no purpose" situation in which the degree of physical or mental impairment will be so great that it is unreasonable to expect a child to endure it; and (5) the "unbearable" situation in which further treatment adds more burdens than can be borne. See Royal College of Paediatrics and Child Health. *Withholding or Withdrawing Life Saving Treatment in Children*. London: Royal College of Paediatrics and Child Health, 1997.

38. See Shewmon DA. The probability of inevitability. The inherent impossibility of validating criteria for brain death or "irreversibility" through clinical studies. *Stat Med* 1987;535–554 and Shewmon DA, De Giorgio CM. Early prognosis in anoxic coma: reliability and rationale. *Neurol Clin* 1989;7:823–843.

39. Lantos JD, Miles SH, Silverstein MD, Stocking CB. Survival after cardiopulmonary resuscitation in babies of very low birth weight: is CPR futile therapy? *N Engl J Med* 1988;318:91–95. See also Lantos JD, Meadow W, Miles SH, et al. Providing and forgoing resuscitative therapy for babies of very low birth weight. *J Clin Ethics* 1992;3:283–287. The concept of medical futility is analyzed in chapter 10.

40. Problems with the three decision-making approaches are discussed further in Caplan A. Cohen CB, eds. *Hastings Cent Rep* 1987:11–12.

41. American Medical Association Council on Ethical and Judicial Affairs. Treatment decisions for seriously ill newborns. In *Code of Medical Ethics of the American Medical Association: Current Opinions with Annotations*, 2006–2007 edition. Chicago: American Medical Association, 2006:103.

42. Rebagliato M, Cuttini M, Broggin L, et al. Neonatal end-of-life decision making: physicians' attitudes and relationship with self-reported practices in 10 European countries. *JAMA* 2000;284:2451–2459 and Cuttini M, Nadai M, Kaminski M, et al. End-of-life decisions in neonatal intensive care. *Lancet* 2000;355: 2112–2118.

43. McHaffie HE, Cuttini M, Brolz-Voit G, et al. Withholding/withdrawing treatment from neonates: legislation and official guidelines across Europe. *J Med Ethics* 1999;25:440–446.

44. Cuttini M, Rebagliato M, Bortoli P, et al. Parental visiting, communication and participation in ethical decisions: a comparison of neonatal unit policies in Europe. *Arch Dis Child Fetal Neonatal Ed* 1999;81:F84-F91.

45. Cuttini M, EURONIC Study Group. The European Union Collaborative Project on Ethical Decision Making in Neonatal Intensive Care (EURONIC): findings from 11 countries. *J Clin Ethics* 2001;12:290–296. For practices elsewhere in the world, see the symposium on international practice of neonatal ethics in *J Clin Ethics* 2001;12:282–318; Burmel J (ed). Caring for newborns: three world views. *Hastings Cent Rep* 1986;16(4):18–23; and Van Leeuwen E, Kimsnia GK. Acting or letting go: medical decision making in neonatology in the Netherlands. *Cambridge Q Healthc Ethics* 1993;2:265–269.

46. Singer P. Sanctity or life or quality of life. *Pediatrics* 1983;72:128–129.

47. For example, see Koop CE. The sanctity of life. *J Med Soc New Jersey* 1978;75:62–69.

48. This position has been defended on moral grounds in Vehmas S. Newborn infants and the moral significance of intellectual disabilities. *J Assoc Sev Handicap* 1999;24:111–121.

49. Saigal S, Stoskopf BL, Feeny D, et al. Differences in preferences for neonatal outcomes among health care professionals, parents, and adolescents. *JAMA* 1999;281:1991–1997.

50. Weir RF, Bale JF Jr. *Neurol Clin* 1989:813–817.

51. The philosopher Peter Singer has forcefully adopted this extreme position against much protest. See Singer P. *Rethinking Life and Death: The Collapse of Our Traditional Ethics.* New York: St. Martin's Press, 1994.

52. Narrative accounts of the painful process of this decision making have been sensitively recorded. See, for example, Jones C, Freeman JM. Decision making in the nursery: an ethical dilemma. *J Clin Ethics* 1998;9:314–322 and the accompanying editorial Howe EG. Treating infants who may die. *J Clin Ethics* 1998;9: 215–224.

53. Those concurring with the superiority of the best interests standard in neonates include: President's Commission for the Study of Ethical Problems in Medicine and Biomedical and Behavioral Research. *Deciding to Forego Life-Sustaining Treatment: Ethical, Medical, and Legal Issues in Treatment Decisions.* Washington, DC: US Government Printing Office, 1983:217–223; Caplan A, Cohen CB, eds. *Hastings Cent Rep* 1987: 17(6):11–12; Weir RF. *Selective Nontreatment of Handicapped Newborns: Moral Dilemmas in Neonatal Medicine,* 1984; Childress JF. Protecting handicapped newborns: who's in charge and who pays? In Milunsky A, Annas GJ, eds. *Genetics and the Law:* Vol 3. New York: Plenum Press, 1985:271–281; and Fost N. Ethical issues in the treatment of critically ill newborns. *Pediatr Ann* 1981;10:16–22. For the most recent analysis and discussion, see Kopelman LM. The best interests standard for incompetent or incapacitated persons of all ages. *J Law Med Ethics* 2007;35:187–196.

54. Walters JW. Approaches to ethical decision making in the neonatal intensive care unit. *Am J Dis Child* 1988; 142:825–830. The best interest standard was debated in Brody H. In the best interests of.... *Hastings Cent Rep* 1988;18:37–39 and Bartholeme W. In the best interests of.... *Hastings Cent Rep* 1988;18:39–40.

55. Lorber J. Ethical problems in the management of meningomyelocele and hydrocephalus. *J Royal Coll Phys* 1975;10(1):47–60, as quoted in Caplan A, Cohen CB, eds. *Hastings Cent Rep* 1987:15.

56. Child Abuse Amendments of 1984 (PL 98–457) [codified as amended at 42 USCA §§5101–5104 (West. Supp. 1985)]. As quoted in Caplan A, Cohen CB, eds. *Hastings Cent Rep* 1987:15.

57. McCormick R. To save or let die: the dilemma of modern medicine. *JAMA* 1974;229:172–176. Quote taken from Caplan A, Cohen CB, eds. *Hastings Cent Rep* 1987:15.

58. Robertson J. Involuntary euthanasia of defective newborns. *Stanford Law Rev* 1975:27:213–269. See also Arras JD. Toward an ethic of ambiguity. *Hastings Cent Rep* 1984;14(2):25–33.

59. Smith GF, Diamond E, Lejeune J, et al. The rights of infants with Down syndrome. *JAMA* 1984;251:229. An analogous situation exists in children with perinatal brain insults that lead to cerebral palsy. School-age children with cerebral palsy rate their own quality of life similarly to the self-ratings by healthy peers. See Dickinson HO, Parkinson KN, Ravens-Sieberer U, et al. Self-reported quality of life of 8–12 year old children with cerebral palsy: a cross-sectional European study. *Lancet* 2007;369:2171–2178.

60. Nelson LJ, Rushton CH, Cranford RE, Nelson RM, Glover JJ, Truog RD. Forgoing medically provided nutrition and hydration in pediatric patients. *J Law Med Ethics* 1995;23:33–46. See also Johnson J, Mitchell C. Responding to parental requests to forego pediatric nutrition and hydration. *J Clin Ethics* 2000;11: 128–132.

61. American Academy of Pediatrics. Joint policy statement: principles of treatment of disabled newborns. *Pediatrics* 1984;73:559–560.

62. Koogler TK, Wilford BS, Ross LF. Lethal language, lethal decisions. *Hastings Cent Rep* 2003;33(2):37–41.

63. Carter BS, Stahlman M. Reflections on neonatal intensive care in the US: limited success or success with limits? *J Clin Ethics* 2001;12:215–222.

64. Smith K, Uphoff ME. Uncharted terrain: dilemmas born in the NICU grow up in the PICU. *J Clin Ethics* 2001;12:231–238.

65. Johnson DE. Thompson TR, Aroskar M, Cranford RE. "Baby Doe" rules: there are alternatives. *Am J Dis Child* 1984;138:523–529.

66. Caplan A, Cohen CB, eds. *Hastings Cent Rep* 1987:17. The unique role of the parents in the model of shared medical decision making in neonatal critical care is discussed in Harrison H. The principles of family centered neonatal care. *Pediatrics* 1993;92:643–650.

67. American Medical Association. *American Medical Association Judicial Council: Opinions and Reviews.* Chicago: American Medical Association, 1982.

68. Walters JW. *Am J Dis Child* 1988:825–830. See also Fost N. *Pediatrics* 1981:321–324.

69. See Vinicky JK, Smith ML, Connors RB Jr, et al. The Jehovah's Witness and blood: new perspectives on an old dilemma. *J Clin Ethics* 1990;1:65–71 and Layon AJ, D'Amico R. Caton D, et al. And the patient chose: medical ethics and the case of the Jehovah's Witness. A*nesthesiology* 1990;73:1258–1262.

70. Peerzada JM, Richardson DK, Burns JP. Delivery room decision making at the threshold of viability. *J Pediatr* 2004;145:492–498.

71. Caplan A, Cohen CB, eds. *Hastings Cent Rep* 1987:18–19. See the data showing the differing attitudes between neonatologists and parents, discussed in note 49.

72. See Miya PA, Boardman KK, Harr KL, Keene A. Ethical issues described by NICU nurses. *J Clin Ethics* 1991;2:253–257 and Hefferman P, Heilig S. Giving "moral distress" a voice: ethical concerns among neonatal intensive care unit personnel. *Camb Q Healthc Ethics* 1999;8:173–178.

73. Harrison H. The principles for family-centered neonatal care. *Pediatrics* 1993;92;643–650. The application of family-centered neonatal care has been illustrated in the film "Dreams and Dilemmas: Parents and the Practice of Neonatal Care" by Richard Kahn. See Little GA, Kahn R, Green RM. Parental dreams, dilemmas, and decision making in *cinéma vérité. J Perinatol* 1999;19:194–196.

74. King NMP. Transparency in neonatal intensive care. *Hastings Cent Rep* 1992;22(3):18–25.

75. American Academy of Pediatrics Committee on Fetus and Newborn, and the American College of Obstetricians and Gynecologists Committee on Obstetrical Practice. Perinatal care at the threshold of viability. *Pediatrics* 1995;96:974–976.

76. Canadian Paediatric Society Fetus and Newborn Committee and Maternal-Fetal Medicine Committee, and the Society of Obstetricians and Gynaecologists of Canada. Management of the woman with threatened birth of an infant of extremely low gestational age. *Can Med Assoc J* 1994;151:547–553.

77. Harrison H. Making lemonade: a parent's view of "quality of life" studies. *J Clin Ethics* 2001;12: 239–250.

78. The reaction of parents to the news that their baby is severely disabled and the duty of physicians to support them emotionally have been described sensitively in several papers. See Silverman WA. Overtreatment of neonates? A personal retrospective. *Pediatrics* 1992;90:971–976; Jellinek MS, Catlin EA, Todres ID, et al. Facing tragic decisions with parents in the neonatal intensive care unit: clinical perspectives. *Pediatrics* 1992;89:119–122; and White MP, Reynolds B, Evans TJ. Handling of death in special care nurseries and parental grief. *Br Med J* 1984;289:167–169.

79. American Academy of Pediatrics Committee on Bioethics. Institutional ethics committees. *Pediatrics* 2001;107:205–209.

80. Nelson RM, Shapiro RS. The role of an ethics committee in resolving conflict in the neonatal intensive care unit. *J Law Med Ethics* 1995;23:27–32.

81. Weir RF. Pediatric ethics committees: ethical advisors or legal watchdogs? *Law Med Health Care* 1987;15(3):99–109. See also Caplan A, Cohen CB, eds. *Hastings Cent Rep* 1987:20–21.

82. Fleming GV, Hud SS, LeBailey SA, et al. Infant care review committees: the response to federal guidelines. *Am J Dis Child* 1990;144:778–881.

83. Carter BS. Neonatologists and bioethics after Baby Doe. *J Perinatol* 1993:13:144–150.

84. Caplan A, Cohen CB, eds. *Hastings Cent Rep* 1987:19–20.

85. Weir RF. *Selective Nontreatment of Handicapped Newborns: Moral Dilemmas in Neonatal Medicine,* 1984.

86. Weir RF. *Selective Nontreatment of Handicapped Newborns: Moral Dilemmas in Neonatal Medicine,* 1984. A similar sequential decision-making model had been outlined earlier in Childress JF. *Who Should Decide?* New York: Oxford University Press, 1982.

87. Catlin A, Carter BS. Creation of a neonatal end-of-life palliative care protocol. *J Clin Ethics* 2001;12: 316–318.

88. Franck L, Lefrak L. For crying out loud: the ethical treatment of infants' pain. *J Clin Ethics* 2001;12:275–281.

89. Reddick BH, Catlin E, Jellinek M. Crisis within crisis: recommendations for defining, preventing, and coping with stressors in the NICU. *J Clin Ethics* 2001;12:254–265.

90. Hulac P. Creation and use of *You are Not Alone*, a video for parents facing difficult decisions. *J Clin Ethics* 2001;12:251–253.

91. For reviews of the legal issues, see Merrick JC. Critically ill newborns and the law: the American experience. *J Legal Med* 1995;16:189–209 and Meisel A, Cerminara KL. *The Right to Die: The Law of End-of-Life Decisionmaking*, 3rd ed. Aspen Publishers, Inc, 2004.

92. Robertson J. Involuntary euthanasia of defective newborns. *Stanford Law Rev* 1975;27:213–269. For general reviews of the legal aspects of termination of treatment of infants, see Weir RF. *Selective Nontreatment of Handicapped Newborns: Moral Dilemmas in Neonatal Medicine*, 1984; Ellis TS III. Letting defective babies die. Who decides? *Am J Law Med* 1982;7:39.3–423; and Skene L. Legal issues in treating critically ill newborn infants. *Camb Q Healthc Ethics* 1993;2:295–308.

93. Two instances in which criminal homicide charges were filed were discussed in Wall SN, Partridge JC. Death in the intensive care nursery: physician practice of withdrawing and withholding life support. *Pediatrics* 1997;99:64–70. These cases were *People of the State of Michigan v Gregory Messenger*, Ingraham County Circuit Court, Lansing, MI, Docket 94–67694FH, February 2, 1995 and *State of Georgia v Eva D Carrizales*, Clayton County Superior Court, Jonesboro, GA, Docket 93-CR-01707–06, November 1, 1994.

94. Weir RF. *Selective Nontreatment of Handicapped Newborns: Moral Dilemmas in Neonatal Medicine*, 1984.

95. See Coplan J. Wrongful life and wrongful birth: new concepts for the pediatrician. *Pediatrics* 1985;75:65–71. See also Shaw MW. To be or not to be? That is the question. *Am J Hum Genet* 1984;36:1–9 and Botkin JR, Mehlman MJ. Wrongful birth: medical, legal, and philosophical issues. *J Law Med Ethics* 1994;22: 21–28.

96. See Botkin JR. The legal concept of wrongful life. *JAMA* 1988;259:1541–1545 and Steinbock B. The logical case for "wrongful life." *Hastings Cent Rep* 1986:16(2):15–20.

97. Facts of the Sidney Miller case were abstracted from Annas GJ. Extremely preterm birth and parental authority to refuse treatment—the case of Sidney Miller. *N Engl J Med* 2004;351:2118–2123. I also relied on discussions in Robertson JA. Extreme prematurity and parental rights after Baby Doe. *Hastings Cent Rep* 2004;34(4):32–39 and Sayeed SA. The marginally viable newborn: legal challenges, conceptual inadequacies, and reasonableness. *J Law Med Ethics* 2006;34:600–610.

98. Annas GJ. Extremely preterm birth and parental authority to refuse treatment–the case of Sidney Miller. *N Engl J Med* 2004;351:2118–2123.

99. For a general account of the Baby Doe case, see Pless JE. The story of Baby Doe. *N Engl J Med* 1983;309;664. For later commentaries, see Stevenson DK, Ariagno RL, Kutner JS, Raffin TA, Young EWD. The "Baby Doe" rule. *JAMA* 1986;256:1909–1912; Angell M. The Baby Doe rules. *N Engl J Med* 1986;314:642–644; and Lantos J. Baby Doe five years later: implications for child health. *N Engl J Med* 1987;317:444–447. For general reviews on the legal and ethical issues raised by the Baby Doe regulations, see Gostin L. A moment in human development: legal protection, ethical standards and social policy on the selective non-treatment of handicapped neonates. *Am J Law Med* 1986;9:455–468 and Lund N. Infanticide, physicians, and the law: the "Baby Doe" amendments to the Child Abuse Prevention and Treatment Act. *Am J Law Med* 1986;9:1–29.

100. U.S. Rehabilitation Act. Public Law 93–112, 29 USC 794 (1973), §504.

101. Department of Health and Human Services. Nondiscrimination on the basis of handicap: interim final rule. *Federal Register* 1983:48:96310–96320 and *Federal Register* 1983:48:30846–30852.

102. See discussion in Angell M. The Baby Doe rules. *N Engl J Med* 1986;314:642–644.

103. For example, see Angell M. Handicapped children: Baby Doe and Uncle Sam. *N Eng J Med* 1983;309: 659–661; Weir RF. The government and selective nontreatment of handicapped infants. *N Eng J Med* 1983;309:661–663; and Shapiro DL, Rosenberg P. The effect of federal regulations regarding handicapped newborns: a case report. *JAMA* 1984;25:2031–2033.

104. Department of Health and Human Services. Nondiscrimination on the basis of handicap: procedures and guideline, relating to health care for handicapped infants. *Federal Register* 1984;49:1622–1654 and Department of Health and Human Services. Office of Human Development Services. Services and treatment for disabled infants: interim model guidelines for health care providers to establish infant care review

committees. *Federal Register* 1984;49:48170–48173. For a commentary, see Murray TH. The final, anticlimactic rule on Baby Doe. *Hastings Cent Rep* 1985;15(3):5–9.

105. See Moskop JC, Saldanha RL. The Baby Doe rule: still a threat. *Hastings Cent Rep* 1986;16(2):8–14.

106. Child Abuse and Neglect Prevention and Treatment Program, final edition. *Federal Register* 1985;50: 14878–14888.

107. Kopelman LM, Irons TG. Kopelman AE. Neonatologists judge the "Baby Doe" regulations. *N Engl J Med* 1988;318:677–683.

108. Todres ID, Guillemin J, Grodin MA, et al. Life-saving therapy for newborns: a questionnaire survey in the state of Massachusetts. *Pediatrics* 1988;81:643–649.

109. Todres ID, Guillemin J, Catlin EA, Marlow A, Nordstrom A. Moral and ethical dilemmas in critically ill newborns: a 20-year follow-up survey of Massachusetts pediatricians. *J Perinatol* 2000;20:6–12.

110. American Academy of Pediatrics Committee on Bioethics. Ethics and the care of critically ill children and newborns. *Pediatrics* 1996;98:149–153.

111. Kopelman LM. Are the 21-year-old Baby Doe rules misunderstood or mistaken? *Pediatrics* 2005;115:797–802.

112. See, for example, Robertson JA. Extreme prematurity and parental rights after Baby Doe. *Hastings Cent Rep* 2004;34(4):32–39 and Sayeed SA. The marginally viable newborn: legal challenges, conceptual inadequacies, and reasonableness. *J Law Med Ethics* 2006;34:600–610.

113. Robertson JA. Extreme prematurity and parental rights after Baby Doe. *Hastings Cent Rep* 2004;34(4):32–39.

114. The general subject of the impact of the severely ill neonate on the family has been considered in Strong C. Defective infants and their impact on families: ethical and legal considerations. *Law Med Health Care* 1983;11(4):168–172. See also Caplan A, Cohen CB. *Hastings Cent Rep* 1987:25–30.

115. Stevenson DK, Ariagno RL, Kutner JS, Raffin TA, Young EWD. The "Baby Doe" rule. *JAMA* 1986;256:1909–1912.

116. Other authors have drafted different guidelines. See, for example, Benitz WE. A paradigm for making difficult choices in the intensive care nursery. *Camb Q Healthc Ethics* 1993;2:281–294 and Weir RF, Bale JF Jr. Selective nontreatment of neurologically impaired neonates. *Neurol Clin* 1989;7:807–821. The Ethics Committee of the International Federation of Gynecology and Obstetrics (FIGO) published guidelines "Ethical aspects of the management of severely malformed newborn infants" and "Ethical aspects in the management of newborn infants at the threshold of viability." See Schenker JG. Codes of perinatal ethics: an international perspective. *Clin Perinatol* 2003;30:45–65.

States of Profound Paralysis with Intact Cognition

14

Challenging ethical issues arise in neurological disorders that produce chronic profound paralysis of voluntary muscles while preserving consciousness and cognition. Disorders that produce this tragic state include the locked-in syndrome, the late stage of amyotrophic lateral sclerosis (ALS), the final stage of Duchenne muscular dystrophy and other progressive neuromuscular diseases, and high-cervical spinal cord transection with ventilator dependency. Medical decision making in these patients is complicated because they cannot move or physically manipulate their environments and have marked communication impairment despite their generally preserved cognitive functioning.

These patients retain the capacity to make health-care decisions because the illnesses producing paralysis usually spare centers controlling consciousness and cognition. Physicians thus have a duty to obtain valid consent for or refusal of life-saving treatment (LST) from the patient, not from a surrogate decision maker. Physicians responding to refusals of LST by profoundly paralyzed patients have a heightened duty to assure the validity of their consent or refusal of treatment by optimizing patients' physical, psychological, communicative, and rehabilitative condition. Physicians responding to treatment decisions of paralyzed patients should: (1) educate patients fully about their disease course, treatment, and rehabilitation; (2) optimize patients' communication abilities to permit them to retain the highest degree of control; (3) fully rehabilitate them using modern therapies of neurorehabilitation; (4) adequately diagnose and

treat concomitant depression; and (5) provide loyal, attentive medical care assuring availability, continuity, emotional support, and encouragement that the physician will support the patient's decision. This chapter focuses on the tragic plight of these patients, the duties of physicians to assist them in making health-care decisions, the compassionate balance of physicians' paternalistic encouragement for them to live against their faithful willingness to stop LST once the patient has refused it validly, and the responsibility of physicians to provide for their rehabilitative, palliative, and terminal care.

PARALYZING NEUROLOGICAL DISORDERS THAT SPARE COGNITION

The paradigmatic chronic neurological conditions causing profound paralysis but sparing cognition that I consider in this chapter are ALS, locked-in syndrome, Duchenne muscular dystrophy, and high-cervical spinal cord transection with ventilator dependency. My analysis applies to other conditions producing the same combination of neurological signs.

Amyotrophic Lateral Sclerosis

ALS is an acquired, progressive, irreversible, paralyzing, incurable, and fatal neuromuscular disease in which affected patients retain relatively normal cognition throughout the illness. Although recent reports stress the presence of cognitive dysfunction as the illness progresses,[1] cognitive impairment usually is not severe enough to interfere with the ability of the ALS patient to provide valid consent to or refusal of treatment. Affected patients develop the subacute onset of progressive, asymmetric muscle weakness leading to diffuse paralysis, muscle atrophy, and fasciculations, with anarthria, aphonia, dysphagia, and progressive respiratory insufficiency. Patients with ALS usually die within several years of disease onset from inexorable respiratory failure, if their ventilation is not supported mechanically. With tracheostomy, gastrostomy, and respiratory support, including tracheostomy positive-pressure ventilation (TPPV), more prolonged survivals are possible.[2] Specific treatments to slow disease progression have only a limited effect.

Locked-In Syndrome

The locked-in syndrome is an acquired state of acute de-efferentation, classically produced by a large infarction or hemorrhage in the pontine tegmentum and base, producing quadriplegia, pseudobulbar palsy, and paralysis of horizontal eye movements. Once the acute encephalopathy resolves, locked-in patients usually remain awake and alert, breathe spontaneously, and have normal cognition, to the extent it can be tested accurately. Inexperienced examiners may incorrectly diagnose them as comatose because of their profound paralysis, pinpoint pupils, and seeming unresponsiveness. They can be taught to communicate with voluntary vertical eye movements and eyelid movements, which typically are the only volitional movements they retain. Most affected patients do not survive longer than a few months, but a small group of otherwise healthy young patients who have suffered basilar artery occlusion can survive for years in a chronic locked-in syndrome.[3] Some chronic locked-in patients have been taught to communicate in Morse code with vertical eye movements or through computerized systems triggered by eye movements, enabling them to communicate complex thoughts successfully.[4] Two young patients in a locked-in syndrome from pontine infarction caused by basilar artery occlusion have "dictated" books poignantly describing their plight and their sources of joy and suffering,

with the assistance of colleagues who carefully recorded and translated their eye movements into words.[5] A narrative of another young locked-in patient, emphasizing the patient's suffering, his difficulties in communication, and the ethical issues in his treatment was featured in the *BMJ* recently.[6] A similar state of locked-in syndrome can result from the final stage of progressive neuromuscular diseases including ALS.[7]

Duchenne Muscular Dystrophy

The muscular dystrophies are a heterogeneous and incurable group of genetic disorders of muscle metabolism in which inexorably progressive muscle weakness develops over many years. Duchenne muscular dystrophy (DMD), affecting 1 in 3,500 boys, is an X-linked recessively transmitted disease that begins in early childhood with weakness of the pelvic and shoulder girdle musculature and progresses to generalized paralysis. Because of progressive weakness, DMD patients usually become confined to a wheelchair by ages 8 to 12 years. At this point they begin to develop progressive paralysis of respiratory muscles that, without ventilatory support, leads to their death, usually between ages 20 and 25 years. Cardiac failure accounts for 10–20% of deaths.[8] Although glucocorticoid therapy may reduce the rate of progression of muscle weakness, DMD patients treated with glucocorticoids survive no longer than those untreated.[9]

Spinal Cord Trauma

Severe trauma to the spinal cord above the fourth cervical segment produces spastic quadriplegia, sensory loss below the level of the lesion, and respiratory paralysis because of damage to the phrenic nerves or nuclei. Not only do such patients lack all motor and sensory function below the neck, they require tracheostomy, endotracheal intubation, and tracheal positive-pressure ventilation (TPPV) for the remainder of their lives. Complete spinal cord transection produces permanent and profound motor, sensory, respiratory, and autonomic deficits. Neurological function from incomplete transactions, spinal cord compressions, and other injuries may spontaneously improve to some extent for up to a year or so and then stabilize.[10]

TELLING PATIENTS THE TRUTH ABOUT DIAGNOSIS AND PROGNOSIS

Once the diagnosis of ALS has been made confidently or once the prognosis for recovery is determined to be poor in the patient with locked-in syndrome or spinal cord transection, physicians are faced with breaking the bad news to patients and families. Most physicians understandably experience psychological discomfort in discussing the diagnosis and the prognosis of hopeless neurological disorders. Most clinicians ultimately choose to state the painful truth, although doing so is difficult.[11]

In the past, some physicians believed that patients with incurable disorders should not be told their diagnosis and prognosis. Instead, these physicians preferred to employ vague euphemisms. In the case of ALS, for example, they may have told their patients that they suffered from a "viral nerve disorder." In an attempt to justify their purposeful deception, they resorted to one or more of the following lines of rationalization: (1) no good is produced by telling the patient the exact diagnosis, because the disease in untreatable; (2) harm is produced in confirming the diagnosis because it removes all the patient's hope for recovery, improvement, or continued life; (3) the patient does not truly wish to know the real diagnosis and would be happier if the stated diagnosis remained a vague euphemism; (4) because there is no way to prove that the clinical diagnosis is correct, it is immoral to make the patient suffer given the physician's uncertainty; and (5) the patient probably would not understand the physician's explanation of the diagnosis and prognosis.[12]

A utilitarian ethical analysis balances the harms and benefits of deceiving patients to test if the harms are justified by the benefits. When patients are deceived about their diagnosis and prognosis, the harms of this deception are numerous and nearly always greatly outweigh the benefits. For example, the fact that ALS may be incurable does not mean it is untreatable. Riluzole may provide a modest prolongation of life.[13] Symptomatic treatments are available for the common complications of ALS, including respiratory failure, dysphagia, and spasticity.[14] The patient can maintain hope by participating as a subject in clinical trials of pharmaceutical agents being tested for their efficacy against ALS. Most significantly, knowing the diagnosis and prognosis permits the patient to make important decisions about marriage, career, financial matters, genetic testing, and end-of-life issues in a timely manner and to make an informed decision whether to consent to TPPV or gastrostomy.

A patient who does not receive a diagnosis from a physician after a reasonable assessment period will visit other physicians, often undergoing repetitive, expensive, wasteful, painful, and potentially dangerous tests until finally he is given a diagnosis. Because of the initial deception, he may distrust physicians and be suspicious about future medical care and honest communication. The patient also will have lost valuable time by undergoing unnecessary repetitive tests, which will unjustifiably delay his opportunity to make adequate plans for the future.

A deontological ethical analysis asks if physicians who advocate deceiving patients about their diagnosis would be willing to state such a policy publicly, have everyone know that they would practice deception in analogous cases, and advocate that all other physicians practice in a similar deceptive pattern. As discussed in chapter 2, neither a utilitarian nor a deontological analysis can justify the paternalism of diagnostic deception in such cases.

Surveys of patients with ALS, multiple sclerosis, and other incurable, chronic neurological disorders reveal that nearly all patients desire to learn their diagnoses and prognoses.[15] Physicians should tell patients the truth about their diagnosis and prognosis, but should tell them in a way that maximizes empathy, hope, and reassurance. Patients should be given the opportunity and encouraged to seek second opinions. As clinicians explain how common complications can be treated, they should also tell their patients to think seriously about what kinds of treatment they would wish to receive in the progressive phases of their illness. The ability of patients to understand and retain control of future treatment decisions is therapeutically beneficial. As Christine Cassel phrased it, "autonomy is therapy" for the ALS patient.[16]

Patients may respond to bad clinical news, such as the diagnosis of ALS, by adopting a sequence of psychological coping strategies that encompass denial, blame, intellectualization, disbelief, and acceptance. They may exhibit one of several affective responses to the news including anger, fear, anxiety, helplessness, hopelessness, shame, relief, or guilt. Timothy Quill and Penny Townsend pointed out that physicians can help a patient adjust to bad clinical news in several ways. They should assure continuity of follow-up care, be available for continuous psychological support, provide necessary information, minimize the patient's isolation, and respond to the patient's physical and emotional discomfort.[17]

The American Academy of Neurology evidence-based practice parameter on the care of ALS patients states that physicians should offer the diagnosis of ALS to the patient who wants to know, or to a family member if the patient prefers.[18] The diagnosis should be communicated in person, not by telephone, in a calm, quiet, unhurried manner and in a supportive environment. The physician should assess the patient's knowledge of the disease and warn the patient that bad news is forthcoming. The physician should acknowledge and explore the patient's emotional reaction to the news. The physician can provide printed material about the disease and instructions on how to contact support and advocacy organizations. In the conversation, the physician should reassure the patient that he or she will continue to provide ongoing medical care, be available to answer questions, provide advice, and treat complications as they occur, will not abandon the patient, and will offer opportunities if available to participate in clinical research. The report of the Robert Wood Johnson Foundation Workgroup on Promoting Excellence in End-of-Life Care in ALS made similar recommendations.[19]

Leo McCluskey and colleagues surveyed ALS patients and their caregivers to assess how well physicians broke the news of the diagnosis. Patients reported that 25% of physicians had below average or poor communication skills. Caregivers were more critical; they rated over 50% of the physicians as having poor or below average communication skills. The authors concluded that there is room for improvement in physicians' communication skills in breaking bad news, and that they need to learn and practice established communication techniques that have been recommended by the American Academy of Neurology and other groups.[20]

EDUCATING PATIENTS ABOUT VENTILATORS AND OTHER FORMS OF LIFE SUPPORT

Neurologists caring for paralyzed, cognitively intact patients have the important duty to educate them about the technological treatment options available to them at different stages of their illness. This information should be presented in an objective, unbiased, and clear manner so patients can understand that each treatment decision ultimately is theirs to make. It is also reassuring for them to know that their neurologist will support them in each decision. For example, many ALS patients who consent to other supportive treatments choose to draw the line at TPPV. They are willing to receive other forms of treatment, but when their respiratory function worsens, they indicate that they would rather die than receive TPPV. Similarly, some ALS patients refuse gastrostomy tube placement, preferring to die at the time they no longer can swallow. The principal technologies about which patients should be instructed are ventilatory options, feeding options, and cardiopulmonary resuscitation.

Many patients and some neurologists incorrectly believe that mechanical ventilation is an "all or none" phenomenon for ALS, muscular dystrophy, and other progressive neuromuscular diseases that cause respiratory failure. They wrongly conceptualize their choice as to accept TPPV or have no ventilatory support at all. In fact, several intermediate ventilatory options are available that usually compensate successfully for lesser states of neuromuscular respiratory failure. ALS patients frequently hypoventilate during sleep ("sleep-disordered breathing") in the early stage of the illness, producing nocturnal awakening, headache, anorexia, lethargy, and daytime drowsiness. Sleep-disordered breathing may be treated successfully by noninvasive nocturnal nasal ventilation using continuous positive airway pressure (CPAP) or bilevel positive airway pressure (BiPAP) by oronasal mask.[21] These devices can be put on and taken off easily and do not require tracheostomy or endotracheal intubation. The noninvasive positive-pressure devices, generally referred to a noninvasive positive-pressure ventilation (NPPV), however, are not capable of compensating for the more severe degrees of ventilatory failure that inevitably occur later in the course of ALS and DMD.[22]

Studies of patients with ALS and DMD show high success rates of using NPPV. Several studies of NPPV in ALS disclosed that its successful use increased patients' survival.[23] The principal problems making patients intolerant of NPPV were bulbar symptoms, especially the sensation of choking from the inability to clear secretions. Patients who are intolerant of NPPV can be offered TPPV.[24] Several studies have shown improved quality of life for ALS patients receiving NPPV.[25] A study of the effect of NPPV on ALS patients and their caregivers found that respiratory muscle weakness had a greater effect than overall ALS severity on patients' rating of their quality of life, that NPPV improved patients' quality of life despite worsening paralysis from ALS, and that NPPV did not significantly increase caregiver burden or stress.[26] However, the relatively low percentage of eligible ALS patients referred for NPPV suggests that many physicians are unaware of its benefits.[27]

Children with early respiratory failure from DMD or spinal muscular atrophy also do well with NPPV. A recent study of children with mild forms of respiratory failure resulting from DMD or spinal muscular atrophy showed that NPPV reduced symptoms of headache and sleepiness, reduced hospitalizations and health-care costs, and had no adverse impact on their quality of life.[28] Nevertheless, in a British survey of physicians' attitudes and practices, 13% of physicians claimed that NPPV resulted in a poor quality of life for DMD patients.[29]

Patients should be told that all mechanical breathing assistive devices including NPPV and TPPV are adaptable for home use, assuming that financial, nursing, and other logistical arrangements are satisfactory.[30] Positive-pressure ventilators that are small, quiet, and easily portable have been developed for home and wheelchair use. Knowing that such technology exists can influence patients in deciding whether they want to receive chronic TPPV treatment.

Many ALS patients and some DMD patients continue to lead highly satisfying lives despite being on long-term home TPPV.[31] Despite their obvious disability, they may be quite satisfied with their life quality. One study showed that ALS patients on long-term TPPV were not more depressed than ALS patients not requiring ventilators.[32] Another study showed that health-care personnel systematically underestimated the quality of life of paralyzed patients on long-term TPPV.[33] In fact, ALS patients' self-assessed quality of life is completely independent of their level of physical functioning.[34] Studies of children receiving home TPPV for respiratory failure from DMD or spinal muscular atrophy show that the technology can be successful and unburdensome.[35] Nevertheless, one survey disclosed that 25% of Canadian physicians did not discuss the option of long-term TPPV with DMD patients.[36]

The adequacy of health-care insurance coverage is the major factor in the patient's decision to maintain home ventilation. Home nursing care represents the greatest component of this expense.[37] Patients should be told that they can be maintained in their home for several years, given sufficient insurance coverage and family support. The renowned British theoretical physicist Stephen Hawking is an unusual example of an ALS patient who has experienced prolonged survival and continues to live successfully at home with a portable positive-pressure ventilator, computerized voice synthesizer, and daily nursing care.

Assisted feeding options include nasogastric tubes, gastrostomy tubes, and jejunostomy tubes. Nasogastric ("Dobhoff") tubes are suitable for temporary use, but they irritate the nasopharynx and esophagus when in place for longer than a month. The feeding gastrostomy tube inserted by percutaneous incision under endoscopic guidance (PEG tube) is an ideal long-term solution for patients who wish to maintain hydration and nutrition when they can no longer swallow. Feeding jejunostomy tubes require a more lengthy and complicated surgical procedure for insertion and more skilled nursing care for maintenance. Jejunostomy tubes avoid the risk of gastroesophageal reflux that complicates the use of some PEG tubes, but they have a smaller gauge than PEG tubes and therefore, require longer daily periods of continuous infusion with a mechanical feeding pump.[38]

For most ALS patients, the PEG tube represents the ideal solution to the problems of maintaining nutritional intake, administering medications, and preventing aspiration. Most ALS patients are satisfied with the use of their PEG device.[39] The PEG tube usually should be inserted at about the time the patient's forced vital capacity falls to 50% of predicted value.[40]

Cardiopulmonary resuscitation (CPR) as a treatment option should be discussed with the patient far in advance of when it might be needed. Many ALS patients refuse to be resuscitated or intubated. They should not be intubated if they develop pulmonary failure, but instead treated with opioid drugs and other medications to reduce air hunger as discussed later in this chapter.

Advance directives can be useful for ALS patients, even if they retain independent decision-making capacity throughout their illness. The directives can formalize patients' decisions about specific treatments and can appoint a legal surrogate decision maker should the patient lose decision-making capacity, even temporarily. In the ALS Patient Care Database, 70% of enrolled patients had completed advance directives.[41] John Bach cautioned that written directives that include preferences for respiratory support could be harmful unless patients are fully informed of all available treatment options.[42] Advance directives also have been used successfully by patients paralyzed by spinal cord injury.[43]

Steven Albert and colleagues studied preferences for LST in 121 ALS patients and compared the decisions they stated earlier in the illness with choices they made a year later when their illnesses had progressed and many had required the modalities in question. They found that patients could clearly express their wishes and that most wishes did not change with increasing disease severity. For example, 20% of the patients who found tracheostomy acceptable underwent the procedure compared with only 3% of those who found it unacceptable. Similarly, 48% of patients who found PEG acceptable underwent the procedure during the study period compared to only 8% of those who found it unacceptable.[44] In a later study, the same investigators found that ALS patients' attitudes toward religion and spirituality were an important factor that influenced their later choices about receiving PEG, tracheostomy, and NPPV.[45]

Cultural factors contribute to ALS patients' decisions to receive TPPV and other forms of LST. In an analysis of attitudes about mechanical ventilation for ALS patients in North America, Europe, and Japan, Gian Borasio and colleagues found cultural differences. In North America, the decision most often was patient-driven and based on a concept of patient autonomy. In Japan, the decision usually was made by the physician, with some physicians ordering ventilators and others not. In Europe, an intermediate situation existed characterized by a balance between patient and physician authority. ALS patients who formerly were not given the option of mechanical ventilation now are given that option in many European countries.[46] Steven Albert and colleagues recently showed that cultural differences in mental health, particularly the presence of pessimism and suffering, affect the will to live and govern the treatment choices of ALS patients at the end of life.[47]

PHYSICIANS' DUTIES TO ENHANCE COMMUNICATION IN PARALYZED PATIENTS

Locked-in patients and ventilator-dependent patients with ALS or high-cervical spinal cord injury have extreme difficulty communicating.

A principal source of their suffering is their inability to make known their feelings, wishes, fears, anxiety, concerns, and decisions. A patient's inability to communicate effectively also creates a serious problem for physicians who are trying to respect and follow the patient's treatment decision. Physicians often cannot know confidently whether patients fully understand the implications of each treatment decision because of their communication impairment. Physicians may even be uncertain about patients' capacity to make decisions because such an assessment is rendered difficult by the profound communication difficulty.

Clinicians have an ethical duty to enhance these patients' communication abilities.[48] Patients can be taught simple communication systems for yes-no responses that require them to make at least rudimentary movements with whatever muscles remain under their control. Whereas, 30 years ago, locked-in patients who retained voluntary motor control only of vertical eye movements could be taught to use Morse code with their eye movements,[49] today, many new high-technology computerized communication systems are available.[50] Physicians should request the services of skilled occupational and speech-language therapists, with training in the use of these communication systems to maximize the patient's ability to consent to treatment.[51] Computerized letter boards, voice synthesizers, and head or eye movement-activated computerized language systems have helped paralyzed patients to overcome profound communication blocks and have permitted them to interact socially using complex language.[52] One of my patients who was locked-in from advanced ALS used a sophisticated communication device activated by laser beam reflections from his cornea that allowed him to write letters and use the Internet and electronic mail.

Many but not all chronically locked-in patients rate their quality of life higher than able-bodied observers might expect.[53] The one factor that correlates with self-reports of adequate quality of life is retaining or learning the ability to communicate.[54] Novel technologies have been employed to assist communication in paralyzed patients, including EEG-based brain-computer interfaces[55] and measurements of salivary pH in response to questions.[56]

PHYSICIANS' DUTIES TO ENHANCE PATIENTS' PSYCHOLOGICAL STATUS

Physicians have a duty to assess the psychological status of their patients to assure that a potentially reversible depression does not unduly influence the patient's decision-making process. This step is necessary to show that the patient's decision is rational; that is, to test if the patient who refuses LST has an adequate reason. It is understandable that a patient dying of ALS or who one who has been left permanently locked-in might develop reactive depression. It is the physician's responsibility to judge the status and relevance of the patient's depression. Depression may be so profound that the patient makes irrational decisions in refusing treatment. In this unusual circumstance, a physician may be ethically justified in overruling a patient's refusal of treatment, at least temporarily. Neurologists should request psychiatric consultation for patients when they suspect that potentially reversible depression may be influencing their refusal of life sustaining treatment (LST).[57]

Physicians should attempt to enhance the psychological status of profoundly paralyzed patients by mastering the principles of care for chronic illness. They should provide continuous care to their patient, be readily available, and exhibit personal inner strength. They should assure the patient that they will do everything possible to prevent him from suffering and to carry out his treatment choices faithfully. Unity of purpose and action among physician, family, and friends creates a milieu of moral support necessary for the patient to cope psychologically with his terminal illness.

The psychological status of patients with ALS is a strong prognostic factor in determining their outcomes. In a cross-sectional, longitudinal prospective study adjusted for confounding factors, E.R. McDonald and investigators found a higher rate of death and a shorter life expectancy in ALS patients who were depressed compared with ALS patients who possessed more healthy psychological profiles at the same stage in their illness.[58] These findings underscore the duty of physicians to identify and treat depression as well as optimize the psychological condition of their chronically ill patients.

Surprisingly, the incidence of major depression in ALS patients is small, even among those in late-stage disease. Judith Rabkin and colleagues found that the prevalence of depression in patients with late-stage ALS was 9% and did not change as death approached, although 19% of patients expressed a wish to die.[59] The depressed patients expressed more pessimism and hopelessness than those who were not depressed. The strongest predictor of depression and anxiety was the degree of social support from spouses, other family members, and friends. ALS patients with poorer family and social supports report greater psychological distress than those who are supported better.[60]

An important factor correlating with depression is the patient's sense of being a burden to the home caregiver. One study showed a positive correlation between the degree of ALS patients' sense of being a burden to their caregivers and their degree of depression and poor quality of life.[61] In an interview study of patient-caregiver pairs, both caregivers and patients reported that the psychosocial stress on the partner was greater than each reported independently: patients reported being a greater burden on caregivers than caregivers perceived, and caregivers reported that the patient shouldered a greater burden from the disease than the patient reported. This disparity in perception contrasted with the otherwise high degree of congruence of both parties' independent reports assessing the patient's level of function, pain level, optimism, and will to live.[62]

In a study of 100 ALS patients and their caregivers, Linda Ganzini and colleagues found that the two major causes of suffering in ALS patients were pain and the feeling of hopelessness.[63] Hopelessness is a classic sign of depression. In a separate study, the same group found that ALS patients' feelings of hopelessness correlated with more favorable attitudes toward physician-assisted suicide.[64] In a study of correlates of the wish to die among end-stage ALS patients, patients who wished to die reported less optimism, less comfort from religion, and greater hopelessness. The authors cautioned that the wish to die in end-stage ALS patients was not simply a feature of depression.[65]

Despite the first impression of some healthy physicians, not all patients in profound states of irreversible paralysis wish to die. In a study of the quality of life experienced by chronically locked-in patients, Anderson and colleagues found that the quality-of-life scores of these chronic patients were lower than the scores of patients with cancer but higher than those of patients with terminal illnesses. Many locked-in patients said that they lived personally meaningful lives and wished to continue despite their severe disability.[66] Neurologists have published detailed accounts of courageous patients who have continued to live active and fruitful lives despite utter paralysis and dependence on TPPV.[67] John Bach reported a series of 89 ALS patients maintained on successful long-term TPPV for a mean of 4.4 years.[68] More recently, Hideaki Hayashi and Edward Oppenheimer reported 70 ALS patients on long-term TPPV, 33 of whom had been on TPPV for more than five years, and eight of whom were totally locked-in. They pointed out that some ALS patients may have long-term survival with TPPV.[69]

MANAGEMENT OF THE CHRONICALLY ILL PARALYZED PATIENT

An often underappreciated duty in the management of the paralyzed patient is to provide optimum medical care for the chronic disease state. As described further in chapter 15, medical care for chronic diseases features both content and process components that differ from medical care for acute diseases.[70] The essence of chronic medical care is to pay careful attention to the seemingly minor symptoms of a patient's illness that impact greatly on quality of life. Concerns such as optimizing bowel and bladder function, assuring nighttime sleep, identifying and treating sources of anxiety and pain, eliminating unpleasant odors, regulating medications carefully to minimize side effects, and improving a patient's appearance are essential components of chronic medical care.[71]

In the process of providing chronic medical care, physicians can demonstrate personal virtues such as devotion, empathy, compassion, conscientiousness, availability, and caring.[72] Physicians should work to optimize their communication skills and ensure continuity of follow-up care by scheduling regular appointments. Physicians should try to be available between appointments for advice by telephone or email. Patients and their families should not be made to feel that they are asking foolish questions or taking too much of the physician's time. The physician's thoughtful attention to the severely disabled patient's medical and nursing needs and to the family's social issues helps improve the patient's quality of life.[73]

Physicians can express devotion to their patients by making an informal pact that no matter how ill the patient becomes, the physician will continue to be available and will never abandon the patient. It is difficult psychologically for physicians to treat and friends to visit a patient with an incurable, inexorably progressive and fatal illness, but it is an essential humane act to conduct with diligence. Many physicians and friends cope with their own fear, frustration, and emotional strain by ceasing to visit the patient. As the illness progresses, the chronically ill patient's fear of being abandoned by physicians, family, and friends becomes a realistic concern.[74]

Physicians caring for chronically ill patients do not have to shoulder the burden alone. They should enlist the assistance of other health-care professionals. Physical, occupational, respiratory, and speech therapists, clinical dietitians, home health nurses, and social workers can provide their unique expertise to help optimize the patient's function and comfort. The physician who provides chronic care should serve as the "captain of the health-care team," coordinating the care provided by the other professionals.

REFUSAL OF LIFE-SUSTAINING TREATMENT

The management of dying, particularly withholding or withdrawing LST, is an important element in the care of patients with ALS, muscular dystrophy, and locked-in syndrome.

In contrast to patients in a vegetative state (chapter 12) or with Alzheimer's disease (chapter 15) who are incompetent to make health-care decisions, patients with ALS, locked-in syndrome, and DMD usually maintain the capacity to consent to life-prolonging medical therapies or to refuse them. Physicians' principal difficulty in carrying out patients' decisions results from the lack of confidence that they constitute valid refusals of treatment because of the extreme difficulty paralyzed patients have in communicating their decisions.

To uphold the ethical concept of respect for autonomy and to fulfill the requirements of valid consent and refusal, patients should be asked whether they wish to begin or continue LST. As described in chapter 2, in all cases of valid consent, patients must be provided with adequate information to make their decisions. Thus, they need detailed accounts of the natural history of their disease and of the effects of intervention with the treatment available. This information should be provided in an unbiased manner. The physician should indicate that he will continue to treat and care for the patient, irrespective of which decision the patient makes. To the fullest extent possible, patients should discuss their decisions with family members and friends.

Physicians should not assume that ALS patients in respiratory failure wish to refuse TPPV. Nor should physicians imply or suggest that termination of LST is the preferred course of action. Experienced clinicians commonly encounter ALS patients with courage and the will to live who wish to be maintained on home TPPV for as long as possible. Some of these patients are able to continue working if their employers are willing to make the necessary workplace adjustments. Such patients should be given maximum encouragement and assistance with the many technical implications of such a decision. David Goldblatt has written moving accounts of the courage and endurance of several such patients.[75]

When a ventilator-dependent patient refuses further LST and wishes to be disconnected from the ventilator, physicians have several duties. They should optimize communication with the patient and eliminating reversible depression as discussed previously. They should ascertain that the patient's treatment refusal is rational and not merely an impulsive reaction to his illness. The physician can assess rationality by examining the consistency of the decision over time and by seeing if it is supported by the patient's family.[76] In acute medical situations, such as acute spinal cord injury causing quadriplegia, it is usually best for the patient to wait several weeks or months before deciding to refuse LST. Waiting permits the physician to clarify the prognosis, rule out reversible disorders, initiate adequate rehabilitative efforts, and assist the patient to accommodate psychologically to his new disability.[77]

Once the physician is convinced that the patient has reached a rational, valid decision, the physician should support him and follow the decision. From the data available on ALS patients who refuse TPPV and die from respiratory failure, only a small minority are offered or request TPPV.[78] Of those who do request TPPV, in my experience, the majority ask to have their ventilators withdrawn later at a more advanced stage of their illness.

It is psychologically difficult for physicians to extubate patients who are awake and who they know will die from respiratory failure.[79] However, physicians must honor this decision when competent patients have made an informed, rational refusal. Four criteria establish the rationality of such a decision: (1) the patient is terminally ill and will die without ventilatory support; (2) the patient's decision to terminate LST has been consistently held over time and is not an impulsive refusal; (3) a potentially reversible depression producing suicidal impulses is not present; and (4) the family supports the decision, agreeing that a more rapid death is a rational alternative to a slower death.[80] In 1993, the American Academy of Neurology published a position paper and editorial asserting this opinion.[81] Later the *Lancet* published an editorial specifically citing and agreeing with the Academy's position.[82]

Family agreement with the patient's decision is a helpful but not essential component of rationality. Sometimes families will disagree vigorously with the patient's decision to terminate medical treatment and urge the physician not to comply with it. But a loving family that concurs with the patient adds validity to

the rationality of his decision. When families disagree, physicians should be especially vigilant to scrutinize the rationality of the patient's decision, search for underlying depression, and treat it. Ultimately, the patient retains the right to refuse life-prolonging therapy, even in the face of family opposition.

Occasionally, family members will disagree with the patient's choice to refuse therapy because they have "hidden agendas" or unresolved psychological issues. If the physician is convinced that the patient's refusal is rational, he should meet with family members to identify the source of the disagreement. For example, do family members oppose the treatment plan because they experience guilt resulting from their inability or unwillingness to manage his care at home? Many of these hidden agendas can be worked through by convening family meetings. The hospital ethics committee, social workers, and hospital clergy may be of assistance to help resolve family conflicts.

Sometimes the attending physician personally finds it morally unacceptable to discontinue ventilatory support when the patient refuses it. In general, physicians should not be compelled to participate in any form of medical care to which they morally object. In cases in which patients have valid reasons for refusing treatment, the physician is obligated, however, to transfer his patient to the care of another physician who is willing to carry out the treatment plan.[83] This duty exists because the right of the patient to refuse treatment is more compelling than the right of the physician to block such action as a result of his own refusal to participate.

Nurses also have complex feelings about participating in procedures to discontinue ventilatory support and administering sedative and depressant drugs that might secondarily accelerate the patient's death.[84] The nursing staff should thoroughly understand that it is the patient's right to refuse treatment and this right forms the basis for the physician's order to discontinue ventilatory support. Ideally, the nursing staff should agree with the decision, realizing that it is the ethically correct course of action. The specific palliative care orders for maintaining patient comfort during the withdrawal of ventilation are discussed in chapter 8.

There is a divergence between the theoretical description of these principles and their application in practice. To investigate how experienced neurologists managed ventilation decisions of ALS patients, David Goldblatt and Jane Greenlaw surveyed 10 directors of neuromuscular disease clinics with large numbers of ALS patients.[85] They found that the majority of the neurologists surveyed recommended initiation of positive pressure ventilatory support in those patients with relatively preserved limb and bulbar motor function. In the patients in whom breathing was the "last to go," the group was split evenly over whether to offer ventilatory support as an option. Similarly, opinion was mixed on whether financial status should be a factor in offering ventilatory assistance. Although all the neurologists were willing to honor a patient's request to remove a ventilator, two required that a court order be obtained first. It should be noted that these opinions were recorded prior to the 1993 publication of the American Academy of Neurology guidelines on termination of ventilator treatment for ALS patients. There now should be greater uniformity in practice, given the existence of these practice guidelines.[86]

PALLIATIVE CARE OF THE DYING PARALYZED PATIENT

Physicians have ethical responsibilities in the management of the paralyzed patient dying of respiratory failure including arranging for hospice care, performing simple humane acts, and writing specific orders designed to minimize the suffering of the dying patient.[87] Hospice referral can provide home assistance for the dying patient and family, as explained in chapter 7. Unfortunately, many ALS patients fail to meet current Medicare hospice eligibility criteria despite the fact that they are dying. Leo McCluskey and Gail Houseman proposed amending hospice eligibility criteria and argued convincingly that the amended criteria should be accepted by Medicare.[88] Their proposed revision of the Medicare hospice eligibility criteria for the dying ALS patient has been supported by the ALS

Association of America and the American Academy of Neurology.

Humane acts include spending time with the patient, talking with him, sitting and holding his hand, and showing him that you, as a physician, are interested to share this experience and care about him. Simple physical presence and caring are all that is required.[89]

The duty to minimize the suffering of the dying patient during the extubation procedure and the dying process requires an understanding of the clinical pharmacology of opioid and benzodiazepine drugs. (See chapter 7.) Pharmaceutical agents should be administered to suppress air hunger and treatment should be given to alleviate all other sources of suffering as the patient dies of respiratory failure. When withdrawing ventilatory support, the physician can disconnect the patient for a brief trial to assess his need for medications. The rate and depth of positive-pressure ventilation can be reduced gradually to minimize air hunger as the patient is weaned from the ventilator. Once severe hypercapnia ensues, the patient becomes comatose and may no longer require much medication to maintain comfort. Patients who are completely dependent on the ventilator usually die within 20 minutes of its removal.

Medications such as morphine sulfate and benzodiazepines (diazepam, lorazepam, midazolam) can be administered parenterally to reduce air, hunger, suffering, and level of awareness. Doses should be chosen to comfort the patient during the dying process without purposely accelerating the moment of death. The ideal dose of morphine and benzodiazepines is the smallest dose that induces adequate patient comfort. It is acceptable to risk accelerating the moment of death as long as the intent of therapy and the dosage prescription are designed for and are appropriate to provide patient comfort.[90]

The primary goal of therapeutics in this setting is to maintain patient comfort. Many physicians have not been sufficiently aggressive in ordering medication doses that are adequate to suppress suffering in the dying patient. The discipline of "aggressive palliative care" holds that, when they prescribe palliative care for terminally ill patients, physicians should practice with the same spirit of aggressiveness that they display when they treat cancer patients with chemotherapy. The Society of Critical Care Medicine Palliative Noninvasive Positive Pressure Ventilation Task Force recently published guidelines for using NPPV for palliative purposes.[91]

For the locked-in patient who refuses hydration, nutrition, and therapeutic medications, the physician has a similar set of duties to minimize subsequent suffering during the dying process. Patients should receive adequate mouth care to prevent parching. Parching can be prevented with mouth swabs and small quantities of water that are insufficient to reverse terminal dehydration. These patients also should receive adequate doses of morphine and benzodiazepines as necessary to assure their comfort as they die. Because of the difficulty in evaluating the degree of discomfort experienced by these dying patients as a result of their communication impairment, physicians should err on the side of providing aggressive palliative care.[92]

The patient who chooses to die at home should formulate a plan for terminal care in advance with the physician.[93] The physician, a visiting nurse, or a hospice volunteer should be on hand to help administer medications if they become necessary. Medications should be prescribed in advance and be available at home for use. The family should be instructed not to call 911 or an emergency squad because emergency medical technicians are trained to begin resuscitative procedures en route to the hospital, whether or not they are requested. Educating the family about how best to treat the agonal symptoms of dying patients permits many terminally ill patients to die at home peacefully.[94] Dying in an inpatient hospice unit, when one is available, is another reasonable option. Caregivers for dying patient require grief support which, one survey showed, often is inadequate.[95]

Patients with ALS comprise a disproportionate percentage of dying people who choose physician-assisted suicide (PAS) in Oregon[96] and PAS and voluntary active euthanasia (VAE) in the Netherlands,[97] where the acts are lawful, as discussed in chapter 9. These high rates suggest that PAS is not being performed solely to

eliminate intractable suffering at the patient's request. Disproportionate rates likely reflect deficiencies in the competence of health-care practitioners caring for ALS patients, patients' lack of access to suitable services, devaluation of the dying patient, or pressures from others to end life prematurely.[98] Irrespective of one's personal opinion on the morality of PAS or the desirability of legalizing it, most supporters believe it should be reserved for use only as a last resort, when optimal palliative measures are unsuccessful.

TERMINAL CARE FOR THE MUSCULAR DYSTROPHY PATIENT

Patients with Duchenne muscular dystrophy (DMD) differ from patients with ALS or locked-in syndrome because DMD begins in childhood and causes death during the teenage years or in early adulthood. Several ethical and practical considerations are unique, therefore, in planning long-term and terminal care for the DMD patient. The issue of a minor providing valid consent becomes relevant when the physician discusses treatment options, such as long-term home TPPV. The emotional reactions of the child's parents to a chronic and terminal illness become relevant, in addition to the patient's own emotional responses. Finally, the ethical and legal duties a physician has to rehabilitate disabled children have certain features distinct from those for adults.

Jerry Mendell and Arthur Vaughn studied the emotional reactions of parents to their children's DMD.[99] Because parents provide home care, their emotional responses are causally related to the level of care they can provide the DMD patient. They found that the parents recapitulated the same sequence of emotional responses when learning of their child's terminal illness as Elizabeth Kubler-Ross found in adults reacting to the death of a loved one.[100] Thus, the parents responded first with denial, followed sequentially by anger, bargaining, depression, and finally acceptance. The emotional needs and responses of the parents must be recognized, considered, and "treated" to promote the best care of the DMD patient.

Chronic care of the DMD patient should be shared among the pediatrician, neurologist, orthopedist, physiatrist, physical therapist, and occupational therapist. The advice of pulmonologists and gastroenterologists may be helpful to plan respiratory and feeding options. Many neuromuscular disease centers have created multispecialty integrated outpatient clinic programs in which DMD patients can visit all the relevant specialists in a single day. Rehabilitation, including use of orthotics to maximize function, should be a constant goal. Children with DMD should be "mainstreamed" into public schools in accordance with the requirements of PL 94-142, the Education for All Handicapped Children Act of 1975.[101]

To the fullest extent possible, the DMD patient should be included in treatment decisions, consistent with the concept of childhood assent discussed in chapter 2. Parents are not necessarily adequate surrogate decision makers for their teenage children because they may not be fully aware of the values and desires of their teenagers. The criteria for valid consent by minors remains an area of controversy.[102] But before important treatment decisions become necessary for most DMD patients, they are at least teenagers; thus their assent is a necessary if not sufficient condition for treatment. However, approximately 30% of all DMD patients have a degree of concomitant mental retardation and this subpopulation requires primary parental consent for all treatment decisions.

The major treatment decision for DMD patients and their parents is whether to initiate TPPV. Tony Hilton and colleagues reported their experience with a group of 14 DMD patients receiving home TPPV.[103] All but one of the ventilated patients was able to be discharged to home. Two of the patients remained alive after home TPPV for eight years. Three patients died after being disconnected from the ventilator accidentally. Half the patients required feeding gastrostomy tubes as well. Half did not require rehospitalization after home TPPV was initiated. The costs for complete home care for each patient ranged from $3,000 to $35,000 per month, which was paid by private and public insurers. Patients and families were given the option of

discontinuing the ventilator at any time. The program was considered successful by both parents and DMD patients.

In a randomized trial of preventive nasal intermittent TPPV in DMD, Jean-Claude Raphael and colleagues found that it did not adequately compensate for respiratory failure or prevent death from respiratory failure. The authors concluded that TPPV was effective for DMD patients only when forced vital capacity was between 20% to 50% of predicted values.[104]

WITHHOLDING AND WITHDRAWING LIFE-SUSTAINING TREATMENT IN THE CHRONICALLY ILL PATIENT

Whether patients who are chronically ill (but not terminally ill) from neurological disorders also have a right to refuse LST is an active area of ethical controversy. Examples include patients with chronic locked-in syndrome, TPPV-dependent quadriplegia as a result of high cervical spinal cord injury, advanced multiple sclerosis, and severe cerebral palsy. These patients are profoundly disabled and dependent on skilled daily medical and nursing care for their survival. Because their illnesses are not progressive and they are in no imminent risk of dying, (assuming the absence of serious comorbidities), they may survive for many months or years with adequate medical and nursing care. Some patients may rate their quality of life as poor and therefore may wish to refuse LST, including artificial hydration and nutrition (AHN).

The fundamental ethical and legal issue to consider when a chronically ill patient refuses LST or AHN and dies as a result is the question of suicide. Is refusal of LST or AHN an act of suicide and, if so, can such suicides be permitted or assisted? (See chapter 9.) There is a higher incidence of suicide among spinal cord injured patients.[105] There is general agreement that terminally ill patients who refuse LST have not committed suicide because they are destined to die soon from their underlying disease, irrespective of treatment. But is the wish to die to escape a life of unmitigated suffering from a chronic disease ever a rational decision? Asked another way, is suicide ever a rational act in a chronically ill patient?[106]

I believe that a chronically ill patient's death resulting from valid refusal of LST does not count as suicide when the death results solely from the effects of the underlying disease or injury and the patient has the right to refuse LST. The most relevant issues are: (1) that the patient's continued life depends on a form of medical therapy; (2) that the patient is competent and his treatment refusal is rational; and (3) that the patient has the right to refuse consent for therapy. Whether the patient is terminally ill is not the critical issue. According to this analysis, the chronically ill ventilator-dependent patient has the same right to refuse further ventilator therapy as the terminally ill ventilator-dependent patient.

The rationality of the decision is crucial. Nearly always it is irrational for a patient to wish to die from a condition that will resolve quickly. Physicians have a nonmaleficence-based duty to dissuade patients from making irrational decisions and to overrule them when they are seriously irrational, as discussed in chapter 2. However, it may be rational for a patient to wish to escape a life of intractable suffering rather than to continue living in a locked-in state. It is essential for physicians to judge whether a patient's depression is affecting the rationality of his treatment refusal and, if it is, physicians should intervene and treat the depression aggressively. But the mere presence of depression, alone, does not automatically invalidate a patient's treatment refusal. Of course, wishing to continue to live despite the locked-in state also is a rational decision.

Physicians have the duty to rehabilitate chronically ill patients physically and psychologically to the fullest extent possible and to advocate and encourage continued life. Some patients who have been rendered suddenly quadriplegic and ventilator dependent may express the unequivocal wish to die during the acute phase of their illness as a result of a reactive depressive response to their great functional loss. Many of these patients later change their mind following a period of rehabilitation and psychological treatment that allows them to adjust to their new life. Once they have been adequately rehabilitated, paraplegic and quadriplegic spinal cord injury patients almost uniformly report that they are glad to be alive and rate their quality of life as high as their physicians rate their own.[107]

One study examined data on life satisfaction following acute spinal cord injury. The investigators found that 92% of quadriplegic spinal cord injury patients reported they were glad to be alive and 86% ranked their quality of life as average or above average. These data contrast strikingly to those of emergency department professionals who reported that, if they became acutely quadriplegic, only 18% would be glad to be alive and 17% would rate their quality of life as average or above average.[108] Another study showed a rate of reported quality of life satisfaction among spinal cord injured quadriplegic patients with ventilator dependency that was nearly equal to that of healthy persons and much higher than that which was predicted by health-care professionals.[109]

As a matter of course, physicians should seriously question the rationality of any patient's decision to refuse LST within the period immediately following such an injury because of a presumption of severe depression.[110] Many physicians would ignore refusals of LST by the newly injured patient on the basis that they were invalid because of depression, but some would respect them as valid refusals of treatment. This remains a highly controversial area in which practice patterns diverge and strong arguments can be made for each course of action.[111]

After maximal physical and psychological rehabilitation have been accomplished, however, competent patients, whether or not they are terminally ill, should retain the right to refuse all forms of treatment, including LST.[112] Physicians should actively oppose a patient's refusal of LST only if they can show that it is an irrational decision. As I argue in chapter 9, the right of patients to refuse LST does not extend to a right to have physicians kill them at their own request or assist in their suicide.

Several heart-wrenching cases have been reported of ventilator-dependent quadriplegic patients who have refused further ventilator treatment and died as a result.[113] In two traumatic spinal cord cases, the patients immediately and consistently refused LST. In both cases, the attending physicians ignored their refusals for weeks to months to permit them to become rehabilitated. The physicians justified their paternalistic behavior by claiming that the patients' immediate refusal of LST was invalid because they were reacting impulsively and irrationally to their tragic plight. The physicians claimed that informed consent was optimized by waiting a period of time before respecting their treatment refusals and stopping the ventilator.[114] Because of the data showing the high quality of life of rehabilitated spinal cord injury patients, paternalism may be justified for brief involuntary treatment in this situation but no one agrees for how long.

An unanswered question is whether the refusal of oral hydration and nutrition by the chronically ill patient should be considered suicide. As I argued in chapter 9, refusal of oral hydration and nutrition (PRHN) represents an acceptable alternative to legalizing physician-assisted suicide for terminally ill patients. In the chronically ill but not terminally patient, however, many people consider PRHN as suicide, as was reported in the celebrated case of Elizabeth Bouvia discussed below.

LEGAL ISSUES

There have been several legal decisions from high courts asserting the right of competent but paralyzed patients to refuse life-prolonging medical therapies, even if they were to die as a result. Such cases have included patients with ALS, locked-in syndrome, spinal cord transections and cerebral palsy. In nearly every case, the courts have ruled that citizens' tangible rights of self-determination were more compelling than the state's abstract right to preserve life. As discussed in chapter 8, in the *Cruzan* ruling in 1990, the U.S. Supreme Court found that all citizens of the United States have a constitutionally protected right to refuse LST, even if death were to result.

The ALS cases of *Perlmutter*, *Farrell*, and *Requena* are noteworthy. In *Perlmutter*, an elderly man with ALS asked his physician to discontinue his positive-pressure ventilator to allow him to die. The Florida Supreme Court affirmed the lower court's approval, ruling

that it was rational for a terminally ill patient to wish to die sooner rather than later and that Mr. Perlmutter was within his rights to refuse permission for therapy. In *Farrell*, the New Jersey Supreme Court ruled that a woman dying of ALS could refuse ventilatory support even though she would die as a result. In *Requena*, the New Jersey Supreme Court ruled that a woman dying of ALS could refuse artificial hydration and nutrition in her community hospital, even though such an act violated the hospital bylaws.[115]

Two locked-in patients were similarly permitted to die when they refused life-sustaining therapy. Hector Rodas was a young man who was chronically locked-in following a brain stem stroke. A Colorado district court found that he had the right to refuse hydration and nutrition because he was "mentally capable of refusing treatment." Under the circumstances, his decision was "rational and reasonable." Murray Putzer also was in a locked-in state and refused hydration and nutrition for the same reason. The New Jersey Supreme Court upheld his right to refuse treatment because it was a rational choice not to want to live in a chronic locked-in state and because refusing therapy in this context did not count as suicide.[116]

Several patients with ventilator-dependent high-cervical spinal cord injuries have asked courts to approve their right to refuse life-prolonging treatment. In *McAfee*, the Georgia Supreme Court upheld the right of a ventilator-dependent man with quadriplegia from a spinal cord injury to die by refusing further mechanical ventilatory support.[117] In the United Kingdom, High Court Judge Dame Elizabeth Butler-Sloss ruled that a 43-year-old woman with high cervical quadriplegia and ventilator dependency could refuse ventilator therapy. The judge said "one must allow for those as severely disabled as Miss B, for some of whom life in that condition may be worse than death." Dr. Michael Wicks, chairman of the British Medical Association's Ethics Committee, said the ruling "reinforces well-established legal and ethical guidelines that every competent adult has the right to refuse medical treatment, even when this may lead to their death."[118]

Although most courts have highlighted the primacy of the right of chronically ill patients to refuse unwanted therapies, even it they die as a result, the opposite conclusion was reached in the *Bouvia* case regarding PRHN. Two courts would not permit Elizabeth Bouvia, a 28-year-old woman with severe debilitating cerebral palsy producing spastic quadriplegia and chronic pain, to refuse oral and parenteral hydration and nutrition. Therefore, she was force-fed by gastrostomy tube during her hospitalizations. Because previously she had been successfully rehabilitated to the point of graduating from college and marrying, her physicians presumed that her current wish to refuse hydration and nutrition was suicidal because she was depressed. Several bioethics commentators decried the illogic of these rulings and their inconsistency with the consensus that had been established in other judiciaries concerning the rights of chronically ill patients to refuse unwanted therapy.[119] However, recent data support critics' claims that her major reason for refusing hydration and nutrition was depression.[120] Heather Dickinson and colleagues showed that the self-reported quality of life in children with cerebral palsy, including those with severe forms, were similar to those in normal children.[121]

In *Conroy*, the highest court in New York permitted an elderly, exceedingly demented, and chronically ill woman to die from cessation of artificial hydration and nutrition when it authorized not replacing the feeding tube she had removed.[122] Because she was incompetent to decide, the substantive issues in her case (discussed further in chapter 15) are dissimilar to those discussed in this chapter, but I cite the case here because in the ruling, the *Conroy* court clearly distinguished a patient's rational refusal of medical treatment from suicide. The judge wrote:

"Declining life-sustaining medical treatments may not properly be viewed as an attempt to commit suicide. Refusing medical intervention merely allows the disease to take its natural course . . . In addition, people who refuse life-sustaining medical treatment may not harbor a specific intent to die, rather, they may fervently wish to live, but to do so free of unwanted medical technology, surgery, or drugs, and without protracted suffering . . . Recognizing the right of a terminally ill person to reject medical treatment respects that person's intent, not to die, but to suspend medical intervention . . . The difference is between self-infliction or self-destruction and self-determination."[123]

NOTES

1. Ringholz GM, Appel SH, Bradshaw M, Cooke NA, Mosnik DM, Schulz PE. Prevalence and patterns of cognitive impairment in sporadic ALS. *Neurology* 2005;65:586–590; Rippon GA, Scarmeas N, Gordon PH, et al. An observational study of cognitive impairment in amyotrophic lateral sclerosis. *Arch Neurol* 2006;63: 345–352; and Murphy JM, Henry RG, Langmore S, Kramer JH, Miller BL, Lomen-Hoerth C. Continuum of frontal lobe impairment in amyotrophic lateral sclerosis. *Arch Neurol* 2007;64:530–534.

2. For reviews of ALS and the comprehensive treatment of the ALS patient, see Rowland LP, Shneider NA. Amyotrophic lateral sclerosis. *N Engl J Med* 2001;344:1688–1700 and Mitchell JD, Borasio GD. Amyotrophic lateral sclerosis. *Lancet* 2007;369:2031–2041.

3. In the largest reported series of chronic locked-in patients, 29 patients survived between 2 and 18 years. See Katz RT, Haig AJ, Clark BB, DiPaola RJ. Long-term survival, prognosis, and life-care planning for 29 patients with chronic locked-in syndrome. *Arch Phys Med Rehabil* 1992;73:403–408. The longest published recorded survival of a locked-in patient is 27 years. See Thadani VM, Rimm DL, Urquhart L, et al. 'Locked-in syndrome' for 27 years following a viral illness: clinical and pathological findings. *Neurology* 1991;41:498–500.

4. For a review of the clinical features of locked-in syndrome, see Smith S, Delargy M. Locked-in syndrome. *BMJ* 2005;330:406–409; Patterson JR, Grabois M. Locked-in syndrome: a review of 139 cases. *Stroke* 1986;17:758–764. For a review of the ethical issues in locked-in syndrome, see Bernat JL. Ethical considerations in the locked-in syndrome. In Culver CM, ed. *Ethics at the Bedside.* Hanover, NH: University Press of New England, 1990:87–98.

5. Bauby JD. *The Diving Bell and the Butterfly*. New York: Alfred A. Knopf, 1997 and Mozersky J. *Locked In: A Young Woman's Battle with Stroke*. Ottawa: The Golden Dog Press, 1996.

6. Chisholm N, Gillett G. The patient's journey: living with locked-in syndrome. *BMJ* 2005;331:94–97.

7. Hayashi H, Oppenheimer EA. ALS patients on TPPV: totally locked-in state, neurologic findings and ethical implications. *Neurology* 2003;61:135–137.

8. For reviews of the medical facts about Duchenne muscular dystrophy, see Biggar WD. Duchenne muscular dystrophy. *Pediatr Rev* 2006;27:83–88. For a careful study of and thoughtful guide to end-of-life care issues in Duchenne muscular dystrophy patients, see Hilton T, Orr RD, Perkin RM, et al. End of life care in Duchenne muscular dystrophy. *Pediatr Neurol* 1993;9:165–177.

9. Moxley RT, Ashwal S, Pandya S, et al. Practice Parameter: Corticosteroid treatment of Duchenne dystrophy. Report of the Quality Standards Subcommittee of the American Academy of Neurology and the Practice Committee of the Child Neurology Society. *Neurology* 2005;64:13–20.

10. For medical facts on high-cervical spinal cord injuries, see Whiteneck CG, Carter RE, Charlifue SW, et al. *A Collaborative Study of High Quadriplegia*. Washington, DC: National Institute of Handicapped Research, 1985.

11. For techniques physicians can use to break bad news to patients, see Quill TE, Townsend P. Bad news: delivery, dialogue, and dilemmas. *Arch Intern Med* 1991;151:463–468; Fallowfield L. Giving sad or bad news. *Lancet* 1993;341:476–478; Buckman R. *How to Break Bad News: A Guide for Health Care Professionals*. Baltimore: Johns Hopkins University Press, 1992; Buckman R, Korsch B, Baile W. *A Practical Guide to Communication Skills in Clinical Practice* on CD ROM. Medical Audio Visual Communications, Inc, 1998; Medical Audio Visual Communications, Inc. Breaking Bad News: Patient, Family, and Professional Perspectives. http://www.mavc.com (Accessed July 4, 2007); and Buckman R. Communication skills in palliative care: a practical guide. *Neurol Clin* 2001;19:989–1004.

12. This argument is presented and rebutted in Bernat JL. Ethical and legal issues in the management of amyotrophic lateral sclerosis. In Belsh JM, Schiffman PL (eds). *Amyotrophic Lateral Sclerosis: Diagnosis and Management for the Clinician*. Armonk, NY: Futura Publishing Co, 1996:357–372.

13. Miller R, Mitchell J, Lyon M, Moore D. Riluzole for amyotrophic lateral sclerosis (ALS)/motor neuron disease (MND). *Cochrane Database Syst Rev* 2007;CD001447.

14. For guidelines on symptom control in ALS, see Miller RG, Rosenberg JA, Gelinas DF, et al. Practice parameter: the care of the patient with amyotrophic lateral sclerosis (an evidence-based review). Report of the Quality Standards Subcommittee of the American Academy of Neurology. *Neurology* 1999;52:1311–1323.

15. See Beisecker AE, Cobb AK, Ziegler DK. Patients' perspectives of the role of care providers in amyotrophic lateral sclerosis. *Arch Neurol* 1988;45:553–556; Silverstein MD, Stocking CB, Antel JP, Beckwith J, Roos RP, Siegler M. Amyotrophic lateral sclerosis and life-sustaining therapy: patients' desires for information, participation in decision making, and life-sustaining therapy. *Mayo Clin Proc* 1991;66:906–913; and Elian M, Dean G. To tell or not to tell the diagnosis of multiple sclerosis. *Lancet* 1985;2:27–128. See also chapter 2, note 91.

16. Cassel C. Patient autonomy as therapy. In Mulder DW, ed. *The Diagnosis and Treatment of Amyotrophic Lateral Sclerosis*. Boston: Houghton Mifflin, 1980:325–332.

17. Quill TE, Townsend P. Bad news: Delivery, dialogue, and dilemmas. *Arch Intern Med* 1991;151:463–468.

18. Miller RG, Rosenberg JA, Gelinas DF, et al. Practice parameter: the care of the patient with amyotrophic lateral sclerosis (an evidence-based review). Report of the Quality Standards Subcommittee of the American Academy of Neurology. *Neurology* 1999;52:1311–1323. The report's section on how to break bad news was adapted from Ptacek JT, Eberhardt TL. Breaking bad news: a review of the literature. *JAMA* 1996:276:496–502.

19. Mitsumoto H, Bromberg M, Johnston W, et al. Promoting excellence in end-of-life care in ALS. *Amyotroph Lateral Scler Other Motor Neuron Disord* 2005;6:145–154. For the longer version of the report, including a CD-ROM with tables and appendices, see ALS Peer Workgroup. *Completing the Continuum of ALS Care: A Consensus Document*. Promoting Excellence in End-of-Life Care and the Robert Wood Johnson Foundation, 2004.

20. McCluskey L, Casarett D, Diderowf A. Breaking the news: a survey of ALS patients and their caregivers. *Amyotroph Lateral Scler Other Motor Neuron Disord* 2004;5:131–135.

21. See Sivak ED, Gipson WT, Hanson MR. Long-term management of respiratory failure in amyotrophic lateral sclerosis. *Ann Neurol* 1992:12:18–23; Meyer TJ, Hill NS. Noninvasive positive pressure ventilation to treat respiratory failure. *Ann Intern Med* 1994;120:760–770; Sherman MS, Paz HL. Review of respiratory care of the patient with amyotrophic lateral sclerosis. *Respiration* 1994;61:61–67; and Hillberg RE, Johnson DC. Noninvasive ventilation. *N Engl J Med* 1997;337:1746–1752. For similar references on respiratory care for

patients with muscular dystrophy, see Smith PEM, Calverley PMA, Edwards RHT, et al. Practical problems in the respiratory care of patients with muscular dystrophy. *N Engl J Med* 1987;316:1197–1205; and Baydur A, Gilgoff I, Carlson M, et al. Decline in respiratory function and experience with long-term assisted ventilation in advanced Duchenne's muscular dystrophy. *Chest* 1990;97:884–889.

22. The Society of Critical Care Medicine Palliative Noninvasive Positive Pressure Ventilation Task Force recently published guidelines for ordering NPPV in critical and palliative settings. See Curtis JR, Cook DJ, Sinuff T, et al. Noninvasive positive pressure ventilation in critical and palliative care settings: understanding the goals of therapy. *Crit Care Med* 2007;35:932–939.

23. See Aboussouan LS, Khan SU, Meeker DP, Stelmach K, Mitsumoto H. Effect of noninvasive positive-pressure ventilation on survival in amyotrophic lateral sclerosis. *Ann Intern Med* 1997;127:450–453; Kleopa KA, Sherman M, Neal B, Romano GJ, Heiman-Patterson T. BiPAP improves survival and rate of pulmonary function decline in patients with ALS. *J Neurol Sci* 1999;164:82–88; Lo Coco D, Marchese S, Pesco MC, La Bella V, Piccoli F, Lo Coco A. Noninvasive positive-pressure ventilation in ALS: predictors of tolerance and survival. *Neurology* 2006;67:761–765; and Bourke SC, Tomlinson M, Williams TL, Bullock RE, Shaw PJ, Gibson GJ. Effects of non-invasive ventilation on survival and quality of life in patients with amyotrophic lateral sclerosis: a randomized controlled trial. *Lancet Neurology* 2006;5:140–147.

24. Bach JR. Amyotrophic lateral sclerosis: predictors for prolongation of life by noninvasive respiratory aids. *Arch Phys Med Rehabil* 1995;76:828–832.

25. Lyall RA, Donaldson N, Fleming T, et al. A prospective study of quality of life in ALS patients treated with noninvasive ventilation. *Neurology* 2001;57:153–156 and Bourke SC, Bullock RE, Williams TL, Shaw PJ, Gibson GJ. Noninvasive ventilation in ALS: indications and effect on quality of life. *Neurology* 2003;61:171–177.

26. Mustfa N, Walsh E, Bryant V, et al. The effect of noninvasive ventilation on ALS patients and their caregivers. *Neurology* 2006;66:1211–1217.

27. Lechtzin N, Wiener CM, Clawson L, et al. Use of noninvasive ventilation in patients with amyotrophic lateral sclerosis. *Amyotroph Lateral Scler Other Motor Neuron Disord* 2004;5:9–15.

28. Young HK, Lowe A, Fitzgerald DA, et al. Outcome of noninvasive ventilation in children with neuromuscular disease. *Neurology* 2007;68:198–201.

29. Kinali M, Manzur AY, Mercuri E, et al. UK physicians' attitudes and practices in long-term non-invasive ventilation of Duchenne muscular dystrophy. *Pediatr Rehabil* 2006;9:351–364.

30. Cazzoli PA, Oppenheimer EA. Home mechanical ventilation for amyotrophic lateral sclerosis: nasal compared to tracheostomy-intermittent positive pressure ventilation. *J Neurol Sci* 1996;139(suppl):123–128.

31. Moss AH, Oppenheimer EA, Casey P, et al. Patients with amyotrophic lateral sclerosis receiving long-term mechanical ventilation: advance care planning and outcomes. *Chest* 1996;110:249–255.

32. McDonald ER, Hillel A, Wiedenfeld SA. Evaluation of the psychological status of ventilator-supported patients with ALS/MND. *Palliat Med* 1996;10:35–41.

33. Bach JR, Campagnolo DI, Hoeman S. Life satisfaction of individuals with Duchenne muscular dystrophy using long-term mechanical ventilatory support. *Am J Phys Med Rehabil* 1991;70:129–135.

34. Robbins RA, Simmons Z, Bremer BA, Walsh SM, Fischer S. Quality of life in ALS is maintained as physical function declines. *Neurology* 2001;56:442–446 and Neudert C, Wasner M, Borasio GD. Individual quality of life is not correlated with health-related quality of life or physical function in patients with amyotrophic lateral sclerosis. *J Palliat Med* 2004;7:551–557. For the design of an instrument that measures quality of life in ALS patients and assesses physical, psychological, and spiritual measures, see Simmons Z, Felgoise SH, Bremer BA, et al. The ALSSQOL: balancing physical and nonphysical factors in assessing quality of life in ALS. *Neurology* 2006;67:1659–1664.

35. Simonds AK. Ethical aspects of home long term ventilation in children with neuromuscular disease. *Paediatr Resp Rev* 2005;6:209–214.

36. Gibson B. Long-term ventilation for patients with Duchenne muscular dystrophy: physicians' beliefs and practices. *Chest* 2001;119:683–684.

37. Moss AH, Casey P, Stocking CB, Roos RP, Brooks BR, Siegler M. Home ventilation for amyotrophic lateral sclerosis patients: outcomes, costs, and patient, family, and physician attitudes. *Neurology* 1993;43;438–443.

38. See, for example, Hull MA, Rawlings J, Murray FE, et al. Audit of long-term enteral nutrition by percutaneous endoscopic gastrostomy. *Lancet* 1993;341:869–872 and Kirby DF. To PEG or not to PEG: that is the costly question. *Mayo Clin Proc* 1992;67:1115–1117.

39. Park RH, Allison MC, Lang J, et al. Randomized comparison of percutaneous endoscopic gastrostomy and nasogastric tube feeding in patients with persisting neurological dysphagia. *BMJ* 1992;304:1406–1409.

40. Mazzini L, Cora T, Zaccala M, Mora G, del Piano M, Gallante M. Percutaneous endoscopic gastrostomy and enteral nutrition in amyotrophic lateral sclerosis. *J Neurol* 1995;242:695–698.

41. Miller RG, Anderson FA Jr, Bradley WG, et al. The ALS Patient Care Database: goals, design, and early results. *Neurology* 2000;54:53–57.

42. Bach JR. Threats to "informed" advance directives for the severely physically challenged? *Arch Phys Med Rehabil* 2003;84 Suppl 2:S23–S28.

43. Blackmer J, Ross L. Awareness and use of advance directives in the spinal cord injured population. *Spinal Cord* 2002;40:581–594.

44. Albert SM, Murphy PL, Del Bene ML, Rowland LP. A prospective study of preferences and actual treatment choices in ALS. *Neurology* 1999;53:278–283.

45. Murphy PL, Albert SM, Weber CM, Del Bene ML, Rowland LP. Impact of spirituality and religiousness on outcomes in patients with ALS. *Neurology* 2000;55:1581–1584.

46. Borasio GD, Gelinas DF, Yanagisawa N. Mechanical ventilation in amyotrophic lateral sclerosis: a cross-cultural perspective. *J Neurol* 1998;245(Suppl 2):S7-S12. Similar findings were reported by Lloyd-Owens SJ, Donaldson GC, Ambrsino N, et al. Patterns of home mechanical ventilation use in Europe: results from the Eurovent survey. *Eur Respir J* 2005;25:1025–1031.

47. Albert SM, Wasner M, Tider T, Drory VE, Borasio GD. Cross-cultural variation in mental health at the end of life in patients with ALS. *Neurology* 2007;68:1058–1061.

48. The American Academy of Neurology published a position statement asserting, this duty: American Academy of Neurology Ethics and Humanities Subcommittee. Position statement: certain aspects of the care and management of profoundly and irreversibly paralyzed patients with retained consciousness and cognition. *Neurology* 1993;43:222–223. An accompanying editorial further explained physicians' duties in this context: Bernat JL, Cranford RE, Kittredge FI Jr, Rosenberg RN. Competent patients with advanced states of permanent paralysis have the right to forego life-sustaining therapy. *Neurology* 1993;43:224–225.

49. Feldman MH. Physiological observations on a chronic case of locked-in syndrome. *Neurology* 1971;21:459–478.

50. For example, see Birbaumer N Ghanayim N, Hinterberger T, et al. A spelling device for the paralyzed. *Nature* 1999;398:297–298.

51. Davis WS, Ross A. Making wishes known: the role of acquired speech and language disorders in clinical ethics. *J Clin Ethics* 2003;14:164–172.

52. See, for example, Newman GC, Sparrow AR, Hospod FE. Two augmentative communication systems for speechless patients. *Am J Occup Ther* 1989;43:529–534.

53. For a story of a chronically locked-in patient expressing his poor quality of life, see Chisholm N, Gillett G. The patient's journey: living with locked-in syndrome. *BMJ* 2005;331:94–97.

54. Laureys S, Pellas F, van Eeckhout P, et al. The locked-in syndrome: what is it like to be conscious but paralyzed and voiceless? *Prog Brain Res* 2005;150:495–511.

55. Hinterberger T, Wilhelm B, Mellinger J, Kotchoubey B, Birbaumer N. A device for detection of cognitive brain functions in completely paralyzed or unresponsive patients. *IEEE* 2005;52;211–220.

56. Wilhelm B, Jordan M, Birbaumer N. Communication in locked-in syndrome: effects of imagery on salivary pH. *Neurology* 2006;67:534–535.

57. See Young EWD, Corby JC, Johnson R. Does depression invalidate competence? Consultants' ethical, psychiatric, and legal considerations. *Camb Q Healthc Ethics* 1993;2:505–515: Ganzini L, Lee MA, Heintz RT, et al. Depression, suicide, and the right to refuse life-sustaining treatment. *J Clin Ethics* 1993;4:337–340; and American Academy of Neurology Ethics and Humanities Subcommittee. *Neurology* 1993;43:221.

58. McDonald ER, Wiedenfeld SA, Hillel A, et al. Survival in amyotrophic lateral sclerosis: the role of psychological factors. *Arch Neurol* 1994;51:17–23.

59. Rabkin JG, Albert SM, Del Bene ML, et al. Prevalence of depressive disorders and change over time in late-stage ALS. *Neurology* 2005;65:62–67.

60. Goldstein LH, Atkins L, Landau S, Brown RG, Leigh PN. Longitudinal predictors of psychological distress and self-esteem in people with ALS. *Neurology* 2006;67:1652–1658.

61. Chiò A, Gauthier A, Calvo A, Ghiglione P, Mutani R. Caregiver burden and patients' perception of being a burden in ALS. *Neurology* 2005;64:1780–1782.

62. Adelman EE, Albert SM, Rabkin JG, et al. Disparities in perceptions of distress and burden in ALS patients and family caregivers. *Neurology* 2004;62:1766–1770.

63. Ganzini L, Johnston WS, Hoffman WH. Correlates of suffering in amyotrophic lateral sclerosis. *Neurology* 1999;52:1434–1440.

64. Ganzini L, Johnston WS, McFarland BH, Tolle SW, Lee MA. Attitudes of patients with amyotrophic lateral sclerosis and their caregivers toward assisted suicide. *N Engl J Med* 1998;339:967–973.

65. Albert SM, Rabkin JG, Del Bene ML, et al. Wish to die in end-stage ALS. *Neurology* 2005;65:68–74.

66. Anderson C, Dillon C, Burns R. Life-sustaining treatment and locked-in syndrome. *Lancet* 1993;342:867–868.

67. Goldblatt D. A life-enhancing condition: the Honourable Mr. Justice Sam N. Filer. *Semin Neurol* 1993;13:375–379 and Bach JR. Threats to "informed" advance directives for the severely physically challenged? *Arch Phys Med Rehabil* 2003;84 Suppl 2:S23–S28.

68. Bach JR. Amyotrophic lateral sclerosis: communication status and survival with ventilatory support. *Am J Phys Med Rehabil* 1993;72:343–349.

69. Hayashi H, Oppenheimer EA. ALS patients on TPPV: totally locked-in state, neurologic findings and ethical implications. *Neurology* 2003;61:135–137.

70. For sources on improving systems of chronic disease care, see Von Korff M, Gruman J, Schaefer J, Curry SJ, Wagner EH. Collaborative model of chronic illness. *Ann Intern Med* 1997;127:1097–1102; Bodenheimer T, Wagner EH, Grumbach K. Improving primary care for patients with chronic illness. *JAMA* 2002;288;1775–1779; Bodenheimer T, Wagner EH, Grumbach K. Improving primary care for patients with chronic illness: the chronic care model, part 2. *JAMA* 2002;288;1909–1914.

71. For a discussion of the ethical principles relevant to chronic medical care, see Jennings B, Callahan D, Caplan AL. Ethical challenges of chronic illness. *Hastings Cent Rep* 1988;18(suppl 1):1–16. For specific information on the chronic care of neurological patients written by a neurologist whose husband had advanced multiple sclerosis, see Seiden MR. *Practical Management of Chronic Neurological Problems*. New York: Appleton-Century-Crofts, 1981.

72. For a beautiful essay by a virtuous clinician illustrating dedicated care to ALS patients, see Goldblatt D. Caring for patients with amyotrophic lateral sclerosis. In Smith RA (ed). *Handbook of Amyotrophic Lateral Sclerosis*. New York: Marcel Dekker, Inc, 1992:271–288.

73. Gelinas DF. Patient and caregiver communications and decisions. *Neurology* 1997;48(Suppl 4):S9–S14.

74. For a poignant account of the impact of abandonment on a physician with ALS, see Rabin D, Rabin PL, Rabin R. Compounding the ordeal of ALS: isolation from my fellow physicians. *N Engl J Med* 1982;307:506–509. See also Munsat TL. Ethical issues. In Mulder DW, ed. *The Diagnosis and Treatment of Amyotrophic Lateral Sclerosis*. Boston: Houghton Mifflin; 1980:321–323.

75. Goldblatt D. A life-enhancing condition: the Honourable Mr. Justice Sam N. Filer. *Semin Neurol* 1993;13:375–379 and Goldblatt D. Decisions about life support in amyotrophic lateral sclerosis. *Semin Neurol* 1984;4:104–110.

76. American Academy of Neurology Ethics and Humanities Subcommittee. Position statement: certain aspects of the care and management of profoundly and irreversibly paralyzed patients with retained consciousness and cognition. *Neurology* 1993;43:222–223.

77. For an argument that physicians should not honor the treatment refusal of a recently spinal-cord-injured patient until many months following rehabilitation, see Patterson DR, Miller-Perrin C, McCormick TR, et al. When life support is questioned early in the care of patients with cervical-level quadriplegia. *N Engl J Med* 1993;328:506–509. For accounts of patients with chronic high-cervical spinal cord injuries who have refused ventilator treatment, see Maynard FM, Muth AS. The choice to end life as a ventilator-dependent quadriplegic. *Arch Phys Med Rehabil* 1987;08:862–864 and Gardner BP, Theocleous F, Watt JWH, et al. Ventilation or dignified death for patients with high tetraplegia. *BMJ* 1985;291:1620–1622.

78. Goldblatt D, Greenlaw J. Starting and stopping the ventilator for patients with amyotrophic lateral sclerosis. *Neurol Clin* 1989;7;789–806.

79. For a beautiful essay illuminating the complex feelings of a physician committed to caring for his ALS patient through the patient's decision to stop his ventilator therapy and die, see Goldblatt D. The gift: when a patient chooses to die. *Perspect Biol Med* 2006;49:537–541.

80. I have discussed these criteria in Bernat JL. Ethical and legal issues in the management of amyotrophic lateral sclerosis. In Belsh JM, Schiffman PL (eds). *Amyotrophic Lateral Sclerosis: Diagnosis and Management for the Clinician*. Armonk, NY: Futura Publishing Co, 1996:357–372.

81. American Academy of Neurology Ethics and Humanities Subcommittee. *Neurology* 1993;43:222–223 and Bernat JL, Cranford RE, Kittredge FI Jr, Rosenberg RN. *Neurology* 1993;43:224–225.

82. Allen CMC. Conscious but paralyzed: releasing the locked-in. *Lancet* 1993;342:130–131.

83. American Academy of Neurology Ethics and Humanities Subcommittee. *Neurology* 1993;43:222–223. For a discussion of the legal protection granted physicians who refuse to participate in medical procedures they

believe are unethical, see Wardle LD. A matter of conscience: legal protection for the rights of conscience of healthcare workers. *Camb Q Healthc Ethics* 1993;2:529–542.

84. See Campbell ML, Carlson RW. Terminal weaning from mechanical ventilation: Ethical and practical considerations for patient management. *Am J Crit Care* 1992;1(3):52–56; Gaul AL, Wilson SF. Should a ventilator be removed at a patient's request'? An ethical analysis. *J Neurosci Nurs* 1990;22:326–329; and Makielski M, Broom C. Administering pain medication for a terminal patient. Part 1. The ethical case. *Dim Crit Care Nurs* 1992;11(3):157–161.

85. Goldblatt D, Greenlaw J. Starting and stopping the ventilator for patients with amyotrophic lateral sclerosis. *Neurol Clin* 1989;7:789–806.

86. American Academy of Neurology Ethics and Humanities Subcommittee. *Neurology* 1993;43:222–223.

87. For general sources on palliative care in ALS, see Voltz R, Borasio GD. Palliative therapy in the terminal stage of neuromuscular disease. *J Neurol* 1997;244(Suppl 4):S2–S10; Borasio GD, Voltz R. Palliative care in amyotrophic lateral sclerosis. *J Neurol* 1997;244(Suppl 4):S11–S17; Oliver D. The quality of care and symptom control: the effects of the terminal phase of ALS/MND. *J Neurol Sci* 1996;139(suppl):134–136; Oliver D, Borasio GD, Walsh D (eds). *Palliative Care in Amyotrophic Lateral Sclerosis*. London: Oxford University Press, 2000; and Misumoto H, Rabkin JG. Palliative care for patients with amyotrophic lateral sclerosis: "prepare for the worst and hope for the best." *JAMA* 2007;298:207–216. See also the evidence-based review or ALS treatment: Miller RG, Rosenberg JA, Gelinas DF, et al. Practice parameter: the care of the patient with amyotrophic lateral sclerosis (an evidence-based review). Report of the Quality Standards Subcommittee of the American Academy of Neurology. *Neurology* 1999;52:1311–1323.

88. McCluskey L, Houseman G. Medicare hospice referral criteria for patients with amyotrophic lateral sclerosis: a need for improvement. *J Palliat Med* 2004;7:47–53.

89. For a moving essay by a compassionate neurologist explaining the impact of sharing a dying ALS patient's experience, see Goldblatt D. Decisions about life support in amyotrophic lateral sclerosis. *Semin Neurol* 1984;4:104–110. For another poignant description of two physicians' feelings on disconnecting a ventilator to allow a patient to die, see Edwards MJ, Tolle SW. Disconnecting a ventilator at the request of a patient who knows he will then die: the doctor's anguish. *Ann Intern Med* 1992;117:254–256.

90. A number of authorities agree that appropriate palliative care during extubation encompasses the administration of morphine and sedatives. For example, see Schneiderman LJ, Spragg RC. Ethical decisions in discontinuing mechanical ventilation. *N Engl J Med* 1988;318:984–988: Smedira NG, Evans BH, Grais LS, et al. Withholding, and withdrawal of life support from the critically ill. *N Engl J Med* 1990;322:309–315; Edwards BS, Ueno WM. Sedation before ventilator withdrawal. *J Clin Ethics* 1991;2:118–122; Wilson WC, Smedira NG, Fink C, et al. Ordering and administration of sedatives and analgesics during the withholding and withdrawal of life support from critically ill patients. *JAMA* 1992;267:949–953; and Truog RD, Berde CB, Mitchell C, et al. Barbiturates in the care of the terminally ill. *N Eng J Med* 1992;327:1678–1682. This topic is considered further in chapter 8.

91. Curtis JR, Cook DJ. Sinuff T, et al. Noninvasive positive pressure ventilation in critical and palliative care settings: understanding the goals of therapy. *Crit Care Med* 2007;35:932–939.

92. For a description of the medical and nursing therapy helpful to maintain the comfort of patients who are dying because they refuse hydration and nutrition, see Bernat JL, Mogielnicki RP, Gert B. Patient refusal of hydration and nutrition: an alternative to physician-assisted suicide or voluntary active euthanasia. *Arch Intern Med* 1993:153:2723–2728.

93. For a discussion of the hurdles in withdrawing a ventilator from an ALS patient at home, see Schwartz JK, Del Bene ML. Withdrawing ventilator support for a home-based amyotrophic lateral sclerosis patient: a case study. *J Clin Ethics* 2004;15:282–290.

94. Most ALS patients receiving palliative care die peacefully. See Ganzini L, Johnston W, Silviera M. The final month of life in patients with ALS. *Neurology* 2002;59:428–431.

95. Hebert RS, Lacomis D, Easter C, Frick V, Shear MK. Grief support for informal caregivers of patients with ALS: a national survey. *Neurology* 2005;64:137–138.

96. During the 8-year period 1998–2006 in Oregon, 2.7% of all ALS patient deaths resulted from physician-assisted suicide, a percentage more than 25 times greater than the mean percentage of all dying patients using physician-assisted suicide. See Oregon Department of Human Services. *Eighth Annual Report on Oregon's Death With Dignity Act*. March 9, 2006 www.deathwithdignity.org (Accessed December 27, 2006). For an account of the earlier experience with physician-assisted suicide by ALS patients in Oregon, see Ganzini L, Johnston WS, McFarland BH, Tolle SW, Lee MA. Attitudes of patients with amyotrophic lateral sclerosis and their caregivers toward assisted suicide. *N Engl J Med* 1998;339:967–973.

97. Disturbingly, 20% of all ALS patients in the Netherlands die as a result of physician-assisted suicide or voluntary active euthanasia. See Veldink JH, Wokke JHJ, van der Wal G, Vianney de Jong JMB, van den Berg LH. Euthanasia and physician-assisted suicide among patients with amyotrophic lateral sclerosis in the Netherlands. *N Engl J Med* 2002;346:1638–1644.

98. Ganzini L, Block S. Physician-assisted death—a last resort? *N Engl J Med* 2002;346:1663–1665.

99. Mendell JR, Vaughn AJ. Duchenne muscular dystrophy: ethical and emotional considerations in long-term management. *Semin Neurol* 1984;4:98–103. See also Gagliardi BA. The family's experience of living with a child with Duchenne muscular dystrophy. *Appl Nurs Res* 1991;4:159–164.

100. Kubler-Ross E. *On Death and Dying*. New York: Macmillan, 1970:38–137. A recent empirical study of grief after death, however, rebutted the sequential stages asserted by Kubler-Ross and found that acceptance was a common initial reaction and that yearning remained present for many years. See Maciejewski PK, Zhang B, Block S, Prigerson HG. An empirical examination of the stage theory of grief. *JAMA* 2007;297:716–723.

101. See Gilgoff IS, Dietrich SL. Neuromuscular diseases. In Hobbs N, Perrin JM, eds. *Issues in the Care of Children with Chronic Illness*. San Francisco: Jossey-Bass, 1985. "Mainstreaming" of handicapped children to comply with the requirements of PL 94–142 is discussed further in chapter 16.

102. See, for example, Holder AR. Minors' right to consent to medical care. *JAMA* 1987;257:3400–3402; King NMP, Cross AW. Children as decision makers: guidelines for pediatricians. *J Pediatr* 1989;115:10–16 and Alderson P. In the genes or in the stars? Children's competence to consent. *J Med Ethics* 1992;18:119–124. See further discussion of the concept of childhood assent in chapter 2.

103. Hilton T, Orr RD, Perkin RM, et al. End of life care in Duchenne muscular dystrophy. *Pediatr Neurol* 1993;9:165–177.

104. Raphael JC, Chevret S, Chastang C, Bouvet F. Randomised trial of preventive nasal ventilation in Duchenne muscular dystrophy. *Lancet* 1994;343:1600–1604.

105. Charlifue S, Gerhart K. Behavioral and demographic predictors of suicide after traumatic spinal cord injury. *Arch Phys Med Rehabil* 1991;72:488–492.

106. Sullivan M, Youngner SJ. Depression, competence, and the right to refuse lifesaving treatment. *Am J Psychiatry* 1994;151:971–978. See the further discussion of this point in chapter 8.

107. Kothari S. Clinical (mis)judgments of quality of life after disability. *J Clin Ethics* 2004;15:300–307.

108. Gerhart KA, Koziol-McLain J, Lowenstein SR, Whiteneck GG. Quality of life following spinal cord injury: knowledge and attitudes of emergency care providers. *Ann Emerg Med* 1994;23:807–812. A recent study of patients rendered paraplegic and quadriplegic by spinal cord injury disclosed self-reported quality of life better than average. Abrantes-Pais FDN, Friedman JK, Lovallo WR. Ross ED. Psychological or physiological: why are tetraplegic patients content? Neurology 2007;69:261–267.

109. Bach JR, Tilton MC. Life satisfaction and well-being measures in ventilator-assisted individuals with traumatic tetraplegia. *Arch Phys Med Rehabil* 1994;75:626–632.

110. The rationality of suicide under any circumstances remains a controversial topic. Advocates of rational suicide see it as an extension of autonomy. Opponents see it as an illness that should be treated. For the spectrum of learned opinion see Childress JF, Roehinger RL, Siegler M, Thorup OA Jr. Voluntary exit: is there a case for rational suicide—a panel discussion. *Pharos* 1982;45(4):25–31; Mayo DJ. The concept of rational suicide. *J Med Philosophy* 1986;11:143–155; Conwell Y, Caine ED. Rational suicide and the right to die: reality and myth. *N Engl J Med* 1991;325:1100–1103; and Clarke DM. Autonomy, rationality and the wish to die. *J Med Ethics* 1999;25:457–462.

111. The most famous such case is that of Dax Cowart, a young man who sustained third degree burns over two-thirds of his body, who repeatedly (and unsuccessfully) begged his physicians to stop his excruciatingly painful cutaneous eschar debridement treatments to allow him to die. His physicians ignored his treatment refusals during the two years of his forced burn treatment. Despite becoming blind and suffering the loss of all his fingers, he was rehabilitated successfully to the point he later graduated from college and law school, and was married. Nevertheless, he continues to strenuously argue that his physicians should have respected his treatment refusals and allowed him to die because no human should have been forced to endure the unspeakable pain he had to suffer. See Kliever L (ed). *Dax's Case: Essays in Medical Ethics and Human Meaning*. Dallas: Southern Methodist University Press, 1989 and Confronting death: who chooses, who controls? A dialogue between Dax Cowart and Robert Burt. *Hastings Center Rep* 1998;28(1):14–24.

112. American Academy of Neurology Ethics and Humanities Subcommittee. *Neurology* 1993:222–223 and Bernat JL, Cranford RE, Kittredge FI Jr, Rosenberg RN. *Neurology* 1993:224–225.

113. Maynard FM, Muth A. The choice to end life as a ventilator-dependent quadriplegic. *Arch Phys Med Rehabil* 1987;68:862–864; Patterson DR, Miller-Perrin C, McCormick TR, et al. When life support is questioned early in the care of patients with cervical-level quadriplegia. *N Engl J Med* 1993;328:506–509; and Powell T, Lowenstein B. Refusing life-sustaining treatment after catastrophic injury: ethical implications. *J Law Med Ethics* 1996;24:54–61.

114. Trevor-Deutsch B, Nelson RF. Refusal of consent leading to death: toward optimization of informed consent. *Ann R Coll Physicians Surg Can* 1996;29:487–489 and Patterson DR, Miller-Perrin C, McCormick TR, et al. When life support is questioned early in the care of patients with cervical-level quadriplegia. *N Engl J Med* 1993;328:506–509.

115. *Satz v Perlmutter*, Fla 362 So 2d 160 (Fla App 1978), Affd Fla Sup Ct 379 So 2d 359, 1980; *In re Farrell*, 108 NJ 335, 529 A 2d 404, 1987; *In re Requena*, 213 NJ Super Ch 475, 1986; *In re Requena*, 213 NJ Super AD 443, 1986.

116. *In re Rodas*, No 86PR139 (Colo Dist Ct Mesa Cty), Jan 22, 1987, as modified Apr 3, 1987; *In re Putzer*, No P-21–87E (Sup Ct NJ Chanc Div, July 9, 1987).

117. *State v McAfee*, 259 GA 579, 385 SE 2d 651 (1989).

118. Hoge W. Paralyzed woman has right to die, a British judge rules. *The New York Times*, March 23, 2002.

119. *Bouvia v Co of Riverside*, No 159780, Sup Ct, Riverside Co, Cal, Dec 16, 1983, Tr 1238–1250 *Bouvia v Glenchur*, LA Sup Ct C 583828, Feb 21, 1986. For commentaries, see Annas GJ. *Judging Medicine*. Clifton, NJ: Humana Press, 1988:290–301 and Kane F. Keeping Elizabeth Bouvia alive for the public good. *Hastings Cent Rep* 1985;15(6):5–8.

120. For an impassioned argument that treating Bouvia against her will was correct because suicide in disabled patients stems largely from social prejudice, written by a disability rights spokesman, who himself has quadriplegia with ventilator-dependency, see Longmore P. Elizabeth Bouvia, assisted suicide, and social prejudice. *Issues Law Med* 1987;3:141–168.

121. Dickinson HO, Parkinson KN, Ravens-Sieberer U, et al. Self-reported quality of life of 8–12 year old children with cerebral palsy: a cross-sectional European study. *Lancet* 2007;369:2171–2178.

122. Curran WJ. Defining appropriate medical care: providing nutrients and hydration for the dying. *N Engl J Med* 1985;313:940–942.

123. *In re Conroy*, 98 NJ 321, 486 A2d 1209 (1985). See further discussion of *Conroy* in chapter 15.

Dementia

15

Challenging ethical problems arise in the management of patients with dementia as a consequence of their inexorably progressive intellectual impairment and of physicians' psychological discomfort in treating patients with cognitive loss. Given the growing prevalence of dementia, these problems will rank among the most common ethical issues that neurologists and other clinicians face in the future. In this chapter, I survey the spectrum of ethical issues in the management of the patient with dementia and end by discussing decisions to withhold and withdraw life-sustaining treatment at the end of life.

The types of ethical issues encountered in the management of patients with dementia vary with its stage.[1] In the early stage, determining decision-making capacity and executing advance directives are common concerns. In the middle and later stages, physicians face questions concerning the appropriate level of medical treatment, whether to restrain agitated patients, how to prevent caregiver burnout, and whether to pursue nursing home placement. End-of-life treatment issues are the principal ethical concerns in the final stage. Problems resulting from impairments in the professional relationship between the neurologist and the demented patient may occur in all stages.

EPIDEMIOLOGY OF DEMENTIA

Dementia is a common condition and one that, because of its increasing incidence with age, will grow in prevalence in the future with

aging of the population in the Western world and increasing life expectancy. Surveys measuring the prevalence of dementia disclose that mild cognitive impairment is present in 2.6% to 15.4% of all persons over age 65 and severe dementia is present in 1.3% to 6.2%. Because the prevalence of dementia increases with advancing age, clinically significant dementia is present in 10.5% of persons 80 to 84 years old and in 20.8% of persons 85 to 89 years old.[2]

Predictions of dementia prevalence in the future are even more sobering. In the United States, it has been estimated that more than 20% of the population will be over 65 years of age by the year 2030, about 10% of whom will have clinically significant intellectual impairment.[3] By 2030, there will be approximately 3.5 million nursing home residents, over half of whom are expected to suffer from at least some degree of cognitive impairment.[4] Worldwide, one recent study conservatively estimated the prevalence of dementia at 24.3 million, a number expected to double every 20 years because of population growth and increasing life expectancy.[5]

Alzheimer's disease (AD) is the most common cause of adult dementia in community, outpatient clinic, and hospital surveys, accounting for over 70% of patients with dementia.[6] Alzheimer's disease is present in 6% to 8% of all persons over 65 years. Its prevalence doubles every five years after the age of 60 so that nearly 30% of all persons over 85 years are affected.[7] The 2000 census recorded 4.5 million people in the United States with AD. By 2050, this number is expected to climb to 13.2 million unless a cure or prevention is found.[8] Vascular dementias, with or without AD, account for another 20% of patients with the syndrome of dementia.[9] The remaining 10% of patients with dementia suffer one of a multitude of disorders, including Parkinson's disease, Huntington's disease, Wernicke-Korsakoff syndrome, head trauma, and metabolic encephalopathies.

Studies of the economic impact of AD reveal the magnitude of the effect of the disease on society, irrespective of the extent of human suffering. Adjusted to 1997 dollars, the annual cost of direct and indirect care for each patient in the United States with AD was estimated to be $35,287 with an aggregate annual cost to society of $141 billion.[10] The Consortium to Establish a Registry for Alzheimer's Disease (CERAD) analyzed the cause of these expenses using Medicare databases.[11] Pharmaceutical success in the arrest or reversal of cognitive impairment or in delaying in the progression of AD (none of which has been accomplished yet[12]) could be translated into substantial cost savings.[13]

One ethical dilemma results from the negative societal attitude toward demented elderly patients. The essential question is, what is the optimal care that society should provide for patients with dementia and how can we maintain humane and dignified care for them given three constraints: (1) the growing public acceptance of the finite resources society has devoted for health care; (2) the low relative value society assigns to expenditures for elderly patients with dementia and total dependency, in comparison to the values assigned to other necessary and meritorious health-care expenditures; and (3) our societal ambivalence toward the demented elderly which results from our psychological difficulty in dealing with patients with permanent cognitive loss?

THE PATIENT-PHYSICIAN RELATIONSHIP

A physician's relationship with a dementia patient has unique features that may interfere with its therapeutic benefit.[14] Consciously or subconsciously, many clinicians regard patients with permanent cognitive loss as undesirable and uninteresting. Early in their training, many physicians develop a sense of failure and frustration in attempting to treat demented patients. A physician may believe that she is powerless to provide any therapeutic benefit to the patient because the syndrome of dementia is inexorably progressive, irreversible, untreatable, and hopeless. A clinician may manifest this overwhelming sense of therapeutic failure through avoidance behavior, spending as little time as possible with the demented patient and thereby overlooking potentially correctable medical problems whose treatment could produce cognitive improvement.[15]

Physicians learn to depersonalize demented patients because they subconsciously equate the loss of intellect with the loss of personhood.[16] As a consequence of their loss of their personhood, the medical subculture has coined a lexicon of pejorative, cynical, and insulting names for demented patients, the most common of which is "gomer." Referring to a patient as a gomer reveals the depth of depersonalization; that is, the patient is no longer a person, she is now a gomer. A gomer no longer possesses the inherent privileges of personhood, namely, human respect and dignity. Therefore, a gomer can be ignored, abused, ridiculed, and neglected.[17] A necessary corrective to this disturbing and insulting depersonalization is to constantly re-emphasize the person behind the illness who deserves our respect, care, and devotion.[18]

Caring for demented patients evokes subconscious fears in physicians because it threatens them with the thought of losing their own intellect, their most prized possession. This subconscious fear is converted into further depersonalization and avoidance behavior to enhance the physician's denial mechanism. This nihilistic and avoidance attitude toward treating patients with dementia creates a self-fulfilling prophesy: the untreatability, irreversibility, and hopelessness of the demented patient. Because nothing possibly can be done to help the patient, nothing should be attempted. Avoidance of demented patients and therapeutic nihilism toward them further reinforce the negative societal stereotypes and fears of aging, dementia, and dependency.[19]

A psychological impediment that some clinicians encounter stems from their failure to shift their therapeutic expectations for demented patients from curing to caring. Some clinicians begin the patient-physician relationship expecting to cure or rehabilitate each patient. This attitude is inappropriate, however, in the management of the demented patient. Only in those rarely encountered cases of "treatable" or "reversible" dementias can a physician reasonably expect significant improvement or cure.[20]

Physicians should adjust their therapeutic goals to caring for the demented patient. According to the model of chronic disease management, "care" requires the physician to attend to the seemingly minor and uninteresting details of the patient's life and health. Some clinicians complain that such an approach resembles the objectives of nursing more than those of medicine. Christine Cassel has observed that the measures of chronic medical care are technically simple and compassionate steps intended to improve the quality of life, but many clinicians may resist and devalue them because they require humane dedication rather than technological virtuosity.[21]

Practical measures of chronic care of the demented patient include careful attention to the maintenance of satisfactory bowel function, peaceful sleep, and adequate dietary intake; correction of urinary incontinence; and compassionate control of agitation. Nursing home staff should permit the patient to keep familiar articles from home in her room and allow her to maintain her own schedule to the fullest extent compatible with institutional policies. For patients living at home, safety is a key objective, particularly around stairs and in the kitchen and bathroom. Patients, whether living at home or in an institution, should be permitted to exert as much control over their lives as possible in keeping with their safe and proper care.[22] Increasing the level of control demented elderly patients exert over their lives improves their physical and psychological status[23] in addition to providing humane benefits.[24]

Another principle in providing effective chronic medical care is to pay conscientious attention to treating the patient's underlying medical illnesses.[25] Functional cognitive impairments in elderly demented patients are due to several concurrent factors: (1) the direct effects of the dementing illnesses; (2) the secondary toxic and metabolic effects on the brain caused by underlying organ failure and comorbid risk factors such as hypertension, diabetes, smoking, and vitamin deficiency; (3) impairments in vision and hearing; and (4) the side effects of medications. All nonessential medications should be withheld and dosages of essential medications carefully monitored to guarantee that the minimum effective dose is prescribed. Many medications, such as digoxin, benzodiazepines, tricyclic antidepressants, and eye drops with anticholinergic properties, may produce toxic encephalopathies in the demented elderly who receive the same dosages that younger patients tolerate well. Controlling hypertension and diabetes, as well as getting demented patients to quit smoking, appears to produce measurable cognitive improvements.[26] Elimination of smoking also removes a serious safety hazard. Improving vision with proper refraction and optimizing hearing by clearing the ear canal of wax and providing professionally prescribed and fitted hearing aids also produces measurable improvement in cognitive function.[27] Optimizing nutrition leads to improved cognitive performance in the elderly as well.[28] Identifying and treating depression in the elderly, which may present cryptically as a "pseudodementia,"[29] improves patient outcomes as does non-pharmacologic and behavioral treatment of depression and behavioral problems.[30]

Physicians need not shoulder the burden alone of managing chronically ill patients with dementia. Specially trained nurse case managers can supervise outpatient care to assure adherence to published guidelines for the optimal treatment of demented patients.[31] A recent study showed that a disease management intervention using a nurse case manager improved AD patients' health-related quality of life, overall quality of life, quality of care by caregivers, social support, and caregivers' needs for assistance.[32] Another study showed that AD outpatients under the care of a nurse case manager showed improvement in their quality of care and a reduction in their behavioral and psychological symptoms without increasing their need for antipsychotic or sedative-hypnotic drugs.[33]

Physicians can overcome the inevitable tendency toward depersonalizing the demented patient by trying to learn about the patient's prior life. Seeing photographs, hearing anecdotes from family members, and trying to appreciate the person prior to the onset of dementia can help diminish the tendency toward depersonalization.

Neurology, psychiatry, geriatrics, internal medicine, and family practice residency programs should teach trainees the principles of caring for patients with chronic diseases. Physicians planning to care for demented elderly patients should understand the importance of paying careful attention to the details of maintaining their patients' health and maximizing the quality of their patients' lives. They should be taught how to develop excellent communication skills and how to recognize and avoid the psychological pitfalls in their relationship with demented elderly patients by converting their therapeutic expectations from "curing to caring."

DISCLOSING THE DIAGNOSIS OF ALZHEIMER'S DISEASE

Some physicians and family members believe that the diagnosis of AD should not be disclosed to the patient, and conveyed only to a family member. They attempt to justify this deception by claiming that the patient who is told the diagnosis is then subjected to unnecessary harms, such as depression and an increased risk of suicide, despite the fact that no evidence supports this assertion. They argue that no good can come of knowing the diagnosis of AD, no diagnostic certainty in AD is ever possible without a brain biopsy or postmortem examination, and on balance it is better to protect the patient from harm.[34]

Studies of cognitively normal patients reveal that the large majority would want to be told the diagnosis of AD once it has been made.[35] One study of AD family members in the United Kingdom found that whereas 71% said they would want to be told if they developed AD, 83% said that the AD patient should not be told.[36] Another study found that 43% of AD family members advocated for a policy of not disclosing the diagnosis of AD.[37]

As discussed in chapter 2, diagnostic deception in this circumstance is a type of paternalism. Despite the beneficent motive, deception is ethically acceptable only if paternalism can be justified. I showed in chapter 2 that paternalism cannot be justified in the overwhelming majority of cases of diagnostic deception. Others have reached the same conclusion and advocate routine disclosure of the diagnosis.[38] Patients may learn of their diagnoses through reading insurance forms, medical bills, or during conversations with other clinicians. Thus, deception is not only unethical but usually unsuccessful.

The American Medical Association Council on Ethical and Judicial Affairs (CEJA) recently stated that it is unethical for physicians to withhold information from patients that they need to make a medical decision, writing, "Withholding medical information for patients without their knowledge or consent is ethically unacceptable."[39] Neurologists should assess patients for their cognitive capacity to understand and the extent to which they wish to know their diagnosis. For patients with both the cognitive capacity to understand and who wish to know their diagnosis, it is wrong to withhold it because, despite the beneficent motive, paternalistic deceptiveness cannot be justified.

How to tell the truth is important. The diagnosis of AD should be communicated compassionately in simple language. Neurologists should discuss available therapies, family support groups, respite admissions, adult day care, and opportunities for research participation. Neurologists should encourage continuity of care with regular appointments and remain available for questions and advice.

DUTIES OF SOCIETY TO DEMENTED PATIENTS

In our current era of global health-care budgeting, competition for scarce resources will become greater as each group of health-care recipients asserts its priority over others. Because macroallocation decisions will be based on mutually held societal values, the future health care of demented elderly patients is precarious. Cost-benefit analyses and econometric models are likely to assign care of the demented elderly a low priority because they no longer are productive citizens. Pure economic analyses may conclude that the demented elderly represent a disproportionate and unjustifiable economic drain.

Ethical concepts of justice, beneficence, and human dignity require, however, that we cannot forget our demented elderly. These patients are entitled to their fair share of health-care resources because of their prior contributions to society, in addition to purely humane considerations. Physicians have a special ethical duty to represent demented patients in macro-allocation decisions because they are no longer able to speak up for themselves. Physicians should advocate for these vulnerable patients in direct proportion to the patients' inability to defend their rights.[40]

In addition to macro-allocation inequities, health-care dollars already earmarked for demented patients are injudiciously distributed. Much of the health-care money currently spent on the elderly pays for high-technology, high-cost tertiary rescue care, such as intensive care unit admissions for dying patients and coronary artery bypass surgery for patients with limited life expectancies. More money should be shifted to low-technology, low-cost amenities, such as hearing aids, eyeglasses, wheelchairs, home health care, and nursing home care, that increase the quality of remaining life of many more elderly and demented patients.[41]

AGE AS A CRITERION FOR HEALTH CARE

Daniel Callahan convincingly argued that public payment for high-cost, high-technology rescue care should be governed by age-based criteria. He argued that our society should be responsible for providing the elderly with decent nursing home and palliative care and low cost amenities that improve the quality of their remaining life. But it is unreasonable and unfair to expect society to provide high-technology, tertiary rescue care, intended only to extend the duration of a person's life, after

the person has outlived her expected life span of approximately 80 years.

Conversely, as a matter of fairness, society has a duty to extend the life span of its younger citizens by all reasonable means to help them achieve a normal life expectancy. Therefore, a greater proportion of health-care resources should be devoted to preventive care and to increasing the availability of health care. For elderly patients who already have achieved their normal life expectancy, their portion of the health-care budget should be devoted to providing more comprehensive chronic, palliative, and supportive care.[42]

Several geriatricians attacked Callahan, accusing him of age discrimination. They argued that advocating age-based criteria for health-care rationing reinforces negative stereotypes of the elderly and implies that older people are less worthy of respect and less deserving of societal resources. They argued that the elderly have just as much right as citizens of any other age to receive high-technology medical care. According to these geriatricians, persons of all ages should share an equal burden in the inevitable rationing of high-cost, high-technology resources.[43]

How should we define society's duty to provide citizens with goods and services equitably? I side with Callahan because I believe that it is most reasonable and fair to expect society to provide all citizens with an equal opportunity to achieve a normal life expectancy. Obviously, this duty is not being exercised currently in the United States. Until it is, I agree that society's principal duty is to provide chronic care, comfort care, and quality of life measures, but not further high-technology, life-prolonging measures for elderly patients who have exceeded their life expectancy. Patients over age 80 could purchase high-technology rescue health care privately if they desired but society does not have the responsibility to provide them given the current inequities in access to medical care.

CONSENT AND COMPETENCE

The extent to which a patient with dementia possesses the capacity to consent to or refuse treatment is an important and changing issue in the patient-physician relationship. In the early stages of AD, patients retain decision-making capacity but thereafter, surrogates must provide consent or refusal on behalf of the patient. Alzheimer's patients comprise a spectrum from the partially competent to the utterly incompetent. Patients in early stage disease often are competent to consent for treatment and complete a valid advance directive for medical care. (See below.) Patients with moderate dementia can be tested reliably for their ability to make a clinical decision by using structured interviews [44] or neuropsychological tests.[45] Bedside instruments have been developed and validated to more precisely assess the capacity of patients with AD to consent to treatment.[46] Laurence McCullough and colleagues refer to what they call the "executive control functions" that are lost progressively in dementia, result in loss of patient autonomy, and require surrogate decision making.[47]

After assessing the patient's degree of decision-making capacity, a dementia patient can be placed into one of three consent/refusal categories as discussed in chapter 2: (1) capable of valid consent or refusal; (2) capable of simple consent or refusal; or (3) unable to provide consent or refusal. Valid consents and refusals are those that are sufficient alone. Simple consents require the corroboration of a surrogate decision maker but simple refusals are sufficient alone. The severely demented patient can make neither a simple consent nor refusal and requires a surrogate for all decisions. Victor Molinari and colleagues adopted the term "assent" from the pediatric usage (discussed in chapter 2) and applied it to the somewhat analogous situation in dementia patients in a concept they termed "geriatric assent."[48] This usage of assent is identical to the concept of simple consent, explained in chapter 2. As in children, assent means that the patient's permission is a necessary but not sufficient condition for consent because it must be corroborated by a surrogate.

Physicians' responses to patients' treatment decisions are straightforward in the mild and severe dementia situations: patients have the independent capacity to provide valid consent and refusal in the former case and no capacity in the latter. Most vexing are the patients with moderate degrees of dementia who lack the capacity to provide independent consent for treatment but retain the capacity to provide independent refusals. Physicians find it difficult to know to what extent they should honor a refusal of treatment in this circumstance. There is no formulaic answer to this question. In practice, it may be useful to seek a psychiatric consultation to determine capacity, request an ethics consultation to determine the rationality of the treatment refusal, or apply one of the standardized bedside neuropsychological instruments to better assess capacity. Joseph Carrese recently described a case, similar to several I have seen as an ethics consultant, in which a demented patient insisted upon leaving the hospital to go home but lacked the physical capacity, financial resources, and social supports to live alone successfully.[49] Ethics consultants must balance the competing considerations of respect for patient autonomy and paternalistic protection of the patient in advising whether the discharge satisfies the usual safe and reasonable criteria.[50]

A recent controversy involving the cognitive capacities of demented patients surrounds the question of whether they should be permitted to vote in public elections. Some commentators believe it is likely that the 2000 United States presidential election turned on the voting preferences of a relatively small group of elderly Florida voters with cognitive impairment.[51] Jason Karlawish and colleagues pointed out that whether demented patients vote depends to a large extent on their caregiver. Patients with AD cared for by a spouse who feels voting is important are more likely to vote.[52] Important ethical, legal, social, and political questions have been raised in this discussion.[53] Should physicians advocate a test of citizen competency to vote? Is such a test constitutional?[54] Should health-care professionals draft guidelines to determine whether and to what extent to encourage or assist demented patients to vote? Should medical societies be involved in this issue? These are broad questions that society and not only physicians must address. Neurologists can inform the discussion by their unique knowledge of AD and the measures available to assess demented patients' capacity to make decisions.

ADVANCE DIRECTIVES

The autonomy and self-determination of a demented patient can be furthered by following the directives for care the patient had executed validly when competent earlier. As discussed in chapter 4, competent patients can execute legally and ethically valid written advance directives and can name a legally authorized surrogate decision maker whose authority is later activated by the incompetence of the patient. As explained in chapter 4, a surrogate appointment generally is more useful than a written statement of preferences alone because the latter is rigid and often ambiguous whereas the former is flexible and permits discretion.[55]

Patients in early stages of dementia can understand and issue valid advance directives.[56] Physicians managing demented patients in the outpatient setting should encourage them to execute advance directives in anticipation of subsequent cognitive incapacity.[57] The directives should be supplemented with detailed discussions with family members, surrogates, and the physician about what types of treatment the patient desires in various clinical circumstances. An advance directive alone without these supplemental discussions is an inadequate advance care plan.[58] Angelo Volandes and colleagues recently found that during advance care planning conversations, showing early-stage dementia patients a video of a patient with advanced dementia increased the percentage of patients who elected comfort care from 50% to 89%.[59]

The most controversial issue in advance directives for demented patients concerns the situation in which a patient's previously executed directive to withhold hydration and nutrition or other life-sustaining treatment conflicts with the demented patient's contemporaneous wish to eat or receive treatment. Which directive should prevail? In general, there is a strong legal tradition for newer directives, such as a more recently executed last will and testament, to trump earlier directives. But should the fact that the earlier directive was made when the patient was competent endow it with special power to trump the later directive because the person is no longer competent?

An earlier directive designed to trump a later conflicting one has been called a "Ulysses contract," referring to Homer's story of Odysseus and the sirens.[60] Anticipating that he would irrationally jeopardize the voyage because of his irresistible attraction to the sirens, Odysseus instructed his men to lash him to the mast and not release him when they sailed passed the sirens, no matter how much he ordered or begged them under the sirens' spell. His sailors therefore ignored his contemporaneous demands to be released, and followed his orders as he had originally instructed them.

Consider the case of a healthy man who has requested that all his medical treatments, including life sustaining hydration and nutrition, should be withheld to permit him to "die with dignity" if he should become demented to such an extent that he could no longer recognize the members of his family. Ten years later the patient, now severely demented, resides in a nursing home, where he appears relatively content. He is hungry, and wishes to eat, but has difficulty swallowing because of advanced AD. Are his physicians bound by the patient's prior directive to withhold his oral feedings or placement of a feeding tube, or are they bound by the patient's present directive, which is to be given food because he is hungry?

Ronald Dworkin had written convincingly that earlier directives executed when a patient was competent should prevail. He pointed out that a patient's interest can be divided into experiential and critical interests, and argues that the latter are worthy of greater respect than the former because they reflect longstanding personal convictions. Experiential interests include the patient's present ephemeral experiences of pain, hunger, pleasure, and satisfaction. Critical interests, by contrast, comprise those longstanding committed convictions about what is important in life that are intrinsic to the individual person's identity and character. Dworkin argued that advance directives mandating withholding treatment permit the critical interest to overrule the experiential interests as they should.[61] Michael Newton concurred with Dworkin that the harms inherent in denying "precedent autonomy" of critical interests exceed those of respecting it.[62]

Other scholars, notably Rebecca Dresser, Sanford Kadish, and Daniel Callahan, take the opposite view. Kadish and Calahan pointed out that the selfhood and identity of the demented person persist even when the patient becomes utterly incompetent from progressive dementia. It is that same self that now is requesting food or treatment and that self should continue to be respected and listened to.[63] Similarly, Dresser argued that an objective balance of burdens and benefits favors providing nutrition and treatment for the demented patient who wishes to receive it, assuming the patient appears relatively content.[64]

Although I respect Dworkin's and Newton's arguments, I believe that contemporaneous directives for food or treatment must be allowed to trump older directives because, with increasing dementia, the clinical circumstance now has changed and the patient's values have changed accordingly. Experienced physicians know that preferences and values established in earlier life about what quality of life is worth living often change with increasing age, infirmity, and illness. Older and sicker patients may become perfectly content with a quality of life that would have seemed unacceptable to the same person when younger and healthier. We always allow for and respect the validity of these changes of perspective because they are part of a normal adaptation to aging and illness.

THE FAMILY CAREGIVER

Family members usually provide the demented patient's primary home care[65] and make treatment decisions for the patient.[66] At some point in the course of the illness, family members no longer can continue to care for the patient at home and institutionalization is required. Factors that determine the duration of successful home care include: (1) the duration, severity, and progression of the dementia; (2) the psychological morbidity of the caregiver, particularly the presence of "burnout" and depression; (3) the presence or absence of caregiver training; (4) the patient's marital status; (5) the functional status of the patient; and (6) the age of the patient.[67] Using these factors, Yaakov

Stern and colleagues validated an algorithm to predict when AD patients will need to enter nursing homes.[68] Other groups have identified similar predictors of institutionalization by using epidemiological studies[69] and surveys of caregivers.[70]

Caregiver training is a critical factor in maintaining successful home care. Once caregivers are taught how to anticipate, manage, and prevent common complications of dementia, patients under their care can continue to function successfully for longer periods before institutionalization becomes necessary. At a minimum, caregivers should purchase and study one of the excellent books that provide facts and advice on home management of the demented patient.[71] Where it is available, caregivers should receive training from visiting nurses or Alzheimer support groups on how to manage patients at home. Assistance from AD nurse care managers is especially useful.

Caregivers need to learn how to recognize and prevent burnout and illness in themselves. Caring for an Alzheimer patient is extremely stressful and contributes to psychiatric and medical illnesses and mortality in the caregiver.[72] Timely psychosocial caregiver interventions and training reduce caregiver illness, dysfunction and burnout.[73] Several studies performed across different racial and ethnic groups showed that programs of caregiver counseling and support significantly delayed nursing home placement of patients with AD and improved patient and caregiver quality of life by preventing caregiver burnout and illness.[74] Surprisingly, the degree of caregiver depression and stress does not diminish following institutionalization of the patient, because most caregivers continue daily visits and care.[75] End-of-life care is especially stressful for caregivers who report being "on duty 24 hours a day." They can benefit from support services including bereavement counseling.[76]

Specific stresses on family caregivers that provoke institutionalization include nighttime awakening and wandering, suspiciousness, accusatory behavior, incontinence, and violence. Of these, nighttime awakening is perhaps the most important. Caregivers need rest. With adequate rest, usually they can cope with whatever unpleasant behavior the patient exhibits during the day. But without adequate rest, they quickly fatigue and no longer can provide proper daily care. Then it is only a short time before institutionalization becomes necessary.[77]

Family caregivers of demented patients should be referred to social workers for evaluation, counseling and assistance in behavioral management, as well as for secondary referral to other appropriate professional services.[78] Families of demented patients need legal and financial counseling to identify sources of available public support and to understand the rules for eligibility for financial assistance and personal services.[79] Visiting nurses can perform home assessments with the intent of arranging periodic visits by home health aides and other necessary professionals. Respite programs, including adult day care and inpatient institutional respite admissions, can be arranged to allow caretakers to have regular rest. These programs were created to prolong the duration of successful home care.

A problem that often complicates the relationship of the physician with the Alzheimer patient living at home is that family caregivers may become the physician's "patient." There are several reasons why this problem occurs. During office visits, the physician's interview usually is directed more to the caregiver than to the patient because demented patients are unreliable respondents. Not only are caregivers more verbal and assertive, but the attending physician relies on them to interpret and communicate the patient's medical and functional status. Some caregivers monopolize the physician's time with accounts of how the daily care of the demented patient stresses them, rather than describing the patient's condition.

Caregivers, thus, can fall into the role of a patient, with the physician attending to their needs over those of the demented patient. Two problems are created when the family caregiver becomes the patient. First, the physician may lose sight of the patient's needs, particularly in those instances in which the needs of the patient conflict with those of the caregiver. Physicians should be alert to signs of neglect or abuse when caregivers appear preoccupied with their own plight over that of the patient.

Second, the caregiver's growing dependency on the physician is harmful because it can reinforce feelings of incompetency in the caregiver and thereby accelerate institutionalization of the patient. Clinicians should not treat family members or other caregivers as patients; rather, they should regard caregivers as their partners in a "joint effort directed at obtaining optimal care for the patient."[80] Although the emotional needs of the caregiver are legitimate, they should remain distinct from the medical needs of the patient.

Family members of patients with AD were interviewed in a series of monthly meetings under the aegis of the Fairhill Center for Aging in Cleveland, Ohio, to determine normative attitudes about care of their demented family members. The results of these conversations were published as a set of guidelines for the care of patients with AD from the family caregiver's perspective.[81] The topics discussed included telling the truth about diagnosis, driving automobiles, respecting choice, controlling behavior, and deciding about death and dying.

NURSING HOME ISSUES

The decision to place a demented patient in a nursing home provides the context for several ethical considerations. An ethical analysis considers the concepts of patient autonomy, nonmaleficence, and beneficence as well as the psychological, social, and financial status of the caregivers. Often, nursing home placement will have occurred following a lengthy and ultimately unsuccessful attempt at home care. In other instances, placement will have occurred before reasonable alternatives have been made at home. Premature nursing home placement may suit the convenience of caregivers, such as middle-aged children who lack the dedication to try to care for an aging demented parent at home. The physician has a difficult role in such cases, in attempting to balance the rights and interests of the dependent, incompetent patient against those of the more assertive and controlling family.

Diane Meier and Christine Cassel performed an ethical analysis of physician and caregiver roles in the process of deciding to institutionalize demented patients.[82] The patient has autonomy-based rights requiring that caregivers and physicians try to the greatest extent possible to follow her previously expressed wishes regarding nursing home placement. Both also have nonmaleficence-based and beneficence-based duties to determine what decision is in the patient's best interest.

Meier and Cassel's ethical analysis generates a checklist for health professionals considering nursing home placement. (1) Health professionals should attempt to determine what the patient wants. If the patient no longer can express herself, the physician should seek some idea of her preferences by inquiring about previous conversations with family, friends, or clergy. Relevant advance directives should be sought. (2) The physician should attempt to analyze the dynamics of the decision for nursing home placement. Is the decision serving the interests of the family more than those of the patient? Has a social worker investigated all reasonable alternatives to nursing home placement? Can the services of home health aides, adult day care, respite admissions, and caretaker training avoid or delay institutionalization? (3) If institutionalization appears inevitable because the patient's needs will be best satisfied in a nursing home or because there are no feasible alternatives, physicians must see that the patient and family continue to receive emotional support, reassurance, security, and freedom from fear of abandonment. If nursing home placement is required because the heath-care system has financial constraints that preclude better alternatives, families can work to change those laws through the political process.[83]

Once the patient has been admitted to a nursing home, the clinician should attend to the fundamental components of nursing home care: palliation, rehabilitation, and management of coexisting illnesses. Palliative care consists of making nursing home life as comfortable as possible for the patient by relieving her physical pain and psychological distress. Palliative measures include optimal design of the physical living space and attention to the emotional responsiveness of the nursing staff. The goal of rehabilitation is to maximize physical and intellectual functioning within the constraints of the patient's illness. Use of physical therapy, prosthetics, orthotics, and cognitive therapies promotes this goal. The importance of careful attention to treating comorbid illnesses and avoiding medication side effects was emphasized previously.[84]

The possibility of admitting the patient to a special nursing care unit dedicated to dementia patients should be investigated. Many nursing homes now have developed special care units for AD patients. It has been estimated that approximately 100,000 long-term special care unit beds were available for demented patients in 1991, although the demand for such beds markedly exceeded the supply.[85] By 1995, 10.4% of all Medicare or Medicaid-certified nursing homes had AD special care units and each facility devoted approximately one quarter of its beds to that unit.[86]

The special care unit for AD patients has a physical plant designed for the safety and ease of 24-hour care of the ambulatory demented patient, in contrast to the "medical" model appropriate for most nonambulatory nursing home patients. The staff receives special training in the treatment of the demented patient, particularly in the means to manage complications of dementia in the most humane and least harmful ways. Additional staff members are available for social stimulation of the patient. Protected outdoor space is available for patient use.[87] Despite the obvious humane aspects of the AD special care units, a controlled study of their use showed no slowing of the functional decline of the AD residents living in them.[88]

Decision making for demented nursing home residents proceeds in the same fashion as decision making for any incompetent patient (see chapters 2, 4, and 8). It is essential to encourage patients to execute advance directives for medical care in the earliest stages of dementia when it still may be possible for them to do so.[89] Treatment plans, including resuscitation status, should be agreed on between the physician and the family at the time of the patient's admission because the plan represents the treatment the patient would wish to receive if she retained the capacity to consent.

Ethical issues arising in the care of the nursing home patient with dementia usually can be resolved by the physician and the family. In those instances in which resolution is not possible, referral to a nursing home ethics committee may be desirable. But because no more than one-fourth of nursing homes have functioning ethics committees, another alternative is to discuss the ethical problem at an open forum of interested nursing home personnel known as "ethics rounds." The rounds consist of a multidisciplinary case presentation followed by an interview of the patient or family, a discussion by the staff, and, when possible, a review by a trained clinical ethicist.[90]

RESTRAINING PATIENTS

The decision to use mechanical or pharmacological restraints to control agitation in demented patients raises medical, nursing, and ethical questions. Mechanical restraints consist, at a minimum, of a cloth jacket ("Posey") tied to the bed or chair to prevent the patient from arising and, at a maximum, leather cuffs applied around each wrist and ankle and tied to the bed ("four-point restraints") to prevent more than a few degrees of limb movement. Pharmacological restraint is achieved by administering psychoactive medications, such as neuroleptics, barbiturates, or benzodiazepines, to sedate or quiet an agitated patient.

The use of mechanical or pharmacological restraints may be justified to better control disruptive and combative behavior that may be harmful to the patient's health, threaten the comfort or safety of other patients, or jeopardize the safety of the nursing staff. The harms caused by ordering restraints include the loss of the patient's personal freedom, the frustration and indignity of being tied down or drugged, the secondary physical injury that may result from improper or injudicious application or prescription of mechanical or pharmacological restraints, the impairment in breathing and in other physiological functions resulting from forced immobility, and the potential for induced worsening of behavioral and cognitive functioning.

Three fundamental ethical questions should be addressed in prescribing restraints: (1) Are the harms produced by restraining a patient justified by the benefits of doing so? (2) Are restraint orders intended more for the patient's good or for the benefit of the nursing staff or institution? (3) Is it ethically justifiable to restrain one patient for the benefit of another? Examining data on the beneficial and harmful effects of restraints and the prevalence of their use helps answer these questions.

The prevalence of mechanical restraint use in hospitalized patients has been estimated at 7% to 22%, and in nursing home patients at 25% to 60%, depending on patient demography, particularly on the percentage of patients who are confused or demented.[91] Studies have shown that older age, disorientation, dependence in dressing, greater participation in social activities, and nonuse of antidepressant drugs are independent predictors of physicians' decisions to order mechanical restraints. The most frequently cited reasons for ordering mechanical restraints were unsteadiness in walking (72%), disruptive behavior such as agitation (41%), and wandering (40%).[92]

Independent risk factors differ for patients restrained mechanically and pharmacologically. Patients for whom mechanical restraints had been ordered were non-ambulatory, dependent on help for transfers, had impaired mental status, a history of hip fracture, and were located in areas of the facility with a high staff-to-patient ratio. By contrast, patients for whom pharmacological restraints had been ordered were physically abusive, had severely impaired mental status, and had frequent family visitation. In comparison to other nursing home units, investigators found that special care units for demented patients were successful in reducing the use of mechanical but not pharmacological restraints.[93] In a later study, investigators found that Alzheimer special care units had the same rate of physical restraint use as traditional units and had a higher rate of using psychotropic medication for pharmacological restraints.[94] In place of sedation or restraints, some institutions have used net beds or devised creative ways to monitor wandering AD patients, such as with the use of electronic tracking devices.[95]

Several studies found that the use of mechanical restraints paradoxically makes patients more likely to sustain injury, In one study of 12 nursing homes, use of mechanical restraints was associated with continued and perhaps increased numbers of fall-related injuries.[96] A study of the effects of mechanical restraints on cognitive function showed that restraints worsened patients' cognitive functioning.[97] Hospitals and nursing homes may encourage the use of restraints on confused or demented patients in an attempt to reduce institutional liability.[98] Confused patients who climb out of bed and suffer hip fractures from falls are common plaintiffs in malpractice litigation against health-care institutions. As a result of liability suits and regulations of the Joint Commission on Accreditation of Healthcare Organizations, most institutions have formulated written policies on the indications, contraindications, and use of restraints.

The following guidelines outline ethically acceptable practices in the use of mechanical or pharmacological restraints on demented nursing home patients.

1. Mechanical restraints should never be ordered routinely or as a substitute for careful patient surveillance.

2. Orders for restraints should trigger a medical investigation aimed at identifying and correcting the patient's medical or psychological problem responsible for the order.

3. The patient's proxy decision maker should consent to the restraints and be given full disclosure of the risks and benefits.

4. When indicated, mechanical restraints should be applied carefully, temporarily, and with the least restrictive device possible.

5. When indicated, pharmacological restraints should be prescribed with the proper agent in the lowest effective dose and with frequent reassessments.[99]

In the United States, legal regulations govern the use of restraints. In 1999, the Health Care Financing Administration (HCFA, now called Centers for Medicare and Medicaid Services) issued regulations that all hospitals receiving Medicare or Medicaid payments include the following standard for the use of restraints. The HCFA standard recapitulates the ethical guidelines cited previously. The HCFA regulations provide:

"(1) The patient has the right to be free from restraints of any form that are not medically necessary or are used as a means of coercion, discipline, convenience, or retaliation by staff . . . (2) A restraint can only be used if needed to improve the patient's well-being and less restrictive interventions have been determined to be ineffective . . . (3) The use of the restraint must be . . . in accordance with the order of a physician or other licensed independent practitioner [and] . . . never written as a standing [or as needed] order . . . (4) The condition of the restrained patient must be continually assessed, monitored, and reevaluated."[100]

END-OF-LIFE MEDICAL TREATMENT

The greatest ethical controversy surrounds decisions at the end of life, particularly decisions to limit or withdraw medical treatment from the patient with severe dementia. It has been a time-honored tradition in medical practice for physicians to allow a failing, elderly patient to die "naturally" when her "time had come." When the elderly patient had severe dementia, it was customary for the physician to allow her to die from inanition when eating became impossible, from pneumonia ("the old man's friend," to paraphrase Sir William Osler), or from other intercurrent illnesses that now can be treated and potentially reversed. Thus, physicians' practices to limit or withdraw medical treatment of elderly demented patients, although now discussed openly and ordered explicitly, are not new.

Several studies in nursing homes have assessed the extent to which current medical practices allow infirm elderly patients to die. In 1979, Brown and Thompson published the first report of nursing home residents who purposely were not treated after developing fever. In 43% of the patients documented to have significant fevers, physicians chose neither to investigate the cause of the fever nor to treat the patients with antibiotics. As a result, 59% of the untreated group died.[101] Other reports described similar practices.[102] Despite the frequency with which physicians limit or withdraw medical treatment, the decision is often a personally painful one for the physician or nurse. The physician may be uncertain of the exact criteria that warrant the decision to forgo treatment and may be unclear about who is authorized to make such a decision. Ambiguity, ambivalence, uncertainty, and guilt are common feelings in physicians who have to decide when to stop potentially life-saving treatment of elderly, demented patients.[103] Cultural factors also are relevant because American physicians are more likely than Dutch physicians to treat pneumonia in demented nursing home residents.[104]

Ethical concepts relevant to a decision not to treat include respect for autonomy, nonmaleficence, and justice. The physician's respect for a patient's autonomy can continue to be exercised despite the patient's dementia if the physician follows the terms of previously executed advance directives. If such a directive stipulated that the patient refuses consent for aggressive medical care if she were to become demented, the physician should respect that wish and not treat the patient aggressively. In the absence of clear advance directives, physicians should seek and follow valid testimony from family members about the patient's wishes and health-care values. Assuming that there is no conflict between the patient's current and past wishes (such as that discussed previously), formal and informal advance directives are valid and should be followed.

The ethical concept of nonmaleficence becomes relevant in the common instance in which the patient has executed no advance directives and no information is available concerning her wishes. In this instance, a benefit-burden analysis is carried out and a best interest standard is applied, as discussed in chapter 4. Given the benefits and burdens of aggressive treatment, is this course in the best interest of the demented patient or is it in her best interest to be permitted to die? Although the benefits of treatment include prolonging life, life of a patient with advanced dementia may be one of suffering without the countervailing pleasures of self-awareness or awareness of family and friends. The burdens of treating a severely demented patient include indignity,

discomfort, and expense. The financial and emotional stress on loved ones is an important factor as well. A strong argument can be made in favor of allowing the severely demented patient to die by purposely not treating intercurrent illnesses or by cessation of tube feedings because this approach seems to be in the patient's best interest.[105]

Concepts of justice also are relevant in these situations. What claim do patients or their surrogate decision makers have to demand high-technology, aggressive treatment for the severely demented patient when society's resources are scarce, particularly because such care has been shown to be futile in outcome studies? Because of society's finite health-care resources, I discuss the argument in chapter 10 that physicians have no ethical duty to provide futile medical care, even if it is requested, and they may have an ethical duty not to provide futile care. Society does have the duty to maintain patients' chronic care, including measures to enhance their comfort and dignity.

Limitation of medical treatment for the patient with severe dementia can be defended on the ethical grounds of respect for autonomy in cases in which advance directives or information about valid health-care preferences is present. In cases in which no advance directives or other information exists, medical treatment can be limited on the ethical grounds of nonmaleficence and justice. Clinicians can provide appropriate medical treatment in patients with advanced dementia by ordering supportive or palliative care. Supportive or palliative care refers to a level of care intended to promote the comfort, hygiene, and dignity of a terminally or chronically ill patient, but which does not necessarily prolong life. Medical conditions that produce discomfort are treated, but conditions that do not produce discomfort are not treated.[106]

Palliative care can be ordered for patients with a terminal illness, an irreversible vegetative states, a chronic irreversible disease (if requested by a competent patient), or a progressive advanced dementia. A palliative care plan should be ordered when the patient is admitted to the hospital or nursing home. The physician should write explicit orders clarifying which therapies should be given and which should be withheld.[107] (See chapter 7.) The nursing staff should understand and concur with the plan because, by following the patient's wishes, it is the ethically correct course of action. Physicians caring for patients with severe dementia can work closely with family members to develop consensus-based treatment plans to determine exactly what elements of palliative care are necessary and desirable in individual cases.[108]

A palliative care plan includes comfort measures, administering oxygen for dyspnea, keeping airways cleared, hygienic measures, including bathing, grooming, skin care, bowel and bladder care, and positioning, and passive range of movement exercises to prevent contractures. Hospital admissions and surgical procedures are avoided unless they are necessary to provide comfort. Do-Not-Resuscitate orders are written. Patients may receive morphine to treat pain or dyspnea and antipyretics to lower uncomfortable fevers. Families are given emotional support as the patient dies. Hydration and nutrition are provided, encouraged, and assisted orally, but they are not administered parenterally or by a feeding tube unless they improve the patient's comfort or are explicitly ordered by a lawful surrogate.[109]

The most common acute ethical issue arising in the nursing home management of the patient with advanced dementia is whether to insert a feeding tube. Patients with progressive AD and other dementing illnesses ultimately lose their ability to chew and swallow, and begin to lose weight.[110] At this point, the question arises whether to maintain hydration and nutrition through a gastrostomy feeding tube. In the past, it was simply accepted that insertion of feeding tubes was indicated and medically appropriate. But over the past two decades, with the accumulation of data showing no benefits of feeding tubes, opinions and practice guidelines on their appropriateness have changed.[111]

The prevalence of tube feeding for patients with advanced dementia has been measured in two studies. In a cross-sectional Medicare database study of nearly 200,000 nursing home residents with advanced dementia, Susan Mitchell and colleagues determined that more than one-third had feeding tubes. Factors correlating with feeding tube use were younger age, male sex, nonwhite race, divorced marital status, lack of advance directives, recent decline in functional status, and no diagnosis of AD.[112] Joan Teno and colleagues, using the 1999 National Repository of the Minimum Data Set of over 385,000 nursing home residents with severe dementia, found that 18.1% had feeding tubes. The rate varied from 3.8% in Nebraska to 44.8% in the District of Columbia. Patients with Do-Not-Resuscitate orders had a markedly reduced utilization of feeding tubes.[113]

Thomas Finucane and colleagues performed an evidence-based review of the effects of feeding tubes in patients with advanced dementia. They were unable to find any data showing benefit of feeding tubes in these patients and found harms from feeding tubes including increased risk of aspiration pneumonia, gastric perforation, and local irritative effects. They concluded that feeding tube placement and use in severely demented patients should be discouraged on clinical grounds.[114] Subsequent editorials, opinion pieces, and reviews in prominent journals concurred with this assessment.[115] A study of hospitalized patients with advanced dementia showed no survival benefit from a feeding tube.[116] An opinion survey of internists found that 84% believed that tube feeding of the patient with advanced dementia was inappropriate.[117] A study of cognitively intact patients over age 65 found that 95% said they would not want tube feedings if they were in a state of severe dementia.[118] One study of 178 nursing home patients with severe dementia found that the patients did not suffer following cessation of hydration and nutrition by gastrostomy tube or parenterally.[119]

One troubling reason for the excessive use of feeding tubes in patients with advanced dementia is that many physicians misunderstand their value. In one survey measuring physician knowledge and beliefs about feeding tube benefits in patients with advanced dementia, 76% of physicians believed that a feeding tube would reduce the risk of aspiration, 75% believed it would accelerate healing of a decubitus ulcer, 61% believed it would prolong survival, and 27% believed it would improve functional status. None of these beliefs can be supported by available data.[120]

The Ethics and Humanities Subcommittee of the American Academy of Neurology published an ethics practice statement about neurologists' ethical duties in managing the patient with dementia. On the topic of feeding tubes in advanced dementia, the Academy stated "Oral hydration and nutrition are offered, assisted, and encouraged, but hydration and nutrition are not provided by artificial enteral or parenteral means unless they contribute to patient comfort or are chosen by the patient or proxy."[121] Two analyses of withholding tube feeding in the patient with severe dementia found that the practice was compatible with traditional Judaism, given that such patients are dying and that they would suffer more with the feeding tube than without it.[122]

In survey studies, the majority of gerontologists, other physicians, and family members of patients with end-stage dementia agreed that a palliative care plan represents the optimum form of medical treatment for the severely demented patient.[123] Yet, there remain some family members and other surrogate decision makers who demand that the severely demented patient receive hospitalization, cardiopulmonary resuscitation, and other similarly aggressive treatments for intercurrent illnesses.[124] How physicians respond to these demands should depend on how rational or futile they appear and to what extent they are consistent with the patient's previously stated wishes and present best interest.

Palliative care plans have been implemented in several special care nursing units for demented patients. Ladislaw Volicer and colleagues reported their experience with administering palliative care to a group of patients with advanced AD. On admission to the unit, patients were assigned to one of five levels of care, which, in retrospect, correlated with the severity of their dementia. At the lowest level, patients received only supportive care without feeding tubes. Interestingly, despite the fact that a total of 62% of the patients in all groups studied were not treated for fever or infection, the mortality rate on the unit did not change from what it had been before the palliative care dementia program was initiated.[125]

Nelda Wray and colleagues reported their experience in instituting a palliative care plan for severely demented patients admitted to an acute care hospital. On admission, care plans based on the severity of dementia and the family wishes were negotiated with the family. The mortality rate of those from whom care was withheld was fivefold higher than on the group that received full care.[126] A recent study found four factors that correlated with healthcare surrogates' satisfaction with the end-of-life care given to patients with advanced dementia: greater communication with staff, better patient comfort, no tube feedings, and care in a specialized dementia unit.[127]

Unfortunately, not all severely demented patients receive proper palliative care at the end of life. Two studies of nursing home patients with advanced dementia showed inadequate palliative care. In one study, physicians predicted that 1.1% of admitted patients with advanced dementia would die within 6 months but 71% of the patients died within that time period. Most dying patients did not receive proper palliative care.[128] Thus, a common barrier to providing palliative care to patients with advanced dementia is that some physicians fail to correctly diagnose them as terminally ill.[129] Susan Mitchell and colleagues developed a risk score for determining the prognosis for survival of nursing home residents admitted with advanced dementia. In their cohort of over 1,900 patients, 28.3% died within six months of admission.[130]

Despite the appropriateness of palliative care in patients with advanced dementia, patients with AD and other primary dementias currently comprise only a small fraction of hospice patients. In a survey of nearly 1,700 hospices in the United States, patients with primary dementia accounted for fewer than 1% of patients and only 21% of hospices even served dementia patients. Because 7% of the patients had secondary dementia, there was no reason why patients with primary dementia could not be served by hospice.[131] As noted, a major barrier to hospice referral is that many physicians do not consider patients with advanced dementia to be terminally ill, despite ample data to the contrary.[132] Specific criteria for identifying advanced dementia patients as terminally ill and enrolling them in hospice have been enumerated.[133] One study showed that hospice referral of dementia patients residing in nursing homes correlated with dying patients' symptoms of pain and dyspnea.[134] In an analysis of government policies and practices that deter hospice use in long-term care, Diane Hoffman and Anita Tarzian suggested restructuring existing incentives to increase the palliative mission of chronic care facilities and lessen concern about overspending the Medicare hospice benefit.[135]

LEGAL ISSUES

Judiciaries and legislatures have addressed the right of dementia patients to refuse life-sustaining medical therapies as well as the procedural issues governing how the decision should be made and by whom.[136] There are parallels between judicial rulings on withholding and withdrawing medical treatment for demented patients and patients in a vegetative state. (See chapters 8 and 12.)

Three Massachusetts cases illustrate this trend. In *Dinnerstein*, the Massachusetts Appeals Court upheld the authority of the physician and family of a man with advanced AD to enter a Do-Not-Resuscitate order without requiring judicial review. In *Spring*, the Massachusetts Supreme Judicial Court authorized a physician, with agreement from the family, to discontinue hemodialysis on an elderly man with AD. In *Hier*, the Massachusetts Appeals Court ruled that physicians were not required to reinsert a feeding tube that an elderly demented woman had repeatedly removed.[137]

The New Jersey Supreme Court decision in *Conroy* was the most influential ruling permitting a severely demented patient to die by purposefully withholding artificial hydration and nutrition. Claire Conroy was an 85-year-old nursing home resident at the time the decision was made. She was severely demented, bedridden, and incontinent. She required tube feedings because she could not eat. Her nephew, who was her legal guardian, petitioned the court to permit not reinserting her feeding tube, which she had removed repeatedly. In its favorable decision, the court provided rule by which feeding, hydration, and other types of life-support measures may be discontinued on

patients who are awake but have "serious and permanent mental and physical impairment . . . who . . . will probably die within one year."[138]

The *Conroy* court articulated three standards that are applicable in three different situations. The first "subjective" standard directed physicians to honor valid advance directives for medical care. In the absence of advance directives, the second "limited objective" standard directed physicians to honor" some trustworthy evidence" provided by family or friends stating that the patient would have refused medical treatment in this situation. Such evidence could be found from previous conversations as well as from inferences that the patient made concerning her attitudes and feelings about dignity. The second standard could be used only if dying would relieve the patient of pain.

In the absence of my reliable evidence, the state would invoke the authority of *parens patriae* to determine the patient's best interest. Here, the third, or "pure objective" standard would be applied, which requires objective proof that the burdens of medical treatment outweighed its benefits. By burdens, the *Conroy* court specifically referred to "recurring, unavoidable, and severe pain," making it "inhumane" to continue treatment.

Although the *Conroy* court was applauded for its substantive achievements, it received criticism for its onerous procedural requirements. The court mandated that physicians who wished to discontinue medical treatment of a nursing home patient must file papers through the state Ombudsman's Office, an office established to investigate allegations of patient abuse in nursing homes. This time-consuming, laborious, and expensive procedural hurdle unjustifiably restricts proper medical decision making and likely will serve to discourage physicians from appropriately terminating medical treatment in demented patients.[139]

The *O'Connor* ruling by the New York Court of Appeals reversed some of the ground gained by the *Conroy* decision and highlighted the difference in evidentiary standards between the states of New York and New Jersey.[140] Mrs. O'Connor suffered several strokes rendering her globally aphasic and hemiplegic but awake. She had previously told her daughters that if she were ever incapacitated by an illness in which she had no hope for recovery, she wished to receive no life-sustaining medical treatment. Accordingly, her daughters petitioned the court to authorize the removal of her feeding tube. The court refused to grant permission, however, citing that Mrs. O'Connor's never specifically stipulated that she included life-sustaining hydration and nutrition as a form of medical treatment that she wished withheld.

As discussed further in chapter 4, the states of New York, Missouri, and Maine have an unusually demanding "clear and convincing" standard for evidence of a person's previous wishes to have medical treatment discontinued before they can be followed. The *O'Connor* court held that the state's clear and convincing standard was not satisfied in this case. Several critics of this decision in the clinical ethics community pointed out that no citizens of New York state who lacked the foresight to stipulate clearly in advance that they considered artificial hydration and nutrition to be forms of medical therapy, could ever have artificial hydration and nutrition withheld under this standard.[141]

It is desirable for patients to execute written and surrogate advance directives for medical care. These directives should also be discussed at length with their family and physicians. It is also desirable for states to enact health-care surrogate laws to provide adequate decision-making procedures for the majority of those elderly patients who lacked the knowledge or foresight to have executed advance directives.[142] Judicial review should be neither necessary nor desirable unless there is unresolvable disagreement on the best course of action within the family or between the family and the physician. As explained in chapter 8, state advance directive statutes vary in the extent to which a lawful surrogate is empowered to discontinue a dying patient's artificial hydration and nutrition in the absence of specific written directions.[143]

RESEARCH ISSUES

How to secure valid consent for a demented patient to serve as a human research subject is the fundamental research ethics issue.[144] As discussed in chapters 2 and 19, approval to begin medical care of or research on incompetent patients requires valid consent of the surrogate decision maker once the patient has lost capacity.[145] When the intent of research is to help the demented patient directly, such as a drug trial of a new pharmaceutical agent designed to improve cognition, obtaining consent from the surrogate usually is a simple matter. The surrogate employs a benefit-burden assessment to weight potential benefits against known risks to the patient to reach a decision.[146] With the potential benefit of a new drug to improve cognition and a small potential risk to the patient, the surrogate usually will provide consent.

Consider, however, a situation in which an investigator requests that a demented patient participate in a research protocol in which the patient probably will not benefit directly, but future patients with her condition may benefit from the knowledge gained. Many surrogate decision makers refuse consent in this situation because they calculate that the risks of participation to the individual patient, even if minimal, exceed the direct benefits. Usually they do not conceptualize their role of patient advocate and protector to encompass a spirit of volunteerism or altruism.

Moreover, guidelines regulating research on dementia patients published by medical societies including the American Academy of Neurology,[147] American College of Physicians,[148] and American Psychiatric Association[149] adopt a paternalistic and protective stance, requiring the research to be of low risk and to offer potential benefit to the human subject. The protective intent of these guidelines is understandable because they were drafted in response to documented instances of abuse of cognitively impaired research subjects to protect them as a class of vulnerable patients from future abuse.[150]

What both surrogate decision makers and medical society guidelines fail to consider, however, is that competent patients with chronic, progressive, untreatable neurological disorders, such as amyotrophic lateral sclerosis and multiple sclerosis, routinely volunteer for research that cannot help them, because it may aid persons who suffer from the disease in the future. These patients volunteer to serve as research subjects as an altruistic and ennobling act to produce good and meaning from their suffering resulting from progressive illnesses.[151] In fulfilling their difficult task, surrogates of cognitively impaired patients have an understandable predisposition to protect the patient and not to foster altruistic goals.

Court rulings and recommendations from national bioethics commissions have further restricted research in cognitively impaired patients by erecting rules and procedural barriers. A New York court ruled that no minor or physically or mentally incapacitated adult could participate in any research protocol that contained a non-therapeutic element, irrespective of the possible benefits to the subject or knowledge to be gained.[152] Similarly, the National Bioethics Advisory Commission recommended tightening the procedural requirements for institutional review boards to "require that an independent, qualified professional assess the potential subject's capacity to consent" for any protocol requiring more than minimal risk, unless the investigator can adequately justify the exception.[153] Several leading neuroscientists and clinicians protested these recommendations, pointing out that they will overprotect cognitively and mentally impaired research subjects and ultimately may do more harm than good by discouraging research that could help them and others with their conditions.[154]

Surrogates should understand that an added benefit to patients serving as human research subjects is the increased intensity of nursing and medical care that they receive. As part of the research protocol, research subjects are examined more frequently and intensively than probably would occur otherwise. As a result of increased professional attention, patient care may be more thorough, potentially improving the patient's functional status.[155]

Surveys in nursing homes confirm that it is difficult to secure surrogate consent for research involving nursing home residents, particularly for those who are cognitively impaired. The surrogates in one study refused consent in 46% of the requests for three reasons: (1) research should not be conducted in nursing homes; (2) the study would disturb the patient unjustifiably; or (3) the patient would have refused were she capable of responding to the request.[156]

Research performed on patients in nursing homes is ethically permissible and should be encouraged if it is conducted under the following guidelines: (1) the nursing home must be associated with a hospital that has an institutional review board; (2) the nursing home must have a record of excellence and have teaching and research as part of its mission; (3) patients and families should share in institutional management decisions to formulate research rules and regulations; (4) appointment of a durable power of attorney for health care should be encouraged to avoid legal complications; and (5) surrogate support groups should be formed to help surrogates cope with their lonely and psychologically difficult task.[157]

The institutional review board (IRB) of a hospital is designed to benefit research subjects by protecting them from various harms, such as dangerous protocols, inadequate safety monitoring, and bad science.[158] (See chapters 5 and 19.) The members of the IRB should take steps, however, not to overprotect cognitively impaired patient by erecting procedural barriers so formidable that research cannot be done in nursing homes.

One possible solution to the problem of surrogates' refusing consent is for patients in early stages of dementia to execute advance directives permitting their later participation as research subjects. These directives could be executed simultaneously with similar advance directives for medical care, thereby providing proxies clear guidelines for future decisions in both areas.[159] Whether executing advance directives is a practical solution remains untested.

In an interview study, Jason Karlawish and colleagues examined why AD patients and their caregivers chose to consent to or refuse entry of the AD patient into a clinical trial. Caregiver-patient pairs who consented to the clinical trial were more likely to include spouse-caregivers who trusted the principal investigator, medical center, or pharmaceutical company. Their trust neutralized their concerns about research risks. Conversely, caregiver-patient pairs who refused entry into the trial were more likely to include adult children-caregivers suffering stress from depression or for whom logistic burdens, such as the difficulty of traveling to the study site, were paramount issues.[160]

Scott Kim and colleagues surveyed people at risk for AD, asking whether they thought the consent of surrogates was sufficient grounds for consent for research. Over 90% of respondents indicated that surrogates properly could consent for studies involving minimal risk or for new therapeutic agents that might improve cognition. A smaller majority approved of more invasive research studies.[161] Jeffrey Berger and Deborah Majerovitz surveyed a small group of older adults about the adequacy of surrogate consent for dementia research. They found that surrogates commonly expressed the motive of lessening the burden on the family, which increased their willingness to consent.[162]

Steven Albert and colleagues found an additional benefit accruing to AD patients who serve as research subjects in clinical trials. In their study comparing outcomes of AD patients who participated or did not participate in clinical trials, they found no difference between the groups in functional endpoints or risk of death. The only significant difference between the groups was that the AD patients who participated in clinical trials had a significantly lower chance of being placed in a nursing home than those who did not participate. The investigators were unclear if the lower rate of nursing home placement was the result of the study drug effect, selection factors, or a beneficial effect of the study on the patients' caregivers.[163]

NOTES

1. Sachs GA, Cassel CK. Ethical aspects of dementia. *Neurol Clin* 1989;7:845–858. For other general reviews of the topic, see Post SG. Key issues in the ethics of dementia care. *Neurol Clin* 2000;18:1011–1022 and Post SG. *The Moral Challenge of Alzheimer Disease: Ethical Issues from Diagnosis to Dying*, 2nd ed. Baltimore: Johns Hopkins University Press, 2000.

2. Mortimer JA, Schuman LM, French LR. Epidemiology of dementing illness. In Mortimer JA, Schuman LM, eds. *The Epidemiology of Dementia*. New York: Oxford University Press; 1981:5. The octagenarian figures are from a meta-analysis of 47 published studies cited in Skoog I, Nilsson L, Palmertz B, et al. A population based study of dementia in 85-year-olds. *N Engl J Med* 1993;328:153–158.

3. Beck JC, Benson DF, Scheibel AB, et al. Dementia in the elderly: the silent epidemic. *Ann Intern Med* 1982;97:231–241.

4. National Nursing Home Survey: United States 1973–1974. Washington, DC: US Government Printing Office, 1977.

5. Ferri CP, Prince M, Brayne C, et al. Global prevalence of dementia: a Delphi consensus study. *Lancet* 2005;366:2112–2117.

6. For reviews of the clinical features and treatment of Alzheimer's disease, see Blennow K, de Leon MJ, Zetterberg H. Alzheimer's disease. *Lancet* 2006;368:387–403 and Clark CM, Karlawish JHT. Alzheimer disease: current concepts and emerging diagnostic and therapeutic strategies. *Ann Intern Med* 2003;138:400–410.

7. These data are derived from Bachman DL, Wolf PA, Linn RT, et al. Incidence of dementia and probable Alzheimer's disease in a general population: the Framingham Study. *Neurology* 1993;43:515–519 and Jorm AF. *The Epidemiology of Alzheimer's Disease and Related Disorders*. London: Chapman & Hall, 1990. See the discussion of these data in Small GW, Rabins PV, Barry PP, et al. Diagnosis and treatment of Alzheimer disease and related disorders: consensus statement of the American Association for Geriatric Psychiatry, the Alzheimer's Association, and the American Geriatrics Society. *JAMA* 1997;278:1363–1371. For a discussion of some of the technical problems in accurately ascertaining AD incidence and prevalence, see Albert MS, Drachman DA. Alzheimer's disease: what is it, how many people have it, and why do we need to know? *Neurology* 2000;55:166–168.

8. Hebert LE, Scherr PA, Bienas JL, Bennett DA, Evans DA. Alzheimer disease in the US population: prevalence estimates using the 2000 census. *Arch Neurol* 2003;60:1119–1122.

9. Mayeux R, Foster NL, Rossor M, et al. The clinical evaluation of patients with dementia. In Whitehouse PJ, ed. *Dementia*. Philadelphia: FA Davis Co, 1993:92.

10. Ernst RL, Hay JW, Fenn C, Tinklenberg J, Yesavage JA. Cognitive function and the costs of Alzheimer's disease: an exploratory study. *Arch Neurol* 1997;54:687–693.

11. For the most recent CERAD publications, see Fillenbaum G, Heyman A, Peterson BL, Pieper CF, Weiman AL. Frequency and duration of hospitalization in patients with AD based on Medicare data: CERAD XX. *Neurology* 2000;54:588–593; Fillenbaum G, Heyman A, Peterson BL, Pieper CF, Weiman AL. Use and cost of hospitalization of patients with AD by stage and living arrangement: CERAD XXI. *Neurology* 2001;56:201–206; and Fillenbaum G, Heyman A, Peterson BL, Pieper CF, Weiman AL. Use and cost of outpatient visits of AD patients: CERAD XXII. *Neurology* 2001;56:1706–1711. The background and purpose of CERAD are explained in Heyman A, Fillenbaum G, Nash F (eds). Consortium to Establish a Registry for Alzheimer's Disease: the CERAD Experience. *Neurology* 1997;49 (suppl 3):S1-S23.

12. For an analysis of the modest treatment benefit of cholinesterase inhibitor drugs in Alzheimer's disease, see Birks J. Cholinesterase inhibitors for Alzheimer's disease. *Cochrane Database Syst Rev* 2006;1:CD005593.

13. Ernst RL, Hay JW, Fenn C, Tinklenberg J, Yesavage JA. Cognitive function and the costs of Alzheimer disease: an exploratory study. *Arch Neurol* 1997;54:687–693.

14. The unique features of the relationship between the demented patient and the physician are discussed further in: Sachs GA, Cassel CK. Ethical aspects of dementia. *Neurol Clin* 1989;7:845–858; Cassel CK. Ethical dilemmas in dementia. *Semin Neurol* 1984;4:92–97; and Cassel CK, Jameton AL. Dementia in the elderly: an analysis of medical responsibility. *Ann Intern Med* 1981:94:802–807.

15. For the importance of treating comorbid illnesses in the demented patient, such as hypertension, diabetes, cardiovascular disease, and osteoporosis, see Brauner DJ, Muir JC, Sachs GA. Treating nondementia illnesses in patients with dementia. *JAMA* 2000;283:3230–3235.

16. The great 19th century British neurologist John Hughlings Jackson wrote in 1894, "Dementia is the fourth state of dissolution . . . At the bottom . . . there is no *person*, but only a living creature." Jackson JH. The factors of insanities. In Adams LB (ed). *Selected Writings of John Hughlings Jackson*. Birmingham, AL: Gryphon Editions, 1985:411–421.

17. For the most egregious example of how demented elderly hospitalized patients are depersonalized by cynical and sadistic medical house officers, see Shem S. *House of God*. New York: Dell Publishers, 1978. For a more scholarly treatment of the problem, see George V, Dundas A. The gomer: a figure of American hospital folk speech. *J Am Folklore* 1978;91:568–577.

18. The spring 1998 issue of the *Journal of Clinical Ethics* was devoted to this topic. See, especially, Kitwood T. Toward a theory of dementia care: ethics and interaction. *J Clin Ethics* 1998;9:23–34; Sabat SR. Voices of Alzheimer's disease sufferers: a call for treatment based on personhood. *J Clin Ethics* 1998;9:35–48; and Lyman KA. Living with Alzheimer's disease: the creation of meaning among persons with dementia. *J Clin Ethics* 1998;9:49–57.

19. Cassel CK. *Semin Neurol* 1984:92–97 and Gorlin R, Zucker HD. Physicians' reactions to patients: a key to teaching humanistic medicine. *N Engl J Med* 1983;108:1059–1063.

20. Arnold SE, Kumar A. Reversible dementias. *Med Clin North Am* 1993;77:215–230.

21. Cassel CK. *Semin Neurol* 1984;4:93. For a discussion of ethical aspects of chronic medical care, see Jennings B, Callahan D, Caplan AL. Ethical challenges of chronic illness. *Hastings Cent Rep* 1988;18(suppl 2):1–16.

22. For reviews of the medical management of the demented patient, see Blennow K, de Leon MJ, Zetterberg H. Alzheimer's disease. *Lancet* 2006;368:387–403 and Clark CM, Karlawish JHT. Alzheimer disease: current concepts and emerging diagnostic and therapeutic strategies. *Ann Intern Med* 2003;138:400–410.

23. Rodin J. Aging and health: effects of the sense of control. *Science* 1986;233:1271–1276.

24. Foley JM. The experience of being demented. In Binstock RH, Post SG, Whitehouse PJ, eds. *Dementia and Aging: Ethics, Values, and Policy Choices*. Baltimore: Johns Hopkins University Press, 1992:30–43.

25. For a study of the frequency of comorbidity in Alzheimer's disease, see Chandra V, Bharucha NE, Schoenberg BS. Conditions associated with Alzheimer's disease at death: case control study. *Neurology* 1986;36:209–211. See also Brauner DJ, Muir JC, Sachs GA. Treating nondementia illnesses in patients with dementia. *JAMA* 2000;283:3230–3235.

26. Meyer JS, Judd BW. Tawakina T, et al. Improved cognition after control of risk factors for multi-infarct dementia. *JAMA* 1986;256 2203–2209. For a recent review of dementia risk factors, see Blennow K, de Leon MJ, Zetterberg H. Alzheimer's disease. *Lancet* 2006;368:387–403.

27. Mulrow CD, Aguilar C, Endicott JE, et al. Quality-of-life changes and hearing impairment: a randomized trial. *Ann Intern Med* 1990;113:188–194.

28. Goodwin JS. Goodwin JM, Garry PJ. Association between nutritional status and cognitive functioning in a healthy elderly population. *JAMA* 1983;249:2917–2921 and Raskind M. Nutrition and cognitive function in the elderly. *JAMA* 1983;249:2939–2940.

29. For prospective series and reviews of how potentially reversible depression may mimic dementia in the elderly patient, see McAllister TW. Overview: pseudodementia. *Am J Psychiatry* 1983;140:528–533; Reding M, Haycox J, Blass J. Depression in patients referred to a dementia clinic: a three-year prospective study. *Arch Neurol* 1985;42:894–896; and Sachdev PS, Smith JS, Angus-Lepan H, et al. Pseudodementia twelve years on. *J Neurol Neurosurg Psychiatry* 1990;53:254–259.

30. Teri L, Gibbons LE, McCurry SM, et al. Exercise plus behavioral management in patients with Alzheimer's disease: a randomized clinical trial. *JAMA* 2003;290:2015–2022.

31. For clinical practice guidelines for the management of the patient with dementia, see Cummings JL, Frank JC, Cherry D, et al. Guidelines for managing Alzheimer's disease: part I. Assessment. *Am Fam Physician* 2002;65:2263–2272; Cummings JL, Frank JC, Cherry D, et al. Guidelines for managing Alzheimer's disease: part II. Treatment. *Am Fam Physician* 2002;65:2525–2234; and Doody RS, Stevens JC, Beck C, et al. Practice parameter: management of dementia (an evidence-based review). Report of the Quality Standards Subcommittee of the American Academy of Neurology. *Neurology* 2001;56:1154–1166.

32. Vickrey BG, Mittman BS, Connor KI, et al. The effect of a disease management intervention on quality and outcomes of dementia care: a randomized, controlled trial. *Ann Intern Med* 2006;145:713–726.

33. Callahan CM, Boustani MA, Unverzagt FW, et al. Effectiveness of collaborative care for older adults with Alzheimer disease in primary care: a randomized, controlled trial. *JAMA* 2006;295:2148–2157.

34. This topic was reviewed in Howard R. Should the diagnosis of Alzheimer's disease always be disclosed? In Zeman A, Emanuel LL, eds. *Ethical Dilemmas in Neurology.* London: W B Saunders Co, 2000:54–60. See also the discussion of diagnostic deception and truth telling in chapter 2.

35. Erde EL, Nadal EC, Scholl TO. On truth telling and the diagnosis of Alzheimer's disease. *J Fam Pract* 1988;26:401–406.

36. Maguire CP, Kirby M, Coen R, Coakley D, Lawlor BA, O'Neill D. Family members' attitudes toward telling the patient with Alzheimer's disease their diagnosis. *BMJ* 1996;313:529–530.

37. Barnes RC. Telling the diagnosis to patients with Alzheimer's disease. *BMJ* 1997;314:375–376.

38. Drickamer MA, Lachs MS. Should patients with Alzheimer's disease be told their diagnosis? *N Engl J Med* 1992;326:947–91 and Meyers BS. Telling patients they have Alzheimer's disease. *BMJ* 1997;341:321–322.

39. Bostick NA, Sade R, McMahon JW, Benjamin R. Report of the American Medical Association Council on Ethical and Judicial Affairs: Withholding information from patients: rethinking the propriety of "therapeutic privilege." *J Clin Ethics* 2006;17:302–306.

40. See Brock DW. Justice and the demented elderly. *J Med Philosophy* 1988;13:73–99; Avorn J. Benefit and cost analysis in geriatric care: turning age discrimination into health policy. *N Engl J Med* 1984;310: 1294–1301; and Kayser-Jones J, Kapp MB. Advocacy for the mentally impaired elderly: a case study analysis. *Am J Law Med* 1989;14:353–376.

41. See Cranford RE, Ashley BZ. Ethical and legal aspects of dementia. *Neurol Clin* 1986;4:479–490 and What do we owe the elderly? Allocating social and health care resources. The Joint International Research Group of the Institute for Bioethics. *Hastings Cent Rep* 1994;24(2):S1-S12.

42. Callahan D. *Setting Limits: Medical Goals in an Aging Society.* New York: Simon & Schuster, 1987 and Callahan D. *What Kind of Life: The Limits of Medical Progress* New York: Simon & Schuster, 1990. A similar argument has been made in Daniels N. *Am I My Parents' Keeper? An Essay on Justice between the Young and the Old.* New York: Oxford University Press, 1988.

43. See the position paper and commentary from the American Geriatric Society: American Geriatric Public Policy Committee. Equitable distribution of limited medical resources. *J Am Geriatr Soc* 1989;37:1063–1064 and Jecker NS, Pearlman RA. Ethical constraints on rationing medical care by age. *J Am Geriatr Soc* 1989;37:1067–1075. For related arguments, see Levinsky NG. Age as a criterion for rationing health care. *N Engl J Med* 1990;322:1813–1816 and Cassell CK. Issues of age and chronic care: another argument for health care reform. *J Am Geriatr Soc* 1992;40:404–409. See also Hunt RW, Callahan D. A critique of using age to ration health care. *J Med Ethics* 1993;19:19–27.

44. Karlawish JHT, Casarett DJ, James BD, Xie SX, Kim SYH. The ability of persons with Alzheimer disease (AD) to make a decision about taking an AD treatment. *Neurology* 2005;64:1514–1519.

45. Gurrera RJ, Moye J, Karel MJ, Azar AR, Armesto JC. Cognitive performance predicts treatment decisional abilities in mild to moderate dementia. *Neurology* 2006;66:1367–1372.

46. Alexander MP. Clinical determination of mental competence: a theory and a retrospective study. *Arch Neurol* 1988;45:23–26; Freedman M, Stuss DT, Gordon M. Assessment of competency: the role of neuro-behavioral deficits. *Ann Intern Med* 1991;115:203–208; Marson DC, Ingram KK, Cody HA, Harrell LE. Assessing the competency of patients with Alzheimer's disease under different legal standards: a prototype instrument. *Arch Neurol* 1995;52:949–954; and Marson DC, Chatterjee A, Ingram KK, Harrell LE. Toward a neurologic model of competency: cognitive predictors of capacity to consent in Alzheimer's disease using three different legal standards. *Neurology* 1996;46:666–672. Daniel Marson and colleagues also have applied the same instrument to test competency in patients with Parkinson's disease. See Dymek MP, Atchison P, Harrell L, Marson DC. Competency to consent to medical treatment in cognitively impaired patients with Parkinson's disease. *Neurology* 2001;56:17–24.

47. McCullough LB, Molinari V, Workman RH. Implications of impaired executive control functions for patient autonomy and surrogate decision making. *J Clin Ethics* 2001;12:397–405.

48. Molinari V, McCollough LB, Workman R, Coverdale J. Geriatric assent. *J Clin Ethics* 2004;15:261–268.

49. Carrese JA. Refusal of care: patient's well-being and physicians' ethical obligations. "But doctor, I want to go home." *JAMA* 2006;296:691–695.

50. For a discussion of the issues ethics consultants should consider, see Swidler RN, Seastrum T, Shelton W. Difficult hospital inpatient discharge decisions: ethical, legal and clinical practice issues. *Am J Bioethics* 2007;7(3):23–28.

51. Henderson VW, Drachman DA. Dementia, butterfly ballots, and voter competence. *Neurology* 2002; 58:995–996.

52. Karlawish JHT, Casarett DA, James BD, et al. Do persons with dementia vote? *Neurology* 2002; 58:1100–1102.

53. For a discussion of these broad questions, see Karlawish JH, Bonnie RJ, Appelbaum PS, et al. Addressing the ethical, legal, and social issues raised by voting by persons with dementia. *JAMA* 2004;292:1345–1350.

54. Keyssar A. *The Right to Vote: The Contested History of Democracy in the United States.* New York: Basic Books, 2000.

55. The President's Council on Bioethics reached this conclusion in a policy recommendation for optimal surrogate decision-making for aging patients. See President's Council on Bioethics. *Taking Care: Ethical Caregiving in our Aging Society.* September 2005. http://www.bioethics.gov/reports/taking_care/chapter5.html (Accessed March 30, 2007).

56. Finucane TE, Beamer BA, Roca RP, et al. Establishing advance medical directives with demented patients: a pilot study. *J Clin Ethics* 1993;4:51–54 and Mezey MD, Mitty EL, Bottrell MM, et al. Advance directives: older adults with dementia. *Clin Geriatr Med* 2000;16:255–268. For how advance directives been accomplished outside the United States, see Lynn J, Teno J, Dresser R, et al. Dementia and advance-care planning: perspectives from three countries on ethics and epidemiology. *J Clin Ethics* 1999;10:271–285.

57. Both the American Academy of Neurology and the Alzheimer's Association believe that demented patients should execute advance directives while they retain capacity. See American Academy of Neurology Ethics and Humanities Subcommittee. Ethical issues in the management of the demented patient. *Neurology* 1996;46:1180–1183 and Alzheimer's Disease and Related Disorders Association. *Ethical Considerations: Issues in Death and Dying.* Chicago: Alzheimer's Disease and Related Disorders Association, 1997. For an essay showing why neurologists have a special duty to encourage advance directives from their patients in anticipation of the progression of their dementia, see Goldblatt D. A messy, necessary end: health care proxies need our support. *Neurology* 2001;56:148–152.

58. Bernat JL. Plan ahead: how neurologists can enhance patient-centered medicine. *Neurology* 2001;56:144–145.

59. Volandes AE, Lehmann LS, Cook EF, Shaykevich S, Abbo ED, Gillick MR. Using video images of dementia in advance care planning. *Arch Intern Med* 2007;167:828–833.

60. Dresser R. Bound to treatment: the Ulysses contract. *Hastings Cent Rep* 1984;14(4):13–16 and Spellecy R. Reviving Ulysses contracts. *Kennedy Inst Ethics J* 2003;13:373–392.

61. Dworkin R. Autonomy and the demented self. *Milbank Q* 1986;64(suppl 2):4–16 and Dworkin R. *Life's Dominion: An Argument about Abortion, Euthanasia, and Individual Freedom.* New York: Alfred A Knopf, 1993. Interestingly, Dworkin's concept of precedent autonomy was cited recently by Dutch advocates of permitting euthanasia and assisted suicide by advance directive for demented patients. See Hertogh CMPM, de Boer ME, Dröes RM, Eefsting JA. Would we rather lose our life than lose our self? Lessons from the Dutch debate on euthanasia for patients with dementia. *Am J Bioethics* 2007;7(4):48–56.

62. Newton MI. Precedent autonomy: life-sustaining intervention and the demented patient. *Camb Q Healthc Ethics* 1999;8:189–199.

63. Callahan D. Terminating life-sustaining treatment of the demented. *Hastings Cent Rep* 1995;25(6):25–31 and Kadish SH. Letting patients die: legal and moral reflections. *Calif Law Rev* 1992;80:857–888.

64. Dresser R. Dworkin on dementia: elegant theory, questionable policy. *Hastings Cent Rep* 1995; 25(6):32–38 and Dresser R, Whitehouse PJ. The incompetent patient on the slippery slope. *Hastings Cent Rep* 1994;24(4):6–12.

65. The role of family members in the care of the demented patient is reviewed in Gwyther LP. Family issues in dementia: finding a new normal. *Neurol Clin* 2000;18:993–1010.

66. That families are willing to permit AD patients to incur significant medical risks resulting from side effects of their treatment was shown in Karlawish JHT, Klocinski JL, Merz J, Clark CM, Asch DA. Caregivers' preferences for the treatment of patients with Alzheimer's disease. *Neurology* 2000;55:1008–1014.

67. These factors were found in four studies: Brodaty H, McGilchrist C, Harris L, et al. Time until institutionalization and death in patients with dementia: role of caregiver training and risk factors. *Arch Neurol* 1993;50:643–650; Severson MA, Smith GE. Tangalos EG, et al. Patterns and predictors of institutionalization in community-based dementia patients. *J Am Geriatr Soc* 1994:42:181–185; Heyman A, Peterson B, Fillenbaum G, Pieper C. Predictors of time to institutionalization of patients with Alzheimer's disease: the CERAD experience, part XVII. *Neurology* 1997;48:1304–1309; and Knopman DS, Berg JD, Thomas R, Grundman M, Thal LJ, Sano M. Nursing home placement is related to dementia progression: experience from a clinical trial. *Neurology* 1999;52:714–718.

68. Stern Y, Tang M-X, Albert MS, et al. Predicting time to nursing home care and death in individuals with Alzheimer disease. *JAMA* 1997;277:806–812.

69. Eaker ED, Vierkant RA, Mickel SF. Predictors of nursing home admission and/or death in incident Alzheimer's disease and other dementia cases compared to controls: a population-based study. *J Clin Epidemiol* 2002;55:462–468.

70. Buhr GT, Kuchibhatla M, Clipp EC. Caregivers' reasons for nursing home placement: clues for improving discussions with families prior to the transition. *Gerontologist* 2006;46:52–61.

71. For example, see Mace NL and Rabins PV. *The 36-Hour Day: A Family Guide for Caring for Persons Alzheimer's Disease, Related Dementing Illnesses, and Memory Loss in Later Life.* Baltimore: Johns Hopkins University Press, 2001; Carrol DL. *When Your Loved One has Alzheimer's: A Caregiver's Guide.* New York: Harper & Row, 1989; Greutzner H. *Alzheimer's. A Caregiver's Guide and Sourcebook,* New York: John Wiley & Sons, 1992; Markin RE. *The Alzheimer's Cope Book: The Complete Care Manual for Patients and their Families.* New York: Carol Publishing Group, 1992; Powell LS, Courtice K. *Alzheimer's Disease: A Guide for Families.* New York: Addison-Wesley, 1992; and Ronch JL. *Alzheimer's Disease. A Practical Guide for Families and Other Caregivers.* New York: Continuum Publishing Co, 1991.

72. Schulz R, Martire LM. Family caregiving of persons with dementia: prevalence, health effects, and support strategies. *Am J Geriatr Psychiatry* 2004;12:240–249 and Schulz R, Beach SR. Caregiving as a risk factor for mortality: the Caregiver Health Effects Study. *JAMA* 1999;282:2215–2219.

73. Brodaty H, Green A, Koschera A. Meta-analysis of psychosocial interventions for caregivers of people with dementia. *J Am Geriatr Soc* 2003;51:657–664.

74. Mittelman MS, Haley WE, Clay OJ, Roth DL. Improving caregiver well-being delays nursing home placement of patients with Alzheimer disease. *Neurology* 2006;67:1592–1599; Schulz R, Martier LM, Klinger JN. Evidence-based caregiver interventions in geriatric psychiatry. *Psychiatr Clin North Am* 2005;28:1007–1038; and Belle SH, Burgio L, Burns R, et al. Enhancing the quality of life of dementia caregivers from different ethnic or racial groups: a randomized, controlled trial. *Ann Intern Med* 2006;145:727–738.

75. Schulz R, Belle SH, Czaja SJ, et al. Long-term care placement of dementia patients and caregiver health and well-being. *JAMA* 2004;292:961–967.

76. Schulz R, Mendelsohn AB, Haley WE, et al. End-of-life care and the effects of bereavement on family caregivers of persons with dementia. *N Engl J Med* 2003;349:1936–1942.

77. See Mohide EA. Informal care of community-dwelling patients with Alzheimer's disease: focus on the family caregiver. *Neurology* 1993;43(suppl 4):S16-S19; Rabins PV. Dementia and the family. *Dan Med Bull* 1985;32(suppl 1):81–83; Rabins PV, Mace NL, Lucas MJ. The impact of dementia on the family. *JAMA* 1982;248:333–335; and Zarit SH, Orr NK. Zarit JM. *The Hidden Victims of Alzheimer's Disease: Families Under Stress.* New York: New York University Press, 1985.

78. See Paveza G.J. Social services and the Alzheimer's disease patient: an overview. *Neurology* 1993:43(suppl 4): S11–S15.

79. See Overman W Jr, Stoudemire A. Guidelines for legal and financial counseling of Alzheimer disease patients and their families. *Am J Psychiatry* 1988:145:1495–1500.

80. Meier DE, Cassel CK. Nursing home placement and the demented patient: a case presentation and ethical analysis. *Ann Intern Med* 1986;104:98–105. The concept of family as patient is also discussed in Christie RJ, Hoffmaster CB. *Ethical Issues in Family Medicine*. New York: Oxford University Press, 1986:68–84. Guidelines for the relationship between physicians and family caregivers are presented in American Medical Association Council on Scientific Affairs. Physicians and family caregivers: a model for partnership. *JAMA* 1993;269:1282–1284.

81. Post SG, Whitehouse PJ. Fairhill guidelines on ethics of the care of people with Alzheimer's disease: a clinical summary. *J Am Geriatr Soc* 1995;43:1423–1429.

82. Meier DE, Cassel CK. Nursing home placement and the demented patient: a case presentation and ethical analysis. *Ann Intern Med* 1986;104:98–105.

83. Meier DE, Cassel CK. *Ann Intern Med* 1986:104.

84. Rango N. The nursing home resident with dementia: clinical care, ethics, and policy implications. *Ann Intern Med* 1985;102:835–841. See also Collopy B, Boyle P, Jennings B. New directions in nursing home ethics. *Hastings Cent Rep* 1991;21(suppl 2):1–15.

85. Williams JK, Trubatch AD. Nursing home care for the patient with Alzheimer's disease: an overview. *Neurology* 1993;43(suppl 4):S20–S24.

86. Mor V, Banaszak-Holl J, Zinn J. The trend toward specialization in nursing care facilities. *Generations* 1996;19(winter):24–29.

87. See Benson DM, Cameron D, Humbach E, et al. Establishment and impact of a dementia unit within the nursing home. *J Am Geriatr Soc* 1987;35:319–323; Ohta R, Ohta B, Special units for AD patients: a critical look. *Gerontologist* 1988;28: 803–808; Coons DH, ed. *Specialized Dementia Care Units*. Baltimore: Johns Hopkins University Press, 1989; and Zinn JS, Mor V. Nursing home special care units. *Gerontologist* 1994;34:371–377.

88. Phillips CD, Sloane PD, Hawes C, et al. Effects of residence in Alzheimer disease special care units on functional outcomes. *JAMA* 1997;278:1340–1344.

89. Finucane TE, Beamer BA, Roca RP, et al. Establishing advance medical directives with demented patients: a pilot study. *J Clin Ethics* 1993;4:51–54.

90. Libow LS, Olson E, Neufeld RR, et al. Ethics rounds at the nursing home: an alternative to an ethics committee. *J Am Geriatr Soc* 1992;40:95–97. The functioning of an ethics committees is discussed in chapter 5.

91. Data on the incidence and prevalence of restraint used on patients in hospitals and nursing homes have been analyzed in Evans LK, Strumpf NE. Tying down the elderly: a review of the literature on physical restraint. *J Am Geriatr Soc* 1989;36:65–74.

92. Tinetti ME, Liu WL, Marotolli RA, et al. Mechanical restraint use among residents of skilled nursing facilities: prevalence, patterns, and predictors. *JAMA* 1991;265:468–471. For data on the frequency and management of wandering by AD nursing home residents, see Hope RA, Fairburn CG. The nature of wandering in dementia: a community based study. *Int J Geriatr Psychiatry* 1990;5:239–245.

93. Sloane PD, Mathew LJ, Scarborough M, et al. Physical and pharmacologic restraint of nursing home patients with dementia: impact of specialized units. *JAMA* 1991;265:1278–1282.

94. Phillips CD, Spry KM, Sloane PD, Hawes C. Use of physical restraints and psychotropic medications in Alzheimer special care units in nursing homes. *Am J Public Health* 2000;90:92–96.

95. McShane R, Hope T, Wilkinson J. Tracking patients who wander: ethics and technology. *Lancet* 1994;343:1274.

96. Tinetti ME, Liu WL, Marotolli RA, et al. *JAMA* 1991:468–471.

97. Burton LC, German PS, Rovner BW, et al. Physical restraint use and cognitive decline among nursing home residents. *J Am Geriatr Soc* 1992;40:811–816. Studies showing that other physiological functions are impaired from the use of restraints are summarized in Evans LK, Strumpf NE. *J Am Geriatr Soc* 1989:65–74.

98. See Johnson SH. The fear of liability and the use of restraints in nursing homes. *Law Med Health Care* 1990:18:263–273.

99. These guidelines are abstracted from Evans LK, Strumpf NE. *J Am Geriatr Soc* 1989:65–74 and Moss RJ, La Puma J. The ethics of mechanical restraints. *Hastings Cent Rep* 1991:21(1):22–25.

100. Health Care Financing Administration, Department of Health and Human Services. Medicare and Medicaid programs: hospital conditions for participation, patients' rights. *Fed Regist* 1998;64(127): 36070–36089. These regulations are described and discussed in Annas GJ. The last resort—the use of physical restraints in medical emergencies. *N Engl J Med* 1999;341:1408–1412.

101. Brown NK, Thompson DJ. Nontreatment of fever in extended-care facilities. *N Engl J Med* 1979: 300:1246–1250.

102. For example, see Lipsky MS, Hickey DP, Browning G. Treatment limitations in nursing homes in north-west Ohio. *Arch Intern Med* 1988;148:1539–1541; Besdine RW. Decisions to withhold treatment from nursing home residents. *J Am Geriatr Soc* 1983;31:602–606.

103. For a poignantly described personal case, see Hilfiker D. Allowing the debilitated to die: facing our ethical choices. *N Engl J Med* 1983;308:716–719. See also Lo B, Dornbrand L. Guiding the hand that feeds: caring for the demented elderly. *N Engl J Med* 1984:311:402–404 and Niemira D. Life on the slippery slope: a bedside view of treating incompetent elderly patients. *Hastings Cent Rep* 1993;23(3):14–17.

104. van der Steen, Kruse RL, Ooms ME, et al. Treatment of nursing home residents with dementia and lower respiratory tract infection in the United States and the Netherlands: an ocean apart. *J Am Geriatr Soc* 2004;52:691–699 and van der Steen, Ooms ME, Ader HJ, Ribbe MW, van der Wal G. Withholding antibiotic treatment in pneumonia patients with dementia: a quantitative observational study. *Arch Intern Med* 2002;162:1753–1760.

105. This argument is developed in Meyers RM, Grodin MA. Decision making regarding the initiation of tube feedings in the severely demented elderly: a review. *J Am Geriatr Soc* 1991;39:526–531 and Arras JD. The severely demented, minimally functional patient: an ethical analysis. *J Am Geriatr Soc* 1988;36:938–944.

106. Task Force on Supportive Care. The supportive care plan—its meaning and application: recommendations and guidelines. *Law Med Health Care* 1984;12:97–102. For an opposing viewpoint, see the rebuttal by Hoyt JD, Davies JM. A response to the Task Force on Supportive Care. *Law Med Health Care* 1984;12:103–105. Palliative care is discussed in chapter 7.

107. For a practical example of how limitation of treatment orders can be written, see O'Toole EE, Youngner SJ, Juknialis BW, et al. Evaluation of a treatment limitation policy with a specific treatment-limiting order page. *Arch Intern Med* 1994;154:425–432.

108. Karlawish JHT, Quill T, Meier DE. A consensus-based approach to providing palliative care to patients who lack decision-making capacity. *Ann Intern Med* 1999;130:835–840.

109. Task Force on Supportive Care. *Law Med Health Care* 1984:99.

110. Otherwise unexplained weight loss may be a warning sign of impending dementia in an elderly patient. See Grendman M. Weight loss in the elderly may be a sign of impending dementia. *Arch Neurol* 2005;62:20–22.

111. For a balanced discussion of the medical and ethical aspects of inserting long-term feeding tubes, see McMahon MM, Hurley DL, Kamath PS, Mueller PS. Medical and ethical aspects of long-term enteral tube feeding. *Mayo Clin Proc* 2005;80:1461–1476.

112. Mitchell SL, Teno JM, Roy J, Kabumoto G, Mor V. Clinical and organizational factors associated with feeding tube use among nursing home residents with advanced cognitive impairment. *JAMA* 2003;290:73–80.

113. Teno JM, Mor V, DeSilva D, Kabumoto G, Roy J, Wetle T. Use of feeding tubes in nursing home residents with severe cognitive impairment. *JAMA* 2002;287:3211–3212.

114. Finucane TE, Christmas C, Travis K. Tube feeding in patients with advanced dementia: a review of the evidence. *JAMA* 1999;282:1365–1370.

115. See Gillick MR. Rethinking the role of tube feeding in patients with advanced dementia. *N Engl J Med* 2000;342:206–210; McCann R. Lack of evidence about tube feeding—food for thought. *JAMA* 1999;282:1380–1381; Post SG. Tube feeding and advanced progressive dementia. *Hastings Cent Rep* 2001;31(1):36–42; and Hurley AC, Volicer L. Alzheimer disease: "it's okay, Mama, if you want to go, it's okay." *JAMA* 2002;288:2324–2331.

116. Meier DE, Aronheim JC, Morris J, Baskin-Lyons S, Morrison RS. High short-term mortality in hospitalized patients with advanced dementia: lack of benefit of tube feeding. *Arch Intern Med* 2001;161:594–599.

117. Hodges MO, Tolle SW, Stocking C, Cassel CK. Tube feeding: internists' attitudes regarding ethical obligations. *Arch Intern Med* 1994;154:1013–1020.

118. Gjerdingen DK, Neff JA, Wang M, et al. Older persons' opinions about life-sustaining procedures in the face of dementia. *Arch Fam Med* 1999;8:421–425.

119. Pasman HRW, Onwuteaka-Philipsen BD, Kriegsman DMW, Ooms ME, Ribbe MW, van der Wal G. Discomfort in nursing home patients with severe dementia in whom artificial nutrition and hydration is forgone. *Arch Intern Med* 2005;165:1729–1735.

120. Shega JW, Hougham GW, Stocking CB, Cox-Haley D, Sachs GA. Barriers to limiting the practice of feeding tube placement in advanced dementia. *J Palliat Med* 2003;6:885–893.

121. American Academy of Neurology Ethics and Humanities Subcommittee. Ethical issues in the management of the demented patient. *Neurology* 1996;46:1180–1183.

122. Gillick MR. Artificial nutrition and hydration in the patient with advanced dementia: is withholding treatment compatible with traditional Judaism? *J Med Ethics* 2001;27:12–15 and Jotkowitz AB, Clarfield AM, Glick S. The care of patients with dementia: a modern Jewish ethical perspective. *J Am Geriatr Soc* 2005;53:881–884.

123. Luchins DJ, Hanrahan P. What is appropriate health care for end-stage dementia? *J Am Geriatr Soc* 1993;41:25–30.

124. Cogen R, Patterson B, Chavin S, et al. Surrogate decision-maker preferences for medical care of severely demented nursing home patients. *Arch Intern Med* 1992;152:1985–1888. One such case was poignantly described in Fried TR, Gillick MR. The limits of proxy decision making: overtreatment. *Camb Q Healthc Ethics* 1995;4:524–529.

125. Volicer L, Rheume Y, Brown J, et al. Hospice approach to the treatment of patients with advanced dementia of the Alzheimer type. *JAMA* 1986;256:2210–2213. Ladislaw Volicer's more recent data are described in Volicer L, Hurley A. *Hospice Care for Patients with Advanced Progressive Dementia*. New York: Springer, 1998.

126. Wray N, Brody B, Bayer J, et al. Withholding medical treatment from the severely demented patient: decisional processes and cost implications. *Arch Intern Med* 1988;148:1980–1984. For a description of a supportive care team that provides terminal care for hopelessly ill hospital patients with varying diagnoses, see Carlson RW, Devich L, Frank RR. Development of a comprehensive supportive care team for the hopelessly ill on a university hospital medical service. *JAMA* 1988;259:378–383.

127. Engel SE, Kiely DK, Mitchell SL. Satisfaction with end-of-life care for nursing home residents with advanced dementia. *J Am Geriatr Soc* 2006;54:1567–1572.

128. Mitchell SL, Kiely DK, Hamel MB. Dying with advanced dementia in the nursing home. *Arch Intern Med* 2004;164:321–326.

129. Mitchell SL, Kiely DK, Hamel MB. Nursing home residents with advanced dementia do not receive optimal palliative care. *Arch Intern Med* 2004;164:321–326 and Aminoff BZ, Adunsky A. Dying dementia patients: too much suffering, too little palliation. *Am J Hospice Palliat Med* 2005;22:344–348.

130. Mitchell SL, Kiely DK, Hamel MB, Park PS, Morris JN, Fries BE. Estimating prognosis for nursing home residents with advanced dementia. *JAMA* 2004;291:2734–2740.

131. Hanrahan P, Luchins DJ. Access to hospice programs in end-stage dementia: a national survey of hospice programs. *J Am Geriatr Soc* 1995;43:56–59.

132. The short-term survival of patients with advanced dementia is limited and their risk of dying after hip surgery or pneumonia is four times higher than non-demented age-matched patients. See Volicer BJ, Hurley A, Fabiszewski KJ, Montgomery P, Volicer L. Predicting short-term survival for patients with advanced Alzheimer's disease. *J Am Geriatr Soc* 1993;41:535–540 and Morrison RS, Siu AL. Survival in end-stage dementia following acute illness. *JAMA* 2000;284:47–52.

133. Luchins DJ, Hanrahan P, Murphy K. Criteria for enrolling dementia patients in hospice. *J Am Geriatr Soc* 1997;45:1054–1059.

134. Munn JC, Hanson LC, Zimmerman S, Sloane PD, Mitchell CM. Is hospice associated with improved end-of-life care in nursing homes and assisted living facilities? *J Am Geriatr Soc* 2006;54:490–495.

135. Hoffman DE, Tarzian AJ. Dying in America—an examination of policies that deter adequate end-of-life care in nursing homes. *J Law Med Ethics* 2005;33:294–309.

136. For an authoritative reference source for all legal questions regarding the right to refuse treatment, see Meisel A, Cerminara KL. *The Right to Die: The Law of End-of-Life Decisionmaking*, 3rd ed. Aspen Publishers, Inc, 2004.

137. See *In re Dinnerstein*, 6 Mass App 466, 380 NE 2d 234 (App Ct Mass 1978); *In re Spring*, 405 NE 2d 115, 120 (Mass 1980); and *In re Hier*, 464 NE 2d 959, review denied, 465 NE 2d 261, 1984. These and other cases are reviewed in Annas GJ, Glantz LH. The right of elderly patients to refuse life-sustaining treatment. *Milbank Q* 1986;64(suppl 2):95–162; and Beresford HR. Legal aspects of termination of treatment decisions. *Neurol Clin* 1989:7:775–789.

138. *In re Conroy*, 98 NJ 321, 486 A 2d 1209, 1985. Much commentary has been written about this case. The discussion in this section relies on Curran WJ. Defining appropriate medical care: providing nutrients and hydration for the dying. *N Engl J Med* 1985;313:940–942.

139. Annas GJ. When procedures limit rights: from Quinlan to Conroy. *Hastings Cent Rep* 1985;15(2):24–26 and Lo B, Dornbrand L. The case of Claire Conroy: will administrative review safeguard incompetent patients? *Ann Intern Med* 1986:104:869–873. For a commentary on the role of the New Jersey ombudsman's office in investigating nursing home medical issues, see Price DM, Armstrong PW. New Jersey's "Granny

Doe" squad: arguments about mechanisms for protection of vulnerable patients. *Law Med Health Care* 1989;17:255–263.

140. *In re O'Connor,* 71 NY 2d 517, 1988.

141. See Gindes D. Judicial postponement of death recognition: the tragic case of Mary O'Connor. *Am J Law Med* 1989;15:301–311 and Annas GJ. Precatory prediction and mindless mimicry: the tragic case of Mary O'Connor. *Hastings Cent Rep* 1988;18(6):31–33. For further commentary on the clear and convincing legal standard, see the discussion of the U.S. Supreme Court *Cruzan* case in chapters 8 and 12.

142. Menikoff JA. Sachs GA, Siegler M. Beyond advance directives—health care surrogate laws. *N Engl Med* 1992;327:1165–1169.

143. For a review of state laws governing physicians' orders to withhold or withdraw artificial hydration and nutrition in terminally ill and permanently unconscious patients, see Larriviere D, Bonnie RJ. Terminating artificial nutrition and hydration in persistent vegetative state patients: current and proposed state laws. *Neurology* 2006;66:1624–1628.

144. For background on ethical issues in research using human subjects with cognitive impairment, see Sachs GA. Cassel CK. Biomedical research involving older subjects. *Law Med Health Care* 1990;18:234–243; Sachs GA, Cassel CK. Ethical aspects of dementia. *Neurol Clin* 1989;7:845–858; High DM. Research with Alzheimer's disease subjects: informed consent and proxy decision making. *J Am Geriatr Soc* 1992,40: 950–957; and Dickens BM, Gostin L, Levine RJ, eds. Research on human populations: national and international guidelines. *Law Med Health Care* 1991;19:157–295.

145. For how to determine the adequacy of a demented patient's capacity to consent to serve as a research subject, see Kim SYH, Caine ED, Currier GW, Leibovici A, Ryan JM. Assessing the competence of persons with Alzheimer's disease in providing informed consent for participation in research. *Am J Psychiatry* 2001;158:712–717.

146. Kim SYH, Appelbaum PS, Jeste DV, Olin JT. Proxy and surrogate consent in geriatric neuropsychiatric research: update and recommendations. *Am J Psychiatry* 2004;161:797–806.

147. American Academy of Neurology Ethics and Humanities Subcommittee. Ethical issues in clinical research in neurology: advancing knowledge and protecting human research subjects. *Neurology* 1998;50:592–595.

148. American College of Physicians. Cognitively impaired subjects. *Ann Intern Med* 1989:111:843–848.

149. Protection of human subjects. In Pincus HA, Lieberman JA, Ferris S (eds). *Ethics in Psychiatric Research.* Washington DC: American Psychiatric Association, 1999.

150. The history of abuses of cognitively impaired research subjects and the delicate balance of public policy necessary to adequately protect but not overprotect these vulnerable patients is presented in Berg JW. Legal and ethical complexities of consent with cognitively impaired research subjects: proposed guidelines. *J Law Med Ethics* 1996;24:18–35; Dresser R. Mentally disabled research subjects: the enduring policy issues. *JAMA* 1996;276:67–72; and Wichman A, Sandler AL. Research involving subjects with dementia and other cognitive impairments: experience at the NIH, and some unresolved ethical considerations. *Neurology* 1995;45:1777–1778.

151. This point is discussed in Cassel CK. *Semin Neurol* 1984:92–97. See also Van den Noort S. Ethical aspects of unproved therapies in multiple sclerosis, amyotrophic lateral sclerosis, and other neurologic diseases. *Semin Neurol* 1984;4:83–85.

152. Haimowitz S, Delano SJ, Oldham JM. Uninformed decisionmaking: the case of surrogate research consent. *Hastings Cent Rep* 1997;27(6):9–16.

153. National Bioethics Advisory Commission. *Research Involving Persons with Mental Disorders that may Affect Decisionmaking Capacity.* Rockville, MD: National Bioethics Advisory Commission, 1998. These guidelines are interpreted and discussed in Capron AM. Ethical and human rights issues in research on mental disorders that may affect decision-making capacity. *N Engl J Med* 1999;340:1430–1434.

154. Michels R. Are research ethics bad for our mental health? *N Engl J Med* 1999;340:1427–1430 and Oldham JM, Haimowitz S, Delano SJ. Protection of persons with mental disorders from research risk: a response to the report of the National Bioethics Advisory Commission. *Arch Gen Psychiatry* 1999;56:688–693.

155. This phenomenon is discussed further in Sachs GA, Cassel CK. Ethical aspects of dementia. *Neurol Clin* 1989;7:845–858.

156. Warren JW, Sobal J, Tenney JH. et al. Informed consent by proxy: an issue in research with elderly patients. *N Engl J Med* 1986;315:1124–1128.

157. Walker JEC, Campion EW. Informed consent by proxy. *N Engl J Med* 1987;316:1028–1029. See also Melnick VL, Dubler NN. Clinical research in senile dementia of the Alzheimer type: suggested guidelines

addressing the ethical and legal issues. *J Am Geriatr Soc* 1984;32:531–536 and Annas GJ, Glantz LH. Rules for research in nursing homes. *N Engl J Med* 1986;315:1157–1158.

158. See President's Commission for the Study of Ethical Problems in Medicine and Biomedical and Behavioral Research. *Protecting Human Subjects: The Adequacy and Uniformity of Federal Rules and their Implementation.* Washington, DC: US Government Printing Office, 1981:92–103. The functioning of the institutional review board is considered further in chapters 5 and 19.

159. For accounts of how advance directives can be employed for consent of demented patients in clinical research, see Dresser R. Advance directives in dementia research: promoting autonomy and protecting subjects. *IRB: Ethics & Human Research.* 2001;23(1):1–6 and Stocking CB, Hougham GW, Danner DD, Patterson MB, Whitehouse PJ, Sachs GA. Speaking of research advance directives: planning for future research participation. *Neurology* 2006;66:1361–1366.

160. Karlawish JHT, Casarett D, Klocinski J, Sankar P. How do AD patients and their caregivers decide whether to enroll in a clinical trial? *Neurology* 2001;56:789–792.

161. Kim SYH, Kim HM, McCallum C, Tariot P. What do people at risk for Alzheimer disease think about surrogate consent for research? *Neurology* 2005;65:1395–1401.

162. Berger JT, Majerovitz SD. Do elderly persons' concerns for family burden influence their preferences for future participation in dementia research? *J Clin Ethics* 2005;16:108–115.

163. Albert SM, Sano M, Marder K, et al. Participation in clinical trials and long-term outcomes in Alzheimer's disease. *Neurology* 1997;49:38–43.

Mental Retardation

16

Ethical issues arise in the care of children and adults with mental retardation as a consequence of retarded patients' irreversible brain damage, limited functional and intellectual potential, incapacity to consent for treatment or research, and need for daily care which must be provided by family members or institutional personnel. These issues are confounded by society's attitude toward mentally retarded and developmentally disabled patients, which ranges from protective to patronizing and discriminatory.

In this chapter, I review basic medical facts about the epidemiology, diagnosis, and treatment of mental retardation. I discuss the fundamental medical-ethical issue in caring for mentally retarded patients: how clinicians can obtain valid consent for treating patients who never have been or ever can be competent to provide consent. I concentrate on three specific consent issues: (1) permission for sterilization; (2) permission for sedation and restraints; and (3) permission to withhold or withdraw life-sustaining medical treatment. Following a brief review of how patients with severe mental retardation affect their families, I explain how the law provides their rights for education and other services and governs surrogates' decisions to withhold or withdraw their life-sustaining treatment. I end by discussing ethical issues that investigators may encounter when using these patients as human research subjects.[1]

The terminology for this group of patients is evolving. The term "non-progressive global developmental delay" describes a syndrome in children with age-specific deficits in adaptation and learning skills caused by various disorders. Affected children are identified because they perform at a level of two or more standard deviations below normal for age in the following skill areas: gross/fine motor, speech/language, cognition, social/personal, and activities of daily living. "Global developmental delay" is the term applied to children under age five years with this profile whereas "mental retardation" is the term applied to children with global developmental cognitive impairment over age five for whom IQ testing is more reliable.[2] Not all children with global developmental delay will later exhibit mental retardation. Many of my comments in this chapter also pertain to the larger class of patients of all ages with developmental disabilities, not all of whom are mentally retarded.[3]

DEFINITIONS AND EPIDEMIOLOGY

In 1983, the American Association on Mental Retardation (AAMR) defined mental retardation as "significantly sub-average general intellectual functioning resulting in or associated with concurrent impairments in adaptive behavior and manifested during the developmental period."[4] In its earlier 1973 report, the AAMR defined "significantly sub-average general intellectual functioning" as performance on psychometric tests that is more than two standard deviations below the mean. Thus, on the Stanford-Binet IQ test, a score below 67 would classify a person as mentally retarded. In 1973, the AAMR also classified the severity of retardation on the basis of IQ scores: mild (52–67), moderate (36–51), severe (20–35), and profound (19 and below).[5]

In its revised report of 1983, the AAMR chose to redefine the boundary separating normal intelligence from mental retardation at an IQ of 70. This score could be extended to as high as 75 in those patients for whom the reliability of the psychometric instrument was questionable, the patient's behavior was impaired, or the clinician deemed that this behavior did not stem from a deficit in reasoning and judgment.[6] In 1992, the AAMR again slightly revised its definition of mental retardation but retained the original essential criteria of "significantly subaverage intellectual functioning" with "limitations in . . . adaptive skill areas."[7]

The AAMR defined "adaptive behavior" as "the effectiveness or degree with which the individual meets the standards of personal independence and social responsibility of his age and cultural group." Measurement of adaptive behavior during infancy and early childhood focused on the development of sensorimotor skills, communication skills, self-help skills, and socialization. During later childhood, adaptive behavior was reflected in academic skills, reasoning and judgment, and socialization. In adolescence and adulthood, performance in vocational and social arenas was the most important measure of adaptive behavior.[8]

Critics attacked the AAMR definition as erecting a boundary between mentally retarded and intellectually normal people where no such boundary exists in human biology. They argued that, rather than comprising a uniform and homogeneous group that is distinct from cognitively normal persons, mentally retarded persons merely occupy one end of a continuous spectrum of intellectual and functional capacities. Within this continuum, there is no distinct boundary but only a gradual blending between the intellectually normal and the mentally retarded. The AAMR definition, they concluded, created an artificial label that encouraged stigmatization and permitted discrimination.[9]

In 2002, the AAMR again revised its definition of mental retardation to the following: "Mental retardation is a disability characterized by significant limitations both in intellectual functioning and in adaptive behavior as expressed in conceptual, social, and practical adaptive skills."[10] In January 2007, the AAMR jettisoned over 130 years of tradition by replacing the term "mental retardation" with "intellectual disability" and changed its own name to the American Association on Intellectual and Developmental Disabilities (AAIDD).[11] These changes were consistent with the World Health Organization's 2001 revision of the International Classification of Functioning, Disability, and Health that "puts the notions of 'health' and 'disability' in a new light. It acknowledges that every human being can experience a decrement in health and thereby experience some degree of disability. Disability is not something that only happens to a minority of humanity. The ICF thus 'mainstreams' the experience of disability and recognises it as a universal human experience."[12] Despite the recent AAMR (AAIDD) recommendation, I use the more familiar term "mental retardation" in this chapter.

The incidence and prevalence of mental retardation have been difficult to quantify because it has not been differentiated from other developmental disabilities, particularly severe states of dyslexia, and because of the confounding effect of illiteracy on the testing paradigm. In an examination of prevalence data in the United States prior to 1962, the President's Panel on Mental Retardation reported that 3% of the American population was mentally retarded. Of this group of approximately 5.4 million people, the panel classified 87% as mildly retarded, 10% as moderately retarded, and 1% as severely retarded.[13]

To discourage citing this 3% figure as a precise measure of the prevalence of mental retardation, the panel stated that the 3% figure represents those people who are mentally retarded "at some time in their lives." Several unverified assumptions have made the 3% figure questionable as a fixed estimate of prevalence: (1) all such patients had an IQ less than 70; (2) mental retardation can be diagnosed accurately in infancy; (3) the diagnosis of mental retardation does not change throughout life; and (4) the mortality rate of retarded patients is identical to that of the general population.[14] In 1997, Nel Roeleveld and colleagues conducted a critical review of the world's literature on the prevalence of mental retardation. Despite variation among countries, they found that the mean of school-age children who are retarded is 3%, with a relatively fixed rate of severe retardation of 3.8/1,000 children.[15]

DIAGNOSIS AND MANAGEMENT

Mental retardation is not a unitary disease but a syndrome in which a range of severity of brain damage or malformation can be produced by a multitude of prenatal, perinatal, and postnatal disorders. The differential diagnosis of a patient with mental retardation includes hundreds of disorders that are most easily understood when classified into groups by pathogenesis. Thus, mental retardation can be produced by prenatal and postnatal infections; birth trauma; metabolic, toxic, nutritional, and endocrine diseases; neurocutaneous and neurodegenerative disorders; congenital malformations; chromosomal aberrations, microdeletions, and mutations; fetal prematurity; and acquired childhood disorders.

A recent epidemiological study of 715 mentally retarded 10-year-old children in Atlanta found prenatal causes in 12%, perinatal causes in 6%, postnatal causes in 4% and no reported cause in 78% of cases.[16] The relative incidence of each of the major diagnostic groups was studied by Allen Crocker in the 1970s in a series of 2,000 patients he examined in the Developmental Evaluation Clinic at the Boston Children's Hospital Medical Center.[17] Crocker found the following breakdown by diagnostic group:

Hereditary (metabolic, neurocutaneous, neurodegenerative)	4%
Embryonic dysgenesis (chromosomal malformations)	33%
Perinatal (birth trauma)	12%
Acquired childhood diseases	4%
Environmental (nutritional deprivation, psychosis, autism)	19%
Unknown (cerebral dysgenesis)	28%

Screening to determine the specific causes of global developmental delay is advocated by the American Academy of Pediatrics,[18] the American Academy of Neurology (AAN), and the Child Neurology Society (CNS). In a recent evidence-based review, the AAN and the CNS offered several guidelines.[19] Because inborn errors of metabolism are currently seen in only about 1% of cases, screening for them is not recommended. Cytogenetic testing is positive in 3.7% and should be carried out even in the absence of dysmorphic features. Fragile X syndrome accounts for 2.6% and may be tested. Rett syndrome and the MECP2 gene may be investigated. Additional genetic testing may be conducted to look for subtelomeric chromosome rearrangements, accounting for 6.6% of cases. If children are at risk for lead poisoning, lead levels should be measured. Hypothyroidism should be excluded if not already screened neonatally. An EEG may be helpful if seizures are present. Neuroimaging by brain CT scan or MRI should be done because it increases diagnostic specificity. Tests of vision and hearing should be performed because they are useful diagnostically. The specific diagnosis should be communicated to the parents or caregivers according to established standards of "breaking bad news" once it is established.[20]

New molecular genetic techniques are revolutionizing diagnostic testing for genetic causes of mental retardation.[21] The genetic etiology of mental retardation currently remains unknown in over half of cases.[22] Innovative techniques such as DNA microarray analysis can identify DNA submicroscopic copy number variations, such as deletions, insertions, duplications, and complex multisite variations, and can pinpoint genetic abnormalities in at least 10% of previously undiagnosed cases, particularly in retarded children with dysmorphic syndromes.[23]

Complete management of the mentally retarded patient requires attention to five general areas: (1) specific medical treatment for the underlying disease; (2) symptomatic treatment for complications resulting from the underlying disease; (3) psychological treatment; (4) educational and vocational counseling; and (5) prevention. Adequate treatment of the retarded patient begins with a thorough medical and neurological examination, including tests of vision and hearing, followed by psychological, social, educational, rehabilitative, and vocational evaluations.[24]

Specific medical treatment to counteract the pathophysiological effects of hereditary metabolic disorders or to replace congenitally absent proteins or enzymes has been modestly successful for only a few of the disorders that produce mental retardation. For example, the combination of erucic and oleic acids ("Lorenzo's oil") has been used with limited success to treat X-linked adrenoleukodystrophy in children,[25] but the benefits of treatment have been overstated by the popular media.[26] Similarly, macrophage-targeted alglucerase and glucocerebrosidase have been used with limited success to treat Gaucher disease[27] and agalsidase-beta treatment can slow the progression of Fabry disease.[28] Despite the equivocal benefits currently resulting from this form of therapy, it is likely that specific therapy targeted to replace absent proteins or enzymes in several of the disorders will be more successful with future advances in technology.

Medical complications of mental retardation include seizures, spasticity, choreoathetosis, and behavioral and attentional disturbances. Seizure disorders can be treated with anticonvulsant medications to optimize control and minimize sedation and psychomotor retardation. Spasticity can be treated with medications, orthotics, physical therapy, and orthopedic surgery to minimize discomfort and maximize motor function. Choreoathetosis and other movement disorders can be suppressed with medications.

Behavioral, attentional, and other psychological disturbances can be treated with medications, psychotherapy, and behavioral modification therapies. The goal of these therapies is to maximize the patient's cognitive function, and not simply to control disruptive behavior to ease the burdens of nursing care. Educational counseling during childhood and vocational training during adolescence are important components of rehabilitation because they maximize the useful function of the retarded patient.

Mental retardation can be prevented through several strategies. The nutrition and general health of pregnant women should be maximized with adequate prenatal medical care. Tobacco, alcohol, street drugs, and all unnecessary medications should be avoided during all stages of pregnancy. Prenatal genetic screening and counseling, newborn diagnostic screening, amniocentesis, and early elective abortion should be more widely available to prevent genetic diseases. Child neglect and abuse should be identified and stopped by timely intervention.

VALID CONSENT FOR TREATMENT IN THE "NEVER-COMPETENT" PATIENT

The essential ethical problem in the medical care of the mentally retarded patient is how to obtain valid consent for diagnosis or treatment. Many of the other clinical-ethical problems arising in the care of these patients stem directly from the consent question. Thus, the ethical issues that surround involuntary sterilization, sedation for frightening medical procedures, prescribing psychotropic medications, behavioral conditioning techniques to modify disruptive behavior, limitation or termination of life-sustaining medical treatment, and research on the retarded patient are all variations of the consent issue.

Respect for human dignity requires that mentally retarded people have the same moral right as cognitively intact people to consent to or refuse tests or therapies.[29] As persons, they also have a legal right that is not extinguished by their cognitive incapacity and that can be exercised by a surrogate decision maker on behalf of the patient.[30] The specific rights of consent of the mentally retarded patient have been codified into law in many countries, as discussed in the section on legal issues later in this chapter. Guardians and other lawful surrogates have authority to consent for or refuse many therapies on behalf of the patient but state statutes and regulations may restrict the authority of guardians and require judicial approval for certain treatments including sterilization, abortion, electroconvulsive therapy and psychosurgery.[31]

The issue of valid consent in the mentally retarded patient has certain features in common with consent issues in other incompetent patients such as elderly demented patients, but it also contains unique aspects. The severely retarded patient not only is incompetent at any given time to provide consent, he never has been and never will be competent to provide consent at any future time. The patient can be thus categorized as "never competent." This circumstance differs in important ways from that of a demented adult who once was competent. Also, there are subtle but important differences between obtaining consent in the mentally retarded patient and obtaining consent in a young child. Although the young child is incompetent, he has the potential to become competent in the future.

A competent adult rendered incompetent by delirium or dementia (chapter 15) has a life history of health-care values that he had expressed verbally or in writing, or that can be gleaned by analyzing his past behavior. These values can be inspected and followed to determine how the patient likely would have responded to questions of consent for a course of medical treatment. Following the standard of substituted judgment, a surrogate decision maker applies the patient's previously expressed values to his current clinical situation to attempt to reproduce the decision that the patient would have made for himself when he was competent (see chapter 4). A process of substituted judgment realistically cannot be used in making decisions for a mentally retarded patient because of the impossibility of his having any history of previously expressed values.[32]

There is a similarity between consent questions in the mentally retarded patient of any age and consent questions in the young child. Because both the very young child and the retarded patient are incompetent and never have been competent, the substituted judgment standard cannot be used for either. Procedurally, consent questions should be handled similarly in both a normal child and a retarded patient of any age with the mental capacity equivalent to that of a normal child. Thus, consent questions are treated substantially in the same manner for a normal 18-month-old and for a retarded adult patient with the mental capacity of a normal 18-month-old.

In both circumstances, the best interest judgment is the preferred decision-making standard. Surrogate decision makers should strive to identify, as objectively as possible, the decision that is in the best interest of the patient. Best interest decisions are less powerful ethically than substituted judgment decisions because surrogate decision makers respect the patient's autonomy in the latter by attempting to follow the course of action that the patient most likely would have chosen. The President's Commission for the Study of Ethical Problems in Medicine and Biomedical and Behavioral Research recommended that the best interest standard should be employed when surrogates make medical decisions for never-competent patients.[33]

A best interest judgment requires balancing the expected benefits of a proposed test or therapy against its expected burdens. This balance is determined by the surrogate decision maker, who employs his or her own assessments and predictions of the burdens and benefits to the patient. In this way, the best interest standard differs from the substituted judgment standard, in which the patient's own balance of burdens and benefits is approximated. If the expected benefits are greater than the burdens, the surrogate consents to the proposed therapy or test. If the burdens exceed the benefits, the best interest standard would rule that a rational surrogate should refuse to provide consent.[34]

The spectrum of cognitive capacity in mentally retarded patients varies as a function of the severity of brain damage in the same way that the spectrum of cognitive capacity in normal children varies as a function of age. No consent other than that of the surrogate is necessary in a profoundly retarded patient or in a child under the age of five years. With lesser degrees of retardation and in older children, the clinician should attempt to obtain the patient's assent by explaining the matter to him to the extent that he can comprehend. To make a patient's assent into valid consent, the surrogate decision maker also must provide consent. The concept of assent was developed for children but is applicable also to patients with less severe forms of dementia and mental retardation.[35]

Applying the best interest standard to a mentally retarded patient and to a child of the same mental age discloses the differences between these two situations. Normal incompetent children are expected to develop into competent adults, whereas incompetent retarded patients will never become competent adults. Therefore, the benefits-to-burdens ratio of a given treatment may be interpreted differently in these two groups.

Consider, for example, a cognitively intact 18-month-old girl with newly diagnosed acute lymphoblastic leukemia (ALL) and a severely retarded 50-year-old woman, with the mental age of an 18-month-old, who also has newly diagnosed ALL. Neither patient can understand the reason that she is being hospitalized and frequently injected with noxious chemotherapeutic drugs. All both know is that they feel violently ill, scream with pain, vomit uncontrollably, and are terribly frightened of doctors, nurses, and needles.

The parents of the child may decide that it is in her best interest to undergo the substantial amount of pain and suffering imposed by chemotherapy because her chances of recovery from this otherwise fatal disease are good, making her life expectancy thereafter relatively normal. Therefore, they consent to the treatment by a best interest standard, accepting the child's suffering as an unpleasant and regrettable but necessary and fully justified price to pay for the intended goal of therapy.

Conversely, the guardian of the retarded woman may decide that it is not in the patient's best interest to undergo substantial pain and suffering accompanying medical treatment because those burdens are not counterbalanced by the expectancy of a normal life thereafter. The guardian may decide that the suffering caused by the treatment cannot be justified by its expected benefits. Although the decision-making procedure may be the same for the two cases, a different substantive decision may have been reached because the prognostic differences significantly influence the surrogate's perception of the balance of the benefits and burdens of treatment to the patient. The close collaboration and shared decision making between the parent or guardian and the physician are essential to reach the decision that is in the patient's best interest.

INVOLUNTARY STERILIZATION

In no area are the ethical conflicts of consent, autonomy, and paternalism brought into clearer focus than in the consideration of involuntary sterilization of a mentally retarded patient. Advocates of this practice point out that mentally retarded patients cannot understand the fundamental facts of sexuality and procreation sufficiently to be responsible for their own sexual behavior. Further, they lack the capacity to raise children that they have conceived irresponsibly or unknowingly. Finally, retarded patients may pass along hereditary diseases to their offspring and thereby perpetuate their medical and social problems into the next generation. In times past, the obvious solution was to sterilize mentally retarded patients involuntarily for their own good and for the good of society.[36]

The social and legal history of involuntary sterilization is colorful but sobering.[37] Eugenic theories were commonly accepted in the United States and England in the late nineteenth and early twentieth centuries. In 1907, Indiana became the first of over 30 states to enact a law authorizing involuntary sterilization of the retarded based on the preceding argument.[38] Implicit in these laws was overt discrimination against and stigmatization of the retarded patient. For example, in the famous 1927 U.S. Supreme Court case of *Buck v Bell,* Justice Oliver Wendell Holmes, Jr. had this to say about the proposed involuntary sterilization of Carrie Buck:

> [She was a] feeble minded white woman who was committed to the state colony . . . the daughter of a feeble minded mother in the same institution, and the mother of an illegitimate feeble minded child. . . . It is better for all the world, if instead of waiting to execute degenerate offspring for crime, or to let them starve for their imbecility, society can prevent those who are manifestly unfit from continuing their kind. The principle that sustains compulsory vaccination is broad

enough to cover cutting the Fallopian tubes. . . . Three generations of imbeciles are enough.[39]

Although the majority of states had enacted sterilization statutes by the 1930s, the U.S. Supreme Court struck down the Oklahoma eugenic sterilization law as unconstitutional in 1942, asserting that procreation was a fundamental right of American citizens. The Court also expressed concern that forced sterilization could "cause races or types which are inimical to the dominant group to wither and disappear."[40] Spurred by the horror of the involuntary sterilization practices in Nazi Germany [41] and the growing civil rights movement in the United States of the 1950s and 1960s, most state legislatures repealed their involuntary sterilization statutes by the 1970s.

In 1979, federal regulations were written barring the use of federal funds to pay for sterilization of mentally retarded patients.[42] As of 1989, twenty states had retained statutes permitting surrogate decision makers to consent to sterilization of a mentally retarded patient, and eight others defined a judicial process for doing so.[43] The laws of the United Kingdom, Australia, and Canada require approval of a high court to permit sterilization of a mentally retarded patient.[44] South Africa has enacted a national statute to provide legal sanction for involuntary sterilization.[45]

Medical societies and scholars have attempted to formulate stringent criteria for the ethical practice of involuntary sterilization. The American College of Obstetricians and Gynecologists (ACOG) published a position paper in 1988 summarizing the relevant medical, ethical, and legal issues of involuntary sterilization. The ACOG stated that the surrogate decision makers should be the parents, immediate family members, or legal guardians of the mentally retarded person. The surrogate should utilize a best interest standard, but the surrogate's decision should be inspected by the physician to assure that there is no conflict of interest. All alternatives to sterilization, such as contraception training, should be considered first. To guarantee that the decision to sterilize is in the patient's best interest, certain facts should be ascertained: (1) the patient's mental incapacity is permanent; (2) the patient

is fertile and likely to engage in sexual intercourse; (3) the pregnancy poses a serious health risk or disproportionate burden to the patient; and (4) the pregnancy would pose a significant risk of a serious congenital disorder in the infant. Relevant laws in the jurisdiction should be followed.[46]

In 1990, the American Academy of Pediatrics reprinted the ACOG report with an accompanying position paper of its own, emphasizing several points. Girls before menarche should not be sterilized. The primary or contributing indications for sterilization based on "presumed or anticipated hardship to others" should be viewed with great skepticism, in light of acceptable alternatives to sterilization such as pharmacological contraception. Determination of "hardship" should be rigorous, and sterilization should not be performed simply as a convenience. Physicians should attempt to obtain informed consent from the patient, and, to the fullest extent possible, they should include the patient in the decision-making process. At all times, physicians should choose the least invasive, least permanent, and safest technique.[47] To these reasonable criteria should be added that newer, less invasive, long-duration hormonal treatments may satisfactorily achieve contraception in some patients without requiring surgical sterilization.[48]

In the less retarded patient, consent for sterilization with a careful explanation of the indications, risks, benefits, and alternatives of the procedure always should be obtained. Failure to obtain the patient's consent should not, itself, be evidence that the patient is incompetent or has made an irrational decision. As Daniel Wikler pointed out, "the fact that some retarded persons pose a threat to their own welfare is not in itself sufficient reason to deny them the liberty to do so."[49] For more severely retarded patients, one philosopher asserted recently "If some of these persons are fertile and sexually active, it may be very well the morally right thing to do to sterilize [them], in their own best interest, but without their consent—if necessary even through coercive means."[50] Between these two extreme positions, the ethical analyses of most scholars have relied on a utilitarian balance of the benefits and risks of sterilization to the patient once necessity has been established.[51]

Joseph Rauh and colleagues, after a review of their own substantial experience with a carefully planned sterilization program, have proposed a model statute they call the "voluntary sterilization act." They believe that the act should be adopted by all states to assure the proper balance of ethical considerations and legal rights for all parties in this debate. Their proposed statute contains the following provisions:

a. The individual is presumed capable of procreation.

b. The individual is, or is likely to be, sexually active.

c. Pregnancy would not usually be intended by a competent person facing analogous choices.

d. All alternative contraceptive methods have proved unworkable or been shown inapplicable.

e. The individual's guardian agrees that sterilization is the best course of action in the case.

f. Comprehensive medical, psychological, and social evaluations recommend sterilization for this individual.

g. The individual is represented by independent legal counsel with demonstrated competence in dealing with the medical, legal, social, and ethical issues involved in sterilization.

h. The individual, regardless of her level of competence, has been informed in full by one able to make her understand, and up to her level of competence shows awareness of the

    1. method of sterilization to be used

    2. nature and consequences of the sterilization

    3. likelihood of success

    4. alternative methods of sterilization

    5. alternative methods of birth control

    6. nature and consequences of pregnancy and parenthood and, after full and fair deliberation of these matters, has given the most complete consent of which she is capable

i. All these determinations are made and true no more than six months before any court proceedings.[52]

In a similar attempt to justify the ethical and legal acceptability of involuntary sterilization to maximally protect the retarded patient, Judith Areen proposed the following list of legal procedural criteria:

1. Those advocating sterilization bear the heavy burden of proving by clear and convincing evidence that sterilization is in the best interest of the incompetent.

2. The incompetent must be afforded a full judicial hearing at which medical testimony is presented and the incompetent, through a guardian appointed for the litigation, is allowed to present proof and cross-examine witnesses.

3. The judge must be assured that a comprehensive medical, psychological, and social evaluation is made of the incompetent.

4. The judge must determine that the individual is legally incompetent to make the decision whether to be sterilized, and that this incapacity is in all likelihood permanent.

5. The incompetent must be capable of reproduction and unable to care for offspring.

6. Sterilization must be the only practicable means of contraception.

7. The proposed operation must be the least restrictive alternative available.

8. To the extent possible, the judge must hear testimony from the incompetent concerning his or her understanding and desire, if any, for the proposed operation and its consequences.

9. The judge must examine the motivation for the request for sterilization.[53]

OTHER CONSENT ISSUES

A group of three related issues involve obtaining consent to control the behavior of mentally retarded patients: (1) sedating retarded women to permit the performance of gynecological examinations; (2) using psychotropic medications to control disruptive and aggressive behavior; and (3) using aversive conditioning techniques to improve maladaptive behavior. All share the goal of reducing the patient's anxiety, improving the patient's health and comfort, and improving the ease of the patient's medical and nursing care. Because these actions all produce some degree of harm to the patient, they require an ethical justification. Under what conditions is the use of involuntary physical or pharmacological restraints ethically acceptable?

Routine gynecological pelvic examinations, including Pap smears, are desirable for preventive purposes. But pelvic examinations often are impossible to perform in moderately to severely retarded women because these women fail to cooperate, as a consequence of fear resulting from their inability to understand the nature and purpose of the examination. Three options to resolve this dilemma are available: (1) the retarded woman can be physically restrained and the examination performed against her will; (2) the examination can be omitted entirely; or (3) the retarded woman can be sedated and the examination performed without resistance.

Physically restraining the patient to perform the examination most likely would produce more intense fear and discomfort. The retarded patient would perceive the examination as a physical assault and likely would resist with all her power. Restraining the patient under these circumstances would be an inhumane act despite the good intent. Omitting the examination altogether would unjustifiably deny the mentally retarded women the health benefits of early disease diagnosis and prevention afforded to other women.

Douglas Brown and colleagues judged that sedating these women was the best option. They used the analogy of young children who also are unable to comprehend the purpose and method of medical examination and treatment. They established a program in which moderately to severely retarded women were administered parenteral ketamine prior to the pelvic examination in much the same way that children have been administered ketamine analgesia to facilitate the performance of successful medical examinations. With ketamine analgesia, these clinicians were able to perform 42 successful pelvic examinations on retarded women who otherwise could not have been examined. Subsequent questionnaire responses from physicians, nurses, and ethics committee members supported the ethical acceptability and medical efficacy of this practice. Respondents believed that this practice was humane, safe, and, on balance, in the patients' best interest.[54]

The use of psychotropic medications and aversive conditioning techniques to control aggressive, combative, and disruptive behavior has been the source of a similar controversy. The goal of prescribing medication and performing aversive conditioning is to make the patient more manageable and less likely to harm himself and others. In the process, he also becomes more functional. Because these techniques have been abused in the past when they have been applied solely for the convenience of the staff, most institutions and agencies now have adopted strict regulations for their use.[55] These regulations are designed to assure that psychotropic medications and aversive therapies will he used only when all other measures fail, that a minimal and humane medication and dosage will be prescribed, and that frequent reassessment will be performed to prove necessity, efficacy, and safety.[56]

WITHHOLDING AND WITHDRAWING MEDICAL TREATMENT

Because of its finality, withholding and withdrawing life-sustaining therapy (LST) is the most vexing ethical decision in the health care of the never-competent, mentally retarded patient. Physicians, families, guardians, and courts have struggled to define the substantive facts and procedures that assure proper respect for human dignity, respect for due process in decision making, and respect for the legitimate rights of individual citizens as balanced with those of society. The ideal balance protects vulnerable patients with severe mental retardation without overprotecting them.

The best interest standard of surrogate decision making is the most plausible process for making end-of-life decisions in the never-competent patient for the reasons I stated earlier about consent for treatment. Surrogate decision makers, such as family members or court-appointed guardians, must make the best interest judgment based on their understanding of the specific facts of the diagnosis and prognosis as explained by the physician. In this way, a shared decision-making, patient-centered model can be followed, in which the value of the patient's life to himself is given maximal emphasis.[57]

The struggles of surrogates to weigh objectively the benefits and burdens of proposed treatments at the end of life most clearly illuminate the advantages and disadvantages of applying a best interest standard. Surrogate decision makers should concentrate on their perception of the risks, benefits, and discomfort the patient would undergo while receiving LST in comparison to that which the patient would experience without LST and with ideal palliative care. If the benefits of continued LST outweigh the burdens of medical risk and suffering, the surrogate should provide consent. However, if the burdens caused by medical risks and suffering from LST outweigh its benefits, a rational surrogate should refuse consent and should provide consent only for palliative care.

Severely retarded patients lack the capacity to comprehend the purpose of invasive and painful medical treatments; they therefore cannot cooperate and passively accept the necessary discomfort. Usually they must be restrained mechanically or pharmacologically to assure that they will not extract their indwelling tubes or otherwise interfere with their treatment. Physical restraints further aggravate their fear, anxiety, discomfort, and suffering. Thus, a profoundly retarded man with chronic renal failure who must undergo hemodialysis three times a week will suffer more than a competent cooperative man who has to undergo the same treatment because of the necessity also to sedate, restrain, or anesthetize the retarded man to accomplish the treatment. The inevitability of the added suffering of the severely retarded patient as a consequence of the sedation and restraints must be considered carefully in the balance of benefits and burdens of any proposed treatments.

Some scholars have justifiably criticized the use of the best interest standard to make end-of-life decisions for a never-competent retarded patient because it relies on an unavoidably subjective determination of the patient's quality of life and, if conducted improperly, may devalue the lives of disabled members of our society.[58] The full appreciation of this risk should infuse an attitude of caution into any surrogate's end-of-life best interest determination.[59] But the alternative of providing LST automatically for these patients, irrespective of the burden placed on them, is unacceptable. Inappropriate treatment, particularly when mechanical restraints are required to carry it out, could be regarded as abuse, despite the benevolent motive.[60] The surrogate and physician must make the hard choice of what is best for the patient. If the default mode were to treat all retarded patients with maximal aggressiveness, they would create more harms than those prevented in many cases.

How surrogates and physicians assess quality of life in disabled patients is critical. A determination of a disabled patient's quality of life never should attempt to estimate the "worth," qualities, or abilities of the person.[61] It should look at the quality of remaining life only as the affected person would live it. It should not view the life through a standard or norm determined by a completely healthy, cognitively intact person because such standards are innately biased against the disabled patient. Susan Martyn described this effort as an attempt to find the unique moral voice of the individual and to practice "best respect" for that person's life.[62]

Unfortunately, some surrogates and physicians make glib and patronizing conclusions about a disabled person's quality of life that systematically undervalue the life because they fail to adequately reflect the person's unique perspective. As a result, they may conduct a biased best interest determination from which they derive a fallacious conclusion. Physically fit and cognitively intact physicians, family members, and friends often view disabled patients as unfortunate and their lives as diminished significantly by their disabilities. But disabled patients usually do not view themselves in that way, especially when their disability is lifelong.[63] To prevent a patronizing and discriminatory outcome, best interest determinations in mentally retarded patients must be conducted with prudence, humility, and caution. Surrogates should attempt to see life from the patient's viewpoint and carefully balance all relevant factors.[64]

One factor intrinsic to surrogate decision making—though addressed only rarely—is the extent to which a surrogate's best interest calculation considers the impact on third parties, particularly family members. Although, ideally, a surrogate's assessment of the benefits and burdens of therapy should be restricted to the direct effects on the patient, concerns about the indirect effects on the family are inescapable and may influence judgment, if only subconsciously. Scholars are divided over whether the impact on third parties is an ethically justified consideration in surrogate decision making.[65] The care of patients with severe mental retardation often places enormous physical, emotional, and financial burdens on families. John Hardwig argued that, on the grounds of fairness, the extreme sacrifices families make to care for a mentally-retarded patient justify considering the family's interests in medical decisions.[66] Whether or not one concedes that such concerns are ethically justified, physicians must recognize the reality that surrogates' decision making using a best interest standard cannot be conducted without considering third-party interests and effects.

Family members, court-appointed guardians, or other surrogates should not be permitted to decide on treatment choices without clinician oversight and counsel. Family members may have conflicts of interest and make an alleged best interest judgment that, in fact, caters more to their own interests than to those of the patient. Physicians should determine whether the surrogate's decision is rational. In those instances in which a physician has evidence that the surrogate is deciding for reasons that clearly oppose the patient's best interests, he should consider seeking judicial assistance to appoint a new surrogate. In most cases, physicians should request assistance from other expert physicians or the institutional ethics committee to help clarify the patient's prognosis and optimize decision-making procedures, thereby ensuring maximal respect for the patient's best interest.[67]

Patients with mild to moderate mental retardation can be granted limited self-determination. They can execute advance directives under physician guidance to stipulate the desired levels of treatment and the extent to which the patient wishes family involvement in medical decisions.[68] Physicians can assess the capacity of patients with mild to moderate mental retardation to provide informed consent and refusal according to accepted standardized tests.[69] Patients' preferences in decision making should be included to whatever extent possible because maximizing retarded patients' sense of self-determination, however limited, improves their ratings of the quality of their lives.[70]

Physicians should not shoulder the burden of supervising these decisions alone. Cases of withholding and withdrawing treatment from patients with mental retardation can be referred to ethics committees or consultants for advice and procedural oversight. The committees can assure that proper diagnosis and prognosis have been determined and that a proper decision-making process has been carried out to protect the patient's interests.[71] Many residential centers for the mentally retarded now have functioning ethics committees.[72] Close collaboration by experienced clinicians, loving family members, lawful surrogates, and ethics consultants can hope to reach consensus and make the correct decision that is truly in the patient's best interest. As is true in all dying patients, dying severely retarded patients require proper palliative care.[73]

In my experience performing ethics consultations for hospitalized severely retarded patients who become critically ill or terminally ill, I have observed an interesting phenomenon. Many public guardians for severely retarded wards of the state are reluctant to follow physicians' recommendations to withhold or withdraw LST. I have found two complementary reasons for their reluctance. Public guardians usually conceptualize their primary role as protectors of the vulnerable patients whom they represent. Guardians do not consider refusing LST as a duty encompassed within their role as protector. As a result, I have found them to be generally more enthusiastic about providing consent for a patient's treatment than about refusing it on behalf of the patient. A second reason for their reluctance to refuse LST stems from compliance requirements to a web of protective regulations within the Office of the Public Guardian or other state agency under which they must operate. In many states, refusing LST for a ward of the state requires a cumbersome bureaucratic process that may take days to weeks before administrative approval can be granted.

As a consequence of the protective attitude of public guardians and the protective rules under which they operate, I have found that it is much more difficult for physicians to discontinue LST for severely retarded, terminally ill patients than for other hospitalized patients who are equally close to death but who have private surrogate decision makers. Some of the mentally retarded patients linger and suffer unnecessarily during the delay caused by this administrative process.[74] In one remarkable case I saw as an ethics consultant, the public guardian forbade removing the ventilator of a brain-dead elderly public ward until state administrative approval could be accomplished. Because this administrative process would have taken several days and the patient had been declared dead under state law, the attending physician unilaterally removed the ventilator without awaiting approval. In these cases, the state regulations written to protect vulnerable patients with mental retardation have accomplished overprotection. In our hospital, physicians routinely request ethics consultations in such cases, both to facilitate decision making and to follow the guidelines of the Office of the Public Guardian.[75]

THE FAMILY OF THE RETARDED PATIENT

Most moderately retarded and many severely retarded patients can be cared for at home rather than in an institution. The benefits of home care in promoting the function and happiness of the majority of retarded patients has been shown in repeated studies.[76] As a result, families may be pressured to care for the retarded patient at home. The impact of the family's responsibility for a patient's care then becomes of direct relevance to the retarded patient's welfare because an adverse effect on the family caused by his presence at home in turn may produce direct harms to the patient.

The family's reaction to the patient is affected greatly by the initial counseling they received from the hospital medical and nursing staff. How and what they are told are potent predictors of how successfully they will relate subsequently to the child at home. Families must understand the diagnosis, prognosis, and ongoing treatment needs of their children as accurately as possible. They should he told the truth in a compassionate and encouraging way. They need to be offered counseling early to help them adjust to their new responsibilities.[77]

Despite popular beliefs to the contrary, the majority of families caring for severely retarded patients at home wish to do so, and they do not feel that they become dysfunctional in the process. Most studies have found that parents in this setting do not become isolated socially. Many parents respond to the handicapped child with guilt and anxiety, but the generation of a little guilt may be adaptive in that it may stimulate the parents to provide the child with the extra attention he needs. Neither the parents nor the other siblings appear to experience harm as a result of the handicapped child's living at home.[78] However, in my experience performing ethics consultations for hospitalized patients with severe mental retardation, I have also seen cases in which the terrible stresses of home care led to divorce of the parents, psychiatric illness in the patient's siblings, and institutionalization of the patient.

Many families of retarded children and young adults successfully incorporate the patient into the family unit. They better understand the needs of the patient and can communicate more effectively with the patient than anyone else. I have several such young adult patients in my practice who function quite well in loving families despite having profound retardation. I have learned to depend on the parents to tell me when the patient is ill by their ability to detect subtle signs. The parents of these patients provide loving and dedicated care to them that seems natural. They are shocked when arrogant, insensitive, and cruel hospital personnel treat the patients as depersonalized objects or worse, as portrayed in a powerful short story by Richard Boyte that should be required reading for all medical students.[79]

Families and retarded patients both need counseling and rehabilitative services to maximize the functioning of the patient and the quality of the care provided by the family. Fortunately, available services for the patient now have been converted from custodial to educational and vocational. Psychological services are widely available for families through community mental health centers. Parent training programs improve the ultimate success that families experience in coping with handicapped patients. Of course it is the patient who becomes the ultimate beneficiary of this success.[80]

LEGAL ISSUES

Law and ethics govern the rights of mentally retarded patients in two general areas: (1) retarded patients as disabled citizens are entitled to the full measure of civil rights enjoyed by all citizens; and (2) retarded patients have the right to refuse unwanted medical therapies, a right that their lawful surrogate decision makers can exercise. These and other areas in which ethics and law affect mentally retarded patients have been the subject of several reviews.[81]

The ethical foundation of laws affording rights to mentally retarded citizens is the concept of justice.[82] All citizens are entitled to a fair share of society's communal resources. The differences in individuals arise from two chance events: the "natural lottery" in which people are endowed with different characteristics, abilities, and capacities through genetic chance; and the "social lottery" in which they receive social standing, wealth, and opportunity through the accident of birth. According to the egalitarian system of justice championed by John Rawls, the essence of justice is fairness, which in this context, requires equal personal opportunity. (See chapter 1.) Principles of justice dictate that society create social systems to compensate for the unfairness of both the natural and social lotteries to equalize opportunity.[83]

Public Laws 94–142 and 101–336

Although there had been many case law precedents asserting the rights of mentally retarded patients as citizens of the United States, the passage of the Education for All Handicapped Children Act of 1975 (PL 94–142) was a landmark event in guaranteeing those rights. The act required "free appropriate public education" to every school-age child, regardless of the severity of his mental retardation. Included in the law was the mandate to provide

> . . . related services [such as] transportation, and such developmental, corrective, and other supportive services (including speech pathology and audiology, psychological services, physical and occupational therapy, recreation and medical and counseling services, except that such medical services shall be for diagnostic and evaluation purposes only) as may be required to assist a handicapped child to benefit from special education, and includes the early identification and assessment of handicapping conditions in children.[84]

A unique feature of PL 94–142 was its requirement that the education of the handicapped child take place in the "least restrictive environment." Thus, children could not be educated in separate institutions or apart from their non-handicapped peers within an institution unless "the nature or severity of the handicap is such that education in regular classes with the use of supplementary aides and services cannot be achieved satisfactorily."[85] This provision mandated a practice of what became known later as "mainstreaming," the default mode in which handicapped children are placed in normal classrooms unless there were compelling reasons why such placement would be bad for the handicapped child.[86] Notably, PL 94–142 did not consider the impact of the handicapped child on the education of his non-handicapped classmates.

The precise public obligations that PL 94–142 imposed on municipal and state agencies and taxpayers have been the subject of a series of cases heard before high state courts and the U.S. Supreme Court. In several decisions in the 1980s, the Supreme

Court backpedaled somewhat on the "rights" imposed by PL 94–142 and on what specific services the law requires local governments to provide in individual cases.[87] Nevertheless, there has been an explosion of services available to handicapped children as a direct result of PL 94–142. The special education budgets of public schools have been markedly increased in many communities to provide these mandated services. Public school boards of directors have sought legal advice to determine their precise liability for required services.

The Americans with Disabilities Act (ADA) of 1990 (PL 101–336) was the second landmark act to protect the interests of mentally retarded patients and all other persons with disabilities. The ADA extended the previous Rehabilitation Act of 1973 to prohibit discrimination against people with disabilities throughout all aspects of life. Its full ramifications continue to evolve through litigation at various levels.[88] The American Academy of Pediatrics (AAP) Committee on Children with Disabilities outlined the duties of pediatricians who care for children with developmental disabilities to adequately comply with this law and the Education for All Handicapped Children Act.[89] The AAP encouraged pediatricians to advocate for their patients with disabilities and increase community sensitivity to the provisions of the ADA in schools, hospitals, physicians' offices, community businesses, and recreational program. The Canadian Charter of Rights and Freedoms grants rights to disabled persons similar to those provided by the ADA.[90]

Withholding and Withdrawing Life-Sustaining Treatment

Influential judicial decisions on the termination of life-sustaining treatment of the never-competent patient began with *Saikewicz* in 1977. In reaching a decision on whether to order chemotherapy for a severely retarded older man with acute leukemia, the *Saikewicz* court ruled that mentally retarded incompetent persons enjoy "the same panoply of rights and choices" as competent persons. The *Saikewicz* court advocated use of the substituted judgment standard of decision making for the incompetent patient but simultaneously acknowledged that "this is an impossible task" in the setting of the never-competent mentally retarded patient. Most controversially, they ruled that these types of decisions cannot be made by surrogates and must be made by courts.[91]

In *Storar*, the highest court in New York applied the best interest standard to decide whether to order blood transfusions for a severely retarded 52-year-old man who was dying of bladder cancer. Although the parents as guardians refused transfusions for him, the court overruled them because it felt that continued medical treatment was in the patient's best interests. The *Storar* court would not permit surrogate refusal of treatment by the patient's parents and required judicial review. They believed that the best interest standard was the most reasonable and powerful standard of decision making for never-competent persons.[92]

Since *Storar*, the best interest standard has been applied widely to medical decision making for the never-competent patient in a number of other high-court decisions.[93] The best interest standard was recommended for decision making in the never-competent patient by the President's Commission for the Study of Ethical Problems in Medicine and Biomedical and Behavioral Research and more recently by the New York State Task Force on Life and the Law.[94]

One exception to the trend of requiring judicial review was the Massachusetts Supreme Judicial Court ruling in *Jane Doe*, approving a family's wish to remove the feeding tube of a woman profoundly retarded by Canavan's disease, to permit her to die. Surprisingly, the court cited *Saikewicz* and ruled on the standard of substituted judgment, ignoring the trend in other jurisdictions and the recommendations from influential commissions to use a best interest standard. As in *Saikewicz*, the court remained unable to explain adequately how a substituted judgment possibly could be conducted in a never-competent patient.[95]

In *Lawrence*, the Indiana Supreme Court ruled that it is more important to permit family members to make medical decisions for retarded patients than to be preoccupied with the standard they use for their decision. In their ruling, the *Lawrence* court cited Nancy Rhoden's law review article in which she advocated that it is more important to emphasize who decides than on how they decide.[96] The *Lawrence* court recommended that the families of patients should be permitted to make decisions regarding life-sustaining treatment for never-competent retarded patients, irrespective of whether they employ a best interest or substituted judgment standard. The court believed that adopting this intuitive and reasonable procedural rule would avoid having to create a legal fiction to bridge the decision-making impasse (such as using substituted judgment for a never-competent patient) and generally would improve decision making for the never-competent patient.[97] In a subsequent commission statement, the New York State Task Force on Life and the Law concurred.[98]

Other states have facilitated surrogate decision making by enacting health-care surrogate acts. (See chapter 4.) These acts automatically appoint a surrogate decision maker, usually from the patient's family, when the patient fulfills certain diagnostic and prognostic preconditions. Whether the mentally retarded patient qualifies to be automatically represented by such an appointment depends on the patient's age and the particular state requirements for disease type and severity.[99]

Despite the requirement in the *Saikewicz* and *Storar* rulings that end-of-life decision making for institutionalized patients with severe mental retardation requires judicial approval, in practice, these cases are referred for judicial review only infrequently. Most commentators on *Saikewicz* and *Storar* found the requirement for routine judicial review utterly unrealistic and unnecessary. Currently, the only treatment issues in institutionalized mentally retarded patients that are commonly referred for judicial review involve consent for organ or tissue donation, sterilization, psychosurgery, or electric shock treatment.[100] End-of-life treatment decisions are made privately by surrogate decision makers, including parents and public and private guardians, in a shared decision-making process with the patient's physician, according to institutional and state guidelines.

RESEARCH ON THE MENTALLY RETARDED PATIENT

Until the past several decades, some researchers believed that the population of institutionalized mentally retarded patients made an ideal group of subjects for research because they were a sequestered "captive population" shielded from public scrutiny, and a group for whom it was not necessary to obtain proper valid consent. The unfortunate Willowbrook State School experiment in New York, discussed in chapter 19, brought to public attention the existence of abusive research practices on institutionalized patients and changed the methods of conducting research on mentally retarded subjects forever. In the Willowbrook State School experiments, institutionalized retarded children were purposely exposed to hepatitis A with parental "consent" obtained by coercive means.[101]

Clearly there are valid experiments that can and should be performed on mentally retarded and other incapacitated institutional residents for their own welfare or for the scientific knowledge gained that may help them or others in the future.[102] The ethical question is how to regulate this practice so that the interests of vulnerable patients remain protected and appropriate and desirable scientific research can be performed. I have culled guidelines that attempt to address both these objectives from two influential reports by the Task Force on Legal and Ethical Issues and the National Commission for the Protection of Human Subjects of Biomedical and Behavioral Research. I also have reviewed guidelines developed by similar committees from other countries.[103]

Although institutionalized retarded patients should be used as research subjects for some studies, they should not be used disproportionately. Retarded persons are institutional inpatients solely to obtain needed medical and nursing care. Neither have they been incarcerated nor have they given presumed consent to serve as research subjects. The burden of serving as research subjects should be shared equitably among all patient groups.[104]

Whenever research on retarded subjects is proposed, it should be conducted in accordance with the requirements of the institutional review board. These requirements include obtaining the full and free valid consent of the patient's surrogate decision maker following a complete disclosure of risks and benefits. The study must be scientifically valid and demonstrate that all reasonable measures are in place to protect the patient at every stage of the research. Surrogate decision makers should have the unequivocal power to refuse consent, and they should exercise this power if they believe the risks to outweigh the benefits. Patients should be included in the consent process to the degree they have the capacity to understand.[105]

Several other criteria must be satisfied. The institution must have the recognized ability to conduct the study properly and to protect the patient. The research cannot interfere with the rehabilitation, education, or proper medical and nursing care of the institutionalized subject. The research itself should relate to the overall health, disease prevention, treatment, or rehabilitation of the mentally retarded patient. Follow-up medical care for any complications acquired from the research protocol should be readily available.[106]

In general, if the proposed research presents more than a minimal risk and no likelihood of direct benefit to the subject, it should be permitted only if the patient is capable of providing independent valid consent.[107] If the patient cannot provide independent consent, the research can be permitted only if the following three conditions are met: (1) the risk to the subject is only slightly greater than a minimal risk; (2) the research is relevant to the subjects' condition; and (3) the research holds the promise of significant benefit in the future, either to the subject or to other patients with similar disorders.[108] The institutional review board should function to protect the retarded child or adult patient from unjustifiably high-risk research protocols.[109]

C.B. Fisher argued that informed consent for research on adults with mental retardation should be reconceptualized as the goodness-of-fit between the research subject's decisional capacity and the consent context to remove an exclusive focus on the research subject's cognitive capacity. Fisher believes that the consent process needs to examine those aspects of the consent setting that create or exacerbate vulnerability and therefore how the consent process can be modified to best protect the hopes, values, concerns, and welfare of the vulnerable research subject.[110] In a study of persons with mild and moderate mental retardation, Fisher and colleagues found that many of the study subjects attained consent scores similar to control subject with normal cognitive capacity. They concluded that investigators should design a consent format tailored for the subject's particular language, memory, and attention deficits.[111]

An unresolved controversy is whether research that cannot possibly help the research subject ("non-therapeutic research") ever should be permitted in institutionalized mentally retarded patients. Can we ascribe altruism to never-competent patients to argue that, like many other suffering patients, had they the capacity to do so, they would volunteer to serve as research subjects as an ennobling act? Or does our duty to protect them as vulnerable patients who are subject to discrimination, exploitation, and abuse ban investigators from using them as subjects for any non-therapeutic research? Do never-competent persons lack the right to "volunteer" for non-therapeutic research that is enjoyed by all competent persons? Should we extend the authority of their surrogates to offer them as non-therapeutic research subjects to fulfill that right?[112] Richard McCormick argued that improving health is such an important goal for society that all citizens, as a matter of social justice, have a shared duty to serve as human subjects. Fulfilling this duty justifies presuming consent for research using never-competent patients.[113]

As I discussed in chapter 15, guidelines from the National Bioethics Advisory Commission (NBAC) have increased the procedural consent requirements for any research using mentally retarded patients as human subjects. The NBAC guidelines were drafted in response to past abuses of this vulnerable research population, such as the Willowbrook experiment, and are intended to prevent future abuses. The guidelines "require that an independent, qualified professional assess the potential subject's capacity to consent" for any protocol requiring more than minimal risk, unless the investigator can adequately justify the exception.[114] This additional procedural requirement to independently assess each potential research subject's capacity to provide valid consent undoubtedly will decrease the number of studies performed on this group of patients. Several leading psychiatrists and neuroscientists protested these guidelines, pointing out that they overprotect cognitively impaired research subjects and ultimately may do more harm than good by discouraging research that could help them and others with their conditions.[115]

NOTES

1. For a scholarly discussion of the conceptual, moral, and legal issues, emphasizing how respect for human dignity is the foundation of decision making for mentally retarded patients, see Cantor NL. *Making Medical Decisions for the Profoundly Mentally Disabled.* Cambridge, MA: MIT Press, 2005.

2. Shevell M, Ashwal S, Donley D, et al. Practice parameter: evaluation of the child with global developmental delay. Report of the Quality Standards Subcommittee of the American Academy of Neurology and the Practice Committee of the Child Neurology Society. *Neurology* 2003;60:367–380.

3. For reviews of the ethical issues in children with developmental disabilities, see Shevell MI. Clinical ethics and developmental delay. *Semin Pediatr Neurol* 1998;15:70–75 and Batshaw ML, Cho MK. Ethical choices: questions of care. In Batshaw ML (ed). *Children With Disabilities*, 4th ed. Baltimore: Paul H. Brooks Publishing Co, 1997:727–742.

4. Grossman H, ed. *Classification in Mental Retardation.* Washington, DC: American Association on Mental Deficiency, 1983:11. The American Association on Mental Deficiency thereafter changed its name to the American Association on Mental Retardation.

5. This classification and the general definitions and history of mental retardation were taken from Scheerenberger RC. *A History of Mental Retardation: A Quarter Century of Promise.* Baltimore: Paul Brookes Publishing Co, 1987:1–17.

6. Grossman H, ed. *Classification in Mental Retardation*, 1983:11,16.

7. American Association on Mental Retardation. *Mental Retardation: Definition, Classification, and Systems of Supports*, 9th ed. Washington, DC: American Association on Mental Retardation, 1992.

8. Grossman H, ed. *Manual on Terminology and Classification in Mental Retardation.* Washington, DC: American Association on Mental Deficiency, 1973.

9. Bourguignon HJ. Mental retardation: the reality behind the label. *Camb Q Healthc Ethics* 1994;3:179–194. See also Kopelman L. Respect and the retarded: issues of valuing and labeling. In Kopelman L, Moskop JC, eds. *Ethics and Mental Retardation.* Dordrecht: D Reidel Co, 1984:65–75.

10. AAMR Definition of Mental Retardation. http://www.aamr.org/Policies/faq_mental_retardation.shtml (Accessed July 2, 2007).

11. World's oldest organization on intellectual disability has a progressive new name. *AAMR News*, November 2, 2006. http://www.aamr.org/About_AAIDD/name_change_PRdreen.htm (Accessed July 2, 2007).

12. World Health Organization. International Classification of Functioning, Disability, and Health. May 22, 2001. http://www.who.int/classifications/icf/en/ (Accessed July 2, 2007).

13. President's Panel on Mental Retardation. *A Proposed Program for National Action to Combat Mental Retardation.* Washington, DC: Superintendent of Documents, 1962.

14. Tarjan G. The next decade: expectations from the biological sciences. *JAMA* 1965;191:160–163.

15. Roeleveld N, Zielhuis GA, Gabreels F. The prevalence of mental retardation: a critical review of recent literature. *Dev Med Child Neurol* 1997;39:125–132.

16. Yeargin-Allsopp M, Murphy CC, Cordero JF, Decoufle P, Holowell JG. Reported biomedical causes and associated medical conditions for mental retardation among 10-year-old children, metropolitan Atlanta, 1985 to 1987. *Dev Med Child Neurol* 1997;39:142–149.

17. Cited in Barlow CF. *Mental Retardation and Related Disorders.* Philadelphia: FA Davis Co, 1978:4.

18. American Academy of Pediatrics Committee on Children with Disabilities. Screening infants and young children for developmental disabilities. *Pediatrics* 1994;93:863–865.

19. Shevell M, Ashwal S, Donley D, et al. Practice parameter: evaluation of the child with global developmental delay. Report of the Quality Standards Subcommittee of the American Academy of Neurology and the Practice Committee of the Child Neurology Society. *Neurology* 2003;60:367–380.
The evidence-based screening recommendations listed are from this article. See also Rydz D, Shevell MI, Majnemer A, Oskoui M. Developmental screening. *J Child Neurol* 2005;20:4–21.

20. How physicians break the news to parents influences their later adjustment to having a child with a cognitive or motor disability. See Dagenais L, Hall N, Majnemer A, et al. Communicating a diagnosis of cerebral palsy: caregiver satisfaction and stress. *Pediatr Neurol* 2006;35:408–414. See chapters 2 and 7 for further discussion on breaking bad news.

21. Speicher MR, Higgins JJ. Hybridize and personalize: the new age of syndromal mental retardation diagnostics. *Neurology* 2007;68:721–722.

22. Moog U. The outcome of diagnostic studies on the etiology of mental retardation: considerations on the classification of causes. *Am J Med Genet A* 2005;137:228–231.

23. Engels H, Brockschmidt A, Hoischen A, et al. DNA microarray analysis identifies candidate regions and genes in unexplained mental retardation. *Neurology* 2007;68:743–750. The molecular biology of submicroscopic copy number variation is described in Redon R, Ishikawa S, Fitch KR, et al. Global variation in copy number in the human genome. *Nature* 2006;444:444–454.

24. These therapies are reviewed in detail in Matson JL, Mulick JA (eds). *Handbook of Mental Retardation*, 2nd ed. New York: Pergamon Press; 1991:347–504. See also Baroff GS. *Mental Retardation: Nature, Cause, and Management.* Philadelphia: Brunner/Mazel, 1999 and Burack JA, Hodapp RM, Zigler E (eds). *Handbook of Mental Retardation and Development.* New York: Cambridge University Press, 1998.

25. Aubourg P, Adamsbaum C, Lavallard-Rousseau MC, et al. A two-year trial of oleic and erucic acids ("Lorenzo's oil") as treatment for adrenomyeloneuropathy. *N Engl J Med* 1993;329:745–752 and Moser HW, Raymond GV, Dubey P. Adrenoleukodystrophy: new approaches to a neurodegenerative disease. *JAMA* 2005;294:3131–3134.

26. Moser HW. Lorenzo oil therapy for adrenoleukodystrophy: a prematurely amplified hope. *Ann Neurol* 1993;34:121–122. The popular movie "Lorenzo's Oil" was particularly misleading. See Jones AH. Medicine and the movies: *Lorenzo's Oil* at century's end. *Ann Intern Med* 2000;133:567–571.

27. Barton NW, Brady RO, Dambrosia JM, et al. Replacement therapy for inherited enzyme deficiency-Macrophage-targeted glucocerebrosidase for Gaucher's disease. *N Engl J Med* 1991;324:1464–1470; Figueroa ML, Rosenbloom BE, Kay AC, et al. A less costly regimen of alglucerase to treat Gaucher's disease. *N Engl J Med* 1992;327:1632–1636; and Lonser RR, Schiffman R, Robison RA, et al. Image-guided, direct convective delivery of glucocerebroside for neuronopathic Gaucher disease. *Neurology* 2007;68:254–261.

28. Banikazemi M, Bultas J, Waldek S, et al. Agalsidase-beta therapy for advanced Fabry disease: a randomized trial. *Ann Intern Med* 2007;146:77–86.

29. For a philosophical discussion of the rights of the mentally retarded, see Murphy J. Rights and borderline cases. In: Kopelman L, Moskop JC, eds. *Ethics and Mental Retardation.* Dordrecht: D Reidel Co, 1984:3–17; Margolis J. Applying moral theory to the retarded. In Kopelman L, Moskop JC, eds. *Ethics and Mental Retardation,* 1984:19–36; and Woozley AD. The rights of the retarded. In Kopelman L, Moskop JC, eds. *Ethics and Mental Retardation,* 1984:47–56. The legal precedents for these rights are outlined in Krais WA. The incompetent developmentally disabled person's right of self-determination: right-to-die, sterilization and institutionalization. *Am J Law Med* 1989;15:333–361.

30. This point is carefully defended in Cantor NL. *Making Medical Decisions for the Profoundly Mentally Disabled.* Cambridge, MA: MIT Press, 2005:33–99. See also the discussions of decision making for incompetent patients in chapters 4 and 8.

31. Cantor NL. *Making Medical Decisions for the Profoundly Mentally Disabled.* Cambridge, MA: MIT Press, 2005:96.

32. In *Guardianship of Jane Doe,* a case in which termination of life-sustaining treatment of a profoundly retarded and essentially vegetative adult with Canavan's disease was being considered, the Massachusetts Supreme Judicial Court stated that using "substituted judgment for a never-competent person is a legal fiction." Nevertheless, the court then proceeded to rely on substituted judgment in its ruling. *Guardianship of Jane Doe,* 583 NE 2d 1263, 1268–1269 (Mass 1992). The relative merits of employing the substituted judgment and best interest standards in the never-competent patient are discussed in Martyn SR. Substituted judgment, best interest, and the need for best respect. *Camb Q Healthc Ethics* 1994;3:195–208.

33. President's Commission for the Study of Ethical Problems in Medicine and Biomedical and Behavioral Research. *Deciding to Forego Life-Sustaining Treatment: Ethical, Medical, and Legal Issues in Treatment Decisions.* Washington, DC: US Government Printing Office, 1983:134–136.

34. Kopelman LM. The best interests standard for incompetent or incapacitated persons of all ages. *J Law Med Ethics* 2007;35:187–196.

35. Molinari V, McCollough LB, Workman R, Coverdale J. Geriatric assent. *J Clin Ethics* 2004;15:261–268. The concept of seeking the assent of children is explained in American Academy of Pediatrics Committee on Bioethics. Informed consent, parental permission, and assent in pediatric practice. *Pediatrics* 1995;95:314–317. See the further discussion of assent in chapter 2.

36. For the most comprehensive reference on this subject, see Macklin R, Gaylin W, eds. *Mental Retardation and Sterilization. A Problem of Competency and Paternalism.* New York: Plenum Press, 1981. For a discussion of the related problem of involuntary sterilization in patients with chronic mental illness, see McCullough LB, Coverdale J, Bayer T, et al. Ethically justified guidelines for family planning interventions to prevent pregnancy in female patients with chronic mental illness. *Am J Obstet Gynecol* 1992;167:19–25.

37. Reilly PR. *The Surgical Solution—A History of Involuntary Sterilization in the United States.* Baltimore: Johns Hopkins University Press, 1991.

38. Quoted in Rauh JL, Dine MS, Biro FM, et al. Sterilization of the mentally retarded adolescent: balancing the equities—the Cincinnati experience. *J Adolesc Health Care* 1989;10:467–472. See also Appelbaum P. The issue of sterilization and the mentally retarded. *Hosp Community Psychiatry* 1982;33:523–524.

39. *Buck v Bell*, 274 US 200, 207 (1927). This controversial opinion has been criticized extensively on moral as well as factual grounds. For critiques, see Macklin R, Gaylin W, eds. *Mental Retardation and Sterilization: A Problem of Competency and Paternalism* 1981:65–69; and Bayles MD. Voluntary and involuntary sterilization: the legal precedents. *Hastings Cent Rep* 1978;8(3):37–41. For historical aspects of this famous case, see Smith JD, Nelson KR. *The Sterilization of Carrie Buck.* Far Hills, NJ: New Horizon, 1989. Following Virginia's 1924 eugenic sterilization law, more than 8,000 state-mandated sterilizations were performed. On May 2, 2002, a historic marker was erected in Charlottesville, Virginia, the home town of Carrie Buck, to commemorate the 75th anniversary of *Buck v Bell*. Virginia Governor Mark Warner sent an official apology that was read at the dedication ceremony, denouncing the role of the Commonwealth of Virginia in the eugenics movement as a "shameful effort." See Lombardo PA. Facing Carrie Buck. *Hastings Cent Rep* 2003;33(2):14–17.

40. *Skinner v Oklahoma*, 316 US 535 (1942) as quoted in Brahams D. Legal power to sterilize incompetent women. *Lancet* 1989;1:854–855. The history of the American eugenics movement is documented in Ludmerer KM. *Genetics and American Society: A Historical Appraisal.* Baltimore: Johns Hopkins University Press, 1972.

41. Sofair AN, Kaldjian LC. Eugenic sterilization and a qualified Nazi analogy: the United States and Germany, 1930–1945. *Ann Intern Med* 2000;132:312–319.

42. 42 *CFR* 50.201–50.210, 1979.

43. Rauh JL, Dine MS, Biro FM, et al. *J Adolesc Health Care* 1989:469.

44. For discussion of the legal status of involuntary sterilization in the United Kingdom and Australia, see Brahams D. *Lancet* 1989:854–855 and Price DPT. Comparative approaches to the nonconsensual sterilization of the mentally retarded. *Med Law* 1990;9:940–949. On the situation in Canada, see Rivet M. Sterilization and medical treatment of the mentally disabled: some legal and ethical reflections. *Med Law* 1990;9:1150–1171.

45. Nash ES, Navias M. The therapeutic sterilization of the mentally handicapped: experience with the Abortion and Sterilization Act of 1975. *S African Med J* 1992;82:437–440.

46. American College of Obstetrics and Gynecology Committee Opinion 63. Sterilization of women who are mentally handicapped. *Pediatrics* 1990;85:869–871.

47. American Academy of Pediatrics Committee on Bioethics. Sterilization of women who are mentally handicapped. *Pediatrics* 1990;85:868.

48. Paransky OI, Zurawain RK. Management of menstrual problems and contraception in adolescents with mental retardation: a medical, legal, and ethical review with new suggested guidelines. *J Pediatr Adolesc Gynecol* 2003;16:223–235.

49. Wikler DI. Paternalism and the mildly retarded. *Philos Public Affairs* 1979;8:377–392.

50. Tannsjo T. Non-voluntary sterilization. *J Med Philosophy* 2006;31:401–415.

51. Denekens JP, Nys H, Stuer H. Sterilisation of incompetent mentally handicapped persons: a model for decision making. *J Med Ethics* 1999;25:237–241 and Diekema DS. Involuntary sterilization of persons with mental retardation: an ethical analysis. *Ment Retard Dev Disabil Res Rev* 2003;9:21–26.

52. Rauh JL, Dine MS. Biro FM, et al. *J Adolesc Health Care* 1989:471.

53. Areen J. Limiting procreation. In Veatch RM (ed). *Medical Ethics.* Boston: Jones & Bartlett, 1989:106–107. For a critical analysis of these criteria, see Applebaum GM, La Puma J. Sterilization and a mentally handicapped minor: providing consent for one who cannot. *Camb Q Healthc Ethics* 1994;3:209–215.

54. Brown D, Rosen D, Elkins TE. Sedating women with mental retardation for routine gynecologic examination: an ethical analysis. *J Clin Ethics* 1992;3:68–75.

55. See the discussion of whether aversive therapies in the retarded patient ever can be employed without abuse, in Murphy G. The use of aversive stimuli in treatment: the issue of consent. *J Intell Disabil Res* 1993;37(Pt 3):211–219.

56. For example, see Rinck C, Guidry J, Calkins CF. Review of states' practices on the use of psychotropic medications. *Am J Ment Retard* 1989;93:657–668; Mulick JA. The ideology and science of punishment in mental retardation. *Am J Ment Retard* 1990;95:142–156; and Schroeder SR, Schroeder CS. The role of the AAMR in the aversives controversy. *Ment Retard* 1989;27:iii–iv. For an overview of this subject, see Scheerenberger RC. *A History of Mental Retardation: A Quarter Century of Promise*, 1987:96–100.

57. McKnight DK, Bellis M. Foregoing life-sustaining treatment for adult, developmentally disabled, public wards: a proposed statute. *Am J Law Med* 1992;18:203–232. See chapters 2 and 4 for a discussion of the shared decision-making model.

58. See, for example, Dresser RS, Robertson JA, Quality of life and non-treatment decisions for incompetent patients: a critique of the orthodox approach. *Law Med Health Care* 1989;17:234–244 and Destro RA. Quality of life, ethics, and constitutional jurisprudence: the demise of natural rights and equal protection for the disabled and incompetent. *J Contemp Health Law Policy* 1986;2:71–126.

59. Pellegrino ED, Thomasma DC. *For the Patient's Good: The Restoration of Beneficence in Health Care*. New York: Oxford University Press, 1988:92–98.

60. See discussion of this point in Rhoden NK. Litigating life and death. *Harvard Law Rev* 1988;102:375–446.

61. For an argument that the "moral worth" of a mentally retarded patient is completely independent of the patient's cognitive capacity, see Byrne P. *Philosophical and Ethical Problems in Mental Handicap*. Basingstoke, UK: Macmillan Press, 2000.

62. Martyn SR. Substituted judgment, best interest, and the need for best respect. *Camb Q Healthc Ethics* 1994;3:195–208.

63. Longmore PK. Medical decision making and people with disabilities: a clash of cultures. *J Law Med Ethics* 1995;23:82–87. One recent study, however, did show a reduction in quality of life ratings made by patients with developmental disabilities. See Sheppard-Jones K, Thompson-Prout H, Kleinert H. Quality of life dimensions for adults with developmental disabilities: a comparative study. *Ment Retard* 2005;43:281–291.

64. Drane JF, Coulehan JL. The best-interest standard: surrogate decision making and quality of life. *J Clin Ethics* 1995;6:20–29. See also Pearlman RA, Jonsen A. The use of quality of life considerations in medical decision-making. *J Am Geriatr Soc* 1985;33:344–352 and the discussion of quality of life in chapter 4. For a review of the quantitative aspects of quality of life determinations in neurological patients, see Meyers AR, Gage H, Hendricks A. Health-related quality of life in neurology. *Arch Neurol* 2000;57:1224–1227.

65. On the breadth of scholarly and judicial opinion concerning the validity of third party interests in surrogate decision making, see Cantor NL. *Making Medical Decisions for the Profoundly Mentally Disabled*. Cambridge, MA: MIT Press, 2005:136–148.

66. Hardwig J. The problem of proxies with interests of their own: toward a better theory of proxy decisions. *J Clin Ethics* 1993;4:20–27.

67. McKnight DK, Bellis M. *Am J Law Med* 1992:230–231.

68. Friedman RI. Use of advance directives: facilitating health care decisions by adults with mental retardation and their families. *Ment Retard* 1998;36:444–456.

69. Morris CD, Niederbuhl JM, Mahr JM. Determining the capability of individuals with mental retardation to give informed consent. *Ment Retard* 1993;98:263–272.

70. Lachapelle Y, Wehmeyer ML, Haelewyck MC, et al. The relationship between quality of life and self-determination: an international study. *J Intellect Disabil Res* 2005;49:74–744.

71. Loewy EH. Limiting but not abandoning treatment in severely mentally impaired patients: a troubling issue for ethics consultants and ethics committees. *Camb Q Healthc Ethics* 1994;3:216–225.

72. Edinger W. Expanding opportunities for ethics committees: residential centers for the mentally retarded and developmentally disabled. *Camb Q Healthc Ethics* 1994;3:226–232.

73. Mentally retarded patients often benefit from receiving palliative care throughout their illness. See Tuffrey-Wijne I. The palliative care needs of people with intellectual disabilities: a literature review. *Palliat Med* 2003;17:55–62.

74. For an extreme example of the over-treatment of a severely retarded, terminally ill patient, who received gastrostomy, tracheostomy, mechanical ventilation, blood transfusions, hemodialysis, and parenteral nutrition

during a 104-day hospitalization before he died, see Lohiya GS, Tan-Figueroa L, Crinella FM. End-of-life care for a man with developmental disabilities. *J Am Board Fam Pract* 2003;16:58–62.

75. Ethics consultation is a reasonable option in cases of discontinuing LST for mentally retarded wards of the state. The ethics consultants can help guarantee that the patient's best interests are protected and due process is followed. For an example of how ethics consultants facilitated a process by which institutionalized, severely mentally retarded patients who developed end-stage renal disease could be permitted to die without receiving chronic hemodialysis, see Kujdych N, Lowe DA, Sparks J, Dottes A, Crook ED. Dignity or denial? Decisions regarding initiation of dialysis and medical therapy in the institutionalized severely mentally retarded. *Am J Med Sci* 2000;320:374–378.

76. Carr J. The effect on the family of a severely mentally handicapped child. In Clarke AM, Clarke ADB, Berg JM (eds). *Mental Deficiency: The Changing Outlook.* 4th ed. New York: Free Press, 1985:512–548. The succeeding discussion was abstracted from Carr's chapter. See also Minnes P. Mental retardation: the impact upon the family. In, Burack JA, Hodapp RM, Zigler E, eds. *Handbook of Mental Retardation and Development.* New York: Cambridge University Press, 1998:693–712.

77. Carr J. *Mental Deficiency: The Changing Outlook,* 1985:513–515.

78. Carr J. *Mental Deficiency: The Changing Outlook,* 1985:515–524.

79. Boyte WR. Pizza ship. *Health Affairs* 2004;23(5):240–241.

80. Carr J. *Mental Deficiency: The Changing Outlook,* 1985:525–538.

81. Scheerenberger RC. *A History of Mental Retardation: A Quarter Century of Promise,* 1987:150–170; Kindred M. The legal rights of mentally retarded persons in twentieth century America. In Kopelman L, Moskop JC, eds. *Ethics and Mental Retardation,* 1984:185–208; Levenbook BB. Examining legal restrictions on the retarded. In Kopelman L, Moskop JC, eds. *Ethics and Mental Retardation,* 1984:209–221; Kunjukrishnan R, Varan LR. Interface between mental subnormality and the law. *Psychiatr J Univ Ottawa* 1989;14:439–452; and Krais WA. *Am J Law Med* 1989:333–361.

82. This argument is developed in Veatch RM. *The Foundations of Justice: Why the Retarded and the Rest of Us Have Claims to Equality.* New York: Oxford University Press, 1986.

83. Rawls J. *A Theory of Justice.* Boston: Harvard University Press, 1971.

84. As quoted in Scheerenberger RC. *A History of Mental Retardation: A Quarter Century of Promise,* 1987:150.

85. Ethical issues in special education for the mentally retarded patient in the United Kingdom are discussed in Alderson P, Goodey C. Doctors, ethics, and special education. *J Med Ethics* 1998;24:49–55.

86. Mainstreaming and its subtle distinction from placement in the "least restrictive environment" are discussed in Gottlieb J, Alter M, Gottlieb BW. Mainstreaming mentally retarded children. In Matson JL, Mulick JA, eds. *Handbook of Mental Retardation.* 2nd ed. New York: Pergamon Press, 1991:63–73.

87. These cases are reviewed in Kindred M. *Ethics and Mental Retardation,* 1984:198–205.

88. These laws and their relevance to retarded and disabled patients are described in Biehl RF. Legislative mandates. In Capute AJ, Accardo PJ (eds). *Developmental Disabilities in Infancy and Childhood,* 2nd ed. Baltimore: Paul H. Brooks Publishing Co., 1996:513–518 and Cooke RE. Ethics, law, and developmental disabilities. In Capute AJ, Accardo PJ (eds). *Developmental Disabilities in Infancy and Childhood,* 2nd ed. 1996:609–618.

89. American Academy of Pediatrics Committee on Children with Disabilities. The role of the pediatrician in implementing the Americans with Disability Act: subject review. *Pediatrics* 1996;98:146–148 and American Academy of Pediatrics Committee on Children with Disabilities. Provision of educationally-related services for children and adolescents with chronic diseases and disabling conditions. *Pediatrics* 2000;105:448–451.

90. The Canadian Charter of Rights and Freedoms is discussed in Shevell MI. Clinical ethics and developmental delay. *Semin Pediatr Neurol* 1998;15:70–75.

91. *Superintendent of Belchertown State School v. Saikewicz,* 373 Mass 728 (1977). The voluminous commentary on the use of the substituted judgment standard in Saikewicz is summarized in Sassaman EA. Ethical considerations in medical treatment. In Matson JL, Mulick JA, eds. *Handbook of Mental Retardation.* 2nd ed. New York: Pergamon Press, 1991:327–335.

92. *In re Storar,* 52 NY 2d, 363;420 NE 2d, 64;439 NYS 2d, 266 (1981).

93. These decisions are reviewed in Weir RF, Gostin L. Decisions to abate life-sustaining treatment for nonautonomous patients: ethical standards and legal liability for physicians after Cruzan. *JAMA* 1990:1848–1853 and in Krais WA. *Am J Law Med* 1989:333–361.

94. President's Commission for the Study of Ethical Problems in Medicine and Biomedical and Behavioral Research. *Deciding to Forego Life-Sustaining Treatment: Ethical, Medical, and Legal Issues in Treatment Decisions,*

1983 and New York State Task Force on Life and the Law. *When Others Must Choose: Deciding for Patients without Capacity*. New York: New York State Task Force on Life and the Law, 1992.

95. *Guardianship of Jane Doe*, 583 NE 2d 1263, 1268–1269 (Mass 1992). See the discussions of this case in Capron AM. Substituting our judgment. *Hastings Cent Rep* 1992;22(2):58–59 and Martyn SR. Substituted judgment, best interest, and the need for best respect. *Camb Q Healthc Ethics* 1994;3:195–208.

96. Rhoden NK. Litigating life and death. *Harvard Law Rev* 1988;102:375–446.

97. *In re Lawrence*, 579 NE 2d 31 (Ind 1991).

98. New York State Task Force on Life and the Law. *When Others Must Choose: Deciding for Patients Without Capacity*, 1992.

99. Menikoff JA, Sachs GA, Siegler M. Beyond advance directives – health care surrogate laws. *N Engl J Med* 1992;327:1165–1169.

100. Cantor NL. *Making Medical Decisions for the Profoundly Mentally Disabled*. Cambridge, MA: MIT Press, 2005:149–201:97–99.

101. This case is described in Goldby S. Experiments at the Willowbrook State School. *Lancet* 1971;1:749. For a retrospective ethical analysis by one of the Willowbrook investigators who attempted to justify his actions, see Krugman S. The Willowbrook hepatitis study revisited: ethical aspects. *Rev Infect Dis* 1986;8:157–162.

102. Freedman RI. Ethical challenges in the conduct of research involving persons with mental retardation. *Ment Retard* 2001;39:130–141 and Weisstub DN, Arboleda-Florez J. Ethical research with the developmentally disabled. *Can J Psychiatry* 1997;42:492–496.

103. Baudoin JL. Biomedical experimentation on the mentally handicapped: ethical and legal dilemmas. *Med Law* 1990;9:1052–1061.

104. Task Force on Legal and Ethical Issues. Experimentation with mentally handicapped subjects. In, Edwards RB, ed. *Psychiatry, and Ethics: Insanity, Rational Autonomy, and Mental Health Care*. Buffalo, NY: Prometheus Books, 1982:224–229.

105. Task Force on Legal and Ethical Issues. *Psychiatry and Ethics: Insanity, Rational Autonomy, and Mental Health Care*, 1982:224.

106. Task Force on Legal and Ethical Issues. *Psychiatry and Ethics: Insanity, Rational Autonomy, and Mental Health Care*, 1982:225–226.

107. Task Force on Legal and Ethical Issues. *Psychiatry and Ethics: Insanity, Rational Autonomy, and Mental Health Care*, 1982:226–227.

108. National Commission for the Protection of Human Subjects of Biomedical and Behavioral Research. *Report and Recommendations: Research Involving Those Institutionalized as Mentally Infirm*. Washington, DC: US Government Printing Office, 1978, as reprinted in President's Commission for the Study of Ethical Issues in Medicine and Biomedical and Behavioral Research. *Protecting Human Subjects: The Adequacy and Uniformity of Federal Rules and Their Implementation*. Washington, DC: US Government Printing Office, 1983:75.

109. The concept of "minimal risk" and the protective role of the institutional review board are discussed in Freedman B, Fuks A, Weijer C. In loco parentis: minimal risk as an ethical threshold for research upon children. *Hastings Cent Rep* 1993;23(2):13–19. The concept of "minimal risk" is discussed and critiqued in chapters 15 and 19.

110. Fisher CB. Goodness-of-fit ethic for informed consent to research involving adults with mental retardation and developmental disabilities. *Ment Retard Dev Disabil Res Rev* 2003;9:27–31.

111. Fisher CB, Cea CD, Davidson PW, Fried AL. Capacity of persons with mental retardation to consent to participate in randomized clinical trials. *Am J Psychiatry* 2006;163:1813–1820.

112. These questions are discussed extensively in Cantor NL. *Making Medical Decisions for the Profoundly Mentally Disabled*. Cambridge, MA: MIT Press, 2005:149–201.

113. McCormick RA. Proxy consent in the experimentation situation. *Perspect Biol Med* 1974;18:2–20.

114. National Bioethics Advisory Commission. *Research Involving Persons with Mental Disorders that may Affect Decisionmaking Capacity*. Rockville, MD: National Bioethics Advisory Commission, 1998. These guidelines were interpreted and discussed in Capron AM. Ethical and human rights issues in research on mental disorders that may affect decision-making capacity. *N Engl J Med* 1999;340:1430–1434. See further discussion of the responses to the NBAC recommendations in chapter 15.

115. Michels R. Are research ethics bad for our mental health? *N Engl J Med* 1999;340:1427–1430 and Oldham JM, Haimowitz S, Delano SJ. Protection of persons with mental disorders from research risk: a response to the report of the National Bioethics Advisory Commission. *Arch Gen Psychiatry* 1999;56:688–693.

Neurogenetic Testing and Treatment

17

The study of ethical issues in neurogenetics has a long history. The field of human biochemical genetics began with the publication of *Inborn Errors of Metabolism* by Sir Archibald Garrod in 1909. Human molecular neurogenetics became established in 1983 when James Gusella and coinvestigators identified a marker for the gene for Huntington's disease on chromosome 4.[1] The importance of addressing ethical issues in human genetics was recognized throughout the 20th century, from the time the first genetic tests were performed for carrier detection, prenatal diagnosis, and presymptomatic diagnosis. In no other branch of clinical or experimental medicine has a more vocal concern been expressed about the ethical and social ramifications of new advances in technology.

Over the past few decades, the pace of technological progress in molecular and clinical genetics has been astonishing. Victor McKusick noted that the number of entries in his magisterial *Mendelian Inheritance in Man* has increased exponentially since the first edition was published in 1966.[2] Hardly a week elapses without announcing that another gene that has been sequenced or cloned. To maintain currency in this rapidly growing field, McKusick and colleagues at Johns Hopkins University created an Internet version of his textbook entitled *Online Mendelian Inheritance in Man* (OMIM). OMIM is a continuously updated and publicly accessible computer database of human genes, gene maps, genetic diseases, statistics, pictures, and comprehensive genetic information maintained by the National Center for Biotechnology Information with references linked to Medline.[3]

The acceleration of advances in molecular genetics was stimulated by the Human Genome Project (HGP), an international cooperative effort from 1990 to 2003 to identify and map the chromosomal location of all 20,000 to 25,000 human genes and to determine the sequence of the three billion chemical base pairs that make up human DNA. The completion of this effort now will allow the identification of each gene's structural and regulatory elements.[4] The HGP was coordinated in the United States by both the National Center for Human Genome Research at the National Institutes of Health and the Department of Energy.[5]

The HGP completed its work far ahead of schedule. By 1996, the genomes of several bacterial species had been completely sequenced. Thereafter, as is now well known, the goal of sequencing the human genome became a race after the dramatic entry of Craig Venter, president of Celera Genomics, a profit-making company that announced publicly that it planned to patent genes it sequenced first. The publicized competition incited by Celera accelerated the progress of the project so that by June 2000, approximately five years ahead of schedule, the directors of the HGP and Celera were able to jointly announce the completion of the first "working draft" of the human genome.[6] Since the initial euphoria over the completion of the HGP in 2003, it has become clear that sequencing the human genome was only the first step in a long scientific path to fully understand the genetic control of disease.

Two principal benefits result from characterizing the structure and function of all human genes: the ability to diagnose all genetic defects at the level of DNA and the ability to manipulate genes involved in human disease for therapeutic purposes. Contemporary microarray technology permits the screening of a large number of genetic diseases due to deletions, duplications, and polymorphisms, confirming the diagnosis of such disorders as Williams disease, Smith-Magenis disease, and velo-cardio-facial syndrome as well as previously undiagnosed genetic causes of mental retardation.[7] Characterization and DNA sequencing of genes allows the identification of defective genes *in vivo*, thereby permitting highly precise genetic counseling, prenatal testing, and identification of carrier states and diseases prior to symptom onset. One review in 2001 identified 146 human genes that have alleles or mutations conferring susceptibility for 168 neurogenetic diseases.[8] (Many new neurogenetic disorders, particularly in young children, have been identified since then.) Sequencing of the genome will permit cloning and pharmaceutical production of gene products as well as somatic and germ-line gene therapy.[9]

In addition to its therapeutic and preventive value, the coding of the human genome is highly relevant to neuroscience research. Studies of human tissue-specific gene expression suggest that as many as 80% of all human genes are expressed in the brain.[10] The HGP has provided a wealth of information for the basic neuroscientist, including data on new receptors, neural membrane proteins, neuron-specific transcription factors, and other neural components amenable to study through molecular genetics.[11]

Ethical issues in contemporary human molecular genetics center on the use and misuse of genetic information learned about individuals. Who should be tested and for which diseases? Should testing information remain confidential or should it be available to third parties? Can testing be mandated by prospective employers or insurers as a condition of employment or insurance? Should neurogenetic prenatal screening information be used as a basis for selective abortion? Should asymptomatic babies and children be tested? Should young persons at risk for adult-onset disorders such as Huntington's disease be tested in the presymptomatic phase? Do others have the right to perform predictive tests on minors who are at risk? To what extent should our society support experiments to correct gene defects with gene therapy? Should germ-line gene therapies be conducted that can affect all future generations?[12] I consider these questions in this chapter.[13]

To address the ethical, social, and legal aspects of sequencing the human genome, 3% to 5% of the total funding for the HGP was designated for the study of nonscientific issues. Using this funding, the United States Human Genome Project Ethical, Legal and Social Implications (ELSI) Research Program and numerous university-based groups worked to answer the ethical questions and to develop guidelines for the optimal use of molecular genetic information to benefit individuals and society.[14]

GENETIC TESTING, SCREENING, AND PREDICTIVE TESTING IN NEUROLOGY

A genetic test is "the analysis of human DNA, RNA, chromosomes, proteins, and certain metabolites in order to detect heritable disease-related genotypes, mutations, phenotypes, or karyotypes for clinical purposes."[15] Henry Paulson pointed out that genetic tests comprise three categories: (1) molecular genetic tests in which segments of DNA can be amplified by the polymerase chain reaction to measure gene mutations, such as the number of CAG trinucleotide repeats in Huntington's disease; (2) biochemical genetic tests in which the molecular product of a defective metabolic pathway can be assayed, such the measurement of elevations of phytanic acid in noninfantile Refsum disease resulting from the mutation in phytanoyl-CoA hydroxylase; and (3) cytogenetic testing of chromosomes such as those used formerly to diagnose fragile X syndrome, Prader-Willi syndrome, and Angelman syndrome,[16] (molecular testing using methylation-sensitive restriction enzymes is the best way currently to test for these imprinting disorders) and that are still used to diagnose Down syndrome, trisomy 13 and 18, Turner syndrome, and Klinefelter syndrome.[17]

Neurologists planning to order genetic tests should be knowledgeable about the mode of inheritance for each neurogenetic disease.[18] (1) Autosomal dominant disorders, such as Huntington's disease, are caused by a single mutation in one allele of the disease gene. Cases occur in succeeding generations, affect males and females equally, and show male-to-male transmission. (2) Autosomal recessive diseases (such as chorea-acanthocytosis) result from mutations in both alleles of the disease gene. Carriers are heterozygous and are unaffected or, in some cases, subtly affected. These disorders usually occur in only one generation. (3) X-linked disorders, such as the X-linked form of Charcot-Marie-Tooth disease (CMT), are caused by mutations on the X chromosome. Most disorders cause disease in males in multiple generations but females also may show signs of the disease.[19] (4) Mitochondrial diseases, such as mitochondrial encephalopathy, lactic acidosis, and stroke-like episodes (MELAS), are caused by mutations in mitochondrial DNA. Inheritance is purely maternal. Siblings are variably affected. (5) Genomic disorders, such as the majority of CMT type 1A, are caused by genetic defects spanning more than a single gene (continuous gene deletion syndromes).

Neurogenetic disorders are seen commonly in neurology practices. Thomas Bird advised clinicians to be alert to the following clues of an underlying neurogenetic disorder: a positive family history for neurologic disease; a similarity of symptoms and signs to a known neurogenetic syndrome; a chronic, progressive course; consanguinity; and the increased frequency of certain disorders within specific ethnic groups. Bird pointed out that some diagnostic syndromes suggest neurogenetic disease and can be considered as "reservoirs" of neurogenetic patients. These syndromes include cerebral palsy, mental retardation, epilepsy, movement disorders, ataxias, dementias, "neuroregressive syndromes" and atypical multiple sclerosis.[20]

The principal diseases of the nervous system under current molecular genetic scrutiny include Huntington's disease, Alzheimer's disease, neurofibromatosis, Duchenne and Becker X-linked muscular dystrophies, myotonic dystrophy, CMT disease, spinocerebellar degenerations, torsion dystonia, Lesch-Nyhan disease, Gaucher's disease, Kennedy's disease, retinitis pigmentosa, malignant hyperthermia, familial amyotrophic lateral sclerosis, tuberous sclerosis, Creutzfeldt-Jakob and other prion diseases, inborn metabolic diseases, mitochondrial encephalomyopathies, Kallman syndrome, Miller-Dieker syndrome, Rett syndrome, and skeletal muscle sodium-channel disease.[21] Published neurological gene maps illustrate and list the location on each chromosome of about 200 genes encoding neurologically relevant proteins, enzymes, and transmitters, including defective genes responsible for many neurogenetic disorders.[22]

Genetic tests are available for symptomatic diagnosis, presymptomatic diagnosis, carrier detection, and prenatal diagnosis of a number of diseases of the nervous system.[23] DNA tests for those disorders in which the gene has been identified have a very high rate of sensitivity and specificity, thus producing high rates of positive and negative predictive values, each approaching 1.0 in the case of Huntington's disease. They are lower in other conditions for which the genetic basis is only partially known due to genetic or locus heterogeneity or mutations in gene regions that are not sequenced, such as the promoter, enhancer, or introns. DNA tests for those disorders in which polymorphic genetic markers tightly linked to the gene have been identified possess a lower sensitivity and specificity, generally in the 0.9 to 0.95 range. With linkage tests, other affected and nonaffected family members must be tested first in order to identify the particular family haplotype. Non-DNA genetic tests have a lower sensitivity and specificity, generally in the 0.5 to 0.95 range. Newborn genetic screening is a growing field. It is likely that in the near future, screening for disorders in addition to those currently performed (phenylketonuria, cystic fibrosis, lysosomal storage disease) will be required.[24] Non-invasive prenatal genetic diagnosis using a maternal blood sample now can be performed for many disorders at no risk to the fetus but this new technique has not been generally accepted by physicians.[25]

As of March 2007, neurologists could order DNA testing or other genetic testing for the large number of neurological disorders listed in Table 17-1. Many non-neurological disorders

TABLE 17-1 Neurological Disorders with Genetic Tests

- Angelman Syndrome
- ARX
- CADASIL
- Canavan disease
- Charcot-Marie-Tooth [CMT 1B]
- Comparative Genomic Hybridization
- Cri-du-chat syndrome
- Deafness, Non-syndromic
  Connexin 26
  Connexin 30
  Deafness (A1555G)
- Dentatorubral-Pallidoluysian Atrophy [DRPLA]
- Duchenne/Becker muscular dystrophy [Diagnosis or Carrier]
- Familial dysautonomia
- Fragile X syndrome
- Friedreich ataxia
- Gaucher disease
- Huntington disease
- Kallman syndrome
- Machado-Joseph Disease (SCA Type III)
- Miller-Dieker syndrome
- Mitochondrial (DNA) Disorders
  All 37 mitochondrial genes
  Chronic Progressive External Ophthalmoplegia (CPEO)
  Kearns-Sayre Syndrome (KSS)
  Leigh syndrome (Mitochondrial)

Leber Hereditary Optic Neuropathy (LHON)
Mitochondrial Encephalomyopathy w/Lactic Acidosis & Stroke-like episodes (MELAS)
Myoclonic Epilepsy w/Ragged-Red Fibers (MERRF)
Neuropathy with Ataxia & Retinitis Pigmentosa (NARP)
- Myotonic muscular dystrophy
- Neurofibromatosis (NF-1)
- Niemann-Pick disease (Type A)
- Pendred syndrome
- Phenylketonuria
- Prader-Willi-Angelman
- Rett Syndrome
- Rett Syndrome-atypical (CDKL5)
- Smith-Lemli-Opitz syndrome
- Spinal muscular atrophy, (Types I, II, III) [Diagnosis or Carrier]
- Spinal and Bulbar Muscular Atrophy (Kennedy disease)
- Spinocerebellar ataxia
- Tay-Sachs disease
- Tuberous Sclerosis 1 or 2
- Von Hippel-Lindau syndrome
- Waardenburg Syndrome (Type 1 PAX3 and Type 2 (MITF only))
- Williams syndrome
- Wilson's disease
- X-linked mental retardation/autism (NLGN3/4)

From Boston University Center for Human Genetics http://www.bumc.bu.edu/Dept/Content.aspx?PageID=2230&DepartmentID=118 (Accessed March 20, 2007).

also can be tested for by DNA analysis in these laboratories. Tests for additional neurogenetic disorders not available commercially may be performed by arrangement in specialized university research laboratories. Many of these research neurogenetic tests likely will be available in commercial laboratories in the future. Direct-to-consumer online genetic testing recently has become available.[26] Patients now may bring genetic testing results to physicians to interpret. I agree with critics who find this type of testing to be unethical and harmful because its interpretation is ambiguous and it

is carried out in the absence of appropriate medical and genetic counseling services.[27]

Preimplantation genetic diagnosis (PGD) is an emerging disease-prevention technology in which embryos created by *in vitro* fertilization are tested for the genetic mutation of a disease in an at-risk family. Only embryos found to be free of the mutation are selected for implantation.[28] PGD has been used to prevent transmission of over 50 hereditary diseases including hereditary cancers,[29] single-gene neurological disorders such as Huntington's disease[30] and familial holoprosencephaly,[31] and multi-gene neurological disorders such as autosomal-dominant Alzheimer's disease.[32] PGD has been generally accepted by those who believe that abortion is acceptable but becomes controversial when used for sex selection.[33] The American Society of Reproductive Medicine Ethics Committee discourages using PGD for sex selection unless its intent is disease prevention, as in the case of preventing Duchenne muscular dystrophy in male offspring.[34] PGD also has been used to create HLA-compatible stem cell donors.[35]

PRESYMPTOMATIC TESTING: HUNTINGTON'S DISEASE

Several challenging ethical issues have been raised by the availability of neurogenetic presymptomatic (predictive) tests to diagnose a disease prior to the onset of symptoms or signs. To illustrate the complexities of these issues, I discuss the most common and carefully studied example in neurology, presymptomatic genetic testing for Huntington's disease (HD).[36] Similar ethical dilemmas arise in the use of presymptomatic testing for other adult-onset neurogenetic disorders such as hereditary ataxia and neuromuscular disorders[37] and hereditary epilepsies.[38] Presymptomatic testing in HD can serve as a model of early diagnostic testing protocols for other late-onset neurodegenerative diseases.[39]

HD is a fatal inherited disease of the central nervous system usually characterized by adult onset of the triad of progressive dementia, emotional disturbance, and involuntary choreiform movements. HD is transmitted as an autosomal dominant disorder with nearly complete penetrance but variable expressivity. All children of a parent with HD carry a 0.5 risk of inheriting the gene and developing the disease. Although varying somewhat from one family to another, overt symptoms of HD usually begin in patients between the ages of 35 and 42 years, and death occurs after a mean of 17 years. Although treatment can reduce the severity of chorea, no therapeutic intervention can reverse the dementia or the inexorably fatal course of the disease.[40] Patients dying of HD require end-of-life and palliative care according to accepted standards.[41]

HD has a prevalence of 0.0001 in white populations, but it affects all races. There are 25,000 to 30,000 HD patients in the United States. The genetic defect has been found to be a mutation on the short arm of chromosome 4 at band 16.3. In the coding region of the gene, there is an unstable, polymorphic trinucleotide CAG repeat, displaying at least 24 alleles, differing only in the number of repeat lengths. The HD gene contains from 37 to 86 repeat CAG lengths, many more than are present normally. In patients in whom the HD gene has more than 55 repeat lengths, the likelihood is 0.89 of paternal disease transmission. As a general rule, the greater the number of repeat lengths in the gene, the earlier the onset of HD symptoms.[42] The well-recognized phenomenon of anticipation, in which succeeding generations show earlier symptom onset than preceding generations, is associated with a greater number of CAG repeats in subsequent generations.[43]

Patients at risk for developing HD are only too familiar with its clinical features, having previously watched affected family members who suffered progressive dementia, chorea, and inanition, with eventual death in an institution. Both at-risk children of affected patients and other family members have clamored for a test to determine which at-risk patients were destined later to develop the disease. Young people at risk must make important decisions about marriage, childbearing, education, and employment before they develop the signs of HD. These decisions may be made differently depending on whether patients will or will not later develop HD.[44] The desire to answer this essential question led to the development of presymptomatic tests for HD.

Some neurologists argued that it was morally wrong to develop and apply predictive tests for HD because of the severe psychological burden a patient must endure, knowing that she will develop an untreatable, fatal disease later in life. For example, C.D. Marsden, a neurologist with extensive experience in managing patients with HD, stated, "It is kinder to ask those at risk of the illness, but lucky enough not to have inherited it, to forego such a test and live with their uncertainty in order to provide the other 50% who carry the lethal gene with some hope during their remaining years."[45]

Nevertheless, numerous surveys of at-risk patients have disclosed that a consistent 75% to 85% of those surveyed want to have predictive tests developed and would use them if they were safe and accurate.[46] Even 50% of the surveyed patients indicated that they would use the ethically and scientifically dubious levodopa provocative test (discussed later) if it were available.[47]

The major reason at-risk patients cite for undergoing testing is to avail themselves of genetic counseling and family planning. In one survey, investigators found that approximately 60% of the at-risk subjects indicated that they would plan fewer or no children if they tested positive for the HD gene. Of the already symptomatic patients, 82% indicated that they would have had fewer or no children had they known for certain that they would develop HD.[48] In another survey of at-risk subjects, investigators found that the percentage who planned to bear children would have decreased from 80% to 42% if the patients had tested positive.[49] These data are especially noteworthy given the known high fecundity rate of HD patients.[50]

Predictive tests should be developed and used according to the highest ethical standards. Thomas outlined the minimal ethical standards that would make a predictive test acceptable for at-risk HD patients or for patients with similar conditions. It should: (1) pose little or no risk to the patient; (2) have no false positives or false negatives, that is, both the positive and negative predictive values should approach 1.0; (3) have no ambiguous results; and (4) have inscrutable results.[51]

Harold Klawans and colleagues performed predictive tests on asymptomatic patients at risk for HD after they observed that oral doses of levodopa transiently exacerbated chorea in symptomatic HD patients. They reasoned that those asymptomatic children of HD parents who are destined to develop HD would be more likely to develop transient chorea following a dose of levodopa than those children without the gene. After administering a single oral dose of levodopa to a group of at-risk patients, Klawans and colleagues observed transient chorea in 36%.[52] When patients in the test

group were followed up, eight years later, the researchers found that 50% of those who earlier tested positive had developed overt HD, as had 5% of those who tested negative.[53] Similar false-negative results have been reported from other groups who have administered this test.[54]

Several ethicists and neurologists attacked the ethical basis of the levodopa provocative test. Stanley Fahn, a neurologist with a sizable experience in treating patients with HD, pointed out its shortcomings. First, patients immediately are aware of the test results and may not be prepared psychologically to handle that information. Indeed, one of Barbeau's patients committed suicide shortly after learning that test results were positive.[55] Second, the test has not been validated, making its positive and negative predictive values unknown. Third, the test is invasive and carries the theoretical risk of precipitating the onset of symptomatic HD sooner than it would have occurred otherwise because of a possible levodopa-induced reduction in striatal neurotransmitters.[56] Klawans's colleagues did not test any additional patients with levodopa but they continue to follow patients tested earlier. Of course, this test has been replaced completely by the more sensitive and specific DNA test described below.

Several other non-DNA presymptomatic tests have been used to attempt to predict which at-risk patients will develop HD.[57] These include electroencephalography, computed tomography, positron emission tomography, measurements of caudate nucleus metabolism, evoked potentials, eye movement and fine motor coordination, neuropsychological function, motor reaction times, cerebrospinal fluid concentrations of GABA, platelet monoamine oxidase levels, and serum IgG levels.[58] Most recently and usefully, tensor-based magnetic resonance morphometry has shown loss of striatal volume in at-risk patients[59] and abnormalities of saccadic eye movements have been recorded in pre-symptomatic patients.[60] Systematic evaluation of presymptomatic patients at risk for HD is underway through the Prospective Huntington At Risk Observational Study (PHAROS).[61] Irrespective of the important scientific information learned from these studies, none of the non-DNA predictive tests can identify the HD gene with a sufficiently high

(>0.95) sensitivity and specificity to achieve ethical acceptability as a predictive test.

The first DNA test, reported in 1983 by James Gusella and colleagues, involved the identification of a polymorphic marker located 5 to 10 centimorgans from the HD gene.[62] Subsequently, investigators in Gusella's group and in other groups found additional genetic markers linked even more tightly to the gene.[63] Finally, in 1993, Gusella and his collaborators culminated their decade-long effort by identifying the HD gene itself.[64]

Testing for the HD gene has the advantages of accuracy and privacy over using a linkage test. First, although linkage tests were believed to have positive and negative predictive values in the 0.95 range—much higher than other putative predictive tests—predictive values of the gene test approach 1.0. Elimination of false-positive and false-negative determinations removes the most serious harm to patients, the harm produced by incorrect prediction. Second, for linkage tests, blood specimens must be obtained from family members with HD and from family members without the disease. Involving other people in the process of testing an at-risk patient raises a separate group of ethical and practical problems.[65] Use of the DNA gene test eliminates this problem because family members need not be tested. Thus, the gene test appears to satisfy Thomas's criteria for an ideal predictive test.

The ethical motive for developing presymptomatic tests is to further the autonomy and self-determination of at-risk patients by providing them with the opportunity to learn if they are destined to suffer HD. These patients usually regard such information as necessary to make important life decisions about marriage, childbearing, and careers. Autonomy is respected when the decision to be tested is totally voluntary. Patients should not be coerced into being tested or tested without their knowledge.[66] Maintaining complete confidentiality of test results is essential. Children under 18 years of age should not be tested unless they are already symptomatic.[67]

A utilitarian ethical analysis balances the benefits and burdens resulting when an at-risk person learns she is destined to develop HD.[68] The benefit of knowing that the test is positive is the facilitation of rational planning of future life decisions. Genetic testing eliminates the burdens that result from an inaccurate test, but may increase the burden of a positive test, because there is virtually no possibility that it is wrong. Patients who learn that they will develop HD might be expected to become depressed from the loss of hope that they can be spared from the disease. Indeed, the rate of suicide in patients with early HD is high.[69] It is essential that all predictive testing be conducted with pre-test and post-test genetic and psychological counseling.[70] It is desirable for the patient to be accompanied by a support person (a spouse or a close friend but not an at-risk relative) throughout the testing process.[71]

A negative test offers the patient immediate relief. She does not have to worry about developing HD or transmitting it to her children. Ironically, however, there is also a psychological burden accompanying a negative test result. Although removing a sword of Damocles from above the head of the at-risk patient might be expected to yield unmitigated joy, studies have shown that some patients suffer "survivor guilt." Like soldiers whose lives were spared in a fierce battle, they feel guilty because they have been saved when their relatives are doomed to die.[72] Thus, ongoing psychological counseling is helpful even for at-risk patients who test negative.

After learning the benefits and risks, some at-risk patients decide not to be tested. Perhaps the most remarkable example of an informed decision not to be tested by a patient at risk for HD is that of Nancy Wexler, Ph.D., Higgins Professor of Neuropsychology in the Departments of Neurology and Psychiatry at Columbia University, President of the Hereditary Disease Foundation (founded by her father, Dr. Milton Wexler), and co-discoverer of the gene for HD. Dr. Wexler's brief explanation echoed the lesson of Sophocles's Oedipus Rex, "If the gods want to drive you mad, first they tell you your future."[73]

In the Canadian Collaborative Study of Predictive Testing for Huntington's Disease, the psychological impact of test results on at-risk patients was studied in a cohort of subjects. Not surprisingly, the investigators found the psychological distress scores lower in those who tested negative as opposed to those who tested positive. Interestingly, the investigators also found that the psychological distress scores were lowered in those at-risk patients who tested positive as compared with those who remained untested. It appears that just knowing for certain (even when the result is positive) relieves much of the anxiety of at-risk patients and diminishes their psychological suffering.[74] Thus, at-risk patients demand presymptomatic testing primarily to relieve the anxiety of not knowing the future. The psychological benefits to the patient and partner persist at three-year followup.[75]

Being diagnosed with HD is a source of shame for many patients and their families. Experienced clinicians can recount poignant instances in which patients with overt signs and positive family histories of HD denied their diagnosis or insisted they had Parkinson's disease or some other condition.[76] This shame causes members of HD families to have varying and conflicting opinions about being tested. Family members should not coerce each other into having tests performed. Nor do family members have a right to know the test results of other members.

Prenatal screening of fetuses for the HD gene is possible now. Some parents request selective abortion if the fetus is affected. Prenatal screening was practiced with the genetic linkage test as well. "Exclusion testing" permits a fetus to be tested without necessarily disclosing the genetic status of the parent.[77] Screening for selective abortion in HD carries ethical implications that are somewhat different from those surrounding infant screening for Tay-Sachs or other infancy-onset or childhood-onset diseases. In HD, patients can be expected to live in a relatively normal state for several decades before symptoms occur. Some physicians refuse to perform requested prenatal HD testing because they argue it raises the same consent objections as in testing a minor.[78]

Prospective parents must make the difficult decision whether such lives should be lived or aborted. Some HD centers expect selective abortion if the gene is discovered prenatally because they believe that the only way to cure HD is to stop gene transmission. One survey, however, disclosed that half the at-risk parents would not choose elective abortion if the fetus

tested positive.[79] Parental ambivalence is common in such circumstances, as exemplified by the statement of Marjorie Guthrie, the widow of the renowned American folksong-writer and singer and HD sufferer, Woody Guthrie, who worked for many years to raise public consciousness about HD and to promote HD prevention: "Does anyone really think it would have been better for Woody not to have come into the world, in spite of everything?"[80]

Several centers have reported their experience over the first few years using the genetic linkage test. The Huntington's Disease Center Without Walls in Boston reported considerable demand for its testing service. When the program was announced in the state's HD society newsletter, the center received over 250 telephone inquiries in the first year, and 47 at-risk patients enrolled in the program. The center found that even though patients were aware of their 50% chance of testing positive, many of those who did test positive were "surprised" or "shocked" by the news. This finding demonstrates the extent of denial mechanisms active in patients at risk for HD. Those who tested negative described their feeling of tremendous relief, an emotion that they continued to report at three-month and nine-month follow-up visits. Over half of those tested expressed relief from anxiety because their genetic status no longer was unknown.[81]

A similar program conducted at Johns Hopkins Hospital involved the experience of 55 at-risk patients. The highly structured protocol of the program mandated that patients have a relatively high educational level, continuous pre-test and post-test counseling, and careful follow-up. In this setting, the researchers found no significant change in psychiatric morbidity between those who tested positive and those who tested negative. Because both the Boston and Johns Hopkins studies required careful patient selection, the generalizability of their findings to unselected patient groups remains unclear.[82]

The HD research group at the University of Wales reported several problems in the course of carrying out its program in nearly 300 at-risk patients who applied to participate. Twenty-eight minors were referred to the program, three adults were referred without their permission, seven adoption agencies requested infant testing, and one insurance company wanted patients tested despite the fact that the program was restricted to adults who consented voluntarily. Ten patients lacked a clear family history of HD and eleven already showed physical signs of HD. Blood specimens were damaged in 20 cases and labeled incorrectly in six.[83]

The Canadian Collaborative Study of Predictive Testing for Huntington's Disease reported a series of ethical and legal problems in the course of conducting its testing program over the first two years. They described confidentiality problems in instances in which siblings arrived together for testing. Although siblings did not wish to share the results of their tests, maintaining their confidentiality became logistically difficult. Several problems resulted when blood specimens had to be obtained from other family members for the linkage test. These problems became moot after the specific DNA gene test was developed. There were difficulties using fetal genetic data to terminate a pregnancy without the mother wishing to know how those data affected her own risk of getting the disease. An employer asked the Canadian Collaborative Study to test an employee without his knowledge. Testing was requested by one at-risk monozygotic twin, but the other twin, whose genetic status was identical, did not wish to know. In this case, to respect the rights of one twin was to deny the rights of the other.[84] In one instance, a married couple requested prenatal exclusion testing. The at-risk prospective father was determined by DNA testing not to have been sired by his HD father; thus, both he and the fetus had no risk of the disease. Should he be told this "good" news despite the fact that he specifically wished not to know his own HD status?[85] Moreover, should he be told the disturbing paternity information that now is known but which he did not seek? Such issues of learning about non-paternity indirectly during DNA testing raise a number of vexing ethical and legal questions, some of which could be mitigated by a more stringent consent process prior to testing that anticipated these issues and provided a level of disclosure preferred by the patient.[86] Discussing the possibility of identifying nonpaternity and stipulating how it will be handled should always be part of pre-test genetic counseling.

Investigators from the University of Leuven recently reported their experience with reproductive decision making by asymptomatic patients found to carry the HD gene. Family planning was an important motive for genetic testing. They found that 58% of asymptomatic carriers chose to have children using prenatal diagnostic techniques or preimplantation genetic diagnosis, 35% decided to have no more children after testing positive, and 7% remained undecided or had no children for other reasons.[87]

In summary, presymptomatic testing for HD is ethically acceptable if the following conditions are met. (1) The test must be safe and have positive and negative predictive values approaching 1. (2) The test should be performed only on adults with their full voluntary informed consent. (3) The test should not be performed at the request or as the result of coercion by third parties. (4) Safeguards should be in place to assure complete patient confidentiality and privacy. (5) Testing should be accompanied by a comprehensive program of pre-test and post-test counseling for patients and their families.[88] The DNA test for the HD gene carried out within an organized genetic counseling program satisfies these conditions.

CARRIER DETECTION AND PRENATAL SCREENING: TAY-SACHS DISEASE

Tay-Sachs disease (TSD) is the quintessential neurogenetic disease for which organized programs of carrier detection and prenatal screening have proved successful in decreasing its incidence. TSD is transmitted as an autosomal recessive trait; thus, heterozygotes are unaffected "carriers" and only "homozygotes"[89] develop the disease. Approximately one-fourth of the infants with two heterozygous parents will inherit one copy of the TSD gene from each parent and develop the disease. One-half of the infants with either one or two heterozygote parents will be carriers.[90]

Ethnicity influences the frequency of the TSD gene. The highest gene frequencies are present in Jews of north-central and eastern European ancestry—the so-called Ashkenazi Jews—in whom the pathologic mutation frequency is 0.032 or approximately 1 in 31. There are several different mutations that show a founder effect. In non-Jewish persons, the pathologic mutation frequency is 0.0036 or approximately 1 in 277.[91] Non-Jewish French Canadians from southeastern Quebec also have an increased TSD gene frequency.[92]

There are three clinical phenotypes of TSD, which depend on the type of gene mutation. In the common (infantile) type, infants at one year of age lose the developmental abilities they have gained since birth. Blindness, dementia, and seizures ensue and death occurs by age three or four years. In the juvenile form, symptoms appear in early childhood and the children die in their mid-teens. The rare adult form is fatal, as well, and often misdiagnosed. Affected patients develop progressive seizures, dementia, and cerebellar ataxia.[93]

TSD is characterized pathologically by neuronal "ballooning" from the massive intralysosomal accumulation of the glycolipid G_{M2} ganglioside, caused by a profound deficiency of the lysosomal hydrolase enzyme β-hexosaminidase A (Hex A). The progressive accumulation of G_{M2} causes neurons to malfunction and die.[94]

Heterozygote TSD screening tests that measure serum or leukocyte Hex A levels are easy to perform, inexpensive, and highly reliable. Prenatal TSD screening requires chorionic villus sampling or amniocentesis. Molecular DNA techniques also have been employed in specialized laboratories to look for one of the nine alpha-chain mutations responsible for infantile TSD. Three of these gene mutations are responsible for over 95% of the Jewish cases.[95] These genetic tests should be performed to confirm positive enzyme tests in non-Jewish carriers and in couples when they are found to be carriers.[96]

Heterozygote screening programs in the Jewish communities of the United States and other countries have been available since 1970 under the auspices of the International Tay-Sachs Disease Testing, Quality Control, and Data Collection Center established by the National Tay-Sachs Disease and Allied Disorders Association. Between 1971 and 2000, over 1.4 million young adults were tested voluntarily throughout the world. Approximately three-fourths of these volunteers resided in the United States. Over 50,000 TSD carriers were detected, including over 1,400 at-risk couples who were found to be TSD carriers.[97]

From the time the first prenatal tests for TSD were available in 1969 through 2000, 3,200 high-risk pregnancies were monitored with amniocentesis or chorionic villus sampling. High-risk pregnancies are those in which both parents are heterozygotes. Of these pregnancies, over 600 fetuses (representing approximately 90% of fetuses testing positive for TSD) were electively aborted. Abortion was not permitted for religious reasons by some ultra-Orthodox Jewish families. These measures have reduced the disease incidence within the Jewish population by more than 90%.[98]

The most striking aspect of the voluntary screening program is its success in decreasing the number of babies born with TSD. In the pre-1970 era, before the beginning of the screening program, approximately 60 new cases of infantile TSD were reported each year in the United States. Cases of Ashkenazi Jewish ethnicity accounted for about 85% of the total TSD births. Currently, there are only about three to five Jewish TSD cases occurring annually in the United States, and the Jewish cases now account for only about 30% of the total cases.[99]

As a result of intermarriage and loss of ethnic identification resulting from assimilation, the question of who is of Ashkenazi Jewish ethnicity may not be as clear as it once was. The American College of Obstetricians and Gynecologists therefore recommends that TSD screening be performed on any couple when one member is identified as Jewish.[100]

A few ethical issues arise in TSD screening programs. Given the psychological burden placed on the carrier, at what age should carrier detection be tested? Many of the patients in the international screening program appear for testing when the partner becomes pregnant. Ideally, testing should be performed sooner. One program in Montreal tests high school students.[101]

When should a known carrier notify a future mate of his or her carrier status? Should engagements be broken if both members of a couple test positive? The Dor Yeshorim Tay-Sachs

Screening Program in Brooklyn, New York, offers anonymous TSD testing for Orthodox Jewish young people and records the results by number. Prospective couples who call the program and provide their code numbers can learn if there is a genetic reason why they should not be wed; that is, if both are TSD heterozygotes. Since the inception of the couples screening program, no TSD babies have been born in this Brooklyn Jewish community.[102]

TSD carrier and prenatal screening has had a high degree of success because it is an entirely voluntary option supported by the at-risk patient community. Screening is incorporated into an educational program with comprehensive genetic counseling. It offers and delivers the hope of preventing a fatal and untreatable disease. Another study reported success in triple disease screening for TSD, type 1 Gaucher disease, and cystic fibrosis. Of the 2,824 Ashkenazi Jewish patients requesting screening for TSD, once the patients were educated about genetic screening, 97% also consented to screening for cystic fibrosis and 95% for type 1 Gaucher disease.[103]

CARRIER DETECTION AND DIAGNOSIS: DUCHENNE MUSCULAR DYSTROPHY

Duchenne muscular dystrophy (DMD) and Becker muscular dystrophy (BMD) are allelic, X-linked recessive myopathies that result from hereditary and spontaneous mutations in the human dystrophin gene. In DMD, which occurs in 1 in 3,500 male births, the defective gene fails to code properly for the muscle protein dystrophin and, as a result, skeletal and cardiac muscles of affected patients contain little or no dystrophin. In BMD, some dystrophin is present but is only partially functional.[104] The absence or decrease of dystrophin in the muscles produces the clinical features of the disease. In the case of DMD, progressive proximal and then distal muscle weakness begins in early childhood and culminates in death in early adulthood from respiratory muscle paralysis, aspiration, cardiac failure, or inanition. Glucocorticoid therapy with prednisone or deflazacort (where available) can improve muscle strength and function but has risks in long-term treatment.[105] In BMD, a less severe chain of events occurs that begins and ends later in life and lasts longer.[106]

The molecular genetics of DMD and BMD is complex. The dystrophin gene is located on the short arm of the X chromosome at Xp21.[107] Approximately 55% of both DMD and BMD case result from partial deletion mutations at this site, 5% of the cases result from gene duplications, and the remaining 40% result from point mutations or no detectable mutations.[108]

Maternal screening programs can detect elevations in serum creatine kinase (CK) levels in some carriers or patients in the early stages of disease. However, only about 70% of the female carriers have serum CK levels above the normal range. Southern analysis or polymerase chain reaction (PCR) techniques can produce a more definitive genetic diagnosis and identify carriers better by detecting deletion mutations or structural inversions of the dystrophin gene. The 40% of DMD cases without a detectable mutation remain a problem for genetic testing and counseling, however. Immunocytochemical analysis of dystrophin in amniocytes, chorionic villus cells, and fibroblasts can assist the prenatal and postnatal diagnosis of DMD in cases in which conventional genetic techniques have failed.[109] PCR techniques also have been applied to identify DMD carriers in families with identified point mutations, but cannot be used to screen for point mutations.[110] Particular patterns of X-chromosome inactivation have been identified in the myonuclei of female carriers of DMD.[111] DMD itself can be diagnosed prenatally using fetal erythrocytes.[112]

Programs of genetic counseling for DMD are more complicated than those for other genetic diseases with a lower incidence of spontaneous mutations. When an isolated patient with DMD does not have a detectable gene mutation or elevated serum CK, the mother has only about a 30% risk of being a carrier.[113] The mother of a DMD patient should be investigated to see if she is a carrier of the DMD gene, but it may be impossible to determine a female carrier status conclusively if she has neither point mutations nor elevated serum CK levels. If she is found to be a carrier, she can enter a genetic counseling program.

The success of carrier detection is further complicated by the presence of germ line mosaicism, in which a percentage of the mother's oocytes are affected by the dystrophin mutation but her somatic cells are not. Prenatal diagnosis of DMD for the purpose of selective abortion is also possible with Southern and PCR techniques that detect linkage or mutation.

USE AND MISUSE OF GENETIC INFORMATION

There is an evolving consensus about the ethical principles for genetic testing.[114] Proper use of genetic information obtained for screening, prenatal testing, carrier identification, or predictive testing enhances patients' opportunities to learn important facts about their personal health and childbearing risks, thereby enabling them to make rational decisions about their lives based on accurate information. Harms also may accrue from genetic testing. Patients may be given misinformation by physicians who do not understand the meaning of the test result. Improper counseling may produce unnecessary psychological suffering. Genetic counselors should be "nondirective," providing adequate information for patients and families to make decisions but not deciding for them.[115] Some clinical geneticists believe that the best model for genetic counseling is shared decision making (see chapter 2) in which physicians help families to identify and achieve their health goals. One common pitfall is overestimation of the predictive value of a test.[116] An inappropriate breach of confidentiality (sharing the information with third parties) may make patients ineligible for health or life insurance, or lead to discrimination in the workplace.[117] Physicians who consider ordering genetic testing should first understand the scientific basis and medical meaning of the test and then conduct a thoughtful assessment of the risks and benefits to the patient in each case.[118]

The patient's valid consent should be secured before testing for genetic information. Consent should be made by a competent person, obtained without coercion, and based on adequate and correct information conveyed by the physician.[119] In many instances, the information necessary for the consent is voluminous and the knowledge the patient acquires from the testing is emotionally charged. In these situations, testing ideally should be conducted through an organized educational program in which genetic and psychological counseling are available throughout the testing process.

With the increased knowledge of molecular genetics resulting from the HGP, in the future it is likely that physicians will be able to order multiple simultaneous genetic tests, some of which may be predictive of future diseases or indicate a heightened risk of future diseases; others may detect carrier states; and still others may diagnose current conditions. A one-time generic consent for such "multiplex" testing raises serious questions concerning the adequacy of the consent process. How can patients be expected to fully understand the implications of multiple tests looking for different genes during a single generic consent process? Physicians need to take the lead in developing consent standards for multiplex testing to assure that patients are adequately educated and protected from harm.[120] In that spirit, the American Medical Association Council on Ethical and Judicial Affairs published guidelines for physicians to help fully inform and protect patients undergoing multiplex genetic testing.[121]

Physicians ordering genetic tests should understand the predictive power of the test and how positive and negative results affect the probabilities that a patient, family member, or potential child has or will develop a particular disease. In neurological practice, this information includes the predictive power of a particular genotype, distinguishing among genotypes that predict diseases with certainty (such as trinucleotide repeat DNA testing in HD) and those that indicate only a heightened probability of diseases, such as tests for the apolipoprotein E $\varepsilon 4$ (*APOE $\varepsilon 4$*) allele in Alzheimer's disease.[122] Unfortunately, several studies have shown that many practicing neurologists and other physicians who order these tests fail to understand the essential medical facts about their predictive value.[123]

For example, the availability of genetic tests for the *APOE $\varepsilon 4$* allele in Alzheimer's disease has been publicized widely and many patients have requested testing. Some physicians have complied with the request with neither a clear understanding of the medical and scientific issues involved nor a comprehension of the meaning of a test result. Three independent ethical-genetic analyses of *APOE ε4* testing for the prediction of Alzheimer's disease all concluded that, aside from the research context, DNA predictive testing is unwarranted in clinical practice, except in the rare instance of the patient from a family with documented early-onset Alzheimer's disease of autosomal dominant inheritance.[124]

Workplace and Insurance Issues

Protecting patient confidentiality and privacy is an essential goal that may be difficult to maintain as institutions and agencies demand more personal genetic data in the future.[125] Physicians should not disclose genetic data to third parties without explicit authorization by patients or their lawful surrogates. Appropriate disclosure of a patient's genetic information to third parties can present a delicate balance between an individual's privacy rights and an institution's or family member's need to know personal medical data. The principal third parties that can contact physicians for genetic information on patients are insurance companies, employers, and family members.[126]

A survey involving 1,122 physicians, 140 medical geneticists, and 137 genetic counselors revealed how they balanced patient confidentiality with their duty to report. Each respondent was presented the following question. If a 35-year-old man at risk for HD tested positive on a genetic test, would you disclose this result to his wife and children (at age of majority), his employer, or his health insurance company without his permission? It was not stated whether the third parties were seeking this information or whether the man had refused to release it. Approximately 20% of the physicians, 11% of the medical geneticists, and 4% of the genetic counselors approved of giving the spouse this information; whereas 29% of the physicians, 19% of the medical geneticists, and 7% of the genetic counselors approved of giving the children this information. Only 0.5%

of the physicians, 0.7% of the medical geneticists, and none of the genetic counselors approved of giving the information to employers, whereas 2.9% of the physicians and none of the medical geneticists or genetic counselors approved of giving the information to health insurance companies.[127]

The most celebrated legal case in which an employer performed a genetic test on employees in a discriminatory fashion involved the Burlington Northern Santa Fe (BNSF) Railroad. Acting on advice from the company physician, BNSF obtained blood from employees who had sought disability for job-related carpal tunnel syndrome and performed DNA testing to detect hereditary liability for pressure palsies. The presumption was that if any employees tested positive, the company could claim that their hereditary condition was responsible for their carpal tunnel syndrome and not employment at BNSF. When it became aware of the testing, the federal Equal Employment Opportunity Commission stopped it and BNSF privately settled monetary claims with affected employees.[128]

In a statement on employer use of genetic testing, the American Medical Association Council on Ethical and Judicial Affairs concluded that it is inappropriate to exclude workers with genetic risks from the workplace simply because of those risks. Because genetic tests do not accurately predict the capacity of workers to perform their jobs properly, the use of such tests to exclude workers counts as unfair discrimination. Possible future unemployability is not in itself an adequate reason to exclude workers with positive genetic tests. The only genetic tests permitted in the workplace are for the rare genetic susceptibility to occupational illnesses. Even for this group, the following conditions must be met: (1) the disease must progress so rapidly and produce such serious and irreversible illness that monitoring would be inadequate to prevent it; (2) genetic testing must be highly accurate; (3) empirical data must strongly associate the genetic abnormality with an employee's increased susceptibility to occupational illness; (4) the cost of protecting the employee from genetic susceptibility to occupational illness must be disproportionately high; and (5) genetic testing must not be undertaken without the informed consent of the employee.[129]

The health insurance industry's appropriate use of genetic test results raises important questions that require examining the concepts of insurance and justice. The concept of insurance is to average the risk of each individual over that of a large group, thereby permitting each subscriber to pay a fixed premium determined actuarily by the average risk of members of the group. Within the large group will be a few members who will require disproportionately large amounts of services and many others who will require relatively few services. Each person pays an equal premium, thus those who need fewer services subsidize those who need many.

Of course, not all members of a large group enter the insurance agreement with the same prospective risk of needing services. Actuarial analysis can identify those members likely to be at greater risk for needing services. One concept of actuarial fairness holds that subscribers with the same degree of risk should pay equal premiums and those with higher risk should pay higher premiums. Although this concept strikes an intuitive chord of fairness, if it were taken to its logical conclusion, the entire concept of insurance—to average risks among large groups of individuals—would disappear because each person would pay only for her personal level of risk.[130]

On the other hand, if the high risks of a few were averaged over a larger group, many subscribers would have to pay a premium larger than their "fair share." The issue can be reduced to one of fairness and public interest. In the United States today, large numbers of high-risk applicants are receiving higher premium ratings or are uninsurable. This unfortunate situation is neither fair nor in the public interest. In contemporary America, a strong argument can be made that the concept of insurance has been subverted because the insurance industry has traveled too far down the continuum of actuarial fairness.[131]

Genetic tests can be considered in this context. If prenatal screening, genetic testing, or predictive testing disclosed the near certainty that a patient would develop a genetic disorder during her life, it is highly likely that such a person would not be able to obtain health-care insurance in our present environment. Some insurance companies, where permitted by law, consider genetic predispositions to be "pre-existing conditions" that are uninsurable.[132] Health-care uninsurability reduces individuals' access to health care. I believe that the public interest is best served if our society provides its citizens with the opportunity to purchase health insurance, so that all can have adequate access to health care. Such a rule will require that some patients "pay more than their share" to provide others who are less fortunate with the opportunity to purchase health insurance. Unless the insurance industry reverses course along the continuum of actuarial fairness in the direction of its original intent, the industry is no longer optimally serving the public interest. Under these circumstances, laws providing public tax support for the insurance industry may need to be re-examined.[133]

In its report, the Task Force on Genetic Information and Insurance of the United States Human Genome Project Working Group on Ethical, Legal, and Social Issues recommended that information about past, present, or future health status, including genetic information, should not be used to deny health-care coverage or access to anyone. Further, the cost to subscribers of health-care coverage for basic health services should not be affected by information about their past, present, or future health status, including genetic information. Until universal access to health care is assured, insurers should consider a moratorium on the use of genetic tests in underwriting.[134]

Legal Issues

American law considers genetic information to require a higher degree of confidentiality protection than other medical information because the linkage between a person's genes and disease propensity provides an opportunity for unjustified and illegal discrimination. Personal genetic information is thus classified as "exceptional" medical data requiring additional legal protections.[135] Some ethics scholars have argued that public laws have an additional indispensable role in the development of practice guidelines and the oversight of genetic testing.[136]

In the United States, over the past two decades, state and federal legislatures have introduced and enacted legislation protecting personal genetic information. As of May 2007, 35 states have enacted laws prohibiting genetic discrimination in employment and 47 states have enacted laws prohibiting genetic discrimination in health insurance.[137] The federal Health Insurance Portability and Accountability Act of 1996 (HIPAA) prohibits group health insurers from applying the "pre-existing condition" exclusion to genetic test results in the absence of symptoms or signs of disease.[138] The Americans with Disabilities Act of 1990 probably further protects the confidentiality and equal opportunity of patients who are carriers of genetic disease or who are destined to develop genetic disease, but this putative right has not been tested in court.[139] Legal scholars have drafted a model genetic privacy act to protect patients in clinical and research contexts but it has not been generally accepted.[140] The law has limits, however, on its power to protect personal genetic information fully.[141]

Enacting federal legislation to protect genetic information has faced greater difficulty. The United States Senate passed the Genetic Information Nondiscrimination Act of 2005 (S. 306) by a vote of 98 to 0. President Bush indicated he would sign the legislation but a compromise bill could not be passed in the House of Representatives. In fact, a similar bill had been introduced in every Congress since 1995 without a final Act being passed.[142] A current House bill (H.R. 493) entitled "To prohibit discrimination on the basis of genetic information with respect to health insurance and employment" was passed in April 2007 with only three representatives voting against it.

International policy-making groups also have drafted regulations. In 2003, the United Nations Educational, Scientific, and Cultural Organization (UNESCO) published the International Declaration on Human Genetic Data. The Declaration requires a high level of confidentiality and privacy of genetic material and data. Among other provisions, it states, "any collection, processing, use, and storage of human genetic data human proteomic data and biological samples shall be consistent with international law and human rights . . . [and that] clear, balanced, adequate, and appropriate information shall be provided to the person whose prior, free, and informed and express consent is sought." The Declaration formulated a list of principles outlining the protection of personal genetic data to maintain confidentiality, privacy, and freedom from discrimination.[143]

A fascinating new medicolegal issue has emerged as a consequence of the impact of a person's genetic test results on the health of family members. A patient's genetic susceptibility to cancers, neurological disorders, other diseases, or genetic polymorphisms may imply an increased risk of disease in the patient's relatives. The debatable question is whether a physician's knowledge of a patient's genetic test results imparts an ethical duty to notify at-risk family members: a "duty to warn." If such an obligation exists, it would pit protecting patient confidentiality against the duty to protect third parties known to be at risk of harm.[144] Several lawsuits against physicians from family members of tested patients have alleged physicians' negligence as a result of their failure to warn at-risk family members once the patient tested positive.

Several medicolegal scholars concluded that health-care professionals have a responsibility to encourage but not to coerce patients to share their genetic data with at-risk family members.[145] The American Medical Association Council on Ethical and Judicial Affairs advised: "At the time patients are considering undergoing genetic testing, physicians should discuss with them whether to invite relatives to participate in the testing process. Physicians also should identify circumstances under which they would expect patients to notify biological relatives of the availability of information related to risk of the disease. During pre-test counseling, some clinical geneticists issue a "genetic Miranda warning" that if the patient does not notify family members of their risk, they will. Physicians should make themselves available to assist patients in communicating with relatives to discuss opportunities for counseling and testing, as appropriate."[146] Some legal scholars have opined that physicians who warn family members do not violate the federal privacy regulations under HIPAA.[147] Other scholars have emphasized that it is the responsibility of patients with genetic diseases to share their genetic test results with at-risk family members because of "relational responsibilities" to them.[148]

Genetic Testing in Children

A consensus has been reached on the ethical acceptability of genetic testing in children. The American Society of Human Genetics and the American College of Medical Genetics jointly impaneled a task force to draft model guidelines for genetic testing of children and adolescents. Potential medical benefits they identified for youngsters include early therapeutic or preventive intervention, increased surveillance, improved diagnosis, clearer prognosis, and better opportunity to avoid or prepare for the birth of a child with a genetic disease. Potential psychosocial benefits included reduction of anxiety and uncertainty, increased opportunity for psychological adjustment and making life plans about important decisions such as education, insurance, employment, and marriage, and alerting other family members to genetic risk. Potential risks they identified included increased anxiety and guilt, distortion of self-image because of knowledge of disease, altered expectations of the child or others for education, employment, or personal relationships, and discrimination in employment or obtaining insurance. They concluded that physicians ordering genetic tests for children should carefully weigh the benefits against the risks in individual cases.[149]

Dorothy Wertz and colleagues balanced the rights of the minor, the rights of the parents, and the benefits and harms of testing in a series of guidelines for presymptomatic testing of children. Tests are acceptable if they detect conditions for which treatment or preventive measures are available or if the tests may be useful to the minor in making reproductive decisions now or in the near future. Tests requested by parents that have neither characteristic should be scrutinized by the physician to decide if they are in the best interest of the child. Testing ordered solely for the benefit of another family member should receive similar scrutiny to test if the overall benefits exceed

the harms.[150] Other scholars studying this problem have reached similar conclusions.[151]

A study of policies in laboratories performing genetic testing of children revealed that 92% requested the patient's age, 46% had policies for presymptomatic testing of late-onset disorders, 33% had policies for testing of carrier status of recessive disorders, and 33% had policies for tests offering no medical benefit within three years. Approximately 22% had tested presymptomatic children under age 12 for HD and most had received requests to test children for carrier status of recessive disorders. A disturbing 45% of laboratories provided testing directly to consumers without a physician's order. There is a need for more uniform guidelines for laboratories performing genetic testing of children. The guidelines should require that only qualified professionals be permitted to order and interpret the test results.[152]

Pascal Borry and colleagues reviewed 27 guidelines published by 31 organizations on presymptomatic and predictive testing in minors.[153] They also reviewed 14 guidelines from 24 professional groups on carrier detection testing in minors.[154] They found that all organizations recommended postponing presymptomatic testing and carrier detection testing until the child could consent as an adult. Lainie Friedman Ross argued that one possible exception can be made for genetic disorders that present later in childhood if the parents favor testing.[155]

There remain a few interesting controversies in the ethics literature about the general context of genetic testing in children. One conflict surrounds the wish of patients with genetic disabilities to bear children who share their particular disability. This unusual problem has been recorded in some parents with achondroplastic dwarfism who regard their unique physiognomy with pride. The conflict has been portrayed as pitting parental autonomy against the child's future autonomy.[156] Ronald Green countered this wish with an argument that all parents have an ethical obligation not to inflict subnormal health on their children.[157]

A second controversy involves the critique of prenatal genetic testing by certain people active in the disability rights political community. These activists have criticized physicians and genetic counselors for unjustifiably discriminating against the disabled in their attempts to suppress genetically transmitted diseases.[158] The extent of the politicization of this conflict can be measured by the language they employ in dialogue. Unjustified discrimination on the basis of genetic endowment has been termed "geneticism" in parallel usage to the well known derogatory term "racism."[159]

GENE THERAPY

A major benefit of the Human Genome Project goal of fully understanding the molecular genetics of human DNA is the potential to provide gene therapy to correct or prevent the development of inherited or sporadic genetic disease. While gene therapy offers the best hope for the cure or prevention of genetic diseases, the very nature of its technology produces unique risks and raises ethical questions that must be addressed before the therapy can be tested and implemented successfully.[160]

Comprehending the ethical issues in gene therapy first requires an understanding of the technology involved. W. French Anderson, a leader in gene therapy research, defined the ultimate goals of gene therapy research as: (1) developing vectors to carry injectable therapeutic genes that target specific cells; (2) creating vectors that accomplish safe and efficient gene transfer into a high percentage of target cells; (3) regulating these new genes by administered agents or by the body's own physiologic signals; (4) developing gene therapy technology that is cost-effective to manufacture; and (5) implementing gene therapy technology that will cure genetic disease.[161]

Ethical issues in gene therapy vary with the intended targets cells and the goals of therapy. The two possible targets are somatic cells and germ-line cells. Somatic gene therapy intends to correct a disease-producing genetic defect in the DNA of somatic cells that affects only the treated patient. Germ-line gene therapy targets an inherited defect in the DNA of a patient's germ cells that can affect the offspring of the treated patient and all future generations.[162]

Goals of gene therapy include the cure or the prevention of genetic disease and the enhancement of desirable traits. Patients already suffering genetic diseases could be cured of the disease by inserting a gene to replace a missing enzyme, structural protein, or other defect. Currently asymptomatic patients destined to suffer an inherited disease later in life could be cured by gene therapy. *In utero* gene therapy on fetuses could prevent the disease in early life. Gene therapy also can be used to enhance desirable characteristics, such as intelligence or height, or to cure purely cosmetic conditions such as baldness.

The history of ethical issues in human gene therapy began with the bold experiment in 1980 by Martin Cline of UCLA in which he attempted to therapeutically manipulate the gene for sickle cell hemoglobin.[163] Although Cline was severely criticized for proceeding with his experiment without institutional peer approval, the publicity surrounding his work stimulated the President's Commission for the Study of Ethical Problems in Medicine and Biomedical and Behavioral Research in 1982 to issue a report on human gene therapy.[164] It also led to empaneling the National Institutes of Health Office of Biotechnology Activities Recombinant DNA Advisory Committee (RAC), and the Human Gene Therapy Subcommittee.

The first RAC-approved somatic cell manipulation experiment toward disease prevention began in 1990 with a protocol designed to cure children born with severe combined immunodeficiency due to congenital absence of the enzyme adenosine deaminase. By 2005, over 500 clinical trial protocols for gene transfer and therapy had been approved by the RAC.[165] The number of trials of gene therapy peaked in 1999 and diminished thereafter as a result of a better appreciation of its risks.[166] Indications for somatic cell therapy in neurology include the repair of single gene defects, such as those causing Tay-Sachs disease, muscle gene therapy for Duchenne muscular dystrophy and Becker's muscular dystrophy, and gene therapy for other inborn neurogenetic errors of metabolism presenting in childhood.[167] Jerry Mendell and Andra Miller explained the current regulatory process for approving and conducting gene therapy clinical trials and provided a comprehensive list of web-based resources for clinicians and investigators planning such trials.[168]

Somatic Cure and Prevention

Somatic cell therapy experiments probably raise no important new ethical issues and therefore can be treated like any other innovative non-genetic therapy.[169] There now is a consensus that somatic cell gene therapy is ethically acceptable.[170] Valid consent of the research subject is required and the experiment must be approved by institutional review boards for scientific merit and adequate human protection. Parents are authorized to provide valid consent for genetic treatment experiments on their children with inborn errors of metabolism or other genetic defects. Mothers are permitted to consent to gene therapy for the fetuses they carry. The American Society of Human Genetics emphasized the critical role played by the investigator in guaranteeing patient protection during any study. The society proposed a "litmus test" for investigational protocols: the investigators should ask themselves whether, if they or a member of their own family had a disease that might benefit from gene therapy, they would enroll their loved one in the gene therapy trial in question.[171]

Theodore Friedmann, the director of the Program in Gene Therapy at the University of California at San Diego and a member of the RAC, outlined the ethical and procedural principles for human gene therapy studies.[172] The impetus for his analysis was the national publicity surrounding the unfortunate death of Jesse Gelsinger, an 18-year-old man with a mild form of ornithine transcarbamylase deficiency, who died of an overwhelming systemic adenovirus infection thought to have been transmitted by the gene therapy viral vector. Hoping for a cure, Gelsinger and his parents consented for the gene therapy protocol under the direction of researchers at the Institute for Gene Therapy at the University of Pennsylvania and the National Children's Medical Center in Washington, DC. As a result of his death, the FDA placed a moratorium on further gene therapy experiments at the Institute for Gene Therapy.[173] Anxiety over the risks of gene therapy was escalated further over the next several years by the publication of reports of T-cell leukemia in two patients with severe combined immunodeficiency disease following retrovirally mediated transfer of the IL2RG gene.[174] "Insertional mutagenesis" was proposed as the mechanism for the development of leukemia after the gene insertional site was found to be adjacent to LMO2, a known human T-cell oncogene.[175]

In an influential article in *Science*, Theodore Friedmann identified seven essential principles for human gene therapy studies:

1. *Human experimentation requires careful patient selection and protection.* Patients or their legally authorized surrogate decision makers must provide voluntary consent. Phase I studies are particularly problematic given the unlikelihood of direct benefit accruing to the research subject. It is debatable how much risk to the research subject is ethically acceptable to learn more about gene therapy for the disease. This problem is particularly knotty when infants are the research subjects.

2. *Human experimentation involves risks.* Irrespective of the extent of planning and care, there are often unanticipated and unavoidable risks of conducting experimental trials.

3. *Adverse results do not invalidate the rationale of gene therapy.* False starts and failures of early experiments contribute to knowledge that helps produce success in future experiments.

4. *Informed consent is crucial to patient protection.* Full disclosure of risks and benefits is crucial. The informed consent process within institutions must be guided by regulations to insure that proper standards of consent are practiced. The public portrayal of the current success of gene therapy should be more realistic and less uncritically optimistic.

5. *Financial conflict of interest must be addressed.* The contemporary reality of gene therapy research is that biotechnology and pharmaceutical companies have entered into financial arrangements with universities and investigators. These financial arrangements create conflicts of interest that can damage public trust in investigators and

their integrity. To minimize conflicts of interest, rules must be created and enforced to require proper disclosure of investigators' financial conflicts. Further, investigators with financial interests in the outcome of the gene therapy studies should not be permitted to participate in patient selection, study direction, or the consent process.

6. *Improvements are needed in review and regulation.* Oversight of previous gene therapy experiments has not been sufficient and needs more strict and consistent regulation.

7. *Gene therapy trials require improved monitoring.* Mechanisms should be implemented to require investigators to report adverse events in a forum that permits other investigators to learn about these events during their performance of their clinical trials.[176]

Other scholars have emphasized that an ethically sound informed consent process must thoroughly explain the known risks and emphasize that other risks are unknown and cannot be anticipated.[177] The risks of neither overwhelming viral vector superinfection nor insertional mutagenesis were fully appreciated until after the subjects who received experimental gene transfers developed these disorders and died.

Fetal Gene Therapy

Human fetal gene therapy is one principal goal of prenatal genetic diagnosis. Performing gene therapy on a fetus offers the opportunity of early prevention or cure of the genetic disease before it creates further damage to the developing organism. It also offers an attractive alternative to selective abortion, the other goal of prenatal genetic diagnosis. Thoughtful utilitarian analyses of the ethical issues involved conclude that fetal gene therapy should be studied and perfected because these benefits outweigh the principal harm of the practice, namely starting down the "slippery slope" toward germ-line gene therapy.[178]

The specific ethical and practice guidelines for fetal gene therapy are similar to those of human gene therapy protocols for infants, and require adequate scientific grounds to proceed,

proper informed and voluntary consent of the parents, resolution of biosafety concerns, and adequate oversight. The only unique ethical feature of fetal gene therapy is that both the fetus and the pregnant woman are patients. Obstetrical ethics has a long history of concern for the health and welfare of the mother-fetus dyad.[179] The medical and ethical goal is to maximize the health of both mother and fetus. But when the medical interests of the two conflict, generally the interest of the mother is afforded primacy. Thus, fetal gene therapy can be regarded ethically as equivalent to neonatal gene therapy unless the mother's health is jeopardized as a result of the protocol.

Enhancement

Somatic human gene therapies to enhance capabilities such as intelligence or height, or to treat cosmetic issues such as baldness, raise an interesting set of ethical issues. Should powerful and potentially dangerous gene therapies be developed to address these relatively minor problems? Are these issues even medical problems which physicians have a professional responsibility to treat?[180] Or does gene therapy for enhancement represent a dangerous example of genetic engineering and eugenics that will create problems for society in the future when the technology becomes extended in ways we now cannot fully imagine?[181] (See chapter 20.)

Analyses of ethical issues in somatic gene therapy for enhancement point out that these therapies are not qualitatively dissimilar to existing pharmaceutical therapies prescribed for baldness or hormonal therapies prescribed for short stature. Moreover, some instances of enhancement may not be as medically trivial as they first appear because of the psychological damage to patients resulting from having socially undesirable physical traits. The risks of genetic therapy for enhancement, once perfected, also may not exceed the risk of alternative treatments with medications.[182] Most commentators agree, however, that scientific attention to and public funds designated for the development of genetic enhancement therapies should be relegated to a priority lower than for those directed against cure or prevention of genetic disease. The American Medical Association Council on Ethical and Judicial Affairs warns, "Efforts to enhance desirable characteristics through the insertion of a modified or additional gene . . . are contrary not only to the ethical tradition of medicine, but also to the egalitarian values of our society."[183]

Germ-Line Gene Therapy

Germ-line gene therapy is qualitatively different from somatic cell therapy because the induced genetic alterations affect not only the treated individual but also all future progeny. The impact on future generations raises a host of difficult questions and unknowns. One critical issue is safety. How can we know what harms might be induced that affect future organisms many generations after the present gene therapy intervention? A second issue is consent. Informed consent is relatively straightforward for gene therapy for an individual patient, or surrogate consent for gene therapy for an infant or fetus. But how can surrogate consent by one individual apply to permitting genetic alterations that affect all future generations?[184]

Germ-line gene therapy might be more ethically acceptable if several additional criteria were fulfilled. (1) It must be shown confidently that the inserted gene will not produce adverse effects on development. (2) The inserted gene must be shown not to cause chromosomal damage to future generations. (3) The method must confidently target specific chromosomal sites. However, our ability to know the answers to these questions confidently is sufficiently limited that these criteria cannot be satisfied for the foreseeable future.[185]

Because of these unsolvable problems, in April 2000, the American Association for the Advancement of Science (AAAS) issued a report calling for a total moratorium on all germ-line gene therapy. Following a two-year series of consultations with experts in the fields of gene therapy, ethics, sociology, and theology, the authors of the report found a strong consensus for the hard-line position of banning all further research. In their proposed moratorium, the AAAS also included related lines of research that might plausibly but accidentally damage germ-line DNA producing alterations affecting future generations.[186] Most bioethics scholars subsequently studying this question have concurred with the AAAS conclusion.[187]

OTHER RESEARCH ISSUES

Neurogenetic research raises ethical issues in addition to those introduced by gene therapy experiments. One longstanding question involves an investigator's duty to disclose genetic research results to experimental subjects, particularly when families are studied. Some scholars have argued that full individual disclosure should be practiced routinely out of respect for the human subject.[188] Other scholars, adopting a more paternalistic approach, have advocated limiting disclosure to selected situations after weighing the benefits and harms of disclosure to each research subject.[189] Federal regulations fail to provide guidance for this question, and institutional review boards (IRBs)[190] and funding agencies[191] have issued varying policies. There is an emerging consensus for an ethical duty of investigators to disclose genetic research results. In a recent review of international ethical guidelines, Bertha Knoppers and colleagues found a consensus that research subjects have a right to know individual results which imparts a duty to disclose, but they found no consensus on who should disclose the results or how and when.[192] They found agreement on the principle that research subjects also have a right not to know results.

Vardit Ravitsky and Benjamin Wilfond recently proposed a method of disclosure that considers the rights of human subjects to know results and provides a means to minimize the harms resulting from disclosure. In their "result-evaluation" approach, they assess the expected information within the context of the study, measure the analytic validity and clinical utility of each specific result, and examine the personal meaning of each research result to determine whether it should be disclosed routinely. They believe that the threshold of clinical utility for disclosing a result in a research study should be lower than that used in clinical practice. They conclude that their individualized approach best enhances the goods and reduces the harms to research subjects and provides a nuanced and flexible system of disclosure.[193]

A related question center on the rights of individuals to know the results of pedigree analysis. Recording pedigree information is an essential step in studying the genetics of multifactorial diseases.[194] Pedigree studies are complicated because individuals may be active or passive participants. Prevailing research ethics models focus on the investigator-subject dyad which does not apply in pedigree studies.[195] Conflicts of interest among family members may occur when some wish to know genetic data and others do not. Family members need to be assured of privacy and confidentiality.[196] To address these concerns, Bradford Worrall and colleagues proposed a "proband-initiated contact" methodology in which the proband or the proband's designate allows the identification of potential families without sacrificing the privacy of individuals within the family. They recommend that IRBs waive the requirements for individual consent by family members in cases in which family history data are collected without direct contact between researchers and individuals in the proband's family.[197]

NOTES

1. Gusella JF, Wexler NS, Conneally FM, et al. A polymorphic marker genetically linked to Huntington's disease. *Nature* 1983;306:234–238. The history of molecular genetics in neurology has been summarized in Rowland LP. The first decade of molecular genetics in neurology: changing clinical thought and practice. *Ann Neurol* 1992;32:207–214 and in Payne CS, Roses AD. The molecular genetic revolution: its impact on clinical neurology. *Arch Neurol* 1988;45:1366–1376.

2. McKusick VA. *Mendelian Inheritance in Man: A Catalog of Human Genes and Genetic Disorders.* 12th ed. Baltimore: Johns Hopkins University Press, 1998. The exponential growth in the number of entries since the first edition of this text is described in McKusick VA. Medical genetics: a 40-year perspective on the evolution of a medical specialty from a basic science. *JAMA* 1993;270:2351–2356.

3. National Center for Biotechnology Information. *Online Mendelian Inheritance in Man.* This indispensable and encyclopedic website maintained by Johns Hopkins University can be accessed at http://www. ncbi.nlm.nih.gov/entrez/query.fcgi?db=OMIM (Accessed March 19, 2007).

4. Collins FS. Shattuck Lecture—Medical and societal consequences of the Human Genome Project. *N Engl J Med* 1999;341:28–37.

5. The Human Genome Project is described in McKusick VA. Mapping and sequencing the human genome. *N Engl J Med* 1989;320:910–915 and Green ED, Waterston RH. The Human Genome Project: prospects and implications for clinical medicine. *JAMA* 1991;266:1966–1975. For a summary of the HGP, see http:// www.ornl.gov/sci/techresources/Human_Genome/home.shtml (Accessed March 27, 2007).

6. McKusick VA, Collins FS. Implications of the human genome project for medical science. *JAMA* 2001;285:540–544. For greater detail on the activities and accomplishments of the HGP, see National Research Council, Committee on Mapping and Sequencing the Human Genome. *Mapping and Sequencing the Human Genome.* Washington, DC: National Academy Press, 2000. For a compelling account of the race to sequence the human genome, see Davies K. *Cracking the Genome: Inside the Race to Unlock Human DNA.* New York: Free Press, 2001.

7. Engels H, Brockschmidt A, Hoischen A, et al. DNA microarray analysis identifies candidate regions and genes in unexplained mental retardation. *Neurology* 2007;68:743–750. See also Sharp FR, Xu H, Lit L, et al. The future of genomic profiling of neurological diseases using blood. *Arch Neurol* 2006;63:1529–1536. For a discussion of the ethical issues in genetic profiling of newborns, see Almond B. Genetic profiling of newborns: ethical and social issues. *Nat Rev Genet* 2006;7:67–71.

8. Cravchik A, Subramanian G, Broder S, Venter JC. Sequence analysis of the human genome: implications for an understanding of nervous system function and disease. *Arch Neurol* 2001;58:1772–1778. The website GeneTests lists the laboratories throughout the world that offer clinical and research testing for those genetic diseases that have a known molecular basis. http://www.genetests.org (Accessed March 24, 2007).

9. Green ED, Waterston RH. *JAMA* 1991:1973–1974.

10. The Allen Institute for Brain Science and the Nature Publishing Group have jointly produced the Allen Brain Atlas which provides maps of the expression of approximately 20,000 genes in the mouse brain (of

the mouse's approximately 25,000 total genes). See Allen Brain Atlas Neuroscience Gateway http://www.brainatlas.org/aba/ (Accessed July 5, 2007).

11. Evans GA. The human genome project: applications in the diagnosis and treatment of neurologic disease. *Arch Neurol* 1998;55:1287–1290.

12. For references addressing the general topic of ethical issues in genetics, see Yesley MS. *ELSI Bibliography: Ethical, Legal, and Social Implications of the Human Genome Project.* U.S. Department of Energy, Office of Energy Research: Washington, DC, 1992; Gert B. *Morality and the New Genetics: A Guide for Students and Health Care Providers.* Jones and Bartlett Publishers: Boston, 1996; Watson JD. *A Passion for DNA: Genes, Genomes, and Society.* Cold Spring Harbor Laboratory Press: Cold Spring Harbor, NY, 2000; Buchanan A, Brock D, Daniels N, Wikler D (eds). *From Chance to Choice: Genetics & Justice.* Cambridge: Cambridge University Press, 2000; and Wertz DC, Fletcher JC, Berg K. World Health Organization Human Genetics Programme. *Review of Ethical Issues in Medical Genetics,* 2003. http://www.who.int/genomics/publications/en/ethical_issuesin_medgenetics%20report.pdf (Accessed April 17, 2007).

13. For short but authoritative reviews on the ethical issues in neurogenetic testing, see Bird TD. Risks and benefits of DNA testing for neurogenetic disorders. *Semin Neurol* 1999;19:243–259 and Ensenauer RE, Michels VV, Reinke SS. Genetic testing: practical, ethical, and genetic counseling considerations. *Mayo Clin Proc* 2005;80:63–73.

14. See Collins FS. Medical and ethical consequences of the Human Genome Project. *J Clin Ethics* 1991;2:260–267 and Durfy SJ. Ethics and the Human Genome Project. *Arch Pathol Lab Med* 1993;117:466–469.

15. Burke W. Genetic testing. *N Engl J Med* 2002;347:1867–1875. On the difference between genetic and nongenetic tests, see Green MJ, Botkin JR. "Genetic exceptionalism in medicine: clarifying the difference between genetic and nongenetic tests. *Ann Intern Med* 2003;138:571–575.

16. Paulson HL. Diagnostic testing in neurogenetics: principles, limitations, and ethical considerations. *Neurol Clin N Am* 2002;20:627–643.

17. Personal communication, Tyler E. Reimschisel, July 4, 2007.

18. These examples were discussed in Paulson HL. Diagnostic testing in neurogenetics: principles, limitations, and ethical considerations. *Neurol Clin N Am* 2002;20:627–643. For a good primer for physicians on using genetic testing in practice, see American College of Medical Genetics. *Genetics for Providers.* (CD-ROM). American College of Medical Genetics Foundation, 2007.

19. The terms "dominant," "recessive," and "carrier state" applied to X-linked disorders recently have fallen out of favor as a result of a growing understanding of the genetics. See Dobyns WB, Filauro A, Tomson BN, et al. Inheritance for most X-linked traits is not dominant or recessive, just X-linked" *Am J Med Genet A* 2004;129:136–143. Females (formerly called carriers) may have formes frustes of X-linked diseases. For example, females with the adrenoleukodystrophy allele may show signs and symptoms of the disease. See Moser HW, Raymond GV, Dubey P. Adrenoleukodystrophy: new approaches to a neurodegenerative disease. *JAMA* 2005;294:3131–3134.

20. Bird TD. Approaches to the patient with neurogenetic disease. *Neurol Clin N Am* 2002;20:619–626.

21. See Rosenberg RN. An introduction to the molecular genetics of neurological disease. *Arch Neurol* 1993;50:1123–1128 and Martin JB. Molecular genetics in neurology. *Ann Neurol* 1993;34:757–773.

22. Rosenberg RN. A neurological gene map. *Arch Neurol* 1993;50:1269–1271.

23. For current descriptions of genetic diseases, genetic tests, and laboratories that perform genetic tests, see the University of Washington and National Library of Medicine-National Human Genome Research Institute website: http://www.genetests.org (Accessed March 24, 2007).

24. Marsden D, Larson C, Levy HL. Newborn screening for metabolic disorders. *J Pediatrics* 2006;148: 577–584.

25. For a current medical and legal review of non-invasive prenatal genetic testing, see Chachkin CJ. What potent blood: non-invasive prenatal genetic diagnosis and the transformation of modern prenatal care. *Am J Law Med* 2007;33:9–54.

26. For example, see DNAdirect. http://www.dnadirect.com/ (Accessed June 12, 2007.)

27. Wasson K, Cook ED, Helzlsouer K. Direct-to-consumer online genetic testing and the four principles: an analysis of the ethical issues. *Ethics Med* 2006;22(2):83–91.

28. Braude P. Preimplantation diagnosis for genetic susceptibility. *N Engl J Med* 2006;355:541–543.

29. Offit K, Sagi M, Hurley K. Preimplantation genetic diagnosis for cancer syndromes: a new challenge to preventive medicine. *JAMA* 2007;296:2727–2730.

30. Moutou C, Gardes N, Viville S. New tools for preimplantation genetic diagnosis of Huntington's disease and their clinical applications. *Eur J Hum Genet* 2004;12:1007–1014.

31. Verlinsky Y, Rechitsky S, Verlinsky O, et al. Preimplantation diagnosis for sonic hedgehog mutation causing familial holoprosecephaly. *N Engl J Med* 2003;348:1449–1454.

32. Verlinsky Y, Rechitsky S, Verlinsky O, Masciangelo C, Lederer K, Kuliev A. Preimplantation diagnosis for early-onset Alzheimer disease caused by V717L mutation. *JAMA* 2002;287:1018–1021.

33. Towner D, Loewy RS. Ethics of preimplantation diagnosis for a woman destined to develop early-onset Alzheimer disease. *JAMA* 2002;287:1038–1040.

34. American Society of Reproductive Medicine Ethics Committee. Sex selection and preimplantation diagnosis. *Fertil Steril* 1999;72:595–598 and American Society of Reproductive Medicine Ethics Committee. Preconception gender selection for nonmedical reasons. *Fertil Steril* 2001;75:861–864.

35. Wolf SM, Kahn JP, Wagner JE. Using preimplantation genetic diagnosis to create a stem cell donor: issues, guidelines & limits. *J Law Med Ethics* 2003;31:327–339.

36. For a recent review of these ethical issues and proposed policy solutions, see Lilani A. Ethical issues and policy analysis for genetic testing: Huntington's disease as a paradigm for diseases with a late onset. *Hum Reprod Genet Ethics* 2005;11(2):28–34.

37. Smith CO, Lipe HP, Bird TD. Impact of presymptomatic genetic testing for hereditary ataxia and neuromuscular disorders. *Arch Neurol* 2004;61:875–880.

38. Shostak S, Ottman. Ethical, legal, and social dimensions of epilepsy genetics. *Epilepsia* 2006;47:1595–1602.

39. Hayden MR. Predictive testing for Huntington's disease: a universal model? *Lancet Neurology* 2003;2:141–142.

40. For a current review on the clinical and genetic aspects of Huntington's disease, see Walker FO. Huntington's disease. *Lancet* 2007;369:218–228.

41. Huntington's Disease Peer Workgroup. *Lifting the Veil of Huntington's Disease: Recommendations to the Field.* Promoting Excellence in End-of-Life Care: a national program of the Robert Wood Johnson Foundation. February, 2004.

42. Gusella JF, MacDonald ME, Ambrose CM, et al. Molecular genetics of Huntington's disease. *Arch Neurol* 1993;50:1157–1163 and Hersch S, Jones R, Koroshetz W, et al. The neurogenetics genie: testing for the Huntington's disease mutation. *Neurology* 1994;44:1369–1373.

43. Kremer B, Goldberg P, Andrew SE, et al. A worldwide study of the Huntington's disease mutation: the sensitivity and specificity of measuring CAG repeats. *N Engl J Med* 1994;330:1401–1406. The clinical and genetic significance of patients having "intermediate alleles" (27–35 CAG repeats) was studied by Semaka A, Creighton S, Warby S, Hayden MR. Predictive testing for Huntington's disease: interpretation and significance of intermediate alleles. *Clin Genet* 2006;70:283–294.

44. These issues are discussed in Bird SJ. Presymptomatic testing for Huntington's disease. *JAMA* 1985;253:3286–3291.

45. Marsden CD. Prediction of Huntington's disease. *Ann Neurol* 1981;10:202–203.

46. These survey data are reviewed in Bird SJ. Genetic testing for neurologic diseases: a rose with thorns. *Neurol Clin* 1989;7:859–870. See, in particular, Mastromauro C, Myers RH, Berkman B. Attitudes toward presymptomatic testing in Huntington's disease. *Am J Med Genet* 1987;26:271–282 and Meissen GJ, Berchek RL. Intended use of predictive testing by those at risk for Huntington's disease. *Am J Med Genet* 1987;26:283–293.

47. McCormack MK, Lazzarini A. Attitudes of those at risk for Huntington's disease toward presymptomatic provocative testing. *N Engl J Med* 1982;307:1406.

48. Tyler A, Harper PS. Attitudes of subjects at risk and their relatives toward genetic counseling in Huntington's chorea. *J Med Genet* 1983;20:179–188.

49. Schoenfeld M, Myers RH, Berkman B, et al. Potential impact of a predictive test on the gene frequency of Huntington's disease. *Am J Med Genet* 1984;18:423–429.

50. Carter CO, Evans KA, Baraitser M. Effect of genetic counseling on the prevalence of Huntington's chorea. *BMJ* 1983;286:281–283.

51. Thomas S. Ethics of a predictive test for Huntington's chorea. *BMJ* 1982;284:1383–1385.

52. Klawans HL, Paulson GW, Ringel SP, Barbeau A. Use of L-Dopa in the detection of presymptomatic Huntington's chorea. *N Engl J Med* 1972;286:1332–1334.

53. Klawans HL, Goetz CG, Paulson GW, Barbeau A. Levodopa and presymptomatic detection of Huntington's disease: eight-year follow-up. *N Engl J Med* 1980;302:1090.

54. Myers RH, Growdon JH, Bird ED, Feldman RG, Martin JB. False-negative results with levodopa for early detection of Huntington's disease. *N Engl J Med* 1982;307:561–562.

55. Personal communication, Dr. Steven P. Ringel, February 12, 1994. Suicide attempts and acute psychiatric decompensation are known complications when at-risk patients test positive for HD. See Almqvist EW, Bloch M, Brinkman R, Crauford D, Hayden MR. A worldwide assessment of the frequency of suicide, suicide attempts, or psychiatric hospitalization after predictive testing for Huntington's disease. *Am J Hum Genet* 1999;64:1293–1304.

56. Fahn S. Levodopa provocative test for Huntington's disease. *N Engl J Med* 1980;303:884.

57. The most recent study of factors predicting the development of HD in at-risk patients found that the combination of subtle motor signs and neuropsychological test results were the most accurate. Langbehn DR, Paulsen JS. Predictors of diagnosis in Huntington disease. *Neurology* 2007;68:1710–1717.

58. For a review of the 1980–1990 literature, see Grafton ST, Mazziotta JC, Pahl JJ, et al. A comparison of neurological, metabolic, structural, and genetic evaluations in persons at risk for Huntington's disease. *Ann Neurol* 1990;28:614–621. Studies since 1990 include Aylward EH, Brandt J, Codori AM, Mangus RS, Barta PE, Harris GJ. Reduced basal ganglia volume associated with the gene for Huntington's disease in asymptomatic at-risk persons. *Neurology* 1994;44:823–828; Giordani B, Berent S, Boivin MJ, et al. Longitudinal neuropsychological and genetic linkage of persons at risk for Huntington's disease. *Arch Neurol* 1995;52:59–64; Foroud T, Siemers E, Kleindorfer D, et al. Cognitive scores of carriers of Huntington's disease gene compared to noncarriers. *Ann Neurol* 1995;37:657–664; Siemers E, Foroud T, Bill DJ, et al. Motor changes in presymptomatic Huntington disease carriers. *Arch Neurol* 1996;53:487–492; Weeks RA, Piccini P, Harding AE, Brooks DJ. Striatal D1 and D2 dopamine receptor loss in asymptomatic mutation carriers of Huntington's disease. *Ann Neurol* 1996;40:49–54; Aylward EH, Codori AM, Barta PE, Pearlson GD, Harris GJ, Brandt J. Basal ganglia volume and proximity to onset in presymptomatic Huntington disease. *Arch Neurol* 1996;53:1293–1296; Kirkwood SC, Siemers E, Stout JC, et al. Longitudinal cognitive and motor changes among presymptomatic Huntington disease carriers. *Arch Neurol* 1999;56:563–568; and Kirkwood SC, Siemers E, Bond C, Conneally PM, Christian JC, Foroud T. Confirmation of subtle motor changes among presymptomatic carriers of the Huntington disease gene. *Arch Neurol* 2000;57:1040–1044.

59. Kipps CM, Duggins AJ, Mahant N, Gomes L, Ashburner J, McCusker EA. Progression of structural neuropathology in preclinical Huntington's disease: a tensor-based morphometry study. *J Neurol Neurosurg Psychiatry* 2005;76:650–655.

60. Blekher T, Johnson SA, Marshall J, et al. Saccades in presymptomatic and early stages of Huntington's disease. *Neurology* 2006;67:394–399.

61. The Huntington Study Group PHAROS Investigators. The PHAROS (Prospective Huntington At Risk Observation Study): Cohort enrolled. *Arch Neurol* 2006;63:991–998.

62. Gusella JF, Wexler NS, Conneally PM, et al. *Nature* 1983:234–238.

63. See, for example, Gilliam TC, Bucan M., MacDonald ME, et al. A DNA segment encoding two genes very tightly linked to Huntington's disease. *Science* 1987;238:950–952 and Wasmuth JJ, Hewitt J, Smith B, et al. A highly polymorphic locus very tightly linked to the Huntington's gene. *Nature* 1988;332:734–735.

64. Huntington's Disease Collaborative Research Group. A novel gene containing a trinucleotide repeat that is expanded and unstable on Huntington's disease chromosomes. *Cell* 1993;72:971–983.

65. These problems are discussed in Smurl JF, Weaver DD. Presymptomatic testing for Huntington's chorea: guidelines for moral and social accountability. *Am J Med Genet* 1987;26:247–257.

66. The voluntariness of HD genetic testing is a prerequisite in all published guidelines. See Commission for the Control of Huntington's Disease. Ethical guidelines for the development and use of a presymptomatic test. In, *Report: Commission for the Control of Huntington's Disease.* Volume 2: Technical Report. Washington, DC: US Department of Health, Education, and Welfare. Public Health Service, National Institutes of Health, 1977:333–341; Huntington's Disease Society of America. *Guidelines for Predictive Testing for Huntington's Disease.* New York: Huntington's Disease Society of America, 1989; and Huntington's Disease Society of America. Ethical issues policy statement on Huntington's disease molecular genetics predictive test. *J Med Genet* 1990;27:34–38.

67. Richards FH. Maturity of judgment in decision making for predictive testing for nontreatable adult-onset neurogenetic conditions: a case against predictive testing of minors. *Clin Genet* 2006;70:396–401. However, there is nothing unethical in testing children who are already symptomatic for diagnostic purposes. For a report of a program in which this testing was successful, see Nance MA. Genetic testing of children at risk for Huntington's disease. *Neurology* 1997;49:1048–1053.

68. Conomy JP, Kanoti G. Ethical aspects of predictive tests in Huntington's disease. *Semin Neurol* 1984;4:73–82. They referred to the ratio of benefits to burdens from testing as the "gain-to-loss" ratio. For other ethical commentary, see DeGrazia D. The ethical justification for minimal paternalism in the use of the predictive test for Huntington's disease. *J Clin Ethics* 1991;2:219–228 and Terrenoire G. Huntington's disease and the ethics of genetic prediction. *J Med Ethics* 1992;18(2):79–85.

69. For a review of data on the risk of suicide among HD patients with and without genetic testing, see Bird TD. Outrageous fortune: the risk of suicide in genetic testing for Huntington disease. *Am J Genet* 1999;64:1289–1292. Suicidal ideation has been reported in 9% of otherwise asymptomatic individuals who are at risk for HD. See Paulsen JS, Hoth KF, Nehl C, Stierman L. Critical periods of suicide risk in Huntington's disease. *Am J Psychiatry* 2005;162:725–731.

70. Most protocols for genetic testing require concomitant counseling. For example, see Craufurd D, Tyler A. Predictive testing for Huntington's disease: protocol of the UK Huntington's Prediction Consortium. *J Med Genet* 1992;29:915–918 and Huntington's Disease Society of America. *Guidelines Predictive Testing for Huntington's Disease,* 1989.

71. Bird TD. Risks and benefits of DNA testing for neurogenetic disorders. *Semin Neurol* 1999;19:243–259.

72. The phenomenon of survivor guilt is discussed in Bird SJ. *JAMA* 1985:3289 and Wexler NS, Conneally PM, Housman D, et al. A DNA polymorphism for Huntington's disease marks the future. *Arch Neurol* 1985;42:20–24.

73. The quotation of Nancy Wexler was cited in the obituary of her father Dr. Milton Wexler. See http://www.nytimes.com/2007/03/24/obituaries/24wexler.html?ref=obituaries (Accessed March 24, 2007.)

74. Wiggins S, Whyte P, Huggins M, et al. The psychological consequences of predictive testing for Huntington's disease. *N Engl J Med* 1992;327:1401–1405. These data confirmed Bates' prediction that even the at-risk patient testing positive would be better off psychologically. See Bates M. Ethics of provocative test for Huntington's disease. *N Engl J Med* 1981;304:175–176.

75. Tibben A, Timman R, Bannick EC, et al. Three-year follow-up after presymptomatic testing for Huntington's disease tested in individuals and partners. *Health Psychol* 1997;16:30–35. For a related study showing the complex and changing psychological issues in tested patients at-risk for HD, see Codori AM, Slavney PR, Young C, et al. Predictors of psychological adjustment to genetic testing for Huntington's disease. *Health Psychol* 1997;16:36–50.

76. For a discussion of family shame in HD, see Hayes CV. Genetic testing for Huntington's disease – a family issue. *N Engl J Med* 1992;327:1449–1450.

77. The technique of exclusion testing is discussed in Quarrell OWJ, Meredith AL, Tyler A, et al. Exclusion testing in Huntington's disease in pregnancy with a closely linked DNA market. *Lancet* 1987;1:1281–1283 and Bird SJ. *Neurol Clin* 1989:864.

78. Duncan RE, Foddy B, Delatycki B. Refusing to provide a prenatal test: can it ever be ethical? *BMJ* 2006;333:1066–1068.

79. Market DS, Young AB, Penney JB. At-risk person's attitudes toward presymptomatic and prenatal testing of Huntington's disease in Michigan. *Am J Med Genet* 1987;26:295–305.

80. Marjorie Guthrie's statement is cited in Rosenfeld A. At risk for Huntington's disease: who should know what and when? *Hastings Cent Rep* 1984;14(3):5–8.

81. Meissen GJ, Myers RH, Mastromauro CA, et al. Predictive testing for Huntington's disease with use of a linked DNA marker. *N Engl J Med* 1988;318:535–542.

82. Brandt J, Quaid KA, Folstein SE, et al. Presymptomatic diagnosis of delayed-onset disease with linked DNA markers: the experience in Huntington's disease. *JAMA* 1989;261:3108–3114.

83. Morris MJ, Tyler A, Lazarou L, et al. Problems in genetic prediction for Huntington's disease. *Lancet* 1989;2:601–603.

84. This topic is discussed further in the symposium: Results of genetic testing: when confidentiality conflicts with a duty to warn relatives. *BMJ* 2000;321:1464–1466.

85. Huggins M, Bloch M, Kanani S, et al. Ethical and legal dilemmas arising during predictive testing for adult-onset disease: the experience of Huntington's disease. *Am J Hum Genet* 1990;47:4–12.

86. Recommendations for the disclosure of nonpaternity in this situation were discussed in President's Commission for the Study of Ethical Problems in Medicine and Biomedical and Behavioral Research. *Screening and Counseling for Genetic Conditions: The Ethical, Social, and Legal Implications of Counseling and Education Programs.* Washington, DC: US Government Printing Office, 1983:59–62.

87. Decruyenaere M, Evers-Kiebooms G, Boogaerts A, et al. The complexity of reproductive decision-making in asymptomatic carriers of the Huntington mutation. *Eur J Hum Genet* 2007;15:453–462.

88. These ethical conditions and a commentary on each consideration are described in the ethical issues policy statement on the predictive test of molecular genetics for Huntington's disease by the Huntington's Disease Society of America. *J Med Genet* 1990;27:34–38. The National Society of Genetic Counselors later published a paper with a similar analysis and similar recommendations: McKinnon WC, Baty BJ, Bennett RL, et al. Predisposition genetic testing for late-onset disorders in adults: a position paper of the National Society of Genetic Counselors. *JAMA* 1997;278:1217–1220. For genetic counseling centers, see the National Society of Genetic Counselors website: http://www.negc.org (Accessed March 24, 2007).

89. Children with Tay-Sachs disease who have two copies of the defective gene usually are not true homozygotes but are compound heterozygotes because each allele has a distinct pathological mutation. Personal communication, Tyler E. Reimschisel, July 5, 2007.

90. Blitzer MG, McDowell GA. Tay-Sachs disease as a model of screening for inborn errors. *Clin Lab Med* 1992;12:463–480.

91. Kaback M, Lim-Steele J, Dabholkar D, et al. Tay-Sachs disease—carrier screening, prenatal diagnosis, and the molecular era: an international perspective, 1970 to 1993. *JAMA* 1993;270:2307–2315.

92. See Myerowitz R, Hogikyan ND. Different mutations in Ashkenazi Jewish and non-Jewish French Canadians with Tay-Sachs disease. *Science* 1986;232:1646–1648 and Blitzer MG, McDowell GA. *Clin Lab Med* 1992:465.

93. Blitzer MG, McDowell GA. *Clin Lab Med* 1992:466.

94. Kaback M, Lim-Steele J, Dabholkar D, et al. *JAMA* 1993:2307 and Blitzer MG, McDowell GA. *Clin Lab Med* 1992:466–467.

95. Triggs-Raine BL, Feigenbaum ASJ, Natowicz M, et al. Screening for carriers of Tay-Sachs disease among Ashkenazi Jews: a comparison of DNA-based enzyme-based tests. *N Engl J Med* 1990;323:6–12.

96. These tests are described in Blitzer MG, McDowell GA. *Clin Lab Med* 1992:468–475. The indications for the DNA tests are from Kaback M, Lim-Steele J, Dabholkar D, et al. *JAMA* 1993:2312–2313.

97. Kaback MM. Population-based genetic screening for reproductive counseling: the Tay-Sachs disease model. *Eur J Pediatr* 2000;159(suppl):S192–S195.

98. Kaback MM. *Eur J Pediatr* 2000;159(suppl):S192–S195. The 90% abortion rate was cited in Kaback M, Lim-Steele J, Dabholkar D, et al. *JAMA* 1993:2309.

99. Kaback M, Lim-Steele J, Dabholkar D, et al. *JAMA* 1993:2309–2310.

100. Committee on Obstetricians. *Screening for Tay-Sachs Disease.* American College of Obstetricians and Gynecologist Committee Opinion Number 93. Chicago: American College of Obstetricians and Gynecologists, 1991.

101. Clow CL, Scriver CR. The adolescent copes with genetic screening: a study of Tay-Sachs screening among high-school students. *Prog Clin Biol Res* 1977;18:381–394.

102. Rosner F. Screening for Tay-Sachs disease: a note of caution. *J Clin Ethics* 1991;2:251–252.

103. Eng CM, Scechter C, Robinowitz J, et al. Prenatal genetic carrier testing using triple disease screening. *JAMA* 1997;278:1268–1272. A carrier screening program in Israel for Gaucher disease found that most couples did not terminate affected pregnancies. The authors believed the findings were a consequence of the low penetrance of Gaucher disease. See Zuckerman S, Lahad A, Shmueli A, et al. Carrier screening for Gaucher disease: lessons for low-penetrance, treatable diseases. *JAMA* 2007;298:1281–1290.

104. Multicenter Study Group. Diagnosis of Duchenne and Becker muscular dystrophies by polymerase chain reaction: a multicenter study. *JAMA* 1992;267:2609–2615.

105. Moxley RT 3rd, Ashwal S, Pandya S, et al. Practice parameter: corticosteroid treatment of Duchenne dystrophy: report of the Quality Standards Subcommittee of the American Academy of Neurology and the Practice Committee of the Child Neurology Society. *Neurology* 2005;64:13–20 and Manzur AY, Kuntzer T, Pike M, Swan A. Glucocorticoid corticosteroids for Duchenne muscular dystrophy. *Cochrane Database Syst Rev* 2004;2:CD003725.

106. For the clinical features of DMD and BMD, see Biggar WD. Duchenne muscular dystrophy. *Pediatr Rev* 2006;27(3):83–88.

107. The clinical-genetic correlations of DMD and BMD are reviewed in Rowland LP. Clinical concepts of Duchenne muscular dystrophy: the impact of molecular genetics. *Brain* 1988;111:479–495 and Gutmann DH, Fischbeck KH. Molecular biology of Duchenne and Becker's muscular dystrophy: clinical applications. *Ann Neurol* 1989;26:189–194.

108. Hoffman EP, Wang J. Duchenne-Becker muscular dystrophy and the nondystrophic myotonias: paradigms for loss of function and change of function of gene products. *Arch Neurol* 1993;50:1227–1237.

109. Sancho S, Mongini T, Tanji K, et al. Analysis of dystrophin expression after activation of myogenesis in amniocytes, chorionic-villus cells, and fibroblasts: a new method for diagnosing Duchenne muscular dystrophy. *N Engl J Med* 1993;329:915–920.

110. Yau S, Roberts RG, Bobrow M, et al. Direct diagnosis of carriers of point mutations in Duchenne muscular dystrophy. *Lancet* 1993;341:273–276 and Fassati A, Tedeschi S, Bordoni A, et al. Rapid detection of deletions of carriers of Duchenne and Becker dystrophies. *Lancet* 1994;344:302–303.

111. Pegoraro E, Schimke RN, Garcia C, et al. Genetic and biochemical normalization in female carriers of Duchenne muscular dystrophy: evidence for failure of dystrophin production in dystrophin-competent myonuclei. *Neurology* 1995;45:677–690.

112. Sekizawa A, Kimura T, Sasaki M, Nakamura S, Kobayashi R, Sato T. Prenatal diagnosis of Duchenne muscular dystrophy using a single fetal nucleated erythrocyte in maternal blood. *Neurology* 1996;46:1350–1353.

113. Hoffman EP, Wang J. *Arch Neurol* 1993:1230.

114. For the most recent and comprehensive guidelines on the ethical basis of medical genetic testing, see Wertz DC, Fletcher JC, Berg K. World Health Organization Human Genetics Programme. *Review of Ethical Issues in Medical Genetics*, 2003. http://www.who.int/genomics/publications/en/ethical_issuesin_medgenetics %20report.pdf (Accessed April 17, 2007).

115. Michie S, Smith JA, Heaversedge J, Read S. Genetic counseling: clinical geneticists' views. *J Genet Couns* 1999;8:275–287. Experienced physicians and clinical geneticists know that patients' deliberations about genetic testing are not always rational. See White MT. Uncertainty and moral judgment: the limits of reason in genetic decision making. *J Clin Ethics* 2007;18:148–155.

116. Hubbard R, Lewontin RC. Pitfalls of genetic testing. *N Engl J Med* 1996;334:1192–1194.

117. See Billings PR, Kohn MA, de Cuevas M, et al. Discrimination as a consequence of genetic testing. *Am J Hum Genet* 1992;50:476–482 and Miller PS. Genetic discrimination in the workplace. *J Law Med Ethics* 1998;26:189–197.

118. The balance of risks and benefits of genetic testing are discussed in Bird TD. Risks and benefits of DNA testing for neurogenetic disorders. *Semin Neurol* 1999;19:253–259 and Bird TD, Bennett RL. Why do DNA testing? Practical and ethical implications of new neurogenetic tests. *Ann Neurol* 1995;38:141–146.

119. The marked similarities in the ethical principles of genetic screening stated in the reports of the President's Commission, the National Academy of Sciences, and the Hastings Center was shown in a table in Wilfond BS, Nolan K. National policy development for the clinical application of genetic diagnostic technologies: lessons from cystic fibrosis. *JAMA* 1993;270:2948–2954.

120. Elias S, Annas GJ. Generic consent for genetic screening. *N Engl J Med* 1994;330:1611–1613.

121. Council on Ethical and Judicial Affairs, American Medical Association. Multiplex genetic testing. *Hastings Cent Rep* 1998;28(4):15–21.

122. Beresford HR, Bernat JL, Brin MF, Ferguson JH, Rosenberg JH, Snyder RD Jr. Practice parameter: genetic testing alert. Statement of the Practice Committee Genetics Testing Task Force of the American Academy of Neurology. *Neurology* 1996;47:1343–1344.

123. See Seshadri S, Drachman DA, Lippa CF. Apolipoprotein E ε4 allele and the lifetime risk of Alzheimer's disease: what physicians know and what they should know. *Arch Neurol* 1995;52:1074–1079 and Hofman KJ, Tambor ES, Chase GA, et al. Physicians' knowledge of genetics and genetic tests. *Acad Med* 1993;68:625–632.

124. American College of Medical Genetics and American Society of Human Genetics Working Group on ApoE and Alzheimer Disease. Statement on using apolipoprotein E testing on Alzheimer disease. *JAMA* 1995;274:1627–1629; Post SG, Whitehouse PJ, Binstock RH, et al. The clinical introduction of genetic testing for Alzheimer's disease: an ethical perspective. *JAMA* 1997;277:832–836; and McConnell LM, Koenig BA, Greely HT, Raffin TA. Genetic testing and Alzheimer's disease: recommendations of the Stanford Program in Genomics, Ethics, and Society. *Genet Test* 1999;3:3–12. These recommendations are discussed in Nusbaum RL, Ellis CE. Alzheimer's disease and Parkinson's disease. *N Engl J Med* 2003;348:1156–1164. For a lucid discussion of the complex genetics in hereditary Alzheimer's disease, see Bird TD. Genetic factors in Alzheimer's disease. *N Engl J Med* 2005;352:862–864.

125. See Gostin LO. Genetic privacy. *J Law Med Ethics* 1995;23:320–330 and Rothstein MA. Genetic privacy and confidentiality: why they are so hard to protect. *J Law Med Ethics* 1998;26:198–204.

126. Legal issues in regulating the misuse of genetic information were discussed in McEwen JE, Reilly PR. State legislative efforts to regulate use and potential misuse of genetic information. *Am J Hum Genet* 1992;51:637–647 and Annas GJ. Privacy rules for DNA databanks: protecting coded "future diaries." *JAMA* 1993;270:2346–2350. For the use and misuse of genetic testing in disability insurance, see Wolf SM, Kahn JP.

Genetic testing and the future of disability insurance: ethics, law & policy. *J Law Med Ethics* 2007;35 (2 Suppl):6–32.

127. Geller G, Tambor ES, Bernhardt BA, et al. Physicians' attitudes toward disclosure of genetic information to third parties. *J Law Med Ethics* 1993;21:238–240.

128. For a discussion of this case and its significance, see Clayton EW. Ethical, legal, and social implications of genomic medicine. *N Engl J Med* 2003;349:562–569.

129. The American Medical Association Council on Ethical and Judicial Affairs. Use of genetic testing by employers. *JAMA* 1991;266:1827–1830.

130. Murray TH. Genetics and the moral mission of health insurance. *Hastings Cent Rep* 1992;22(6):12–17. The concept of actuarial fairness is also considered in Clifford KA, Iuculano RP. AIDS and insurance: the rationale for AIDS-related testing. *Harvard Law Rev* 1997;100:1806–1824.

131. See Kass NE. Insurance for the insurers: the use of genetic tests. *Hastings Cent Rep* 1992;22(6):6–11 and Harper PS. Insurance and genetic testing. *Lancet* 1993;341:224–227.

132. Glazier AK. Genetic predispositions, prophylactic treatments and private health insurance: nothing is better than a good pair of genes. *Am J Law Med* 1997;23:45–68.

133. These social policy questions are examined comprehensively in the genetics-life insurance circumstance in Rothstein MA (ed). *Genetics and Life Insurance: Medical Underwriting and Social Policy.* Cambridge, MA: MIT Press, 2004.

134. Task Force on Genetic Information and Insurance. *Genetic Information and Health Insurance.* Bethesda, MD: National Center for Human Genome Research, 1993. The recommendations of the task force were reprinted in Murray TH. Genetics and just health care: a Genome Task Force report. *Kennedy Inst Ethics J* 1993;3:327–331.

135. Hellman D. What makes genetic discrimination exceptional? *Am J Law Med* 2003;29:77–116.

136. Parker M, Lucassen A. Working towards ethical management of genetic testing. *Lancet* 2005;360:1685–1688.

137. Hudson KL. Prohibiting genetic discrimination. *N Engl J Med* 2007;356:2021–2023.

138. Health Insurance Portability and Accountability Act, PL 104–191, 110 Stat, 1936 (1996).

139. Alper JS. Does the ADA provide protection against discrimination on the basis of genotype? *J Law Med Ethics* 1995;23:167–172. The ADA citation is 42 USC §§ 12101–12213 (1990).

140. Annas GJ, Glantz LH, Roche PA. Drafting the Genetic Privacy Act: science, policy, and practical considerations. *J Law Med Ethics* 1995;23:360–366.

141. Annas GJ. The limits of state laws to protect genetic information. *N Engl J Med* 2001;345:385–388.

142. Greely HT. Banning genetic discrimination. *N Engl J Med* 2005;353:865–867.

143. UNESCO International Declaration on Human Genetic Data. October 16, 2003. http://portal.unesco .org/en/ev.php-URL_ID=17720&URL_DO=DO_TOPIC&URL_SECTION=201.html (Accessed March 22, 2007). The Declaration is discussed in Coupland R, Martin S, Dutli MT. Protecting everybody's genetic data. *Lancet* 2005;365:1754–1756.

144. Symposium. Results of genetic testing: when confidentiality conflicts with a duty to warn relatives. *BMJ* 2000;321:1464–1466.

145. These opinions are discussed in Offit K, Groeger E, Turner S, Wadsworth EA, Weiser MA. The "duty to warn" a patient's family members about hereditary disease risks. *JAMA* 2004;292:1469–1473.

146. American Medical Association Council on Ethical and Judicial Affairs. Opinion 8-I-03. Disclosure of familial risk in genetic testing. http://www.ama-assn.org/ama1/pub/upload/mm/369/ceja_1203j.pdf (Accessed March 22, 2007).

147. Fleisher LD, Cole LJ. Health Insurance Portability and Accountability Act is here: what price privacy? *Genet Med* 2001;3:286–289.

148. Burgess MM, d'Agincourt-Canning L. Genetic testing for hereditary disease: attending to relational responsibilities. *J Clin Ethics* 2001;12:361–372.

149. American Society of Human Genetics Board of Directors and the American Society of Medical Genetics Board of Directors. Points to consider: ethical, legal, and psychosocial implications of genetic testing in children and adolescents. *Am J Hum Genet* 1995;57:1233–1241.

150. Wertz DC, Fanos JH, Reilly PR. Genetic testing for children and adolescents: who decides? *JAMA* 1994;272:875–881.

151. Hoffman DE, Wulfsberg EA. Testing children for genetic predispositions: is it in their best interest? *J Law Med Ethics* 1995;23:331–344 and Ross LF, Moon MR. Ethical issues in genetic testing in children. *Arch Pediatr Adolesc Med* 2000;154:873–879.

152. Wertz DC, Reilly PR. Laboratory policies and practices for the genetic testing of children: a survey of the Helix Network. *Am J Hum Genet* 1997;61:1163–1168.

153. Borry P, Stultiens L, Nys H, Cassiman JJ, Dierickx K. Presymptomatic and predictive genetic testing in minors: a systematic review of guidelines and position papers. *Clin Genet* 2006;70:374–381. Despite this consensus, a majority of Swiss medical and law students believe that the age for independent consent for genetic testing should be lowered to 16 years. See Elger BS, Harding TW. Should children and adolescents be tested for Huntington's disease? Attitudes of future lawyers and physicians in Switzerland. *Bioethics* 2006;20:158–167.

154. Borry P, Fryns JP, Schotsmans P, Dierickx K. Carrier testing in minors: a systematic review of guidelines and position papers. *Eur J Hum Genet* 2006;14:133–138.

155. Ross LF. Predictive genetic testing for conditions that present in childhood. *Kennedy Inst Ethics J* 2002;12:225–244.

156. See Davis DS. Genetic dilemmas and the child's right to an open future. *Hastings Cent Rep* 1997;27(2):7–15 and McGee G. Parenting in an era of genetics. *Hastings Cent Rep* 1997;27(2):16–22.

157. Green RM. Parental autonomy and the obligation not to harm one's child genetically. *J Law Med Ethics* 1997;25:5–15.

158. See Parens E, Asch A, eds. The disability rights critique of prenatal genetic testing: reflections and recommendations. *Hastings Cent Rep* 1999;29(5):S1–S22.

159. Wolf SM. Beyond "genetic discrimination": toward the broader harm of geneticism. *J Law Med Ethics* 1995;23:345–353.

160. For a review of ethical issues in gene therapy, see Smith KR. Gene therapy: theoretical and bioethical concepts. *Arch Med Res* 2003;34:247–268.

161. Anderson WF. Human gene therapy. *Nature* 1998;392(Suppl):25–30. This section was modified from Bernat JL. Ethical Issues in Gene Therapy. Presented at the American Academy of Neurology Annual Meeting, Philadelphia, PA, May 9, 2001. © American Academy of Neurology.

162. Walters L. Ethical issues in human gene therapy. *J Clin Ethics* 1991;2:267–274.

163. Walters L. *J Clin Ethics* 1991:267–274.

164. President's Commission for the Study of Ethical Problems in Medicine and Biomedical and Behavioral Research. *Splicing Life: The Social and Ethical Issues of Genetic Engineering with Human Beings*. Washington, DC: U S Government Printing Office, 1982.

165. Mendell J, Miller A. Gene transfer for neurologic disease: agencies, policies, and process. *Neurology* 2004;63:2225–2232.

166. Kimmelman J. Recent developments in gene transfer: risk and ethics. *BMJ* 2005;330:79–82.

167. Morsy MA, Mitani K, Clemens P, Caskey CT. Progress toward human gene therapy. *JAMA* 1993;270:2338–2345. For example, myoblast transfer of the dystrophin gene has been conducted for the treatment of DMD. See Mendell JR, Kissel JT, Amato AA, et al. Myoblast transfer in the treatment of Duchenne's muscular dystrophy. *N Engl J Med* 1995;333:832–838.

168. Mendell J, Miller A. Gene transfer for neurologic disease: agencies, policies, and process. *Neurology* 2004;63:2225–2232.

169. MacKay CR. Discussion points to consider in research related to the human genome. *Human Gene Ther* 1993;4:77–95 and Holtug N. Altering humans—the case for and against human gene therapy. *Camb Q Healthc Ethics* 1997;6:157–174.

170. McDonough PG. The ethics of somatic and germline gene therapy. *Ann N Y Acad Sci* 1997;816:378–382 and Anderson WF. *Nature* 1998:25–30.

171. Board of Directors of the American Society of Human Genetics. Statement on gene therapy, April 2000. *Am J Hum Genet* 2000;67:272–273.

172. Friedmann T. Principles for human gene therapy studies. *Science* 2000;287:2163–2165.

173. The Gelsinger tragedy and its aftermath are described in Verma IM. A tumultuous year for gene therapy. *Mol Ther* 2000;2:415–416.

174. Hacein-Bey-Abina S, Von Kalle C, Schmidt M, et al. LMO2-associated clonal T cell proliferation in two patients after gene therapy for SCID-X1. *Science* 2003;302:415–419.

175. Davé UP, Jenkins NA, Copeland NG. Gene therapy insertional mutagenesis insights. *Science* 2004;303:333.

176. Friedmann T. *Science* 2000:2163–2165.

177. Kim SY. Assessing and communicating the risks and benefits of gene transfer trials. *Curr Opin Mol Ther* 2006;8:384–389 and Chan S, Harris J. The ethics of gene therapy. *Curr Opin Mol Ther* 2006;8:377–383.

178. Fletcher JC, Richter G. Human fetal gene therapy: moral and ethical questions. *Human Gene Ther* 1996;7:1605–1614.

179. Mattingly SS. The maternal-fetal dyad: exploring the two-patient obstetrical model. *Hastings Cent Rep* 1992;22(1):13–18.

180. Chatterjee A. Cosmetic neurology: the controversy over enhancing movement, mentation, and mood. *Neurology* 2004;63:968–974.

181. Anderson WF. Genetics and human malleability. *Hastings Cent Rep* 1990;20(1):21–24.

182. Miller HI. Gene therapy for enhancement. *Lancet* 1994;344:316–317.

183. American Medical Association Council on Ethical and Judicial Affairs. Gene therapy. In, *Code of Medical Ethics of the American Medical Association: Current Opinions with Annotations*, 2006–2007 edition. Chicago: American Medical Association, 2006:42–43.

184. Wivel NA, Walters L. Germ-line gene modification and disease prevention: some medical and ethical perspectives. *Science* 1993;262:533–538.

185. Fletcher JC, Anderson WF. Germ-line gene therapy: a new stage of debate. *Law Med Health Care* 1992;20:26–38.

186. Marshall E. Moratorium urged on germ line gene therapy. *Science* 2000;289:2023.

187. For example, see Frankel MS. Inheritable genetic modification and a brave new world: did Huxley have it wrong? *Hastings Cent Rep* 2003;33(2):31–36 and King NMP. Accident and desire: inadvertent germline effects in clinical research. *Hastings Cent Rep* 2003;33(2):23–30.

188. See Partridge AH, Winer EP. Informing clinical trial participants about study results. *JAMA* 2002;288:363–365 and Shalowitz DI, Miller FG. Disclosing individual results of clinical research: implications of respect for participants. *JAMA* 2005;294:737–740.

189. See Fuller BP, Kahn MJ, Barr PA, et al. Privacy in genetics research. *Science* 1999;285:1359–1361; National Bioethics Advisory Commission. *Research Involving Human Biological Materials: Ethical issues and Policy Guidance*. Rockville, MD: National Bioethics Advisory Commission, 1999; and Beskow LM, Burke W, Merz JF, et al. Informed consent for population-based research involving genetics. *JAMA* 2001;286:2315–2321.

190. Hull SC, Gooding H, Klein AP, Warshauer-Baker E, Metosky S, Wilfond BS. Genetic research involving human biological materials: a need to tailor current consent forms. *IRB* 2004;26(3):1–7.

191. Bookman EB, Langhorne AA, Eckfeldt JH, et al. Reporting genetic results in research studies: summary and recommendations of an NHLBI working group. *Am J Med Genet A* 2006;140:1033–1040.

192. Knoppers BM, Joly Y, Simard J, Durocher F. The emergence of an ethical duty to disclose genetic research results: international perspectives. *Eur J Hum Genet* 2006;14:1170–1178.

193. Ravitsky V, Wilfond BS. Disclosing individual genetic results to research participants. *Am J Bioethics* 2006;6:8–17.

194. Scheuner MT, Wang SJ, Raffel LJ, Larabell SK, Rotter JI. Family history: a comprehensive genetic risk assessment method for the chronic conditions of adulthood. *Am J Med Genet* 1997;71:315–324.

195. See the discussions of the unique features of pedigree research ethics in Frankel MS, Teich AH. *Ethical and Legal Issues in Pedigree Research*. Washington, DC: American Association for the Advancement of Science, 1993 and American Society of Human Genetics. ASHG report: statement on informed consent for genetics research. *Am J Hum Genet* 1996;59:471–474.

196. Botkin JR. Protecting the privacy of family members in survey and pedigree research. *JAMA* 2001;285:207–211.

197. Worrall BB, Chen DT, Meschia JF. Ethical and methodological issues in pedigree stroke research. *Stroke* 2001;32:1242–1249.

HIV and AIDS

18

Despite its familiarity, acquired immunodeficiency syndrome (AIDS) has been recognized as a clinical entity only since 1981. In slightly more than a quarter-century, AIDS has grown from a clinical curiosity to a "pandemic [that is] undoubtedly the defining public health crisis of our time."[1] Although, in developed countries, the availability of highly active antiretroviral therapy (HAART) and comprehensive treatment has converted human immunodeficiency virus (HIV) infection to a chronic disease,[2] it remains a terminal disease throughout most of the developing world. Because there is neither a cure nor a vaccine and because primitive public health measures in many parts of the world are inadequate to provide proper treatment or to prevent its spread, HIV/AIDS promises to become a greater public health threat during the 21st century, primarily in the poor and developing world.

The human immunodeficiency virus, transmitted from an infected person, causes AIDS.[3] Disease transmission requires intimate exposure to an infected person's body fluid, particularly blood, semen, and cervicovaginal secretions. HIV transmission occurs most often through heterosexual or homosexual intercourse, intravenous injections performed with shared needles, transfusions of infected blood and blood products, and from mother to fetus or neonate.[4]

A "clinical latent period" of 4 to 12 years separates the acute HIV infection and the conversion to AIDS. Although few outward symptoms are present during the latent period, the peripheral blood CD4[+] T-lymphocyte count becomes progressively depleted. In untreated people, the duration of the latent period varies as a function of the baseline CD4[+] count and HIV viral load in combination with host genetic and immunological factors.[5] The latent period may be shorter in cases of massive viral infection from blood transfusion. The latent period also may be longer. There are documented cases of persons infected with HIV for decades who have developed neither declining CD4[+] counts nor AIDS.[6]

AIDS can be diagnosed in two ways: (1) by the presence of HIV antibodies and a peripheral blood CD4[+] cell count of <200 cells/μL; or (2) by HIV seropositivity and evidence of one or more "indicator diseases," such as *Pneumocystis carinii* pneumonia, *Cryptococcus neoformans* meningitis, *Toxoplasma gondii* encephalitis, Kaposi's sarcoma, primary central nervous system lymphoma, pulmonary tuberculosis, recurrent bacterial pneumonia, or cervical cancer among others.[7]

As of January 1, 2006, more than 25 million persons worldwide already had died of AIDS and over 40 million persons had HIV infection or AIDS, of whom approximately 1.1 million were residents of the United States. The epidemic remains worst in sub-Saharan Africa and other tropical regions of the developing world where infection rates continue to rise far more rapidly than in the developed world and where the prevalence of HIV infection in several countries exceeds 25%. Of the 4.3 million new HIV cases occurring worldwide in 2006, over 95% occurred in developing countries. In the developing world, HIV spreads primarily through heterosexual intercourse whereas in the United States and Europe, a major mode of HIV transmission is men who have sex with men. The HIV epidemic in the developing world is further accelerated by lack of preventive services, social stigma, government denial, labor migration, concurrent sexual partnerships, gender inequalities, limited availability of condoms, and lack of circumcision.[8] HIV infection is the fourth leading cause of death worldwide, resulting in 2.9 million deaths in 2006.[9]

The Centers for Disease Control and Prevention (CDC) estimated that as of January 1, 2006, over 988,000 cumulative cases of AIDS had occurred in the United States with over 550,000 AIDS-related deaths. The actual figure may be higher because of inaccurate diagnoses on death certificates. By January 1, 2006, over 438,000 persons in the United States were living with AIDS, there were over 46,000 new HIV infections annually, and over 17,000 people died annually from AIDS. Approximately one-fourth of the 1.04 to 1.19 million Americans infected with HIV as of January 1, 2004, were unaware of their infection.[10] In 1992, AIDS became the leading cause of death in the United States in men between the ages of 25 and 44 years. African-Americans and Hispanic-Americans are affected disproportionately, with infection rates eight and three times higher respectively than in Caucasian-Americans.[11] In 2005, AIDS patient ethnicity in the United States had the following composition: African-American 48%, Caucasian 28%, Hispanic 18%, and other ethnicity 6%.[12]

Beginning in 1996, the annual death rates from HIV in the United States began to fall as a consequence of widespread treatment of AIDS patients with HAART.[13] The trend of increased survival times also has been observed in other parts of the developed world, including western Europe and Australia. Decreasing AIDS death rates in the developed world are attributed primarily to the availability of antiretroviral drugs and secondarily to improved prophylaxis against opportunistic infections, improved overall treatment of the HIV patient, improved access to health care, post-exposure prophylaxis, and decreased numbers of new HIV cases resulting from successful preventive efforts.[14]

Unfortunately, this promising trend is conspicuously absent in the developing world where the large majority of HIV patients reside and where most new infections occur. The death rates from HIV in sub-Saharan Africa and other parts of the tropical developing world continue to rise, largely because of poverty and its consequences, particularly the inability of HIV patients to afford antiretroviral, antibacterial, and antifungal drugs, social and cultural factors, and the absence of an effective public health infrastructure to implement preventive efforts and provide basic medical care.[15]

AIDS can be considered as a neurological disease although HIV is not classified as a neurotropic virus like rabies or poliovirus. Although HIV does not directly invade neurons, it is considered "neuroinvasive" because, when it enters the body, it infects the parenchyma of the brain and spinal cord and the cerebrospinal fluid. Infected macrophages and other monocytes are believed to carry the virus to the nervous system.[16] Primary parenchymal invasion of the brain and spinal cord produces the AIDS-dementia complex and HIV myelopathy.

Many infections, neoplasms, and other secondary complications of AIDS affect the nervous system. Thus, neurologists may examine HIV/AIDS patients to diagnose and treat seizures, headaches, dementia, confusion, stupor, coma, stroke, meningitis, or movement disorders, and may diagnose HIV infection of the brain and spinal cord, cryptococcal meningitis, toxoplasma encephalitis, primary central nervous system lymphoma, progressive multifocal leukoencephalopathy, and various myelo-pathies, radiculopathies, neuropathies, and myopathies.[17] As many as two-thirds of adults and 90% of children with AIDS eventually develop overt, symptomatic neurological disorders.[18]

Patients with HIV infection pose challenging ethical, social, and legal dilemmas.[19] A gradual consensus has emerged over the past two decades that has rendered some of the original issues less controversial. The evidence for this consensus is that scholarly debate over them has largely ceased. However, the resolved dilemmas have been superseded by more urgent international ethical issues. I discuss the historical account of the original ethical dilemmas because understanding how a consensus over them was achieved offers important lessons that may help to resolve emerging ethical problems.

The ethical issues in patients with HIV/AIDS during the early stage of the pandemic challenged decision makers in our society to re-examine the fundamental assumptions underlying the care physicians and nurses give AIDS patients and the extent of the patients' rights. What are the professional duties of physicians and nurses to treat AIDS patients if they risk becoming infected accidentally? Under what circumstances can or should physicians breach their duty to maintain a patient's confidentiality and privacy by disclosing HIV status to protect his sexual partners from becoming infected? Who should be screened for HIV infections? Is HIV an exceptional disorder requiring a higher level of confidentiality than other diseases? In what ways can or should the civil rights of AIDS patients be compromised to halt the spread of the disease? Should physicians and other health-care workers be screened routinely for HIV? How much claim do patients dying with AIDS have on scarce medical resources, such as intensive care units, cardiovascular surgery, cardiopulmonary resuscitation, and hemodialysis? Should the scientific and public safety rules ordinarily required for the testing of new pharmaceuticals be relaxed for "compassionate" reasons in the treatment of AIDS patients?

A newer set of ethical questions stems from the global pandemic of HIV sweeping the developing world and causing untold suffering and early death, destroying families, and ruining economies. What is the ethical duty of the developed world to try to halt the epidemic by helping to provide therapy to patients in the developing world?[20] Is the global inequality of life expectancy between the developed and developing world resulting from HIV/AIDS an ethical issue?[21] To what extent should assistance be provided by governments and by private citizens? To what extent can the developing world dictate safe practices to members of the developing world that they may resist for cultural reasons? Does research using human subjects with HIV/AIDS performed in the developing world require equal, greater, or lesser human subject protection than in the developed world?

IMPEDIMENTS IN THE PHYSICIAN-PATIENT RELATIONSHIP

The relationship between physicians and patients with HIV/AIDS may become strained by physicians' fear, prejudice, hatred, and burnout. The fear of contracting HIV from the patient during medical care can negatively affect a physician's attitude toward the patient. Physicians may harbor prejudice and hatred, blaming gay men or intravenous drug abusers with AIDS for having engaged in avoidable unhealthy behaviors. Finally, physicians may develop burnout from the rigors of providing continuous care to a dying patient.[22]

Is a physician's fear of contracting AIDS from an infected patient rational? Physicians and other health-care workers who treat HIV-infected patients risk being injured from contaminated needles or other sharp instruments or being exposed to blood or other bodily fluids through their mucous membranes. Although this risk has been estimated, its exact extent remains imprecise because the rates of HIV-seropositivity in patients vary in different communities and the chance of being injured in practice differs among various medical specialists. The risk to most physicians who employ universal precautions is extremely low in the absence of a needlestick accident.

The CDC estimated that a health-care worker has a 0.003 annual risk of becoming HIV-seropositive as the result of an accidental injury from a hollow-bore needle containing HIV-seropositive blood.[23] Physicians who do not perform surgery suffer an accidental needlestick or other sharp injury about once every two years, and surgeons suffer them about four times as often. If we assumed that all needles and sharps were contaminated with HIV-seropositive blood, the annual risk of seroconversion would be approximately 0.0015 for a generalist or internist and would be about 0.006 for a surgeon.

These figures are artificially high because not all needles and sharps involved in accidents are contaminated with HIV-seropositive blood and not all blood-contaminated sharps carry equal risks of transmitting HIV. For example, transmission of HIV has been documented in injuries from hollow-bore needles used in venipuncture but not from solid needles, such as those used for surgical suturing. In a case-control study, Denise Cardo and colleagues identified the following risk factors for needle-stick HIV seroconversion: deep injury, injury with a device visibly contaminated with the infected patient's blood, injury occurring during attempted arterial puncture or venipuncture, and exposure to a source patient who died within two months of AIDS.[24] For most physicians who treat relatively few HIV-positive patients, the risk is minuscule. For example, if an internist's practice consisted of 5% HIV-seropositive patients, his annual risk for accident-induced seroconversion would be no higher than 0.000075. The risk can be lowered further by immediate post-exposure chemoprophylaxis with antiretroviral drugs which are highly effective in preventing HIV seroconversion if administered to exposed caregivers within 48 hours.[25]

For at-risk physicians whose practice consists of higher percentages of HIV-seropositive patients, particularly if they perform procedures, the risks become more significant. If a surgeon's practice consisted of 50% HIV-seropositive patients, his annual risk for accident-induced seroconversion would be as high as 0.003. This is a highly significant risk for contracting what could become a fatal disease. To place these risk data into perspective, the annual risk of death faced by firefighters is approximately 0.002.[26]

Physicians have responded to the real and perceived risk of HIV infection by devising several strategies. The most rational response has been to adhere strictly to protocols of universal precautions, such as appropriate gloving, shielding, and recapping of needles after injection. Some physicians also formulated regulations and practices that restricted HIV-seropositive patients from undergoing certain procedures in which the risk of HIV transmission is great. Hemodialysis, plasma exchange, cardiovascular surgery, orthopedic surgery, and neurosurgery are examples of such high-risk procedures. This practice becomes of questionable morality, however, when the reason to limit or prohibit these treatment modalities in AIDS patients is disguised misleadingly as "medical appropriateness" or "medical judgment."

Denial of certain forms of therapy for HIV-seropositive patients should be based on the real risk to the health-care provider, without being a covert action. Each therapeutic modality should be selected on the basis of its efficacy in a given clinical situation. Although the risks of transmission from each therapeutic modality are not irrelevant, they should be considered honestly and directly. Conscious attempts should be made to reduce the risks. If the risks remain too great after reasonable attempts to minimize them, physicians can refuse to perform the therapeutic procedure, although the actual reason should be cited.

In a recent review of performing surgery on HIV patients, Darin Saltzman and colleagues pointed out that, in the past 20 years, restrictive practices have nearly ceased because of improved surgical outcomes, more accurate data showing a low risk to the surgical team, more uniform use of universal precautions, and the availability of effective post-exposure chemoprophylaxis.[27] Greater health-care worker risk in treating HIV patients exists in developing countries where HIV prevalence rates are high and where disposable syringes, sterilized equipment, universal precautions supplies, and post-exposure prophylaxis medication are less available.[28]

Prejudice and hatred can confound the physician-patient relationship if physicians blame patients, such as gay men or intravenous drug abusers, for contracting AIDS because of risky practices. Patients with AIDS from these groups have been stigmatized because of their homosexuality or drug abuse, and may be unfairly perceived as having diminished social value and even as a threat to society.[29] Unfortunate public proclamations by a few religious leaders that AIDS represents divine retribution for sinful behavior have exaggerated this stigma.[30] Further, a disproportionate percentage of HIV/AIDS patients are already disenfranchised by society because of their minority and socioeconomic status.

The extent to which physicians expressed prejudicial attitudes toward gay male AIDS patients was revealed in a case vignette survey. The physicians were presented with two identical case histories, the only difference being that one was a homosexual man with AIDS and the other a heterosexual man with leukemia. The responding physicians were questioned about their feelings and attitudes after reading the cases. Analysis of these responses disclosed that significantly more physicians blamed the AIDS patient for his disease and felt less sympathy for him, less willingness to talk to him, less interest in attending a party if he were present, and less willingness to work in the same office with him.[31] It requires little imagination to extrapolate the damaging effects that these negative attitudes have on a physician's relationship with an AIDS patient.

In a remarkable but disheartening book entitled *Getting Rid of Patients*, Terry Mizrahi graphically described the negative attitudes and unprofessional behavior of resident physicians when they were faced with the obligation to care for patients they found unpleasant, hateful, or uninteresting. One such group was composed of patients whom the residents blamed for their condition. Another comprised patients with chronic illnesses whom the residents believed they could not cure. The anger, frustration, depersonalization, and outright discrimination these residents exhibited in their clinical encounters with these patients illustrates the damage that prejudices can wreak on the physician-patient relationship.[32]

Physician burnout during the chronic care of AIDS inpatients also exerts a negative impact on the physician-patient relationship. In the pre-HAART era when a diagnosis of AIDS was a death sentence, residents on medical wards containing many AIDS patients often cared for severely ill and inexorably dying patients largely of their own age. This care required engaging in a series of emotionally stressful battles in the course of treating acute, life-threatening complications of AIDS when they knew they would ultimately lose the war. Repeated episodes of this frustrating and seemingly futile experience led to physician burnout, similar to that seen in physicians and nurses on inpatient oncology and bone marrow transplantation wards. Burnout is characterized by depression, emotional blunting, overwhelming sense of failure, and nihilistic attitudes toward therapeutic endeavors. A quintessential symptom that health-care workers experience with burnout is losing the sense of caring about the patient.[33] When physicians have burnout, it is highly unlikely that they can sustain a successful physician-patient relationship.[34] Fortunately, these problems are much less common in the HAART era because of markedly increased life expectancies.

There is now a legal remedy in the United States for unjustified discrimination against patients with HIV or AIDS. In their 1998 ruling in *Bragdon v. Abbott*, the U.S. Supreme Court found that the American With Disabilities Act of 1990 provided antidiscrimination protection to citizens infected with HIV because HIV infection counts as a disability.[35] Although judicial rulings may not change people's prejudicial attitudes or erase their negative stereotypes, *Bragdon v. Abbott* clearly provides a legal remedy for overt and unjustified instances of discrimination against patients with HIV in housing, employment, and education.

THE PHYSICIAN'S DUTY TO TREAT

Do physicians have the right to refuse to treat an HIV/AIDS patient or do they have a professional duty to treat the patient even at their own personal risk? This question has engaged much thoughtful discussion since the risk to physicians was first described. The issue has been approached from several perspectives. For example, historical accounts of physicians' behaviors and duties in previous epidemics have shown some who have conducted courageous acts of dedication and altruism, and some who have performed acts of self-protection and cowardice.[36] Other scholars have emphasized that physicians as professionals have ethical duties to treat the ill that include assuming risks of incurring personal harm.[37] Medical societies' codes of professional conduct have formalized duties of dedication to sick patients.[38] The physician's legal duty to treat illness has been analyzed,[39] and virtue-based theories of physician behaviors have been cited to demand that physicians show courage in the face of danger.[40] Each of these perspectives sheds some light on the answer.

Historians have recorded physicians' behaviors during epidemics such as the Black Death of Europe in the 14th century, the Great Plague of London in the 17th century, and the yellow fever epidemic of Philadelphia in the 18th century. During each of these epidemics, some dedicated physicians remained to care for the sick and dying, greatly risking their own health and lives, while others fled. Fleeing physicians provided several justifications for their behavior: (1) the duty to care for their patients who also were fleeing the city; (2) the duty to maintain their own health in order to treat other patients; and (3) the responsibility of self-preservation, which compelled them not to carry out suicidal missions.[41] Of course, these justifications may be viewed simply as self-serving rationalizations motivated by the primary goal of self-protection.

Ezekiel Emanuel explained the fundamental reason why physicians have a duty to treat AIDS patients. Medicine, as a learned profession and not a trade, creates binding ethical obligations on its members. Were medicine simply a commercial enterprise whose objective was the accumulation of wealth, no such binding obligations to others would exist. Medicine, however, is a learned profession dedicated to the moral ideal of promoting the welfare of patients as its highest professional ethic, not the betterment of its practitioners' financial status. When a person enrolls, trains, and becomes socialized into the profession of medicine, he takes an explicit and implicit oath to uphold this commitment to treat the sick, even at some risk to his own health.[42]

Codes of medical professional conduct provide physicians with the freedom to decide whom to treat, within bounds. (See chapter 3.) To the best of their ability, physicians should treat all patients in an emergency situation. They are neither required nor should they be expected to provide treatment that lies outside the scope of their training. However, if physicians possess the requisite training, it would be unethical to refuse to treat HIV patients solely on the basis of their diagnosis because prejudicial behavior on these grounds counts as unjustified discrimination.

How does the concept of personal risk to the physician fit into this discussion? An irreducible degree of personal risk is implicit in the treatment of sick patients. Physicians over the years have contracted countless cases of infectious diseases from their patients, including plague, tuberculosis, hepatitis, leprosy, and the common cold. The assumption of a certain degree of risk in acquiring infectious diseases is intrinsic to the medical and nursing professions. The willingness to enter these professions entails the willingness to endure these risks.[43]

Yet there should be a reasonable limit to such risks. No one should require physicians or anyone else to endure risks in their practices that are tantamount to suicide. Extreme risks can be assumed voluntarily as a supererogatory act, but they should not be mandated as a professional duty. At what degree of personal risk do physicians lose their professional duty to continue caring for patients?

The annual risk of physicians acquiring HIV from their patients in most settings has been quantified as less than 0.001. In general, this risk is not sufficiently high to justify a physician's refusal to care for an HIV/AIDS patient because the risk is not excessive by accepted social standards in other professions entailing personal risk. For surgeons whose practices consist largely of HIV/AIDS patients, a more significant danger exists. In this case, it is reasonable for physicians and hospital administrators to devise mechanisms to lower the risk, such as arranging for a group of surgeons to share equally in the treatment of high-risk patients. Pregnant physicians whose clinical practice could put them at significant risk of HIV seroconversion should be suspended from this duty to treat because maternal infection produces a 50% chance of fetal infection.[44] All health-care workers should be thoroughly trained in universal precautions to which they should adhere at all times and they should receive prompt post-exposure chemoprophylaxis.[45]

Medical societies have concurred unanimously that physicians have an ethical duty to treat HIV/AIDS patients. This duty has been affirmed in formal pronouncements by a number of societies, including the American Medical Association, the American College of Physicians, the Infectious Diseases Society of America, the American Academy of Neurology, the American College of Obstetrics and Gynecology, and the Surgeon General of the United States.[46]

PRIVACY AND CONFIDENTIALITY

The laudable goal of maintaining the privacy and confidentiality of HIV/AIDS patients becomes an ethical dilemma if other persons are harmed in the process. The privacy rights of the patient and the right of third parties in jeopardy of harm from the infected patient may conflict in two related areas: providing consent for HIV testing and the notification of a sexual partner without the patient's consent. Over the past decade, the aura of exceptionalism for HIV testing that required an added layer of confidentiality protection is in the process of being reversed with the introduction of programs of routine screening and mandatory partner notification.

HIV Testing

When the serum test for the HIV antibody first became available and was validated in 1985, a consensus emerged that the test should be performed only with a patient's informed and voluntary consent, except in a few well-defined circumstances.[47] Mandatory screening without consent was permitted only for the following groups: prospective blood, organ, or tissue donors; military personnel; prisoners; and life insurance applicants.[48] Hospitals drafted rules to protect the confidentiality of patients who were tested to safeguard them from harm. These rules required a patient's written informed consent before the test could be performed.

The justification for classifying HIV infection an "exceptional" disease that required a level of consent and confidentiality exceeding that necessary in other conditions was to prevent the feared outcomes of stigmatization and unjustified discrimination against the patient. Harms to HIV patients, including

infringement of liberties and outright discrimination in employment, housing, and education, were amply recorded in the early days of the pandemic.[49] These harms could be prevented by requiring voluntary consent and absolute confidentiality of HIV testing.[50] The public health argument was widely accepted that a democratic society should favor voluntary rather than mandatory public health programs for disease control.[51] HIV was thus granted an exceptional status requiring explicit, written consent and extreme confidentiality of test results in medical records.

Serological data initially supported selective HIV screening. Mandatory HIV screening of low-risk populations was regarded as undesirable because of the relatively high rate of false-positive results in comparison with those obtained from screening high-risk populations.[52] Both serum tests for HIV—the enzyme-linked immunosorbent assay (ELISA) and the Western blot test—have a very high sensitivity and specificity for detecting HIV antibodies (specificities of 0.998 and 0.994, respectively), but, according to Bayes' Theorem, their positive predictive value depends on the prevalence of HIV in the population screened.

When both tests are used, the false-positive rate has been estimated to fall between 0.0001 and 0.00001.[53] A false-positive rate of 0.0001 would be perfectly acceptable for a screening test if the population screened had a disease prevalence of 0.1, because there would be only one false positive for each 1,000 true positives. But the same false-positive rate would be unacceptably high if the population screened had a disease prevalence of 0.00003, because the number of false positives and true positives would be about equal. Thus, for example, the positive predictive value of a positive HIV serology in a homosexual man, intravenous drug abuser, or woman prostitute is 0.999, but it is only 0.647 in a woman who is a first-time blood donor with no HIV risk factors.[54]

There was an early consensus among scholars and public officials that screening high-risk patients was valuable, but routine screening was rejected by most institutions and in most jurisdictions. Even in the earlier phase of the pandemic, some commentators advocated voluntary screening of all patients on hospital admission if they lived in communities with high seroprevalence rates. In this way, hospital inpatients, who probably represent a high-risk group, could receive immediate treatment following diagnosis.[55] In this spirit, the CDC recommended that hospitals treating patients in communities with high rates of HIV infection should offer voluntary HIV serum testing and counseling to all patients aged 15 to 54.[56] This policy seemed justified by the results of a subsequent study showing that mandatory inpatient HIV testing was not cost-effective unless the hospital seroprevalence rate exceeded 1%.[57] However, subsequent studies performed in the HAART era showed that HIV screening was cost-effective even in relatively low prevalence populations.[58] These data helped spur the CDC to abandon their longstanding selective policy and to advocate broad routine screening (see below).

Prior to the 1990s, asymptomatic HIV-seropositive patients who were identified early benefited from being followed medically at intervals and from receiving preventive counseling on how to halt the spread of HIV to others. However, the identification that an asymptomatic patient was HIV-seropositive could be perceived as a social liability because the patients could be unjustifiably discriminated against in employment, education, or housing. These two opposite effects were generally perceived as more or less balancing each other; therefore, the patients themselves were permitted to make the decision about whether they would undergo early testing.

This balance has been disturbed now that there is compelling evidence that patients receive health benefits by early determination of HIV seropositivity. Patients found to be infected with HIV, before it has progressed to AIDS, can undergo preventive treatment for infectious diseases that later could become florid and difficult to treat. Tuberculin tests can be performed on HIV-seropositive patients before they become anergic, and inactive tuberculosis can be eradicated to prevent its activation later in the course of AIDS. Similarly, before anergy occurs, HIV-positive patients can be immunized against *Haemophilus influenzae*, pneumococcus, and hepatitis A and B. Furthermore if identified in

a timely fashion, life-saving prophylactic treatment can be given to prevent infection with *Pneumocystis carinii*, *Mycobacterium avium* complex, and *Toxoplasma gondii*, among others. Further, patients can be screened for common complicating co-infections such as syphilis, gonorrhea, chlamydia, viral hepatitis and human papilloma virus.[59]

A major benefit of early HIV diagnosis is the early institution of HAART. HAART dramatically prolongs life expectancy of patients with AIDS, and earlier institution of HAART prolongs life in comparison to HAART started during HIV-related immunodeficiency.[60] One reason for this effect is the prevention of AIDS-related opportunistic infections.[61] Moreover, by lowering the HIV viral load, HAART can prevent transmission to uninfected sexual contacts of patients on therapy.[62] Thus, the benefits of early diagnosis of a patient's HIV-seropositivity now clearly exceed its harms.

In response to recent recommendations from the United States Preventive Services Task Force[63] and the publication of cost-effectiveness data from the HAART era showing benefits of HIV screening in low-risk situations,[64] in September 2006, the CDC issued a sweeping revision of its earlier testing guidelines. Whereas the CDC previously recommended routine HIV testing only for persons at high risk or for persons in health-care environments with high seroprevalence rates, the new CDC guidelines recommended routine HIV screening for all persons aged 13 to 64 years irrespective of risk factors, HIV seroprevalence, or other factors.[65] The CDC policy contains an "opt-out" provision that permits patients to refuse HIV testing, but its default mode is to permit testing in the absence of explicit refusal.[66] No longer is there a requirement for the patient to sign a separate consent; general consents are sufficient. Commentators have pointed out that the new CDC policy is evidence of the "end of HIV exceptionalism" in which HIV testing now is considered to be identical to that of any other diagnostic testing.[67] State and local policy-makers now must decide whether and how to change existing laws to incorporate this recommendation.

The new CDC guidelines also have impacted on approaches to formerly contentious HIV ethical and legal consent issues. One important issue is whether HIV testing ethically can be conducted on critically ill patients from whom consent cannot be obtained. The new CDC guideline will support hospitals in the design of policies permitting clinicians to test critically ill patients for HIV without explicit consent when the physician determines that testing is likely to alter the patient's diagnostic or therapeutic management in a meaningful way.[68] A second issue is whether patients can be compelled to undergo HIV testing after a health-care worker caring for the patient has sustained a needlestick injury.[69] Whereas most patients readily consent, I have performed ethics consultations in instances in which consents were not given or possible. In one case, the patient refused testing. In the second, the patient died and post-mortem testing was requested. Hospital lawyers were divided on the question of whether state law banned post-mortem HIV testing without prior consent. In the new paradigm of non-exceptionalism, these questions would be easier to resolve because the elevated standard of explicit consent demanded by HIV exceptionalism no longer would be required.

I believe that the CDC revision will facilitate an appropriate revision of protective laws that have overprotected patients at the risk of health-care workers. A strong argument can be made that health-care workers suffering needlestick injuries have a right to know if they have been exposed to HIV and other pathogens. They should not be forced to undergo the risks of chemoprophylaxis and worrying because laws enacted to protect patients from discrimination have unreasonably interfered with the appropriate medical care of health-care workers.

Partner Notification

Until the mid 1990s, the law in the United States was curiously ambivalent regarding public health surveillance of HIV and AIDS. Beginning in 1983, the law mandated that AIDS be reported in all states, but there was no similar uniform mandatory HIV reporting.

Throughout the 1980s, most states did not classify HIV infection as a sexually transmitted, communicable disease; thus, the sexual contacts of HIV-seropositive patients without AIDS were not traced systematically. Partner notification was considered as an entirely voluntary pursuit.[70]

This seemingly paradoxical situation was largely the result of the influence of politically well-organized gay organizations that understandably feared that mandatory HIV reporting and partner notification laws could compromise their privacy and confidentiality and lead to a series of discriminatory practices. Thus, HIV infection without AIDS became an exception to the public health rules governing other sexually transmitted diseases. Throughout the 1980s, medical groups attempted unsuccessfully to have HIV classified as a sexually transmitted, communicable disease.[71]

Public attitudes about HIV as an "exceptional" disease began to change in the early 1990s with the publication of data showing that HIV-seropositive patients without AIDS benefited directly from early comorbid disease prevention and antiretroviral treatment. When these data became widely publicized, the organized opposition to reporting the HIV-positive status of patients began to diminish. Thereafter, both the number of states requiring that HIV infection be reported by name and the number permitting or requiring partner notification increased.[72] A 1999 review found 31 states with laws mandating that public health officials be notified of positive HIV status with patients' names.[73] Contrary to fears, the introduction of mandatory reporting by name did not diminish the use of voluntary HIV testing in publicly funded programs.[74] The current public health regulation trend to increasingly require HIV patient reporting by name has been described as the social change "from exceptionalism to normalism."[75] Some scholars have argued that only a national HIV surveillance system can adequately monitor the epidemic, and they have proposed a model national system.[76]

Voluntary partner notification schemes have had mixed results.[77] In the only randomized trial undertaken, the responsibility for partner notification was left to the index patient in one group and to the health-care provider in the other. Despite a state law that required the HIV-infected patient to notify his partner(s), the investigators found that index patients were unsuccessful in doing so whereas public health counselors were highly effective.[78] A successful partner notification program run by public health workers has been in effect in Sweden since 1985.[79]

Although physicians ordinarily have an ethical and legal duty to maintain patient confidentiality, that duty may be superseded by the ethical duty to protect other persons known to be at risk. The duty not to disclose the diagnosis of HIV may need to be abrogated to protect the health and safety of partners of HIV-seropositive patients known to be at risk for unknowingly contracting the disease.[80] Some state courts have found a legal duty for clinicians to disclose a patient's HIV-positive status to at-risk persons and public health officials.[81]

If a physician practices in a state that requires HIV infections to be reported and partners to be notified, he should report this information to responsible public health officials. If a physician practices in a state that does not require this information, he should assess the degree of risk his patient poses to his partners. If this risk is substantial, the physician should urge the patient to notify his partners voluntarily. Given the value of maintaining a long-term clinical relationship with patients with HIV infection, every effort should be made to facilitate partner notification in a collaborative fashion. However, if the patient's partner remains at risk and the patient steadfastly refuses to notify him or her or take proper precautions against HIV transmission, the physician should take the necessary steps to report this to a public health official. If the public health official refuses to warn the partner, the physician should notify the partner directly because, in this case, the duty to warn trumps the duty to preserve patient confidentiality.[82] In the United Kingdom, the Home Office suggested criminalizing HIV transmission without adequate warning when the subject knowingly and negligently infects another person. An ethical analysis shows an unequivocal duty of the infected patient to warn and protect a partner at risk.[83]

THE HIV-INFECTED PHYSICIAN

Another ethical and legal controversy centered on the appropriate restrictions that should be placed on an HIV-infected physician. The prevalence of HIV-infected physicians is unknown, but the essential issues would remain the same even if the number were small. Do HIV-infected physicians endanger their patients? Should they be permitted to practice? What aspects of their medical practice pose a risk to patients? Do patients have a right to know if their physician is HIV-seropositive? Should physicians or other health-care workers be screened for HIV? How can we balance the rights of physicians with HIV to practice against the rights of patients to be protected from unnecessary harm?

These questions first reached public attention through several newspaper reports about surgeons dying of AIDS. Despite the fact that there had been no reported instances of surgeon-to-patient transmission of HIV, public fear and outcry was immediate. The overwhelming majority of people surveyed in several polls indicated that they would not want to be treated by an HIV-infected physician. They also believed that they had the right to know the HIV status of their physician.[84] Public concern reached hysterical proportions when a report was confirmed that a Florida dentist with AIDS had transmitted HIV to six of his patients.[85]

The only plausible mechanism for an HIV-infected physician to transmit HIV to his patient is for his infected blood to enter the patient's bloodstream. Theoretically, such transmission could occur during surgery if a physician's finger was cut by a needle or sharp instrument and his blood absorbed by the patient's body. The CDC estimated the risk of this event to be between 1 in 42,000 and 1 in 420,000 surgical operations. Based on the number of operations in the United States and the estimated number of HIV-seropositive surgeons, the CDC estimated that surgeons could have infected between 3 and 28 patients as of 1991.[86]

However, practicing surgeons subsequently presented convincing data showing that the CDC prediction was an overestimate for most surgical settings.[87]

Numerous epidemiologic "look-back" studies on the HIV status of patients who underwent surgical procedures performed by HIV-seropositive surgeons have failed to disclose a single case of documented transmission.[88] In the largest such study, the CDC followed 22,171 patients of 64 HIV-positive clinicians and found not a single case of clinician-to-patient transmission of HIV infection.[89] Moreover, epidemiologic models predict a minuscule theoretical risk of physician-to-patient HIV transmission.[90]

Thus, the Florida dentist case appears to be unique and inexplicable. Detailed epidemiological studies of this case have failed to elucidate the mode by which HIV was transmitted to the six patients infected.[91] Because of the apparent uniqueness of this case, the fact that six patients were infected, and the lack of a clear mechanism for transmission, intentional infection has been entertained as a plausible explanation.

Despite the improbability of physician-to-patient HIV transmission, medical societies, hospitals, and governmental agencies have formulated positions and regulations governing the professional activities of HIV-infected physicians. The American Medical Association (AMA) initially stated that "a physician who knows that he or she is seropositive should not engage in any activity that creates a risk of transmission of the disease to others."[92] Subsequently, the AMA clarified that its proscription was limited to those invasive procedures that "pose an identifiable risk" to patients.[93]

The American Academy of Orthopedic Surgeons recommended voluntary, confidential HIV testing for orthopedic surgeons. The Academy stated that HIV-infected orthopedic surgeons should not perform surgical procedures in which there is a high probability of injuries from sharps, such as those using internal fixation devices and wires.[94] Yet, a carefully performed 13-year look-back study of the HIV-seropositivity status of 2,317 patients operated on by an HIV-infected orthopedic surgeon disclosed not a single

case of surgeon-to-patient transmission of HIV.[95]

CDC regulations in this area have inspired controversy since their publication in 1991. Among other provisions, the CDC requires the identification of "exposure-prone" procedures that present a "recognized risk of percutaneous injury to the health-care worker and . . . the health care worker's blood is likely to contact the patient's body cavity, subcutaneous tissues and/or mucous membranes." Physicians and dentists performing exposure-prone procedures should know their HIV status. HIV-infected physicians and dentists should not perform exposure-prone procedures unless an expert review panel has given them permission.[96] In a later minor modification of the guidelines, the CDC eliminated the requirement for listing exposure-prone procedures and referred to them collectively as "invasive procedures."[97]

In the ethical analysis of this problem, it is axiomatic that the welfare of the patient should remain paramount.[98] If, while undergoing surgery or dentistry, patients are exposed to a potential risk from an HIV-infected professional, they need to understand the magnitude of the risk in order to provide valid consent. Unfortunately, most patients' concept of the risk exaggerates its true size by several magnitudes. It has been estimated that the risk of contracting HIV from a surgeon during an operation is one-tenth the risk of dying from general anesthesia administered for the operation itself, a risk that all patients accept who consent to surgery. Further, the risk of contracting HIV during surgery is comparable to the risk of contracting fatal hepatitis B from a surgeon, which has not produced a similar public outcry for physician testing or regulation. The risk is also similar to that of contracting HIV from a blood transfusion after the blood has been tested negative for HIV.[99]

Despite the minuscule risk of contracting HIV from a surgeon, the desire to avoid it is rational. Patients routinely bank their own blood preoperatively to avoid an identical risk from heterologous blood transfusion. Therefore, the CDC recommendations attempting to minimize this tiny risk are reasonable.

Surgeons and other physicians who engage in exposure-prone, invasive procedures that provide an opportunity for the transmission of HIV should volunteer to be tested. All physicians who have risk factors for HIV should volunteer to be tested. If they are seropositive, they should consult with an expert panel to judge whether it is safe for them to continue to perform certain operative procedures. The protection of patients should remain the highest ethic.

Patients have the right to know if their physician is HIV-seropositive only if the physician poses a risk to them. Otherwise, there is no ethical duty for physicians to be tested or to disclose their antibody status to their patients. Two legal analyses similarly concluded that no legal duty exists for physicians to disclose their HIV status in the absence of demonstrable risk to the patient.[100]

Most office and hospital encounters with an HIV-infected physician pose essentially zero risk to patients, just as most similar encounters with an HIV-infected patient pose essentially no risk to physicians. Moreover, two studies showed that it is not cost-effective to routinely screen physicians, surgeons, or dentists for HIV.[101] Thus, to mandate mass HIV screening of physicians and other health-care professionals would be a misguided policy based more on fear than on reason. Such mass screening would produce financial and human costs that would exceed its benefits.[102]

HIV-seropositive physicians or surgeons have a right to practice in most clinical settings. They should cease only those exposure-prone, invasive procedures that produce a risk of transmission to patients. If they are qualified, they should be permitted to practice in other areas of medicine in which they do not pose a risk to patients.[103] I believe that, as a condition of employment, physicians should be given the opportunity to purchase disability insurance to protect them financially in a future situation in which they may be prevented from practicing their profession.[104]

Supervisors of HIV-infected physicians should act rationally and responsibly. Hospital administrators should avoid tragic overreactions, such as that which destroyed the career of the resident physician, Dr. Hacib Aoun.[105]

Similarly, legal overreaction should be shunned, such as that demonstrated by the hospital that summarily revoked all surgical privileges from an otorhinolaryngologist with AIDS.[106] With guidance from the expert panel, the HIV-infected physician and his supervisor need to work out a practice arrangement that fully protects patients but does not unjustifiably discriminate against physicians.

UNORTHODOX THERAPIES

A vexing ethical issue in treatment that was common in the 1980s involved HIV patients who used "nonvalidated therapies." In the AIDS subculture of several American urban communities, unusual substances alleged to have efficacy against HIV were self administered routinely in the hope that they would be effective. Bernard Lo described the smuggling of "compound Q" into the United States from China and its illicit use by AIDS patients in San Francisco. This substance, derived from the roots of the Chinese cucumber, had been touted by some AIDS patients as a cure despite the fact that there was no scientific evidence of its efficacy. Illicit use of compound Q resulted in serious complications, including seizures, coma, and death.[107]

Benjamin Freedman defined nonvalidated therapies as "those drugs, medical, and surgical interventions, and regimens that are offered to and accepted by a patient on the basis of potential benefit, and that have neither been accepted nor discredited by the scientific community."[108] Freedman observed ironically that many more patients were prepared to accept the risks of nonvalidated therapies than those willing to participate in controlled scientific trials. In some well-educated and affluent gay AIDS communities, use of unorthodox substances was widespread.

Informed consent becomes an issue when unorthodox substances are used. If a patient chooses to try an unknown substance because he has heard through his friends that it active against HIV, is such consent truly voluntary when he feels that he has no choice because he is dying of AIDS? How can the decision be informed when the knowledge of side effects is scanty or absent? And as the unfortunate experience with compound Q proved, simply because a person with AIDS believed that he was beyond help, it does not necessarily follow that he was beyond being hurt.[109]

The best solution to the unorthodox substance problem is to optimize the patient's trust in his relationship with his physician. Unfortunately, many physicians may find it difficult to earn that trust. Patients with HIV/AIDS have been discriminated against and stigmatized publicly. As a result, they may distrust organized medicine and have implicit faith only in their own subculture. Physicians need to prove to HIV/AIDS patients that they are committed to caring for them and wish to work with them to fight the disease together.

In the setting of a trusting relationship, the physician can inspect the unorthodox medications that the patient is taking. The physician should approve of those that are harmless, such as many vitamins and herbs, but the patient who is taking unorthodox substances known to be harmful should be counseled that this behavior is irrational and dangerous. If the patient wishes to try a new agent, the physician can help him get access to one in a treatment protocol or on a parallel track. Ideally, the patient should be encouraged to enroll in a treatment study so that his experience can be used to further scientific knowledge and help future patients. It is generally believed that because of the efficacy of HAART, the use of unorthodox substances has diminished.

END-OF-LIFE ISSUES

Medical treatment of the AIDS patient at the end of life raises ethical issues involving the use of intensive care and palliative care.[110] The decision whether to provide curative (disease-specific) or palliative (symptom-specific) care to patients with HIV/AIDS has evolved dramatically with changes in prognosis resulting from HAART and the accumulation of data showing improved outcomes after aggressive treatment of opportunistic infections. Peter Selwyn and Marshall Forstein pointed out that the "curative vs. palliative care" decision in patients with late-stage HIV/AIDS represents a false dichotomy because HAART has transformed HIV into a chronic disease and comprehensive late-stage treatment should embrace both elements simultaneously.[111]

Not only in the terminal phase of their illness can AIDS patients become critically ill. Florid pulmonary failure from *Pneumocystis carinii* pneumonia (PCP) is a common occurrence that warrants intensive care treatment during the midcourse of AIDS. With proper aggressive treatment today, many critically ill patients with PCP can be successfully discharged from the hospital. Several clinical issues involving decisions to treat AIDS patients in intensive care units (ICUs) have ethical dimensions. How confidently can we state the prognosis of critically ill AIDS patients? What kinds of treatment are they offered and what kind do they want? How do physician attitudes toward AIDS patients influence their treatment? How does society's attitude toward them influence their treatment?

Early reports in the pre-HAART era indicated that AIDS patients required intensive care primarily for treatment of pulmonary failure from PCP. AIDS patients also were admitted to ICUs for seizures, cardiovascular instability, sepsis, coma, or organ system failure, or to perform special procedures. Numerous reports suggested that the prognosis of AIDS patients in pulmonary failure from PCP was very poor. As a result, trends in the 1980s showed a continuing decrease in ICU treatment because patients and physicians believed such therapy to be futile.[112]

A turning point occurred in the late 1980s, when improved therapy for PCP improved prognosis. In a 1992 review of published outcome studies of critical care for patients with AIDS, Robert Wachter and colleagues at San Francisco General Hospital found that the reported survival rates of patients with AIDS complicated by PCP-induced respiratory failure increased from 0% to 14% in the mid-1980s to 36% to 55% by the early 1990s. They concluded that PCP-induced respiratory failure in AIDS patients no longer could be considered a medically untreatable complication.[113] Similarly, better treatment protocols improved the prognoses of central nervous system toxoplasmosis and cryptococcal meningitis in AIDS patients.

The third era of PCP treatment occurred during the 1990s. Wachter and colleagues showed that the cost-effectiveness of PCP treatment of AIDS patients had fallen to a level lower than that of many other accepted medical interventions, such as intensive care unit admissions for patients with cancer. Two reasons they cited for this change were a greater use of DNR orders among AIDS patients yielding a generally sicker group of patients undergoing aggressive treatment, and a marked increase in ICU costs and lengths of stay for treatment.[114]

AIDS patients' attitudes about receiving intensive care treatment also have evolved with improvements in outcomes. In a study performed in the 1980s when patient outcomes from PCP-induced pulmonary failure were poor, Robert Steinbrook and colleagues at San Francisco General Hospital surveyed 188 homosexual AIDS patients about their treatment preferences. They found that 95% of the patients desired antibiotics and hospital admission for PCP, but only 55% would consent to ICU admission and 46% to cardiopulmonary resuscitation (CPR).[115] These generally well-educated AIDS patients were aware of the dismal statistics on AIDS patients once they required ICU care. They considered pulmonary failure from PCP as a marker for imminent death; therefore, many chose to die without life-sustaining treatment once this complication ensued. The same nihilistic attitudes about PCP in AIDS patients were found among residents and attending physicians caring for them. When the physicians communicated the poor prognosis, they agreed with their patients that ICU care for severe PCP was not indicated.[116]

With the inception of HAART, the prognosis of HIV infection and even the most devastating opportunistic infections has changed dramatically. Given the changes in the prognosis of PCP with new forms of treatment, both AIDS patients and their physicians should alter their obsolete attitudes and make decisions about intensive care based on contemporary data. The decisions made in this context are nonetheless extremely complex, and can test both physician and patient concepts of the nature of their relationship.[117]

Some patients with HIV/AIDS request physician-assisted suicide or euthanasia. (See chapter 9.) Euthanasia and physician-assisted suicide now are practiced widely in the Netherlands. A Dutch study recently reported that homosexual men with AIDS comprised a disproportionate percentage of patients requesting and undergoing euthanasia and physician-assisted suicide.[118] In the United States, physician-assisted suicide has been explicitly legalized only in the state of Oregon. During the first nine years of the law, the Oregon Health Division reported that the percentage of AIDS patients requesting and conducting physician-assisted suicide was 30 times greater than that of the mean of all dying patients in Oregon.[119]

HIV/AIDS patients should be encouraged to complete advance directives for medical care before they become critically ill. Studies in the 1990s found that patients with HIV/AIDS were less likely than other patients to prepare advance directives and discuss end-of-life treatment wishes with physicians.[120] The situation improved a decade later (see below). Patients' decisions about these directives should be based on contemporary information regarding treatment and prognosis. Directives should stipulate the patient's wish for life-sustaining ICU care as well as for CPR. It is particularly important for AIDS patients to complete advance directives early in the course of their illness because they may become incompetent because of neurological complications as the disease progresses. Ideally, patients should name a health-care agent to make medical decisions for them should they become incompetent.[121]

Neil Wenger and colleagues studied the prevalence of end-of-life discussions, use of advance directives, and preferences of end-of-life treatment in a cross-sectional survey of over 230,000 adults with HIV from whom 2,864 patients were sampled randomly. They found that only 50% of patients had discussed some aspect of end-of-life care with their practitioner and that 38% had completed an advance directive. Black and Latino patients were less likely than Caucasian patients to discuss preferences. Women and patients with children in the household were most likely to discuss preferences. Patients who had acquired HIV by intravenous drug abuse and those with less education were least likely to have prior end-of-life discussions with practitioners. The groups underutilizing advance care planning should receive targeted interventions in HIV treatment programs.[122]

Dying patients with AIDS need proper palliative care.[123] But, as in other chronic treatable but ultimately fatal diseases, striking a balance between curative and palliative care can be difficult in the setting of progressive illness. With the advent of HAART, AIDS has been converted most commonly to a chronic disease that ultimately is fatal. But given the markedly increased longevities with HAART, some HIV patients die of unrelated conditions before they die of AIDS or HIV complications. As is true in other chronic diseases, curative and palliative approaches are mutually compatible and can be provided simultaneously.[124] A recent critique of the outcomes of palliative care in HIV/AIDS patients concluded that "home palliative care and inpatient hospice care significantly improved patient outcomes in the domains of pain and symptom control, anxiety, insight, and spiritual wellbeing."[125]

PEDIATRIC ISSUES

Children born of mothers infected with HIV have a high risk of contracting the disease. The risk of transmission can be dramatically reduced by maternal treatment with antiretroviral drugs and omission of breast feeding.[126] Most mothers willingly take antiretroviral drugs and omit breast feeding to protect their unborn child from infection. Occasionally, mothers refuse: I was an ethics consultant in one case in which an HIV-infected mother refused to believe the data on transmission and feared toxicity from the drugs. The actions of obstetricians and pediatricians in such cases have legal and ethical dimensions. In some cases, physicians who are unable to convince the mother have pursued legal action to secure a judicial order mandating maternal treatment.[127] In many jurisdictions, however, no legal remedy is possible until after the child is born. This and other ethical and legal issues involving pregnant women with HIV arising in the perinatal period have been the subject of scholarly discourse.[128]

An emerging medical and ethical issue that affects the female partner (and potentially the child) of an HIV-infected man is whether to permit the use of reproductive technologies to reduce the risk of paternal HIV transmission. In cases in which the man is HIV-infected but the woman is not ("discordant couple"), in vitro fertilization using the man's washed sperm can reduce the rate of HIV transmission to the woman, and thereby to the child. Ethical analyses of this practice conclude that because it achieves pregnancy more safely than sexual intercourse, it produces more benefit than harm and violates no ethical principles.[129] Baker and colleagues described a program that safely and successfully used this technology when the HIV-infected man had an undetectable viral load.[130] The unique ethical considerations of using reproductive technology to treat infertility when the mother is infected with HIV also have been analyzed.[131]

The ethical conundrums raised by the risk of transmission of HIV from mother to child do not end at childbirth: breastfeeding remains a major source of HIV transmission to children around the world today.[132] Because breastfeeding lasts longer than parturition, antiretroviral therapy to prevent transmission is more complex and less well studied. Furthermore, breastfeeding is the major if not the only source of safe infant nutrition in many parts of the world. Thus, counseling women to avoid HIV transmission by eschewing breastfeeding is a complex and evolving topic.[133]

A common ethical question affecting older children and adolescents infected with HIV is when and how to disclose their diagnosis. Now that HAART has permitted HIV-infected babies to survive to older childhood and adolescence, informing children of their diagnosis becomes necessary at some point. Some scholars have made the analogy of the duty to disclose a child's HIV infection to the duty to disclose a child's diagnosis of cancer. The two diagnoses have different meanings to the parents, however, that may influence their willingness to disclose the diagnosis. Unlike cancer, childhood HIV is imbued with social stigma, discrimination, and parental guilt over transmission.[134]

The American Academy of Pediatrics (AAP) *encourages* developmentally appropriate disclosure to school-age children and *strongly recommends* disclosure to adolescent patients.[135]

There is less controversy over the need for disclosure than over when and how to disclose. Erin Flanagan-Klygis and colleagues performed surveys of pediatricians and parents just prior to publication of the AAP guideline. They found what other researchers had found earlier, that pediatricians reported a high rate of not disclosing the diagnosis of HIV to children aged 4 to 12. The rate of pediatricians' willingness not to disclose at the parents' request fell as the child got older but was 30% even for children over age 12. Physicians reported ambiguity over the proper course of action in the face of parental nondisclosure in children over age 8: over 50% of pediatricians responded "undecided." The investigators found that 65% of parents did not disclose the diagnosis to their child. To explain their reasons, parents cited concerns over the child's capacity to understand, their fear that the child would become depressed, and their fear of creating social stigma and discrimination. The investigators recommended that physicians help parents develop a plan of when to disclose and how much to disclose as the child matures that is individually determined and that respects the particular needs and interests of the parents and child.[136] One technique to assist determining these needs that also helps to make treatment decisions later in the illness is conducting a "values history" of parents with HIV-infected children.[137]

RESEARCH ISSUES

Several research ethics issues arise in patients with HIV/AIDS. Should HIV/AIDS patients be granted an exception to the usual strict rules for research in therapeutics? Should unvalidated therapies be permitted for use in treating AIDS patients? How can we encourage participation in HIV research by underrepresented groups? How can prisoners with HIV/AIDS serve as human research subjects? How can HIV/AIDS research be conducted ethically in developing countries?[138]

In the days before HIV/AIDS became a chronic disease, activists argued that therapeutic agents believed to be effective against HIV should be exempt from the rigorous scrutiny ordinarily required of new pharmaceuticals to demonstrate safety and efficacy. Activists pointed out that patients were dying while research on therapeutic agents was being carried out in a leisurely manner. They believed that it was morally wrong to withhold any possibly effective therapy from dying patients. They lobbied vigorously to relax the Food and Drug Administration (FDA) rules that govern investigational new drugs (IND) in the treatment of HIV. A similar level of activism in cancer patients to lobby for access to unapproved cancer drugs through a high-profile lawsuit against the FDA was rejected in August 2007 by the Court of Appeals for the District of Columbia Circuit.[139]

As a result of lobbying and public sympathy, AIDS activists were successful in modifying the FDA rules that apply to testing of agents believed to be effective for HIV by the passage of the Treatment Investigational New Drug (IND) Rule.[140] This rule permits the clinical use of drugs on AIDS patients before testing shows them to be effective if three conditions have been satisfied: (1) the FDA finds some evidence that the agent "may be effective"; (2) the risks of the agent are not "unreasonable and significant"; and (3) the agent is used to treat only an immediate life-threatening condition. As a result of the Treatment IND Rule, experimental agents for HIV have become available sooner to the general public.[141]

The second major accomplishment by the AIDS activists was to modify the requirement for randomized clinical trials (RCT) to prove drug efficacy in AIDS and HIV patients. In many studies, the highly rigorous RCTs have been replaced with less rigorous "community studies." With enrollment in a community study, each patient is given the authority to specify which drug he wishes to take. Investigators observe and record the effects of the agent on the course of each patient's disease in a standardized format without controls or blinds.[142] Additionally, randomized clinical trials have been designed and executed using surrogate markers.

AIDS activists also spurred the development of the "parallel track" mechanism that allows patients to receive INDs. The parallel track permits patients with AIDS and HIV to receive investigational drugs despite not being enrolled in a formal study protocol. Those eligible to receive INDs on a parallel track include patients who cannot tolerate standard therapies, patients who have not responded to standard therapies, patients who reside at too great a distance from the study site, and patients who are ineligible to enroll or, for other reasons, cannot enroll in a research protocol.[143]

Disagreement between scientists and AIDS activists over patient access to experimental drugs results partially from contradictory views about the purposes of clinical trials. Clinical investigators and scientists view the trials as research; that is, as means to obtain scientific knowledge about the efficacy and safety of pharmaceuticals in different clinical situations. Conversely, patients view clinical trials as therapy designed to benefit the patient directly. Although investigators also want the experimental subjects to benefit, that is not the primary goal of the clinical trial.[144]

To some extent, changes in FDA policy have resulted from necessity and not simply from political activism and public compassion. There have been major problems in enrolling AIDS patients in phase three clinical trials of new pharmaceutical agents. Many patients who believed they had been randomized to placebo or control groups dropped out of the studies. Some patients purposely broke the study rules by consuming illicit substances or obtaining the study drug through clandestine sources. Other patients took greater doses of study drugs than were permitted in the protocol. Each of these noncompliant behaviors resulted from the patients' primary motivation, which was to give themselves the greatest probability of cure, not necessarily to further scientific research.[145]

The IND rules attempted to salvage scientific research in the setting of epidemic noncompliance by HIV-seropositive research subjects.[146] However, the new rules exacted a cost on the science of therapeutics research and on the welfare of the HIV-seropositive community. The ability to bypass RCTs diminished the scientific value of pharmaceutical studies because researchers could not guarantee that they would be able to exclude confounding variables systematically. The design

and implementation of the RCT was a major advance in clinical therapeutics. Compromise on scientific integrity hamstrung the interpretation of data from community studies on the efficacy of new agents because investigators were not able to draw confident conclusions about which agents were effective and which were not in various clinical circumstances. Nevertheless, some investigators argued that RCTs could be abandoned in some scientific studies without a great loss of validity.[147]

One commentator observed that by bowing to the *realpolitik* of the research marketplace, the FDA may have "set back rather than advanced the search for better therapies for AIDS."[148] This was an unfortunate outcome because future HIV-seropositive patients would suffer the most harm from the lack of scientific evidence for the efficacy of pharmaceuticals, despite years of use. Benjamin Freedman concluded "more lives will be saved, in the end, by aiming accurately than by aiming early."[149] Yet, the parallel track has been useful as a mechanism to study patients not available otherwise for scientific study.

Some ethnic and demographic groups are underrepresented among patients volunteering for HIV clinical trials. Several studies in the 1990s showed fewer minority groups and women as human subjects.[150] Allen Gifford and colleagues performed a large survey in the United States in which 2,864 subjects were chosen randomly from 231,400 adults with HIV infection. They found that 14% of patients participated in a medication trial or study, 24% had received experimental medications, and 8% had tried and failed to receive experimental treatments. Blacks and Hispanics were less likely to participate in clinical trials, as were patients enrolled in health maintenance organizations, but women were not underrepresented. The authors believed that negative attitudes of Blacks and Hispanics about serving as research subjects and their distrust of researchers were responsible.[151] The ethical and legal barriers to permitting incarcerated prisoners with HIV to serve as research subjects have been examined, with model guidelines proposed.[152]

An area of continuing controversy surrounds the question of whether HIV research in developing countries should be conducted under the same ethical rules as those required in developed countries. As described further in chapter 19, on ongoing tension exists between the requirements of the Declaration of Helsinki and the needs of citizens in developing countries. The Declaration of Helsinki requires that: "The benefits, risks, burdens and effectiveness of the new method should be tested against those of the best current prophylactic, diagnostic and therapeutic methods . . . At the conclusion of the study, every patient entered into the study should be assured of access to the best prophylactic, diagnostic and therapeutic methods identified by the study."[153] However, these requirements are often unrealistic in countries so poor that they cannot afford medications or do not possess a health-care infrastructure sufficient to provide the "best" treatments identified.

Harold Shapiro and Eric Meslin, representing the U.S. National Bioethics Advisory Commission, argued that clinical trials carried out in developing countries by research groups or companies in the United States should be bound by American ethical standards. We never should exploit vulnerable populations and we should limit trials to those that are responsive to host countries' needs and their abilities to provide to their populations.[154] But often, representatives of the affected developing countries believe that their citizens would derive benefit from conducting the trials and charge developed countries with "ethical imperialism" by trying to forcibly export their ethical standards. The solution is to create a collaboration between IRBs in the developed world and representatives of the host countries to produce research guidelines that are both ethically sound and provide for the needs and best interests of the citizens of the host countries.[155] The resulting research is best conceptualized as a "partnership" between researchers and citizens of the host countries.[156]

PUBLIC POLICY ISSUES

One factor affecting the treatment for HIV/ AIDS patients results from the attitude of society, given that AIDS is a chronic and ultimately terminal illness that consumes substantial amounts of money and medical resources. The cumulative direct cost of medical care for HIV patients is staggering. In a recent study in the United States, using current therapy guidelines, the lifetime cost of medical care was $618,000 for an HIV-infected adult with a CD4+ count of <350 cells/μL, whose projected life expectancy was 24.2 years. The lifetime cost was $567,000 for a patient with a CD4+ count of <200 cells/μL, whose projected life expectancy was 22.5 years.[157] In the current era of HAART, the cost profile has evolved from predominantly inpatient hospital costs to predominantly outpatient pharmaceutical costs. In a 2001 study of the costs of treating HIV infections, the annual direct costs were found to have decreased from $20,300 to $18,300 between 1996 and 1998, reflecting less inpatient care.[158]

In the United States, 40% to 50% of patients with AIDS are covered by Medicaid.[159] State Medicaid programs pay varying amounts for the expensive antiretroviral drugs but more than 20% of patients with AIDS lack Medicare, Medicaid, and private insurance and cannot afford to buy the drugs. The federally funded, state-administered AIDS Drug Assistance Programs (ADAPs) were created as part of Title II of the Ryan White Comprehensive AIDS Resources Emergency Act (CARE) to fulfill this need.[160] Over 100,000 people with HIV received payment for antiretroviral medications through this program in 2000.[161] Although coverage for antiretroviral drugs currently is adequate in most states, coverage for drugs to treat opportunistic infections remains uneven.[162]

Pharmacoeconomic models predict overall public cost savings with full insurance payment of HAART costs because of an anticipated concomitant reduction in inpatient and outpatient care expenses.[163] But in addition to purely economic considerations, moral considerations dictate that our affluent society should provide antiretroviral therapy to all patients who could benefit from it. This moral duty challenges those in the developed world to solve the global problem of how to provide proper therapy to the vast majority of HIV patients dying in impoverished countries from the utter lack of adequate health care and treatment.[164]

In many urban medical centers in the United States, there remains a disproportionate burden on emergency room and inpatient services from patients with AIDS. I use the term disproportionate only to indicate that AIDS patients who require emergency services or hospitalization are very ill and, as a result, generally need more high-technology and skilled, labor-intensive services than patients with other diseases.[165]

Some observers view this strain on the medical system as competition for finite hospital resources between HIV/AIDS patients and patients with other disorders, both of whom are very ill. The increasing demand on ICU beds indicates that these beds will need to be increasingly rationed in the future. Because of the competition for scarce medical resources, prospective utilization strategies must be developed for intensive care unit beds.[166] Those who draft these strategies have an ethical duty to scrutinize outcome studies and employ concepts of justice. Utilization strategies should not be influenced by irrational fears, prejudice, or unjustified discrimination against HIV/AIDS patients. Those who develop strategies for use of ICU beds should take into account the young age of most HIV/AIDS patients who potentially have more years to live than comparably ill older patients with heart disease or stroke. Policy makers designing a national health-care system should employ concepts of justice in the design of rules for the rationing of ICU beds and other scarce medical resources.

NOTES

1. Simon V, Ho DD, Abdool Karim Q. HIV/AIDS epidemiology, pathogenesis, prevention, and treatment. *Lancet* 2006;368:489–504.

2. A recent study in Denmark showed that the mean survival of an HIV-infected adult was more than 35 years from the time of infection to death. See Lohse N, Hansen AB, Pederson G, et al. Survival of persons with and without HIV infection in Denmark, 1995–2005. *Ann Intern Med* 2007;146:87–95.

3. Two human immunodeficiency viruses, known as HIV-1 and HIV-2, have been identified as the causative agents of AIDS. The overwhelming majority of AIDS cases in the United States are caused by HIV-1. For simplicity, I refer to both viruses as HIV throughout the chapter.

4. Friedland GH, Klein RS. Transmission of the human immunodeficiency virus. *N Engl J Med* 1987; 317:1125–1135.

5. Pantaleo G, Graziosi C, Fauci AS. The immunopathogenesis of human immunodeficiency virus infection. *N Engl J Med* 1993;328:327–335.

6. Lifson AR, Buchbinder SP, Sheppard HW, et al. Long-term human immunodeficiency virus infection in asymptomatic homosexual and bisexual men with normal CD4+ lymphocyte counts: immunologic and virologic characteristics. *J Infect Dis* 1991;163:959–965.

7. Centers for Disease Control 1993 revised classification system for HIV infection and expanded surveillance case definition for AIDS among adolescents and adults. *MMWR* 1992;41:1–10. The adoption of this new definition increased the official prevalence of AIDS in the United States. See Chaisson RE, Stanton DL, Gallant JE, et al. Impact of the 1993 revision of the AIDS case definition on the prevalence of AIDS in a clinical setting. *AIDS* 1993;7:857–862.

8. Beyrer C. HIV epidemiology update and transmission factors: risks and risk contexts—16th International AIDS Conference epidemiology plenary. *Clin Infect Dis* 2007;44:981–987.

9. World Health Organization. *Global Summary of the AIDS Epidemic, December 2006.* http://www.who.int/hiv/mediacentre/02-Global_Summary_2006_EpiUpdate_eng.pdf (Accessed April 13, 2007). For a learned commentary on the worldwide epidemiology of AIDS, see Fauci AS. The AIDS epidemic: considerations for the 21st century. *N Engl J Med* 1999;341:1046–1050.

10. Department of Health and Human Services. Centers for Disease Control and Prevention. *HIV/AIDS Surveillance Report* Vol 17. Cases of HIV infection and AIDS in the United States and dependent areas, 2005. http://www.cdc.gov/HIV/topics/surveillance/basic.htm#hivest (Accessed March 31, 2007).

11. *HIV/AIDS Surveillance Report.* Vol 10, No 2. Atlanta: Centers for Disease Control and Prevention, 1998:1–43 and Update: mortality attributable to HIV infection among persons aged 25–44 years—United States, 1991 and 1992. *MMWR* 1993;42:869–872.

12. Department of Health and Human Services. Centers for Disease Control and Prevention. *HIV/AIDS Surveillance Report* Vol 17. Cases of HIV infection and AIDS in the United States and dependent areas, 2005. http://www.cdc.gov/HIV/topics/surveillance/basic.htm#hivest (Accessed March 31, 2007).

13. Lee LM, Karon JM, Selik R, Neal JJ, Fleming PL. Survival after AIDS diagnosis in adolescents and adults during the treatment era, United States, 1984–1997. *JAMA* 2001;285:1308–1315. The principles of antiretroviral drug use in HIV are discussed in Feinberg MB, Carpenter CC, Fauci AS, et al. Report of the NIH Panel to Define Principles of Therapy of HIV Infection. *Ann Intern Med* 1998;128:1057–1078. The latest guidelines for the use of highly active antiretroviral therapy (HAART) in HIV in varying stages were published in 2006 by the International AIDS Society—USA Panel. See Hammer SM, Saag MS, Schechter M, et al. Treatment for adult HIV infection. 2006 recommendations of the International AIDS Society–USA Panel. *JAMA* 2006;296:827–843. For these and other treatment guidelines, see Rathbun RC, Lockhart SM, Stephens JR. Current HIV treatment guidelines—an overview. *Curr Pharm Des* 2006;12:1045–1063 and the HIV/AIDS Treatment Information Service (ATIS) website http://www.hivatis.org/(Accessed March 31, 2007).

14. Fauci AS. *N Engl J Med* 1999:1047–1048. For a recent review of the efficacy of antiretroviral therapy to prevent the sexual transmission of HIV, including post-exposure prophylaxis, see Cohen MS, Gay C, Kashuba ADM, Blower S, Paxton L. Narrative review: antiretroviral therapy to prevent the sexual transmission of HIV-1. *Ann Intern Med* 2007;146:591–601.

15. For thoughtful commentaries by Jonathan Mann on the ethical issues of HIV treatment and prevention in the Third World, see Mann JM. Medicine and public health: ethics and human rights. *Hastings Cent Rep* 1997;27(3):6–13 and Mann J, Tarantola D, O'Malley J. Toward a new health strategy to control the HIV/AIDS pandemic. *J Law Med Ethics* 1994;22:41–52.

16. Epstein LG, Gendelman HE. Human immunodeficiency virus type 1 infection of the nervous system: pathogenetic mechanisms. *Ann Neurol* 1993;33:429–436.

17. The neurological complications of AIDS have been the subject of several reviews. See Brew BJ. *HIV Neurology*, 2nd ed. New York: Oxford University Press, 2007; Berger JR (ed). Neurological complications of AIDS. *Semin Neurol* 1999;19:101–234; and McArthur JC, Brew BJ, Nath A. Neurological complications of HIV infection. *Lancet Neurology* 2005;4:543–555.

18. American Academy of Neurology AIDS Task Force. Human immunodeficiency virus (HIV) infection and the nervous system. *Neurology* 1989;29:119–122.

19. There is a large literature on the ethical issues in patients with HIV/AIDS. General sources to consult include Reamer FG, ed. *AIDS & Ethics*. New York: Columbia University Press, 1991; Manuel C, Enel P, Charrel J, et al. The ethical approach to AIDS: a bibliographic review. *J Med Ethics* 1990;16:14–27; Simberkoff MS. Ethical aspects in the care of patients with AIDS. *Neurol Clin* 1989;7:871–882; and Walters L. Ethical issues in the prevention and treatment of HIV infection and AIDS. *Science* 1988;239:597–603. The specific ethical duties neurologists have toward AIDS patients were outlined in the American Academy of Neurology Ethics and Humanities Subcommittee. The ethical role of neurologists in the AIDS epidemic. *Neurology* 1992;42:1116–1117. The legal issues concerning AIDS patient have been reviewed in Dickens BM. Legal rights and duties in the AIDS epidemic. *Science* 1988;239:580–586 and Gostin LO. The AIDS Litigation Project: a national review of court and human rights commission decisions. Parts 1 and 2. *JAMA* 1990;263:1961–1970, 2086–2093.

20. See Gostin LO. Why rich countries should care about the world's least healthy people. *JAMA* 2007;298:89–92 and World Health Organization and UNAIDS. *Guidance on Ethics and Equitable Access to HIV Treatment and Care*, 2004. http://www.who.int/ethics/en/ethics_equity_HIV_e.pdf (Accessed April 9, 2007).

21. Dorling D, Shaw M, Smith GD. Global inequality of life expectancy due to AIDS. *BMJ* 2006;332:662–664.

22. Levine RJ. AIDS and the physician-patient relationship, In: Reamer FG, ed. *AIDS & Ethics*. New York: Columbia University Press, 1991:199–204.

23. Henderson DK, Fahey BJ. Willy M, et al. Risk for occupational transmission of human immunodeficiency virus type 1 (HIV-1) associated with clinical exposures: a prospective evaluation. *Ann Intern Med* 1990;113:740–746. The risk of seroconversion of 0.0036 after needlestick injury is documented in Tokars JI, Marcus R, Culver DH, et al. Surveillance of HIV infection and zidovudine use among health care workers after occupational exposure to HIV-infected blood. *Ann Intern Med* 1993;118:913–919.

24. Cardo DM, Culver DH, Ciesielski CA, et al. A case-control study of HIV seroconversion in health care workers after percutaneous exposure. *N Engl J Med* 1997;337:1485–1490.

25. Henderson DK. Postexposure chemoprophylaxis of occupational exposures to the human immunodeficiency virus. *JAMA* 1999;281:931–936. The same treatment can be administered after nonoccupational HIV exposure through sexual intercourse or shared needles. Considerations for the use of such treatment

were discussed in Lurie P, Miller S, Hecht F, Chesney M, Lo B. Postexposure prophylaxis after nonoccupational HIV exposure: clinical, ethical, and policy considerations. *JAMA* 1998;280:1769–1773.

26. The estimated incidence of needlestick injuries sustained by medical practitioners and its analogy to the risk of death of firefighters is from Emanuel EJ. Do physicians have an obligation to treat patients with AIDS? *N Engl J Med* 1988;318:1686–1690. These data may be underestimates. A recent study of needlestick injuries in surgical residents and fellows found that many injuries were unreported. See Makary MA, Al-Attar A, Holzmueller CG, et al. Needlestick injuries among surgeons in training. *N Engl J Med* 2007; 356:2693–2699.

27. Saltzman DJ, Williams RA, Gelfand DV, Wilson SE. The surgeon and AIDS: twenty years later. *Arch Surg* 2005;140:961–967.

28. Sagoe-Moses C, Pearson RD, Perry J, Jagger J. Risks to health care workers in developing countries. *N Engl J Med* 2001;345:538–541.

29. Jonsen AR. The duty to treat patients with AIDS and HIV infection. In: Gostin LO, ed. *AIDS and the Health Care System*. New Haven: Yale University Press, 1990:155–168. Albert Jonsen pointed out that the word "stigma" is derived from the Greek word describing the mark used to brand a criminal, explicitly identifying him as one who does not deserve the rights of other members of society.

30. Data on negative public attitudes toward AIDS patients during the early years of the epidemic were summarized in Blendon RJ, Donelan K. Discrimination against people with AIDS: the public perspective. *N Engl J Med* 1988;319:1022–1026.

31. Kelly JA, St. Lawrence JS, Snith S Jr, Hood HV, Cook DJ. Stigmatization of AIDS patients by physicians. *Am J Public Health* 1987;77:789–791.

32. Mizrahi T. *Getting Rid of Patients: Contradictions in the Socialization of Physicians*. New Brunswick, NJ: Rutgers University Press, 1986:70–78. See also an earlier work on the same subject: Groves JE. Taking care of the hateful patient. *N Engl J Med* 1978;298:883–887. Formal surveys of resident physicians have also disclosed their negatives attitudes toward AIDS patients. See Shapiro MF, Hayward RA, Guillemot D, et al. Residents' experiences in, and attitudes toward, the care of persons with AIDS in Canada, France, and the United States. *JAMA* 1992;268:510–515.

33. Zuger A. AIDS on the wards: a residency in medical ethics. *Hastings Cent Rep* 1987:17(3):16–20.

34. Spickard A, Gabbe SG, Christensen JF. Mid-career burnout in generalist and specialist physicians. *JAMA* 2002;288:1447–1450.

35. See Annas GJ. Protecting patients from discrimination—the Americans With Disabilities Act and HIV infection. *N Engl J Med* 1998;339:1255–1259 and Parmet WE. The Supreme Court confronts HIV: reflections on *Bragdon v. Abbott*. *J Law Med Ethics* 1998;26:225–240.

36. Zuger A, Miles SH, Physicians, AIDS, and occupational risk: historic traditions and ethical obligations. *JAMA* 1987;258:1924–1928; Zuger A. AIDS and the obligations of health care professionals. In Reamer FG, ed. *AIDS & Ethics*. New York: Columbia University Press, 1991; and Fox DM. The politics of physicians' responsibility in epidemics: a note on history. *Hastings Cent Rep* 1988;18(2):5–10.

37. Emanuel EJ. *N Engl J Med* 1988;318:1686–1690 and Daniels N. Duty to treat or right to refuse? *Hastings Cent Rep* 1991;21(2):36–46.

38. Freedman B. Health professions, codes, and the right to refuse to treat HIV-infectious patients. *Hastings Cent Rep* 1988;18(2):20–25.

39. Annas GJ. Legal risks and responsibilities of physicians in the AIDS epidemic. *Hastings Cent Rep* 1988;18(2):26–32 and Cohen J. Access to medical care for HIV infected individuals under the Americans with Disabilities Act: a duty to treat. *Am J Law Med* 1992;18:233–250.

40. Arras JD. The fragile web of responsibility: AIDS and the duty to treat. *Hastings Cent Rep* 1988;18(2):10–20 and Angoff NR. Do physicians have an ethical obligation to care for patients with AIDS? *Yale J Biol Med* 1991;64:207–246. The opposite conclusion, namely that physicians do not have an ethical duty to treat AIDS patients, was reached in Tegtmeier JW. Ethics and AIDS: a summary of the law and a critical analysis of the individual physician's ethical duty to treat. *Am J Law Med* 1990;16:249–265.

41. Zuger A, Miles SH. *JAMA* 1987:1924–1926.

42. Emanuel EJ. *N Engl J Med* 1988:1686.

43. See Kim JH, Perfect JR. To help the sick: a historical and ethical essay concerning the refusal to care for patients with AIDS. *Am J Med* 1988;84:135–138.

44. Emanuel E. *N Engl J Med* 1988:1690.

45. For a description of the measures to limit the risk of HIV transmissibility in the health-care setting, see Conte JE Jr. Infection with human immunodeficiency virus in the hospital: epidemiology, infection

control, and biosafety considerations. *Ann Intern Med* 1986;105:730–736. The "universal precautions" promulgated by the Centers for Disease Control and Prevention are outlined in Centers for Disease Control. Universal precautions for prevention of transmission of human immunodeficiency virus, hepatitis B virus, and other blood-borne pathogens in health-care settings. *MMWR* 1988;37:377–382, 387–388. The health-care workplace precautions mandated by the Occupational Health and Safety Administration are stated in Department of Labor and Department of Health and Human Services. Joint advisory notice: protection against occupational exposures to hepatitis B virus (HBV) and human immunodeficiency virus (HIV). *Federal Register* 1987;52:41818–41823. The American Medical Association Council on Scientific Affairs published guidelines to prevent needlestick injuries. Tan L, Hawk JC III, Sterling ML. Report of the Council of Scientific Affairs: Preventing needlestick injuries in health care settings. *Arch Intern Med* 2001;161:929–936.

46. American Medical Association Council on Ethical and Judicial Affairs. Ethical Issues involved in the growing AIDS crisis. *JAMA* 1988;259:1360–1361; American College of Physicians Health and Public Policy Committee. The acquired immunodeficiency syndrome (AIDS) and infection with human immunodeficiency virus (HIV). *Ann Intern Med* 1988;108:460–469; American College of Physicians and Infectious Diseases Society of America. Human immunodeficiency virus (HIV) infection. *Ann Intern Med* 1994;120:310–319; American Academy of Neurology Ethics and Humanities Subcommittee. The ethical role of neurologists in the AIDS epidemic. *Neurology* 1992;42:1116–1117; and American College of Obstetrics and Gynecology. Human immunodeficiency virus infection: physicians' responsibilities. ACOG Committee Opinion: Committee on Ethics, No 130—November, 1993. *Int J Gynecol Obstet* 1994;44:88–91. The Surgeon General's pronouncement was cited in Simberkoff MS. *Neurol Clin* 1989:873.

47. Bayer R. Public policy and the AIDS epidemic: an end to AIDS exceptionalism? *N Engl J Med* 1991;324:1500–1504 and Dresser R. Should consent be required for an HIV test? In, Zeman A. Emanuel L (eds). *Ethical Dilemmas in Neurology.* London: W B Saunders, 2000:13–21.

48. Lo B, Steinbrook RL, Cooke M, et al. Voluntary screening for human immunodeficiency virus (HIV) infection: weighing the benefits and harms. *Ann Intern Med* 1989;110:727–733.

49. Van Brakel WH. Measuring health-related stigma: a literature review. *Psychol Health Med* 2006; 11:307–334.

50. Bayer R, Levine C, Wolf SM. HIV antibody screening: an ethical framework for evaluating proposed programs. *JAMA* 1986;256:1768–1774. Some of the detrimental social consequences of HIV testing were reported in Gunderson M, Mayo D, Rhame F. Routine HIV testing of hospital patients and pregnant women: informed consent in the real world. *Kennedy Inst Ethics J* 1996;6:161–183.

51. Walters L. *Science* 1988:599; Macklin R. Predicting dangerousness and the public health response to AIDS. *Hastings Cent Rep* 1986;16(suppl 6):16–23; Eickhoff TC. Hospital policies on HIV antibody testing. *JAMA* 1988;259:1861–1862; and Gostin LO, Curran WJ, Clark ME. The case against compulsory case finding in controlling AIDS—testing, screening and reporting. *Am J Law Med* l987;12:7–53

52. Cleary PD, Barry MJ, Mayer KH, et al. Compulsory premarital screening for the human immunodeficiency virus: technical and public health considerations. *JAMA* 1987;258:1757–1762.

53. Hagen MD, Meyer KB, Pauker SG. Routine preoperative screening for HIV: does the risk to the surgeon outweigh the risk to the patient? *JAMA* 1988;259:1357–1359.

54. Lo B, Steinbrook RL, Cooke M, et al. *Ann Intern Med* 1989:729.

55. Rhame FS, Maki DG. The case for wider use of testing for HIV infection. *N Engl J Med* 1989; 320:1248–1254. The American Medical Association also called for more "routine" use of HIV testing. See American Medical Association. Report to the Board of Trustees: HIV testing. In *Proceedings of the House of Delegates of the American Medical Association.* Chicago: American Medical Association, 1991:140–144.

56. Centers for Disease Control. Recommendations for HIV testing services for inpatients and outpatients in acute-care hospital settings. *MMWR* 1993;42:1–6.

57. Lurie P, Avins AL, Phillips KA, Kahn JG, Lowe RA, Ciccarone D. The cost-effectiveness of voluntary counseling and testing of hospital inpatients for HIV infection. *JAMA* 1994;272:1832–1838.

58. Sanders GD, Bayoumi AM, Sundaram V, et al. Cost-effectiveness of screening for HIV in the era of highly active antiretroviral therapy. *N Engl J Med* 2005;352:570–585 and Paltiel AD, Weinstein MC, Kimmel AD, et al. Expanded screening for HIV in the United States—an analysis of cost-effectiveness. *N Engl J Med* 2005;352:586–595.

59. Jewitt JF, Hecht FM. Preventive health care for adults with HIV infection. *JAMA* 1993;269:1144–1153 and Gallant JE, Moore RD, Chaisson RE. Prophylaxis for opportunistic infections in patients with HIV infection. *Ann Intern Med* 1994;120:932–944.

60. Egger M, May M, Chêne G, et al. Prognosis of HIV-1-infected patients starting highly active antiretroviral therapy: a collaborative analysis of prospective studies. *Lancet* 2002;360:119–129.

61. Hirsch MS, D'Aquila RT. Therapy for human immunodeficiency virus infection. *N Engl J Med* 1993;328:1686–1695. Although zidovudine delays the onset of AIDS, it simultaneously decreases the quality of life because of its side effects. See Lenderking WR, Gelber RD, Cotton DJ. Evaluation of the quality of life associated with zidovudine treatment in asymptomatic human immunodeficiency virus infection. *N Engl J Med* 1994;330:738–743.

62. Cohen MS, Gay C, Kashuba AD, Blower S, Paxton L. Narrative review: antiretroviral therapy to prevent the sexual transmission of HIV-1. *Ann Intern Med* 2007;146:591–601.

63. U.S. Preventive Services Task Force. Screening for HIV: recommendation statement. *Ann Intern Med* 2005;143:32–37 and Chou R, Huffman LH, Fu R, Smits AK, Korthuis PT. Screening for HIV: a review of the evidence for the U.S. Preventive Services Task Force. *Ann Intern Med* 2005;143:55–73.

64. Branson BM. To screen or not to screen: is that really the question? *Ann Intern Med* 2006;145:857–859. The authors reviewed data on recent cost-effectiveness studies such as those cited in note 58.

65. Gostin LO. HIV screening in health care settings: public health and civil liberties in conflict? *JAMA* 2006;296:2023–2025.

66. Lifson AR, Rybicki SL. Routine opt-out testing. *Lancet* 2007;369:539–540.

67. Bayer R, Fairchild AL. Changing paradigm for HIV testing—the end of exceptionalism. *N Engl J Med* 2006;355:647–549 and Wynia MK. Routine screening: informed consent, stigma and the waning of HIV exceptionalism. *Am J Bioethics* 2006;6(4):5–8.

68. Halpern SD. HIV testing without consent in critically ill patients. *JAMA* 2005;294:734–737.

69. Ross JJ, Levangie D, Worthington MG. Should patients be compelled to undergo HIV testing after a needlestick injury involving a health care worker? *The Pharos* 2006;69:32–36.

70. Bayer R. *N Engl J Med* 1991:1501 and Angell M. A dual approach to the AIDS epidemic. *N Engl J Med* 1991:1498–1500.

71. Bayer R. *N Engl J Med* 1991:1501.

72. Bayer R. *N Engl J Med* 1991:1502–1503.

73. Osmond DH, Bindman AB, Vranizan K. Name-based surveillance and public health interventions for persons with HIV infection. *Ann Intern Med* 1999;131:775–779. For a summary of which infectious diseases mandate unconsented reporting in each state, see Roush S, Birkhead G, Koo D, Cobb A, Fleming D. Mandatory reporting of diseases and conditions by health care professionals and laboratories. *JAMA* 1999;282:164–170.

74. Nakashima AK, Horsley R, Frey RL, Sweeney PA, Weber JT, Fleming PL. Effect of HIV reporting by name on use of HIV testing in publicly funded counseling and testing programs. *JAMA* 1998;280:1421–1426.

75. De Cock KM, Johnson AM. From exceptionalism to normalism: a reappraisal of attitudes and practice around HIV testing. *Br Med J* 1998;316:290–293. For a related argument, see Casarett DJ, Lantos JD. Have we treated AIDS too well? Rationing and the future of AIDS exceptionalism. *Ann Intern Med* 1998;128:756–759.

76. Gostin LO, Ward JW, Baker AC. National HIV case reporting for the United States: a defining moment in the history of the epidemic. *N Engl J Med* 1997;337:1162–1167.

77. Lo B. Ethical dilemmas in HIV infection: what have we learned? *Law Med Health Care* 1992;20:92–103.

78. Landis SE, Schoenbach VJ, Weber DJ, et al. Results of a randomized trial of partner notification in cases of HIV infection in North Carolina. *N Engl J Med* 1993;320:101–106.

79. Giesecke J, Ramstedt K, Granath F, et al. Efficacy of partner notification for HIV infection. *Lancet* 1991;338:1096–1100.

80. The ethical duty to protect third parties known to be at risk and the applicability of the California *Tarasoff* decision to the requirement for notification are discussed in chapter 3. The ordinary ethical duty of protecting patient confidentiality is discussed in Boyd KM. HIV infection and AIDS: the ethics of medical confidentiality. *J Med Ethics* 1992;18:173–179. For a statement by two medical societies affirming the precedence of the protection of third parties known to be at risk over maintaining patient confidentiality when the duties to each conflict, see American College of Physicians and Infectious Diseases Society of America. Human immunodeficiency virus (HIV) infection. *Ann Intern Med* 1994;120:316–317.

81. Gostin LO, Webber DW. HIV infection and AIDS in the public health and health care systems. *JAMA* 1998;279:1108–1113.

82. This decision tree was formulated in the report of the American Medical Association Council on Ethical and Judicial Affairs. *JAMA* 1988:1361. See also Brennan TA. AIDS and the limits of confidentiality: the physician's duty to warn contacts of seropositive individuals. *J Gen Intern Med* 1989;4:242–246.

83. Bennett R, Draper H, Frith L. Ignorance is bliss? HIV and moral duties and legal duties to forewarn. *J Med Ethics* 2000;26:9–15.

84. These data are discussed in Gostin L. HIV-infected physicians and the practice of seriously invasive procedures. *Hastings Cent Rep* 1989;19(1):32–39 and in Daniels N. HIV-infected professionals, patient rights, and the "switching dilemma." *JAMA* 1992;267:1368–1371.

85. Centers for Disease Control. Update Transmission of HIV infection during an invasive dental procedure—Florida. *MMWR* 1991;40:21–27 and Centers for Disease Control. Update: investigations of persons treated by HIV-infected health care workers—United States. *MMWR* 1993;42:329–337.

86. Centers for Disease Control. *Estimates of the Risk of Endemic Transmission of Hepatitis B Virus and Human Immunodeficiency Virus to Patients by the Percutaneous Route during Invasive Surgical and Dental Procedures.* Atlanta: Centers for Disease Control, 1991.

87. Gerberding JL, Littell C, Tarkington A, et al. Risk of exposure of surgical personnel to patients' blood during surgery at San Francisco General Hospital. *N Engl J Med* 1990;322:1788–1793.

88. These studies are reviewed in Mishu B, Schaffner W. HIV-infected surgeons and dentists: looking back and looking forward. *JAMA* 1993;269:1843–1844.

89. Robert LM, Chamberland ME, Cleveland JL, et al. Investigations of patients of health care workers infected with HIV: the Centers for Disease Control and Prevention database. *Ann Intern Med* 1995;122:653–657.

90. Schulman KA, McDonald RC, Lynn LA, Frank I, Christakis NA, Schwartz JS. Screening surgeons for HIV infection: assessment of a potential public health program. *Infect Control Hosp Epidemiol* 1994;15:147–155.

91. The epidemiologic facts of this case suggest that the dentist infected six of his patients but the exact mode of transmission remains unknown. See Ciesielski CA, Marianos DW, Schochetman G, Witte JJ, Jaffe HW. The 1990 Florida dental investigation: the press and the science. *Ann Intern Med* 1994;121:886–888. Alternative explanations are offered in Barr S. The 1990 Florida dental investigation: is the case really closed? *Ann Intern Med* 1996;124:250–254. These explanations are refuted in Brown D. The 1990 Florida dental investigation: theory and fact. *Ann Intern Med* 1996;124:255–256.

92. American Medical Association Council on Ethical and Judicial Affairs. *JAMA* 1988:1361.

93. American Medical Association. *AMA Statement on HIV-Infected Physicians.* Chicago: American Medical Association, 1991.

94. American Academy of Orthopedic Surgeons Task Force on AIDS and Orthopedic Surgery. *Recommendations for the Prevention of Human Immunodeficiency Virus Transmission in the Practice of Orthopedic Surgery.* Park Ridge, IL: American Academy of Orthopedic Surgeons, 1989.

95. von Reyn CF, Gilbert TT, Shaw FE Jr, et al. Absence of HIV transmission from an infected orthopedic surgeon: a 13-year look-back study. *JAMA* 1993;269:1807–1811.

96. Centers for Disease Control. Recommendations for preventing transmission of human immunodeficiency virus, hepatitis B virus to patients during exposure-prone invasive procedures. *MMWR* 1991;40:1–9, as reprinted in *JAMA* 1991;266:771–776.

97. The history of the CDC regulations is described in Lo B, Steinbrook R. Health care workers infected with the human immunodeficiency virus: the next steps. *JAMA* 1992;267:1100–1105.

98. Gostin L. The HIV infected health care professional: public policy, discrimination, and public safety. *Law Med Health Care* 1990;18:303–310.

99. Lo B, Steinbrook R. *JAMA* 1992:1100–1101.

100. DiMaggio SL. State regulations and the HIV-positive health care professional: a response to a problem that does not exist. *Am J Law Med* 1993;19:497–522 and De Ville KA. Nothing to fear but fear itself: HIV-infected physicians and the law of informed consent. *J Law Med Ethics* 1994;22:163–175.

101. Phillips KA, Lowe RA, Kahn JG, Lurie P, Avins AL, Ciccarone D. The cost-effectiveness of HIV testing of physicians and dentists in the United States. *JAMA* 1994;271:851–858 and Owens DK, Harris RA, Scott PM, Nease RF Jr. Screening surgeons for HIV infection: a cost-effectiveness analysis. *Ann Intern Med* 1995;122:641–652.

102. Gostin L. *Law Med Health Care* 1990:306–307.

103. Brennan TA. Transmission of the human immunodeficiency virus in the health care setting: time for action. *N Engl J Med* 1991;324:1504–1509.

104. Lo B, Steinbrook R. *JAMA* 1992:1103–1104.

105. See Dr. Aoun's autobiographical accounts in Aoun H. When a house officer gets AIDS. *N Engl J Med* 1989;321:693–696 and Aoun H. From the eye of the storm, with the eyes of a physician. *Ann Intern Med* 1992; 116:335–338.

106. Orentlicher D. HIV-infected surgeons: *Behringer v Medical Center. JAMA* 1991; 266:1134–1137.

107. Lo B. Ethical dilemmas in HIV infection: what have we learned? *Law Med Health Care* 1992;20:92–103.

108. Freedman B. Nonvalidated therapies and HIV disease. *Hastings Cent Rep* 1989;19(3):14–20.

109. Freedman B. *Hastings Cent Rep* 1989:16.

110. For an overview of the issues in intensive care of HIV/AIDS patients, see Morris A, Masur H, Huang L. Current issues in critical care of the human immunodeficiency virus-infected patient. *Crit Care Med* 2006;34:42–49. For an overview of palliative care of HIV/AIDS patients, see Selwyn PA. Palliative care for patients with human immunodeficiency virus/acquired immunodeficiency syndrome. *J Palliat Med* 2005;8:1248–1268.

111. Selwyn PA, Forstein M. Overcoming the false dichotomy of curative vs palliative care for late-stage HIV/AIDS. "Let me live the way I want to live, until I can't." *JAMA* 2003;290:806–814.

112. See, for example, Rogers PL, Lane HC, Henderson DK, et al. Admission of AIDS patients to a medical intensive care unit: causes and outcome. *Crit Care Med* 1989;17:113–117. The data from the early studies showing a dismal outcome from PCP are summarized in Wachter RM, Luce JM, Lo B, et al. Life-sustaining treatment for patients with AIDS. *Chest* 1989;95:647–652 and in Simberkoff MS. *Neurol Clin* 1989:878.

113. Wachter RM, Luce JM, Hopewell PC. Critical care of patients with AIDS. *JAMA* 1992;267:541–547. The same conclusions were reached by Rosen MJ, De Palo VA. Outcome of intensive care for patients with AIDS. *Crit Care Clin* 1993;9:107–114 and by Rosner F, Kark PR, Bennett AJ, et al. Medical futility. Committee on Bioethical Issues of the Medical Society of the State of New York. *NY State Med J* 1992:92:485–488. The improvement in the prognosis of other opportunistic infections is discussed in Lane HC (moderator). Recent advances in the management of AIDS-related opportunistic infections. *Ann Intern Med* 1994;120:945–955.

114. Wachter RM, Luce JM, Safrin S, Berrios DC, Charlebois E, Scitovsky AA. Cost and outcome of intensive care for patients with AIDS, *Pneumocystis carinii* pneumonia, and severe respiratory failure. *JAMA* 1995;273:230–235.

115. Steinbrook R, Lo B, Moulton J, et al. Preferences of homosexual men with AIDS for life-sustaining treatment. *N Engl J Med* 1986;314:457–460.

116. Wachter RM, Cooke M, Hopewell VC, et al. Attitudes of medical residents regarding intensive care for patients with acquired immunodeficiency syndrome. *Arch Intern Med* 1988;148:149–152 and Wachter RM, Luce JM, Hearst N, et al. Decisions about resuscitation: inequities among patients with different diseases but similar prognoses. *Ann Intern Med* 1989;111:525–532.

117. Karasz A, Dyche L, Selwyn P. Physicians' experiences of caring for late-stage HIV patients in the post-HAART era: challenges and adaptations. *Soc Sci Med* 2003;57:1609–1620.

118. Bindels PJE, Krol A, van Ameijden E, et al. Euthanasia and physician-assisted suicide in homosexual men with AIDS. *Lancet* 1996;347:499–504. See further discussion in chapter 9.

119. See Oregon Department of Human Services. *Ninth Annual Report on Oregon's Death with Dignity Act.* March 2007 available at http://egov.oregon.gov/DHS/ph/pas/ar-index.shtml and www.deathwithdignity .org (Accessed March 31, 2007). See further discussion in chapter 9.

120. Curtis JR, Patrick DL. Barriers to communication about end-of-life care in AIDS patients. *J Gen Intern Med* 1997;12:736–741.

121. Wachter RM, Lo B. Advance directives for patients with human immunodeficiency virus infection. *Crit Care Clin* 1993;9:125–136.

122. Wenger NS, Kanouse DE, Collins RL, et al. End-of-life discussions and preferences among persons with HIV. *JAMA* 2001;285:2880–2887.

123. Kuhl DR. Ethical issues near the end of life: a physician's perspective on caring for persons with AIDS. *J Palliative Care* 1994;10:117–121.

124. Selwyn PA, Arnold R. From fate to tragedy: the changing meanings of life, death, and AIDS. *Ann Intern Med* 1998;129:899–902 and Selwyn PA, Forstein M. Overcoming the false dichotomy of curative vs palliative care for late-stage HIV/AIDS. "Let me live the way I want to live, until I can't." *JAMA* 2003;290:806–814.

125. Harding R, Karus D, Easterbrook P, Raveis VH, Higginson IJ, Marconi K. Does palliative care improve outcomes for patients with HIV/AIDS? A systematic review of the evidence. *Sex Transm Infect* 2005;81:5–14.

126. Stoto MA, Almario DA, McCormick MC. *Reducing the Odds: Preventing Perinatal Transmission of HIV in the United States.* Committee on Perinatal Transmission of HIV, Institute of Medicine and Board on Children, Youth and Families of the National Research Council. Washington, DC: National Academy Press, 1999.

127. Wolf LE, Lo B, Beckerman KP, Dorenbaum A, Kilpatrick SJ, Weintrub PS. When patients reject interventions to reduce postnatal human immunodeficiency virus transmission. *Arch Pediatr Adolesc Med* 2001; 155:927–933.

128. Powderly K. Ethical and legal issues in perinatal HIV. *Clin Obstet Gynecol* 2001;44:300–311.

129. Spriggs M, Charles T. Should HIV discordant couples have access to assisted reproductive technologies? *J Med Ethics* 2003;29:325–329.

130. Baker HWG, Mijch A, Garland S, et al. Use of reproductive technology to reduce the risk of transmission of HIV in discordant couples wishing to have their own children where the male partner is seropositive with an undetectable viral load. *J Med Ethics* 2003;29:315–320.

131. Minkoff H, Santoro N. Ethical considerations in the treatment of infertility in women with human immunodeficiency virus infection. *N Engl J Med* 2000;342:1748–1750.

132. Kourtis AP, Lee FK, Abrams EJ, Jamieson DJ, Bulterys M. Mother-to-child transmission of HIV-1: timing and implications for prevention. *Lancet Infect Dis* 2006;6:726–732.

133. John-Stewart GC. Breast-feeding and HIV-1 transmission—how risky for how long? *J Infect Dis* 2007;196:1–3.

134. Lipson M. Disclosure of diagnosis to children with human immunodeficiency virus or acquired immunodeficiency syndrome. *Devel Behav Pediatr* 1994;15:S61–S65.

135. American Academy of Pediatrics Committee on Pediatric AIDS. Disclosure of illness to children and adolescents with HIV infection. *Pediatrics* 1999;103:164–166.

136. Flanagan-Klygis E, Ross LF, Lantos J, Yogev R. Disclosing the diagnosis of HIV in pediatrics. *J Clin Ethics* 2001;12:150–157.

137. Wissow LS, Hutton N, Kass N. Preliminary study of a values-history advance directive interview in a pediatric HIV clinic. *J Clin Ethics* 2001;12:161–172.

138. For a recent review of this topic, see Muthuswamy V. Ethical issues in HIV/AIDS research. *Indian J Med Res* 2005;121:601–610.

139. See Jaconson PD, Parmet WE. A new era of unapproved drugs: the case of *Abigail Alliance v Von Eschenbach*. *JAMA* 2007;297:205–208 and Okie S. Access before approval—a right to take experimental drugs? *N Engl J Med* 2006;355:437–440. The constitutional issues in this case are analyzed in Annas GJ. Cancer and the constitution—choice at life's end. *N Engl J Med* 2007;357:408–413.

140. Food and Drug Administration: Investigational new drug, antibiotic, and biological drug product regulations: treatment use and sale: final rule. *Federal Register* 1987;52:19466–19477. This rule is discussed in Young FE, Norris JA, Levitt JA, et al. The FDA's new procedures for the use of investigational drugs in treatment. *JAMA* 1988;259:2267–2270.

141. Freedman B. Nonvalidated therapies and HIV disease. *Hastings Cent Rep* 1989;19(3):14–20.

142. Stolley PD. The hazards of misguided compassion. *Ann Intern Med* 1993;118:822–823. The ethical issues in randomized controlled clinical trials are discussed in chapter 19.

143. Public Health Service, Department of Health and Human Services. Expanded availability of investigational new drugs through a parallel track mechanism for people with AIDS and HIV-related disease. *Federal Register* 1990;55:20856–20860. The parallel track is discussed in Lo B. *Law Med Health Care* 1992:95–96.

144. Levine C. AIDS and the ethics of human subjects research. In, Reamer FG, ed. *AIDS & Ethics*. New York: Columbia University Press, 1991:77–104. See also Appelbaum PS, Roth LH, Lidz CW. False hopes and best data—consent to research and the therapeutic misconception. *Hastings Cent Rep* 1987;17(2):20–24.

145. Arras JD. Noncompliance in AIDS research. *Hastings Cent Rep* 1990;20(5):24–32. For a scholarly analysis of the subject of patient noncompliance. See Lerner BH. From careless consumptives to recalcitrant patients: the historical construction of noncompliance. *Soc Sci Med* 1997;45:1423–1431. For a specific application of this theory to AIDS patients, see Lerner BH, Gulick RM, Dubler NN. Rethinking nonadherence: historical perspectives on triple-drug therapy for HIV disease. *Ann Intern Med* 1998;129:573–578.

146. Edgar H, Rothman DJ. New rules for new drugs: the challenge of AIDS to the regulatory process. *Milbank Q* 1990;68(suppl 1):111–142.

147. Byar DP, Schoenfeld DA, Green SB, et al. Design considerations for AIDS trials. *N Engl J Med* 1990;323:1343–1348. For a debate on the ethics of randomized clinical trials, see Hellman S, Hellman D. Of mice but not men: problems of the randomized clinical trial. *N Engl J Med* 1991;324:1585–1589 and Passamani E. Clinical trials: are they ethical? *N Engl J Med* 1991;324:1589–1592. The current controversy on using RCTs in developing countries is discussed in chapter 19.

148. Stolley PD. *Ann Intern Med* 1993:823.

149. Freedman B. *Hastings Cent Rep* 1989:17.

150. For example, see Stone VE, Mauch MY, Steger K, Janas SF, Craven DE. Race, gender, drug use, and participation in AIDS clinical trials: lessons from a municipal hospital cohort. *J Gen Intern Med* 1997;12:150–157.

151. Gifford AL, Cunningham WE, Heslin KC, et al. Participation in research and access to experimental treatments by HIV-infected patients. *N Engl J Med* 2002;346:1373–1382.

152. Lazzarini Z, Altice FL. A review of the legal and ethical issues for the conduct of HIV-related research in prisons. *AIDS Public Policy J* 2000;15:105–135.

153. World Medical Association Declaration of Helsinki (2004). http://www.wma.net/e/policy/b3.htm (Accessed April 7, 2007). For a discussion of the tension these rules have caused in developing countries, and how the research establishment in the United States has addressed it, see Lurie P, Greco DB. U.S. exceptionalism comes to research ethics. *Lancet* 2005;356:1117–1119.

154. Shapiro HT, Meslin EM. Ethical issues in the design and conduct of clinical trials in developing countries. *N Engl J Med* 2001;345:139–142.

155. Lo B, Bayer R. Establishing ethical trials for treatment and prevention of AIDS in developing countries. *BMJ* 2003;327:337–339 and Participants in the 2001 conference on ethical aspects of research in developing countries. Moral standards of research in developing countries: from "reasonable availability" to "fair benefits." *Hastings Cent Rep* 2004;34(3):17–27.

156. UNAIDS. Creating effective partnerships for HIV prevention trials: report of a UNAIDS consultation, Geneva 20–21 June 2005. *AIDS* 2006;20(6)W1–W11.

157. Schackman BR, Gebo KA, Walensky RP, et al. The lifetime cost of current human immunodeficiency virus care in the United States. *Med Care* 2006;44:990–997.

158. Bozzette SA, Joyce G, McCaffrey DF, et al. Expenditures for the care of HIV-infected patients in the era of highly active antiretroviral therapy. *N Engl J Med* 2001;344:817–823.

159. Diaz T, Chu SY, Conti L, et al. Health insurance coverage among persons with AIDS: results from a multistate surveillance project. *Am J Public Health* 1994;84:1015–1018.

160. Bayer R, Stryker J. Ethical challenges posed by clinical progress in AIDS. *Am J Public Health* 1997;87:1599–1602.

161. Steinbrook R. Providing antiretroviral therapy for HIV infection. *N Engl J Med* 2001;344:844–45.

162. Steinbrook R. *N Engl J Med* 2001:845.

163. Moore RD, Bartlett JG. Combination antiretroviral therapy in HIV infection. *PharmacoEconomics* 1996;10:109–113.

164. Steinbrook R. *N Engl J Med* 2001:845.

165. Cotton DJ. The impact of AIDS on the medical care system. *JAMA* 1988;260:519–523.

166. See Kalb PE, Miller DH. Utilization strategies for intensive care units. JAMA 1989;261:2389–2395 and Zoloth-Dorfman L, Carney B. The AIDS patient and the last ICU bed: scarcity, medical futility, and ethics. *QRB* 1991;17:175–181.

ETHICAL ISSUES IN RESEARCH

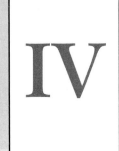

Clinical Research

19

The conduct of clinical research introduces a unique set of ethical issues that stem from using humans as research subjects.[1] An ethical maxim of human dignity famously emphasized by Immanuel Kant is that humans always should be treated as an end in themselves and never as a means of achieving another end.[2] The essential ethical problem in using humans as research subjects is that it violates Kant's ethical axiom because they are employed as the means to the end of answering a scientific question. Justifying the violation of Kant's maxim imparts a series of ethical obligations on the clinical investigator to maximally protect the interests and welfare of the human research subject. Investigators must obtain the subject's voluntary consent and protect the subject from exploitation, unnecessary suffering, and other harms. Directly or indirectly, all the ethical issues I discuss in this chapter result from the use of the human subject as a means to the end of conducting clinical research.

Clinical investigators using human subjects in research develop a relationship with them that shares some features of the patient-physician relationship. The investigator-subject relationship imparts ethical duties to the investigator because the investigator intervenes in subjects' lives and creates potential harms to them. These ethical duties comprise a responsibility to protect and guard the subjects' welfare throughout the trial. Some ethicists have argued that medical researchers owe human subjects the same level of care that physicians owe patients, a quantity exceeding that which is stipulated in the research protocol.[3] Other scholars hold that the ethical requirements of physicians providing medical care cannot translate fully to investigators conducting clinical research[4] and investigators therefore lack the fiduciary duty to research subjects that physicians have to patients.[5]

Clinical research is a systematic investigation designed to create generalizable knowledge to advance science and ultimately to benefit mankind. Without the potential good that may result from clinical research, no risk of harm to the human subject could be justified. The use of humans as research subjects can be conceptualized as permitting an acceptable risk of harm to one person with consent in exchange for greater benefits to others in the future (and possibly for the subject now). A person's decision to serve as a research subject may be an act of altruism or an attempt to improve his or her health by receiving the latest treatment. At a minimum, the human subject's participation should be voluntary and undertaken only after a full disclosure of the attendant risks and possible benefits. The disclosure-consent ethical requirement is the research equivalent of the clinical doctrine of informed consent.

To fully understand the concept of clinical research, it is useful to distinguish it from related endeavors.[6] These distinctions are important because related endeavors that are not research may not require the degree of regulation and informed consent required for the ethical conduct of research. Therapeutic innovation is related to research but is intended to benefit an individual patient, not necessarily to develop generalizable knowledge.[7] Therapeutic innovation, unlike research, may not be intended for publication. The distinction between research and quality improvement is subtle with much overlap. Although the intent of quality improvement initiatives originally was local, now they are being viewed more as research because their results are being generalized into practice standards.[8]

One element of an ethical analysis of clinical research is the ratio of scientific knowledge gained to harms risked by the human subject. The design and execution of a clinical trial may be considered an ethical matter because a poorly designed or executed trial will generate invalid results and thus render as unjustifiable even trivial risks to the study subjects. Professional conduct issues are also important. To maintain scientific integrity, the investigators must not have conflicts of interest or must adequately disclose those than cannot be eliminated.

Ezekiel Emanuel and his colleagues epitomized the seven requirements that make clinical research ethical: (1) value—the research must yield enhancements of health or knowledge; (2) scientific validity—methodological rigor is required to make the results valid; (3) fair subject selection—subject selection should be based upon scientific objectives and should not unfairly exploit vulnerability or award privilege; (4) favorable risk-benefit ratio—the totality of benefits to the individual and society should outweigh the risks to the study subject; (5) independent review—a body of responsible reviewers should scrutinize the study and approve it only if it meets stringent scientific and ethical criteria; (6) informed consent—the free, informed, and voluntary consent of the research subject is essential; and (7) respect for enrolled subjects—the investigators are responsible for protecting the welfare of the subject throughout the study and subjects may withdraw from the study at any time without repercussion.[9] Because of the risks and time devoted to participating in the study, human subjects also have a right to know the aggregate conclusions of the research.[10]

In a survey of over 300 physicians and nurses involved in clinical investigation at the National Institutes of Health, Gordon DuVal and colleagues studied the incidence and types of ethical dilemmas encountered in clinical research. They found that 95% of investigators could identify their most difficult type of ethical problem and 76% could recall a recent ethical dilemma. Nearly half the surveyed clinical investigators reported requesting an ethics consultation to help resolve an intractable ethical problem. They scored the value of the consultation at a mean of 8 out of 10. The extent of their training and experience in ethics predicted the likelihood that they would request an ethics consultation but was not predictive of their satisfaction with the consultation. The investigators acknowledged that most hospital ethics consultation services do not provide research ethics consultations.[11]

HISTORY AND DEVELOPMENT OF CODES OF RESEARCH ETHICS

The history of research ethics begins with shameful examples of investigators' unethical behavior and ends with the development of an international consensus on the ethical standards of human subjects research design and conduct as embodied in established codes of research ethics. In the United States, a number of clinical trials and other experiments were performed on patients in the 19th and early 20th centuries without their consent.[12] In a controversial article in 1966, Henry K. Beecher, a Harvard anesthesiology professor and pioneer in American research ethics, chronicled 22 examples of unethical research performed in American institutions during the 20th century.[13]

The most widely publicized examples of unethical clinical research in the United States were the Tuskegee syphilis study, the Willowbrook hepatitis experiment, and the Jewish Chronic Disease Hospital cancer study, probably because they took place in the second half of the 20th century, after international codes of clinical research had been accepted. The Tuskegee syphilis study was begun in 1932 by the United States Public Health Service (USPHS) to examine the natural history of untreated (or undertreated[14]) syphilis in a group of 399 poor black male sharecroppers from Macon County, Georgia.

Following World War II when penicillin became widely available, the men remained untreated and some remained unaware that a treatment existed that might help them. Amazingly, the study continued until 1972 when Peter Buxton, a USPHS official who was frustrated at having his ethical concerns about the study ignored by more senior USPHS officials, alerted reporters who subsequently published exposés of the study in the *New York Times* and the *Washington Star*. Public outrage generated by these articles prompted the USPHS to terminate the study in 1972. In 2000, on behalf of the United States government, President Clinton formally apologized to the few Tuskegee research subjects remaining alive.[15]

The Willowbrook State School hepatitis study involved the purposeful induction of hepatitis A virus (and other enteric pathogens) in institutionalized mentally retarded children. The goal of the study was to understand the spread of enteric pathogens within institutions and thereby reduce the risk of hepatitis spread through institutionalized patients, a serious medical problem in all such institutions. Although Saul Krugman, one of the principal investigators, later explained that parental consent for the study had been obtained, the extent to which the children's parents were informed of risks or alternatives was a point of criticism and remains unclear.[16]

The Jewish Chronic Disease Hospital of Brooklyn cancer study, spearheaded in 1964 by Chester Southam, a noted Memorial Sloan-Kettering Cancer Center investigator, involved the injection of live cancer cells into 22 hospitalized patients without their knowledge to study the immunology of cancer. Patients were told that they would receive injections of a "cell suspension" but the word "cancer" was omitted because Southam believed that the chance that these cells actually would produce a cancer was minimal and he feared that the word "cancer" would frighten patients unnecessarily. Some staff physicians refused to participate because they believed it was wrong. When a member of the hospital board of directors learned of the research, he sued to have it stopped. The cessation of the research was accomplished through the resulting publicity.[17]

Without comparison, the medical experiments provoking the greatest worldwide public outrage were the infamous human experiments conducted during the Third Reich. These sadistic medical studies were carried out by German physicians on victims of Nazi death camps, with no attempt to obtain consent and, remarkably, with no reluctance on the part of the physicians.[18] Worldwide horror and disgust provoked by public reporting of these experiments and the unspeakable suffering of their victims led to the development of codes of research ethics, beginning with the Nuremberg Code of 1947.

In Nuremberg, Germany, in 1947, following the trials of Nazi physicians who had conducted the despicable human experiments, American jurists formulated the Nuremberg Code. Its authors are believed to have been Judge Harold Sebring and Drs. Leo Alexander and Andrew Ivy. The Nuremberg Code stated axiomatically that no research should be conducted on human subjects without their full and voluntary consent. The Code stipulated further that all clinical experiments should be designed to minimize unnecessary suffering and excessive risk. Human research subjects should be protected at all times and free to terminate participation in the study at will.[19]

In 1964, the World Medical Association meeting in Helsinki formulated an international code of research ethics called the Declaration of Helsinki and amended it in six subsequent revisions through 2004. The Declaration of Helsinki provides 32 ethical principles to guide physicians in all biomedical research that involves human subjects. The Declaration reasserts the principles of the Nuremberg Code and places additional ethical duties on the investigator to insure the welfare of the human research subject at all times during the study.[20]

Commissions in the United States drafted reports stipulating additional standards of ethical conduct of research involving human subjects. The most noteworthy of these are the *Belmont Report* and *Protecting Human Subjects*. The *Belmont Report* was published in 1978 by the United States National Commission for the Protection of Human Subjects of Biomedical and Behavioral Research. The unique feature of the *Belmont Report* was its emphasis on the ethical principles of respect for persons, beneficence, and justice in the realm of human experimentation, and its explanation of how the rules for protecting human research subjects were derived from ethical principles.[21]

In 1981, the United States President's Commission for the Study of Ethical Problems in Medicine and Biomedical and Behavioral Research published *Protecting Human Subjects.* This report reiterated the principles embodied in the Nuremberg Code and the *Belmont Report.* It further required a favorable assessment of risks and benefits of the research and stipulated fair procedures in the selection of subjects.[22] It suggested a heightened role for the institutional review board (IRB), which had been mandated in American law by the National Research Act of 1974, to better oversee and protect human research subjects. IRB approval now is mandatory. In a study of clinical trials published in major medical journals, investigators reported subjects' consent or IRB approval in 91% of trials.[23]

IRBs exist because of the general acknowledgement that neither the full protection of human research subjects nor the responsibility for determining whether research fulfills ethical standards should be left solely to the investigator. The functions of the IRB are stipulated in federal regulations.[24] Approval by the local IRB is a federally mandated prerequisite for any research involving human subjects under the "common rule," so named because the regulations have been adopted by all agencies that conduct or fund human subjects research.[25] The IRB has three principal roles: (1) to certify and document that the patient's full and free informed consent has been obtained; (2) to demonstrate that the risks to the research subject are outweighed by the totality of potential benefits to the subject and future patients; and (3) to protect the privacy, confidentiality, dignity, and welfare of the human research subject.[26]

The functioning of the contemporary IRB is governed by both federal regulations and local practices. Variation in IRB daily operations among institutions is permissible. In many academic medical centers, the IRB agenda and personnel are overwhelmed with the volume of experimental protocols to review. The constant pressure to expedite approval of protocols at times may make review less careful than is optimal. Multicenter trials are another stress on IRBs. Some IRBs provide only a casual review if the study has been approved previously by another institution's IRB.[27] In a comprehensive analysis from the Consortium to Examine Clinical Research Ethics, Ezekiel Emanuel and colleagues identified these among 15 systemic problems of contemporary IRB structure, function, and oversight, and proposed recommendations for improvements.[28] (See further discussion in chapter 5.)

Additional national and international agencies have propounded research guidelines.[29] In 1993, the Council for International Organizations of Medical Sciences and the World Health Organization published *International Ethical Guidelines for Biomedical Research Involving Human Subjects.*[30] In the United States, the National Institutes of Health (NIH) Office for Human Research Protection (OHRP, formerly known as the Office for the Protection from Research Risks or OPRR) publishes and updates guidelines on protecting human subjects that govern all research projects receiving federal funding.[31] The United States National Bioethics Advisory Commission proposed recommendations for heightening consent and competency requirements when investigators perform clinical trials on vulnerable research subjects.[32] The Association of American Medical Colleges formulated a guide to scientific societies for developing codes of ethics in research.[33] The American Association for the Advancement of Science now publishes a newsletter with guidelines on ethical conduct for scientists.[34] Franklin Miller and Alan Wertheimer recently pointed out that the paternalism inherent in research ethics guidelines is fully justified and does not conflict with the primacy of obtaining subjects' informed consent.[35]

VALID CONSENT

Since the drafting of the Nuremberg Code 60 years ago, the necessity of obtaining the full, free and informed consent of the research subject has been elevated to an axiom of clinical research. Implicit in the doctrine of consent is the right of the research subject to refuse entrance into the study or to withdraw from the study at any time. As is true in the doctrine of informed consent for clinical treatment, a subject's consent for research becomes valid only after there has been complete disclosure of the risks and benefits of the various treatment arms and their alternatives. The subject must have the cognitive capacity to accept or refuse, and there must be no coercion by individuals or agencies. The formalization of the consent process by the subject's signing of a written document is essential. Patients volunteering as research subjects must be provided a written summary of the proposed research containing an accurate account of the consequences of their participation drafted in clear, understandable language, and including contact information for any questions or problems.[36]

Valid consent for serving as a subject in a clinical trial is an ideal that often is not realized in practice.[37] Busy investigators often spend insufficient time on the process of education of the patient in the details of their participation in the clinical trial. Even when much time has been spent, there is evidence that many research subjects simply fail to understand the information in consent forms,[38] misunderstand the concept of randomization,[39] fail to appreciate the difference between a clinical trial and ordinary therapy, or cannot comprehend the language of the consent form.[40] Some subjects summarily decide to enroll and do not pay attention to the wealth of information presented to them and contained in the consent form.

A research subject's failure to understand that participation in a clinical trial is primarily for the purpose of research and not therapy is an intractable problem in research ethics that Paul Applebaum and colleagues called the "therapeutic misconception."[41] Many patients consent to participate in a clinical trial because they believe that the trial represents their best chance to receive the latest and best treatment.[42] Despite the investigator's efforts to explain the research nature of the clinical trial, the patient continues to conceptualize

participation as an opportunity to receive therapy. Some patients erroneously assume that the newest experimental treatment is necessarily the best treatment and therefore simply wish to have access to it. The therapeutic framing of most clinical trials of pharmaceuticals further aggravates the therapeutic misconception[43] as does the circumstance of dual agency in which the clinical investigator also is the patient's physician.[44]

Volunteering as a subject in a phase I oncology trial raises several ethical concerns. Subjects should not be coerced into consenting for clinical trials because coercion violates the freedom criterion for valid consent. However, some patients with widespread cancer for whom no known therapy is effective conceptualize their choice as either enrolling in a phase I oncology trial or dying. They automatically conclude that they have no real choice and therefore must enroll. As a result, during the consent process, they neither seek to learn nor attend to the described details of treatment side effects or other adverse consequences. Some scholars have called this circumstance "implicit coercion of desperate volunteers" and believe that it raises doubts about whether such a subject's consent ever can be truly voluntary.[45] A study from the National Institutes of Health showed that as patients became sicker, they understood less of the consent document and more frequently misunderstood the experimental purpose of the clinical trial. The authors pointed out that "research patients with life-threatening illnesses continue to view themselves primarily as patients seeking treatments."[46]

In the consent process, investigators (particularly in phase I oncology trials) have a heightened duty to be unambiguously clear about the research basis of the clinical trial and its true benefits to patient-subjects and society.[47] Interventional attempts to improve subjects' understanding and enhance voluntariness have had mixed results.[48] The actual magnitude of the ethical problem of desperate volunteers may be overstated because the benefit to patients from participating in phase I oncology trials is greater than that formerly assumed and usually is sufficient to satisfy the ethical requirement of a favorable risk-benefit ratio.[49]

Moreover, investigators make offers of participation to prospective research subjects, not threats; therefore overt coercion usually is not practiced.[50] The ethical problems of phase I oncology trials are further mitigated because consent forms almost never promise benefit and usually communicate serious risks.[51] Another problem faced by patients who volunteer for a phase I study is that current Medicare regulations deny hospice benefits to any terminally ill patient enrolled in a phase I oncology trial. This perverse disincentive should be eliminated.[52]

In a recent study of subjects offered participation in a phase I gene transfer therapy trial for Parkinson's disease, Scott Kim and colleagues examined the differences between equal groups of prospective subjects who volunteered and who refused. They found that those subjects willing to participate tended to perceive a lower probability of risk, were tolerant of greater risk, were more optimistic about the benefits of the research to society, and were more decisive and action-oriented.[53]

Some patients prefer to defer the decision to enroll in a clinical trial to their physicians whom they trust implicitly. When the clinical investigator also serves as the patient's physician, this double agency further compounds the confusion in the patient's mind between research and therapy and also creates a conflict of interest.[54] In some cases, patients consent to participate in a clinical trial out of gratitude to their physicians because their participation may be the most demonstrable way patients can express their gratitude. Although there is nothing wrong with expressing gratitude, some patients may fear retaliation from their physician if they refuse to participate, a condition that raises the question of true voluntary consent. In a recent article, the physician-attorney-ethicist David Orentlicher boldly suggested that when the preferred course of treatment for a particular condition is unknown, patients' treatment should be conditional on their willingness to participate as a research subject in a clinical trial to fulfill the societal goal of learning the best treatment.[55]

A practicing physician may conduct research consisting of an experimental or innovative therapy on a single patient, an "n-of-1" experiment, that is not part of an IRB-approved study.[56] Physicians conducting ad hoc experimental therapy should assure themselves that a scientific basis exists for the experiment and that the patient has provided full valid consent with an understanding that the therapy is experimental. In those instances in which the experimental therapy poses a significant risk to the patient, before beginning the physician should discuss the advisability of proceeding with the experiment with knowledgeable colleagues.[57]

Whether to pay research subjects remains controversial. Some scholars have worried that subjects enrolling in a clinical trial may be subjected to "undue inducement" if payments were offered. The same fear has been raised in research in developing countries (see below) in which participating in the research may be the only means for impoverished citizens to obtain a particular therapy.[58] Although a few scholars have argued that paying research subjects is inherently unethical because it may motivate a patient to take risks that he or she otherwise never would take,[59] most commentators agree that it is acceptable in some cases if it is regulated by careful attention to the intersection of ethical considerations and market forces.[60] Federal regulations leave the matter of payments to IRBs to decide, but the "common rule" regulation prohibits "undue inducement."[61] In a survey of 32 research organizations, Neal Dickert and colleagues found that most organizations paid research subjects for their time (87%), inconvenience (84%), travel (68%), as an incentive (58%), or for risks incurred (32%), but only 37% had written policies governing payments.[62] Ezekiel Emanuel pointed out that inducements are a normal part of life and human motivation and are not inherently unethical. He believes that proper informed consent and IRB oversight of the risk-benefit ratio can prevent inducements from becoming undue.[63]

Robert Truog and colleagues provocatively argued that subjects' informed consent is not always necessary for their participation in clinical trials. The authors pointed out that physicians are authorized to treat individual patients with experimental therapies in a clinical context with general consent and require specific consent for the same therapy only when it is part of a clinical trial. They offered criteria exempting informed consent in clinical trials, the first of which is that all treatments in the trial must be available outside the trial without specific informed consent.[64] But here they confounded the ethical and legal requirements for consent. If an experimental therapy is proposed, ethically it should require the same degree of consent, irrespective of whether it is in a clinical trial. However, they were correct in asserting that there is a marked difference between the ideal and real consent-obtaining behaviors of physicians in the two circumstances.

Whether institutions have an ethical responsibility to provide compensation or medical care to subjects who sustain research injuries remains controversial. Some scholars assert that institutions have an ethical duty to provide care or compensation regardless of blame and whether the subjects have been paid or not. Other scholars disagree, claiming that compensation or care for research injuries is not ethically required because the subjects were made aware of the risks and accepted them during the informed consent process.[65] Academic medical centers have varying policies on providing compensation and care of subjects who sustain research injuries, with slightly more than half not providing free care.[66] Irrespective of a particular institution's policy on payment, each research protocol should clearly stipulate the plan for handling research-related injuries, so that during the consent process, the subject is aware of and concurs with how this contingency will be handled.

Consent for Vulnerable Subjects

The principal remaining controversies in obtaining consent for research surround obtaining the consent of a "vulnerable subject." Subjects are classified as vulnerable when they reasonably cannot be expected to provide independent valid consent, as a consequence of treatment urgency or of physical or cognitive incapacity, and thus they require surrogates to provide consent on their behalf.

Vulnerable subjects deserve special procedural protections because they have been the victims of past research abuses resulting from deficient or absent surrogate consent. But neither should they be overprotected to the point that research cannot be done at all because research on their conditions is desirable. Thus, reasonable guidelines should be formulated for conducting research on vulnerable subjects that adequately protect but do not overprotect them. The major categories of vulnerable subjects are those with emergency conditions, children, and patients with cognitive impairments. Carol Levine and colleagues decried the recent tendency to expand the class of vulnerable patients to include people residing in economically disadvantaged countries, members of lower socioeconomic groups, and other large groups because the concept loses meaning and force when applied to too many people.[67]

Emergency Research. Often it is impossible to obtain valid consent for a clinical trial to study an emergency treatment. The problem is how a clinical trial ever can be administered in a setting in which it may not feasible to obtain consent because of the obvious time constraints of emergency treatment and the frequent unavailability of surrogates. Some scholars have advocated that the doctrine of implied (waived) consent could be applied in this circumstance, arguing by analogy that the emergency treatment doctrine permitting physicians to provide standard emergency therapy without consent also should pertain to conducting emergency research. However, given that the standard for obtaining consent for serving as a research subject is more stringent than consent for clinical care, and that many patients refuse to enter clinical trials, it is not clear that consent for an emergency clinical trial can be merely presumed.[68]

Unless the consent issue can be handled successfully, no ethically acceptable clinical trials can be conducted for studying emergency treatments.[69] The Coalition Conference of Acute Resuscitation and Critical Care Researchers pointed out that patients with emergency conditions not only are vulnerable to being victimized by their incapacity but also are vulnerable to being denied potentially life-saving treatments if those treatments cannot be studied adequately. They urged the development of federal guidelines to permit and regulate such studies.[70]

Federal regulations propounded by the United States Food and Drug Administration (FDA) and the United States Department of Health and Human Services (DHHS) address the situation of informed consent in emergency research.[71] The regulations stipulate those emergency circumstances in which it is acceptable for a clinical trial to be performed without the consent of the research subject. The FDA criteria[72] permit the use of an investigational drug in an emergency instance if: (1) the human subject is confronted by a life-threatening situation necessitating the use of the test article; (2) informed consent cannot be obtained from the subject because of an inability to communicate; (3) time is insufficient to obtain consent from the subject's legal representative; and (4) there is no available alternative method of approved or generally recognized therapy that provides an equal or greater likelihood of saving the life of the subject.[73]

Similarly, the DHSS regulations to waive informed consent[74] require that: (1) the research involves no more than minimal risk to the subject; (2) the waiver will not adversely affect the rights and welfare of subjects; (3) the research could not be practicably carried out without the waiver; and (4) whenever appropriate, the subjects will be provided with additional pertinent information after participation.[75] Alison Wichman and Alan Sandler tabulated the specific FDA and DHHS criteria for designing an acceptable clinical trial using the consent waiver.[76]

These federal regulations were written because of the shared belief that individuals and society would be best served if emergency research took place. Authority has been vested in the IRB to guarantee that the approved clinical trials are justified by their scientific validity, safety, and proper patient protections. Members of the public mandated to serve on IRBs have a responsibility to define normative risks. They and the other IRB members have the additional difficult task of determining

whether the proposed research falls within the definition of "minimal risk."[77] Minimal risk usually refers to a probability and magnitude of harm not greater than that ordinarily encountered in daily life.[78] David Wendler criticized this definition as flawed because many people choose to undergo significant risks in their daily lives.[79] Two respected research ethics scholars, Robert Levine and Jay Katz, wondered whether IRB members will be able to adequately interpret and apply these criteria to successfully approve randomized clinical trials of emergency medications.[80]

Children. The participation of a minor in a clinical trial raises vexing questions that attempt to balance the opposing goals of paternalistic protection of vulnerable minors against their appropriate access to clinical trials to establish efficacy and safety of therapy.[81] A minor's participation requires consent of the minor's surrogate decision maker (usually the parent) and the assent of the minor, provided the minor is capable of understanding the proposed clinical trial.[82] "Assent" is the term referring to the child's permission to proceed with treatment or experimental therapy. Although assent does not replace the legal duty of parental or other surrogate consent, it is an ethical prerequisite for treatment of children, especially for experimental purposes. The Committee on Bioethics of the American Academy of Pediatrics issued recommendations for obtaining assent in children of various ages.[83] Nancy Ondrusek and colleagues determined that children under the age of nine years lacked the capacity to understand the fundamental characteristics of a research study. They proposed that the concept of assent for research in children should be implemented only once children are at least nine years old.[84]

Federal regulations from the DHSS and FDA and overseen by the NIH Office of Human Research Protection (OHRP) permit certain research in children and other vulnerable human subject populations for whom there is no prospect of direct benefit only if the research involves no greater than minimal risk.[85] Federal regulations define minimal risk as the risk for which " . . . the probability and magnitude of the harm or discomfort anticipated in the research are not greater in and of themselves than those ordinarily encountered in daily life or during the performance of routine physical or psychological examinations or tests."[86] However, this seemingly straightforward concept implying a very low absolute risk has been subject to varying interpretations and considerable disagreement. Charles Weijer, a leader in research ethics, has provided a comprehensive analysis of the ethical and legal concepts of risk in clinical trials.[87]

For example, applying the concept to research on children, Benjamin Freedman and colleagues pointed out that children and teenagers frequently conduct highly risky behaviors in the course of their normal daily lives, such as riding bicycles without helmets, driving automobiles recklessly and without using seatbelts, and engaging in unprotected sexual intercourse.[88] Thus, they ponder, is the concept of minimal risk meant to entail a magnitude of risks such as these simply because they are encountered in daily life? Because what counts as minimal risk is subject to such varying interpretations, it is no surprise that IRBs have struggled with the task of assessing whether the risks of a clinical trial for which they are considering approval are or are not greater than minimal risk and applying the regulations consistently and correctly.[89]

David Wendler and colleagues quantified risks that children experience in everyday life. They found that the risk of injury or death from automobile trips and participation in sports were greater than that produced by experimental therapeutic agents that many IRBs dismissed on the grounds of posing risks greater than those encountered in ordinary life.[90] Loretta Kopelman advocated a plausible sliding scale analysis to more reasonably interpret the federal regulations.[91] Because of the intractable ambiguity of the language of federal regulations and their inconsistent application, some scholars have called for the creation of a national consensus on the interpretation of the regulations.[92]

Researchers wishing to seek IRB approval of a clinical trial have a great incentive to seek minimal risk status to comply with the statute even when the risks arguably are greater than minimal. Indeed, the OHRP catalogued a series of risk misstatements or misjudgments in funded protocols. In its first year of operation, the OHRP restricted or suspended research activities at eight institutions because of failure to accurately assess risks in consent forms or provide safeguards for vulnerable subjects.[93]

Patients with Cognitive Impairment. Research on patients with cognitive impairment is discussed in chapter 15.

Privacy and the HIPAA Regulations

The United States Congress enacted the Health Insurance Portability and Accountability Act (HIPAA) in 1996 to protect citizens' health information. In December 2000, the Department of Health and Human Services issued the Privacy Rule establishing standards for protecting health information. Staff members of hospitals, physicians' offices, and other health sites have been instructed in how to comply with the lengthy and cumbersome new privacy and confidentiality regulations that took effect in April 2003 (see chapter 3). Although the Privacy Rule was intended primarily to protect clinical information, its broad application to "covered entities" encompassed medical information collected in the context of human subjects research.[94]

The Privacy Rule concerns all "individually identifiable" health information created or maintained by a covered entity including a research enterprise. The HIPAA regulations heighten the requirements for obtaining informed consent from research subjects over those already required by the United States federal research consent requirements. The prolixity and complexity of the regulatory language has spawned an industry of consultants to interpret the regulations and of compliance officers to assure that they are followed correctly. IRBs have struggled to understand the precise requirements of the new law, particularly as it applies to research involving data registries, and in defining those situations in which waivers or exemptions may be permissible.[95]

Commentators have opined that the regulations have hampered research because of the logistical hurdles they impose, the added expense of compliance, the fear and intimidation that IRB members and investigators have experienced over their own liability for possibly violating a regulation, and the fact that alternative means of protecting research subjects' privacy could be accomplished without the problems caused by HIPAA. IRB members have required that investigators add complex and lengthy text to research consent forms to comply fully with HIPAA regulations. This additional text is likely to confuse research subjects and is unlikely to improve their understanding of the study.[96] Clearly, the HIPAA regulations, intended to improve privacy protection of confidential medical information, have had a perverse effect of impeding clinical research while providing no obvious benefit.

THE RANDOMIZED CLINICAL TRIAL

The randomized clinical trial (RCT) is the ultimate scientifically rigorous clinical investigation.[97] The RCT is an experiment testing a hypothesis in which the investigator randomly assigns patients to groups experiencing different exposures to interventions. By carefully controlling the intervention arms to assure that the groups are otherwise identical in composition and treatment, the investigator can reasonably conclude that any measured difference in the outcomes of the groups resulted from the difference in exposures because that was the only difference among them.[98]

Investigators have ethical duties to patients serving as subjects in a RCT that exceeds their duty to subjects in an observational study. The RCT investigator's intervention into the subject's life creates a relationship between investigator and patient-subject that imparts an ethical duty to the investigator to protect the subject's welfare.[99] The investigator's duty to protect the research subject forms the ethical foundation for research on human subjects. Some have argued that physicians' ethical imperative to try to improve health care of all patients confers an ethical imperative to encourage patient participation in RCTs.[100]

The RCT has several scientific benefits. Without a controlled study it may be impossible to evaluate the efficacy of a specific therapy, unless the benefit is clinically obvious. The RCT design minimizes investigator bias and confounding variables. It is the experimental method most likely to yield reliable clinical knowledge with a minimum of methodological error and observer bias.[101] Additionally, it can yield cost savings to society and safety benefits to future patients by eliminating ineffective therapies.[102] Patients enrolling in RCTs frequently fare better medically than comparably ill patients treated outside RCTs because of the increased monitoring of study patients required by the protocol.[103]

Because of its rigid designs, the RCT also has several shortcomings. First, it may not conform to the particular desires of a patient or physician for a treatment tailored to a patient's specific clinical needs. Second, it may introduce bias by promoting violations of the study design including nonrandom selection, subversion of randomization,[104] patient dropout, or patient noncompliance. Finally, a RCT may yield inadequate enrollment and therefore fail as a valid study.[105] Although the RCT remains the purest standard of scientific study design, its design may be unnecessary to accomplish certain scientific goals. For example, historical controls may suffice in some studies, thereby avoiding the ethical problems of a placebo control arm.[106]

The fundamental basis for the initiation and continuation of a clinical trial is the maintenance of the state of clinical equipoise. Charles Fried defined theoretical equipoise as a state of genuine uncertainly regarding the relative merits of the arms of a protocol such that the evidence is balanced.[107] In true equipoise there is complete ignorance of which arm is superior, thus satisfying the null hypothesis. Because the findings from even a single case could eliminate theoretical equipoise and thereby make a RCT unethical, Benjamin Freedman modified the concept to the clinical arena. Freedman defined clinical equipoise as a state in which there exists an honest, professional disagreement among experts in the clinical community concerning the comparative merits of two or more forms of treatment for a condition.[108] Jason Karlawish and John Lantos suggested that the concept of clinical equipoise should be expanded further to incorporate the opinions of a community of physicians and patients, a concept they call community equipoise.[109]

For a RCT to be ethical, it must be designed, implemented, and carried out in a state of clinical equipoise. Because the trial is intended to answer the question of which treatment arm is superior, it should be designed to disturb the state of clinical equipoise at its conclusion. However, if within the course of a RCT equipoise is disturbed, the ethically correct course of action is to terminate the trial and provide all patients with the superior therapy. The question of to what extent clinical equipoise must be disturbed before terminating the trial was addressed in a survey. Most investigators concurred that in a two-armed study, once clinical equipoise had been disturbed to levels greater than 70:30 the trial should be stopped.[110] Data monitoring committees have an important responsibility to continuously monitor results and to terminate trials once clinical equipoise has been disturbed sufficiently to produce unequivocal results.[111] These committees have an important responsibility because premature termination of a RCT creates its own set of ethical problems.[112]

The determination of clinical equipoise in each study, however, is not as straightforward as it first might appear. Data from separate studies often conflict and the resolution of the conflict may not be clarified even through meta-analysis.[113] Expert opinion may differ as a function of discipline. For example, epidemiologists and urologists appear to differ by discipline on the utility of screening with serum levels of prostate-specific antigen for the diagnosis and treatment of prostate cancer.[114] Specialty societies and other expert bodies may publish guidelines based on learned opinion rather than data. These guidelines then may be regarded as defining the standard of care and, despite the absence of an evidence base, they may be difficult for investigators to ignore. Individual physicians also may express a strong opinion about which arm of a RCT may be better for an individual patient based on specific details of the patient's illness and patient preferences.[115]

The RCT has come under criticism for several other potential ethical shortcomings.[116]

The RCT in which the patient's treating physician also serves as the investigator creates a state of double agency in which the two professional roles may conflict. Treating physicians have a fiduciary duty always to put the welfare of their patient first. The investigator, conversely, is concerned primarily with a scientific question for which the patient as a research subject is a means to an end. These conflicting responsibilities can damage a physician's fiduciary duty to the patient by creating a conflict of responsibility.

Enrollment in a RCT may diminish a patient's autonomy. True autonomy can be exercised only when the patient has the freedom to choose which arm of the protocol to enroll in.[117] The unique value system and personal preferences of a patient may make one arm appear more desirable even though there is no evidence that the outcome from that arm is superior.[118] Some scholars even have suggested that this problem could be avoided by obtaining consent after randomization. Consent would be necessary only if the patient was randomized to the experimental arm. Explicit consent would be unnecessary if the patient was randomized to the control arm because the patient then would receive standard therapy.[119] However, self-selection introduces a new variable that may be relevant in outcome. The fate of all "eligible refusers" must be followed to provide information about whether self-selection has affected the generalizability of results.

The RCT may limit physicians' authority. If the physician has reason to believe that one arm of a protocol is superior to another for a given patient, the physician's ethical duty to see that the patient is enrolled in that arm is thwarted by the randomized study design.[120] But because these clinical judgments often are influenced heavily by nonscientific factors such as last case bias, physicians should exercise caution and not base a conclusion about which arm may be superior for a given patient on insufficient evidence.

More recent critics have argued that clinical equipoise fails as a concept. Deborah Hellman claims that clinical equipoise is a belief unrelated to a decision and sick people need to make decisions.[121] Franklin Miller and Howard Brody claim that the ethical foundation for clinical equipoise is flawed because it wrongly conflates research ethics with clinical ethics; what is ethically required is to prevent patient exploitation.[122] Lynn Jansen counters that the Miller-Brody position fails because it would permit clinical trials that are not in the best medical interest of research subjects which she calls "bad trial deals."[123] Winston Chiong disagrees with the Miller-Brody account and suggests replacing it with the Kantian universalizability test for the reasonable partiality that physicians should show their patients.[124] Despite some merits in these arguments, clinical equipoise has remained a durable foundation for the ethics of clinical trials that has been widely understood and accepted. I doubt that it will be abandoned soon.

Once the RCT is concluded, the trial results should be reported accurately and honestly, with a clear account of the patient accrual, randomization process, and statistical analysis, according to accepted practices and guidelines.[125] The Consolidated Standards of Reporting Trials (CONSORT) committee has published guidelines for the ethically correct reporting of RCTs.[126]

Pharmaceutical companies, which sponsor many clinical trials, have been criticized for not making public the details of trial results to volunteer research subjects and others. In 1997, the United States Congress enacted the Food and Drug Modernization Act, one feature of which was the creation of a public registry for clinical trials (ClinicalTrials.gov) under the FDA Investigational New Drug regulations.[127] In 2004, the International Committee of Medical Journal Editors announced that its journals would no longer publish the results of any clinical trial that had not been entered into the ClinicalTrials.gov registry or another qualified public registry.[128] This move led to a striking increase in the number of clinical trials registered in 2005.[129] All clinical trial sponsors should enter the trial details into the registry in fairness to the research subjects who, by dint of volunteering and accepting risks, have a right to know the results and to benefit from the ethical principle of transparency.

The Placebo in Trials of Medication or Surgery

The placebo has achieved an important if controversial place in the design and execution of clinical trials. The RCT, the most robust method to test the efficacy of newly discovered pharmaceuticals, often employs a placebo-control arm to rigorously test if the drug in question exerts beneficial effects or side effects significantly greater than placebo. The use of placebo controls in RCTs raises both scientific and ethical issues worthy of consideration.

Ethical analyses generally conclude that using a placebo control in a RCT is acceptable when there is no known therapy of proven effectiveness for the condition in question.[130] The principle of clinical equipoise holds that placebo-controlled or active-controlled RCTs are ethical when there exists genuine uncertainty in the scientific community regarding the efficacy of competing arms of a clinical trial.[131] Franklin Miller and Howard Brody defended the use of placebos in RCTs while attacking the principle of clinical equipoise as mistaken and unnecessary. They argued that a placebo arm in a RCT is justified ethically when it is supported by a sound methodology and when it does not expose research subjects to excessive risks of harm.[132]

The ethical debate currently centers on those RCTs in which a therapy of proven effectiveness exists for the condition in question but a placebo control is employed nevertheless. In a much quoted article, Kenneth Rothman and Karin Michels decry as unethical the continued practice of using placebo controls in studies in which treatment of proven effectiveness exists, and they assert that only active controls should be used.[133] Rothman and Michels cite the passage in the Declaration of Helsinki that states "every patient—including those of a control group, if any—should be assured of the best proven diagnostic and therapeutic method."[134]

In a rebuttal of this position, Robert Temple and Susan Ellenberg defended the use of placebo controls in RCTs that test conditions in which effective therapy exists. Temple and Ellenberg concurred with Rothman and Michels that the use of placebo controls would be unethical for conditions for which delay or omission of available treatments would increase mortality or irreversible morbidity in the population studied. However, they argued that for conditions in which delay or omission of available treatments would not produce any of these serious harms, placebo controls can remain ethical if the patient is fully informed of the availability of alternative therapy. Temple and Ellenberg further contended that the framers of the Declaration of Helsinki did not intend the phrase cited by Rothman and Michels to categorically eliminate the use of placebo controls.[135]

A patient's decision to enroll as a human subject of a RCT involves many considerations. Some patients prefer to receive standard therapy when RCT entry creates the risk that they may be randomized to a placebo arm. Some accept that risk because they have reason to believe that the tested pharmaceutical is superior and RCT entry at least gives them a chance to receive it. Baruch Brody pointed out that other factors motivate research subjects to enroll in RCTs, including the patient's interest in being treated and monitored by the experts involved in the research protocol, curiosity about the research, disenchantment with the efficacy of existing therapies, and altruism.[136]

Regulatory agencies also influence the scientific decision as to whether a RCT uses placebo controls or active controls. In an editorial discussing the use of placebo-controlled studies in the testing of new anticonvulsant drugs, David Chadwick and Michael Privitera pointed out that the FDA requires new anticonvulsant drugs to be tested against placebo controls and is unwilling to grant evidence of efficacy if the drug is tested only against a standard anticonvulsant and found to be equivalent. They understand the FDA's rationale that equivalency also could mean that both drugs are equally ineffective or that a potentially effective drug might appear ineffective depending upon the dose chosen, the population of patients studied, and other factors. Chadwick and Privitera explained that testing one anticonvulsant drug against another also would provide comparative efficacy information that clinicians value. After all, clinicians must decide which anticonvulsant drug to use in each case, not whether to use an anticonvulsant drug or a placebo.[137]

While the use of a placebo arm in a RCT has become standard practice in the evaluation of new pharmaceuticals, a placebo arm has not been a tradition in the development of new surgical procedures. Development and acceptance of new operations are based upon plausibility, feasibility, and results in animal studies and in small, uncontrolled studies of patients. These uncontrolled trials therefore can introduce biases and placebo effects that raise serious questions about the actual efficacy of the surgical procedures.[138] Surgery itself has a clear placebo effect.[139] A number of previously accepted surgical procedures have been abandoned once careful controlled studies demonstrated their lack of efficacy or safety. Only about 7% of surgical investigators employ a randomized study design of any type.[140]

The issue of placebo surgery was brought to public attention by the NIH-funded, placebo-controlled, clinical trial of fetal nigral dopamine neuron transplantation for the treatment of Parkinson's disease.[141] To control for all variables, half of the study patients received sham surgery without instillation of the fetal nigral dopamine neurons. This protocol received approval by the NIH study section and the IRBs of the participating institutions. All reviewers concurred that absent a placebo arm with sham surgery, it would impossible to know if the procedure was effective. A major benefit of this study was to prevent harm to future patients if the procedure was shown to be ineffective.[142] The investigators understood that the risks to the patient in the placebo arm might not be justified by the benefit to them but argued that this situation is no different from the risks incurred in a pharmaceutical study. They pointed out that there are clear risks of new pharmaceuticals and that this study design minimized the surgical risks to the subjects. They also believed that a rigorous informed consent procedure was sufficient to insure voluntary participation.[143]

Some medical ethicists rejected these justifications and argued that it was unethical to conduct sham surgery—because of the attendant risks—even for the goal of developing generalizable knowledge. For example, Ruth Macklin posed the problem as tension between the highest standard of research design and the highest standard of ethics.[144] When these two important goals come into conflict, which should prevail? She explained that the magnitude of the risks of anesthesia and surgery for the placebo arm never would be permitted by a safety committee in a clinical trial of a pharmaceutical agent.

Macklin was particularly concerned that the usual practice of informed consent may be inadequate to protect vulnerable patient-subjects volunteering because of their strong belief in the efficacy of the transplantation procedure and their hope to be randomized to the active treatment group. She wondered to what extent paternalism would be ethically justified to create regulations that protect overeager patients from undergoing unnecessary risk.[145]

I believe that some surgical procedures for which the benefit is not obvious require proper clinical trials including, if necessary, a trial arm with placebo surgery. I view the consent for such surgery as an essential protection for the patient-subject. But I would not overprotect the patient-subject. Because a RCT often is necessary to prove efficacy, I would allow patients, after full disclosure, to make an ennobling gesture by volunteering to contribute to research that may improve the lives of future patients. I have heard this sentiment expressed by patients to whom the opportunity to participate in the study was profoundly important and imparted transcendent meaning to the suffering they endured from their illness. While I agree with Macklin that the risks may be disproportionate for the benefit, I believe that a spirit of volunteerism also should be permitted and respected. Franklin Miller provided an ethical analysis supporting the use of sham surgery in RCTs that emphasized its methodological necessity, favorable risk-benefit assessment, and mitigation of harms to subject through informed consent.[146]

Developing Countries

An ongoing controversy in the execution of RCTs in developing countries involves whether it is ethical to carry out placebo-controlled trials for preventable disorders when the cure is unaffordable in that country. The controversy began over NIH-sponsored trials in developing countries to reduce maternal-to-fetal transmission of HIV. These trials were designed with control arms that did not include antiretroviral drug treatment, even though providing this treatment could have prevented some deaths, because such treatment is not affordable in the countries being studied. Several ethicists attacked the NIH claiming that because the investigators had the opportunity to prevent deaths and because the control groups would have been given antiretroviral drugs if the study had been performed in the developed world, this practice was unethical.[147]

In a response to these attacks, the directors of the NIH and the U.S. Centers for Disease Control and Prevention defended their decisions by justifying the design of these trials.[148] They pointed out that the placebo-controlled group experienced a risk no greater than they would have experienced without the study because antiretroviral drugs were not available. Most importantly, they explained that this particular study design answered a question about the safety and value of an intervention that could be made available in the local setting in which it was performed. The goal was to improve the quality of medical care in that particular developing country and the study was essential to answer the question of whether the intervention would succeed. Moreover, despite the ethical criticism from scholars in the developed world, the studies enjoyed the sponsorship of officials within the countries who agreed that the particular study design would satisfactorily and usefully answer the question and ultimately improve the health of the local citizens.

This controversy highlighted a larger question: if the practice is ethical, perhaps the Declaration of Helsinki should be revised to permit developing countries to carry out RCTs incorporating placebo-controlled arms for preventable or otherwise treatable diseases, such as the HIV perinatal transmission situation. The Declaration of Helsinki requires that: "The benefits, risks, burdens and effectiveness of the new method should be tested against those of the best current prophylactic, diagnostic and therapeutic methods . . . At the conclusion of the study, every patient entered into the study should be assured of access to the best prophylactic, diagnostic and therapeutic methods identified by the study."[149]

Robert Levine argued that the Declaration should be modified to incorporate the concept of the "highest attainable and sustainable therapy."[150] This concept refers to the highest standard of therapy the host country could reasonably be expected to sustain following the completion of the trial.[151] When a developing host country cannot be expected to provide continued antiretroviral therapy because it cannot afford it, a RCT in that country should not be required to provide these drugs to all patients during the trial. Other commentators, however, believed that such modifications of the Declaration of Helsinki were misdirected because they would weaken accepted international ethical standards protecting human research subjects.[152]

Physicians and scientists living in Third World communities adopted varying positions on the question. For example, in Uganda in 1997, the National Consensus Conference in Bioethics and Health Research adopted the *Guidelines for the Conduct of Health Research involving Human Subjects in Uganda*. These guidelines provided a series of protections to human research subjects but permitted placebo-controlled studies in which "the placebo arm is provided with the treatment or diagnosis product or device that is considered to be the normal standard of care in the community in which the trial is being conducted."[153] Conversely, in Thailand, an AIDS physician working for the Thai Red Cross Society opined that placebo-controlled studies of maternal-to-fetal HIV transmission that did not provide antiretroviral drugs were unethical.[154]

More recently, the United States National Bioethics Advisory Commission argued that clinical trials carried out in developing countries by research groups or companies in the United States should be bound by American ethical standards. They held that researchers in the developed world never should exploit vulnerable populations and should limit trials to those that are responsive to host countries' needs and their abilities to provide the drug or device to their own populations.[155] Research guidelines derived from these principles that are ethically

sound and provide for the needs and best interests of the citizens of the host countries have been proposed in collaboration with representatives of the host countries. These guidelines emphasize: (1) the provision of fair benefits to research subjects and the host population, availability of the intervention to the population, appropriate public health measures, and financial rewards to the test population; (2) the creation of a collaborative partnership emphasizing informed consent of research subjects and approval of the protocol by the population; and (3) the maintenance of transparency with a central repository of benefits agreements and community consultation about the research.[156] Research satisfying these criteria can be ethically acceptable when it is carried out as a partnership between researchers and citizens of the host countries.[157]

CONFLICTS OF INTEREST

Over the past several decades, the formerly scholarly pursuit of clinical investigation has become an industry some have called the "academic-industrial complex."[158] Corporate sponsorship by pharmaceutical and medical device manufacturers long ago eclipsed federal scientific sponsorship (e.g., NIH, NSF) as the principal source of funding for clinical trials and now accounts for approximately 70% of all clinical drug trials in the United States [159] and 57% of all biomedical research funding.[160] In most clinical trials, investigators are compensated by capitated payments on the basis of the numbers of patients enrolled or patient visits, or by an institutional block grant. The amount of these payments is budgeted in advance to compensate the investigators and institutions for incurred expenses, but the sums provided by the corporate study sponsors routinely exceed expenses.[161] The generous level of reimbursement is designed to provide an incentive to enroll patients. Indeed, many academic departments and some practices have grown to depend on the profits accrued from these trials to provide operational income. They often regard guaranteed corporate income as a welcome alternative to the uncertain game of applying for peer-reviewed federal funding.

A conflict of interest can occur when a physician-investigator, in an attempt to generate income, urges a patient to enroll in a study that may not be in the patient's best interest. For example, a better form of treatment for a patient's medical condition may be available but the financial incentive leads the physician-investigator to recommend that the patient enroll in the trial. As is true in most conflicts of interest, the involved professional likely would vigorously deny that the financial incentive plays any role in the recommendation to enroll. However, the influence may be exerted subconsciously.[162] Because of usually inadequate disclosure, most patients enrolled in clinical trials remain unaware of the financial arrangements and monetary incentives that may motivate their physicians to enroll them.

This conflict is aggravated by the dual roles many physician-investigators play, simultaneously serving as the patient's physician and the study clinical investigator. In this state of double agency, the physician's fiduciary duty to place the patient's interests first can be compromised by the competing scientific or financial interests of the investigator.[163] The immutable reality of clinical investigation, however, is that in many circumstances the roles cannot be separated. The dual role has become even more common given the recent trend for physicians in private practice to serve as participating "clinical investigators" in community-based multi-center drug trials.[164] The conflict implicit in the dual role imparts an even higher standard of ethical behavior on the physician-investigator to guarantee that the best interests of the patient are not compromised by the concurrent investigator role, particularly given the profit incentive. The philosopher Hans Jonas stated one resolution to this type of conflict over 30 years ago: "The physician is obligated to the patient and to no one else. He is neither the agent of society, nor of the interests of medical science."[165]

Several concrete steps can reduce this conflict of interest.[166] (1) The "finder's fee," a commission paid for finding and enrolling a patient, should be eliminated because it aggravates the financial conflict by creating further monetary incentives to recruit patients.[167] (2) Patients should be notified about the precise financial relationship between the study sponsor and the physician-investigator. Although full disclosure does not eliminate the conflict, it mitigates it by making patients aware that physicians may have a nonscientific motive.[168] (3) Payments to physician-investigators and institutions should be commensurate with their expenses and not excessive to reduce the overt profit inducement to enroll patients. (4) The income from study sponsors should be redistributed to minimize the direct financial incentive to enroll patients. For example, the money could pass through an office that pays direct study expenses first, then places any remaining funds in an institution-wide pool to which investigators can apply for additional funds but which they do not control.[169] (5) Monetary payments to compensate research subjects should be structured on a wage-payment model in which payments are made as a standard wage for unskilled labor. A wage-payment model fairly and appropriately reimburses the research subject for time and effort but lessens excessive inducement and the creation of an economic underclass of subjects who disproportionately bear the risks of clinical trials.[170]

Conflicts Between Academic Institutions and Industry

Conflicts of obligation and financial conflicts of interest may coexist when physicians have simultaneous relationships with academic institutions and industry.[171] A 1994 survey of companies conducting life-sciences research revealed that approximately 90% already had established relationships with academic institutions.[172] Academic institutions benefit from these relationships because corporate partners can provide increased support for academic research, generate income for academic health centers, increase the potential for greater scientific and commercial productivity in both universities and industry, and enhance the opportunity for undergraduate and postgraduate education.[173] But such relationships also produce risks including the requirement of increased secrecy in an otherwise open academic environment[174] and a concomitant diminution of public sector support for life sciences research.[175] Industrial sponsors also may dictate the direction of academic research to be more applied ("translational") than basic.

Physicians with dual loyalties to academic institutions and industry may have conflicting duties in their attempts to serve both masters. The corporate sponsor may impose certain restrictions on the university investigator on the publication, communication, or other free use of research results. These restrictions on the usual activities of an researcher may create the perception that the investigator has been "bought" by the sponsor.[176] And the corporate sponsor may exert irresistible pressure on the researcher to publish only those results the company believes are beneficial to its commercial success.[177]

Harms of the relationship also may affect the academic institution.[178] These risks include a reluctance of investigators to freely share research results among colleagues; damage to the institution's public relations resulting from the public's perception that the institution is seeking profits; and uncompensated use of institutional facilities.[179] A survey of funded investigators showed that these harms are not merely theoretical. The survey disclosed an alarmingly high number of cases of publication embargoes and refusals to share research results with other investigators, both actions intended to protect patent applications, protect the research group's scientific lead over its competitors, or facilitate the resolution of disputes over ownership of intellectual property.[180] A more recent survey of academic medical centers offered more promising findings. Over 85% of respondents reported that they would not approve contractual provisions giving industry sponsors the authority to revise manuscripts or decide whether results should be published.[181]

Even more complex relationships and conflicts may result from academic institutions that have a direct financial stake in research conducted within their own laboratories, in the context of a financial agreement with a biotechnology company. In these increasingly common relationships, academic institutions hold equity positions in biotechnology companies, often owning hundreds of thousands or millions of the company's shares. One survey found that approximately two-thirds of academic institutions held equity positions in start-up high-technology firms that sponsored research at those institutions.[182] Members of university faculties often create these companies and, with the university, share equity positions in the corporations. These relationships create the potential for both individual and institutional conflicts of interest.[183]

Institutional conflicts of interest may be created when the interests of the biotechnology company, partially owned by the university and its faculty, diverge from the missions of the university. These conflicts may produce unique harms to the academic center and to its faculty. There may be overt or subtle pressure to streamline the process of patient-subjects' consent for clinical trials of the product of the jointly owned biotechnology company. There may be pressure to minimize side effects or other shortcomings of the proposed therapy during the consent process. There may be pressure on postdoctoral trainees or students to assist in research to advance these products that may not be beneficial to the trainees' academic development. Investigators within the university may develop a subconscious bias toward the product's success during the clinical trial that compromises their scientific integrity. And, most seriously, once the public becomes aware that the institution is conducting research in which there is a financial conflict of interest, such knowledge may erode confidence in the integrity of the biomedical research establishment and lessen its public support.[184]

IRB members who approve human subjects research also have conflicts of interest arising from their relationships with industry. A recent study found that 36% of IRB members at 100 academic institutions had at least one relationship with an industrial research sponsor during the previous year.[185] About 15% of IRB members reported that they had reviewed at least one protocol within the past year from a company with whom they had a financial relationship. Only 58% reported that they always disclosed the relationship to an IRB official and about two-thirds recused themselves from voting on the protocol as is appropriate to mitigate conflicts of interest.[186]

Several scholars and organizations have proposed regulatory solutions to prevent or mitigate these conflicts.[187] The simplest is to recognize that the decision to engage in such a conflicting relationship represents a voluntary choice. Therefore, a faculty member or university simply may opt out of such a relationship.[188] However, the monetary benefits to faculty members and the university are sufficiently seductive that opting out is an uncommon solution. Disclosure of conflicts of interest does not eliminate them but can mitigate them to some degree. To be effective, however, disclosure must be made publicly and to the patients who serve as research subjects.[189] Enhanced internal oversight by IRBs of investigators' relationships can help prevent or regulate the most serious conflicts.[190] Otherwise, external regulation of the conflicts by governmental agencies will be inevitable.[191]

Nearly everyone agrees that universities should draft and enforce strict policies regulating the relationship of the university and its faculty to industry. A survey of all 127 American medical schools and 170 other research institutions, however, showed that the rules of the disclosure policies varied widely. The authors of the study urged universities to adopt stricter standards of disclosure and enforcement to protect academic and scientific integrity.[192] Another survey of all American medical schools found that the median annual number of contracts with clinical trial sponsors was 103 per school but compliance with guidelines published by the International Committee of Medical Journal Editors governing study design, access to data, and control over publication was under 10%.[193]

In a related survey of the 10 universities receiving the largest amount of research funding from the NIH, Bernard Lo and colleagues found the same wide variation in disclosure requirements and rules of equity ownership. They suggested that rules should uniformly prohibit university investigators and research staff from owning stock, holding stock options, or having positions of responsibility within the company that could plausibly affect research results.[194] In an accompanying opinion piece, the two chief academic officers of the Harvard Medical School discussed the benefits and risks of industry–university relationships and offered ideas to create a "just and prudent balance" between the two entities.[195]

Hamilton Moses and Joseph Martin proposed a series of principles and remedies to regulate the conflicts of interest inherent in university-industry relationships. They offered the following principles: (1) veracity of results of basic research and of clinical trials should not be compromised; (2) oversight by a disinterested party should occur; (3) proprietary rights and control of intellectual property ought to be acknowledged at the outset and assurances made regarding the right to publish; and (4) financial and nonfinancial incentives should be designed to address institutional, senior investigator, and junior faculty needs. They suggested several possible remedies: (1) universities and their industrial sponsors might create separate research institutes; (2) external oversight should be enhanced, perhaps by empowering independent boards, such as IRBs, to examine research conflicts of interest; and (3) a new entity should be created, separate from the university, to hold equity and receive royalties.[196]

In 2001, the Association of American Medical Colleges published a series of detailed guidelines regulating individual and institutional conflicts of interest in human subjects research. The guidelines require full prior reporting of an individual's significant financial interests, the development of institutional policies of transparency, the empaneling of an institutional conflicts of interest committee to review and rule on potential conflicts, and a rebuttable presumption banning individuals from conducting any research in which they have significant financial interests.[197] Most academic medical centers have drafted institutional guidelines to comply with these and other national guidelines.[198] The NIH recently passed strict and controversial guidelines preventing conflicts of interest in intramural NIH researchers that some scholars fear will make recruitment and retention of NIH scientists more difficult.[199]

SCIENTIFIC MISCONDUCT

The professional conduct of scientists and clinical investigators performing research has been much in the news over the past two decades, with scandals reported in the popular press of research data falsification and fraudulent publication, misrepresentation of credentials, and plagiarism.[200] Any analysis of scientific misconduct should begin with its definition. The United States Public Health Service (USPHS) stated that scientific misconduct encompasses "fabrication, falsification, plagiarism, or other practices that seriously deviate from those that are commonly accepted within the scientific community for proposing, conducting, or reporting research." These categories specifically excluded "honest error" and "honest difference in interpretation or judgments of data." The NSF uses a similar definition.[201]

The National Academy of Sciences (NAS) tightened the definition, responding to valid criticisms that the USPHS inclusion of the phrase "other practices that seriously deviate from those that are commonly accepted . . ." might unwisely broaden the definition to include unorthodox but legitimate research activities. The NAS definition limits misconduct to "fabrication, falsification, or plagiarism in proposing, performing, or reporting research." They classified "questionable research practices" including insufficient supervision of laboratory personnel and "honorary coauthorship" as separate and less severe offenses.[202] Rebecca Dresser pointed out that the intent of the scientist who performed misconduct should be incorporated into the definition because more severe punishments should be administered to a scientist who intended to deceive than to a scientist who was merely lazy or sloppy, or took short cuts.[203] Her separation of willful dishonesty from inadvertent negligence also is consistent with the intuition of surveyed scientists about the seriousness and appropriate punishment of various types of scientific misconduct.[204]

The process of investigating an allegation of misconduct should follow established legal doctrines with regard to the behavior of the investigators, procuring of evidence, convening the hearing, and releasing information to the public.[205] Unfortunately, the current scientific misconduct disciplinary processes in place at most universities are suboptimal.[206] University policies, federal law, and court precedents should be rigorously followed.[207] Whistleblowers should receive adequate protection from retaliation.[208] The greater use of proper legal due process will more adequately protect the scientist accused of misconduct.[209] Educational programs in scientific ethics developed to clarify the difference between appropriate and inappropriate professional scientific behaviors should be made part of required medical and scientific curricula.[210]

Federal oversight of allegations of research misconduct in the United States is performed by the DHHS Office of Research Integrity (ORI). The ORI provides a process to investigate allegations of scientific misconduct and an appeals process in which researchers accused of scientific misconduct can challenge the government's findings in a hearing before the Research Integrity Adjudications Panel. The due process followed in such cases is clearly delineated and extensive.[211] Professional journal editors also have created administrative processes to handle allegations of breaches of publication ethics and criteria for retracting published articles when author misconduct has been demonstrated.[212] Assuring scientific integrity and maintaining public confidence are essential for continued public support of the research enterprise.

NOTES

1. For general references reviewing the topic of ethical issues in clinical research, see Emanuel EJ, Crouch RA, Arras JD, Moreno JD, Grady C (eds). *Ethical and Regulatory Aspects of Clinical Research: Readings and Commentary.* Baltimore: Johns Hopkins University Press, 2003; Vanderpool HY (ed). *The Ethics of Research Involving Human Subjects.* Frederick, MD: University Publishing Group, 1996; and Levine RJ. *Ethics and the Regulation of Clinical Research,* 2nd ed. New Haven: Yale University Press, 1988. For a brief review of this topic as it pertains to neurology, see American Academy of Neurology Ethics and Humanities Subcommittee. Ethical issues in clinical research in neurology: advancing knowledge and protecting human research subjects. *Neurology* 1998;50:592–595.

2. Kant I. *Groundwork of the Metaphysics of Morals,* 3rd ed. Ellington JW, transl. Indianapolis: Hackett Publishing Co., Inc., 1981:36 [Ak. 436–439]. Kant's axiom forms the ethical basis for outlawing slavery.

3. Richardson HS, Belsky L. The ancillary-care responsibilities of medical researchers: an ethical framework for thinking about the clinical care that researchers owe their subjects. *Hastings Cent Rep* 2004;34(1):25–33.

4. Miller FG. Research ethics and misguided moral intuition. *J Law Med Ethics* 2004;32:111–116.

5. Morreim EH. The clinical investigator as fiduciary: discarding a misguided idea. *J Law Med Ethics* 2005;33:586–598.

6. The boundary concepts are discussed in Brody BA, McCullough LB, Sharp RR. Consensus and controversy in clinical research ethics. *JAMA* 2005;294;1411–1414.

7. For an analysis of the distinction between innovation and research that proposes criteria for determining when institutional review board review is necessary, see Bernstein M, Bampoe J. Surgical innovation or surgical evolution: an ethical and practical guide to handling novel neurosurgical procedures. *J Neurosurg* 2004;100:2–7.

8. Casarett D, Karlawish JH, Sugarman J. Determining when quality improvement initiatives should be considered research: proposed criteria and potential implications. *JAMA* 2000;283:2275–2280.

9. Emanuel EJ, Wendler D, Grady C. What makes clinical research ethical? *JAMA* 2000;283:2701–2711.

10. Shalowitz DI, Miller FG. Disclosing individual results of clinical research: implications of respect for participants. *JAMA* 2005;294:737–740.

11. DuVal G, Gensler G, Danis M. Ethical dilemmas encountered by clinical researchers. *J Clin Ethics* 2005;16:267–276.

12. This remarkable history is outlined in Lock S. Research ethics—a brief historical review to 1965. *J Intern Med* 1995;238:513–520.

13. Beecher HK. Ethics and clinical research. *N Engl J Med* 1966;274:1354–1360. For a fascinating historical account and follow-up of the cases Beecher reported, see Rothman DJ. Ethics and human experimentation: Henry Beecher revisited. *N Engl J Med* 1987;317:1195–1199.

14. Reverby SM. More fact than fiction: cultural memory and the Tuskegee Syphilis Study. *Hastings Cent Rep* 2001;31(5):22–28.

15. For a contemporaneous account of the Tuskegee study, see Curran WJ. The Tuskegee syphilis study. *N Engl J Med* 1973;289:730–731. For a series of essays on the social and historical context of the Tuskegee study, see Crigger B-J (ed). Twenty years after: the legacy of the Tuskegee syphilis study. *Hastings Cent Rep* 1992;22(6):29–40. For a comprehensive historical account viewing the study in the context of American racism, see Reverby SM (ed). *Tuskegee's Truths: Rethinking the Tuskegee Syphilis Study*. Chapel Hill, NC: University of North Carolina Press, 2000.

16. This case is described in Goldby S. Experiments at the Willowbrook State School. *Lancet* 1971;1:749. For a retrospective ethical analysis and defense by one of the Willowbrook investigators, see Krugman S. The Willowbrook hepatitis study revisited: ethical aspects. *Rev Infect Dis* 1986;8:157–162.

17. This episode is discussed in Lerner BH. Sins of omission – cancer research without informed consent. *N Engl J Med* 2004;351:628–630 and Preminger BA. The case of Chester M. Southam: research ethics and the limits of professional responsibility. *The Pharos* 2002;65(2):4–9.

18. See Lifton RJ. *The Nazi Doctors: Medical Killing and the Psychology of Genocide*. New York: Basic Books, 1986 and Caplan AL ed. *When Medicine Went Mad: Bioethics and the Holocaust*. Totowa, NJ: Human Press, 1992.

19. Much commentary has been written about the Nuremberg Code. See Annas GJ. *The Nazi Doctors and the Nuremberg Code: Human Rights in Human Experimentation*. New York: Oxford University Press, 1992; Shuster E. Fifty years later: the significance of the Nuremberg Code. *N Engl J Med* 1997;337:1436–1440; and Moreno JD. Reassessing the influence of the Nuremberg Code on American medical ethics. *J Contemp Health Law Policy* 1997;13:347–360.

20. World Medical Association Declaration of Helsinki: ethical principles for medical and research involving human subjects. *JAMA* 2000;284:3043–3045 and World Medical Association Declaration of Helsinki (2004). http://www.wma.net/e/policy/b3.htm (Accessed April 7, 2007).

21. The National Commission for the Protection of Human Subjects of Biomedical and Behavioral Research. *The Belmont Report: Ethical Principles and Guidelines for the Protection of Human Subjects of Research*. US Department of Health, Education and Welfare, DHEW Publication No. (OS) 78-0012, 1978. See the retrospective commentary by Cassell EJ. The principles of the Belmont Report: how have respect for persons, beneficence, and justice been applied to clinical medicine? *Hastings Cent Rep* 2000;30(4):12–21.

22. President's Commission for the Study of Ethical Problems in Medicine and Biomedical and Behavioral Research. *Protecting Human Subjects: The Adequacy and Uniformity of Federal Rules and their Implementation*. Washington, DC: US Government Printing Office, 1981.

23. Yank V, Rennie D. Reporting of informed consent and ethics committee approval in clinical trials. *JAMA* 2002;287:2835–2838.

24. 45 *Code of Federal Regulations* § 46. Department of Health and Human Services Regulations for the Protection of Human Subjects. Revised June 18, 1991.

25. Steinbrook R. Improving protection for research subjects. *N Engl J Med* 2002;346:1425–1430.

26. For a comprehensive and succinct summary of how IRBs function to protect human subjects, see Wagner RM. Ethical review of research involving human subjects: when and why is IRB review necessary? *Muscle Nerve* 2003;28:27–39. For a more detailed account directed at educating new IRB members, see Mazur DJ. *Evaluating the Science and Ethics of Research on Humans. A Guide for IRB Members.* Baltimore: Johns Hopkins University Press, 2007.

27. See the further discussion of these problems in Woodward B. Challenges to human subjects protections in US medical research. *JAMA* 1999;282:1947–1952.

28. Emanuel EJ, Wood A, Fleischman A, et al. Oversight of human participants research: identifying problems to evaluate reform proposals. *Ann Intern Med* 2004;141:282–291. One indicator of current IRB dysfunction is the rise of litigation against IRBs and investigators. See Mello MM, Studdert DM, Brennan TA. The rise of litigation in human subjects research. *Ann Intern Med* 2003;139:40–45.

29. For the interrelationship and status of international codes, see Fluss SS. The evolution of research ethics: the current international configuration. *J Law Med Ethics* 2004;32:596–603.

30. Council for International Organizations of Medical Sciences and World Health Organization. *International Ethical Guidelines for Biomedical Research Involving Human Subjects.* Geneva: World Health Organizations, 1993. These recommendations are discussed in Levine RJ. New international guidelines for research involving human subjects. *Ann Intern Med* 1993;119:339–341.

31. National Institutes of Health Office for Human Research Protection. http://www.hhs.gov/ohrp/ (Accessed May 7, 2007).

32. The National Bioethics Advisory Commission published several works that involve research consent. See, for example, National Bioethics Advisory Commission. *Research Involving Persons with Mental Disorders That May Affect Decision Making Capacity.* Vol 1. Rockville, MD: National Bioethics Advisory Commission, 1998. http://www.georgetown.edu/research/nrcbl/nbac/ (Accessed May 9, 2007).

33. Association of American Medical Colleges. *Developing a Code of Ethics in Research: A Guide for Scientific Societies.* Washington, DC: Association of American Medical Colleges, 1997.

34. American Association for the Advancement of Science. *AAAS Professional Ethics Report.* Washington, DC, 2007. http://www.aaas.org/spp/sfrl/per/per48.pdf. (Accessed May 1, 2007).

35. Miller FG, Wertheimer A. Facing up to paternalism in research ethics. *Hastings Cent Rep* 2007;37(3):24–34.

36. For an analysis of the legal standards of informed consent for human subjects research, see Noah L. Informed consent and the elusive dichotomy between standard and experimental therapy. *Am J Law Med* 2002;28:361–408.

37. For a discussion of the shortcomings of the consent process in practice, see Lantos J. Informed consent: the whole truth for patients? *Cancer* 1993;72:2811–2815.

38. Lavelle-Jones C, Byrne DJ, Rice P, Cuschieri A. Factors affecting quality of informed consent. *Br Med J* 1993;306:885–890.

39. Snowdon C, Garcia J, Elbourne D. Making sense of randomization: responses of parents of critically ill babies to random allocation of treatment in a clinical trial. *Soc Sci Med* 1997;45:1337–1355.

40. Paasche-Orlow MK, Taylor HA, Brancati FL. Readability standards for informed-consent forms as compared with actual readability. *N Engl J Med* 2003;348:721–726.

41. Appelbaum PS, Roth LH, Lidz CW, et al. False hopes and best data: consent to research and the therapeutic misconception. *Hastings Cent Rep* 1987;17(2):20–24. Not only patient-subjects are unclear about when a given therapy counts as an experiment or a treatment, some physicians are also confused. See King NMP. Experimental treatment: oxymoron or aspiration? *Hastings Cent Rep* 1995;25(4):6–15.

42. The confusion between scientific experiment and treatment in many patients' minds, leading them to enroll in clinical trials, is discussed in Miller M. Phase I cancer trials: a collusion of misunderstanding. *Hastings Cent Rep* 2000;30(4):34–42.

43. Miller FG, Rosenstein DL. The therapeutic orientation to clinical trials. *N Engl J Med* 2003;348:1383–1386.

44. Lidz CW, Appelbaum PS, Grisso T, Renaud M. Therapeutic misconception and the appreciation of risk in clinical trials. *Soc Sci Med* 2004;58:1689–1697.

45. Implicit coercion of "desperate volunteers" is discussed in Minogue BP, Palmer-Fernandez G, Udell L, Waller BN. Individual autonomy and the double-blind controlled experiment: the case of desperate volunteers. *J Med Philosophy* 1995;20:43–55 and Logue G, Wear S. A desperate solution: individual autonomy and the double-blind controlled experiment. *J Med Philosophy* 1995;20:57–64.

46. Schaeffer MH, Krantz DS, Wichman A, Masur H, Reed E, Vinicky JK. The impact of disease severity on the informed consent process in clinical research. *Am J Med* 1996;100:261–268.

47. King NMP. Defining and describing benefit appropriately in clinical trials. *J Law Med Ethics* 2000;28:332–343.

48. Flory J, Emanuel E. Interventions to improve research participants' understanding in informed consent for research: a systematic review. *JAMA* 2004;292:1593–1601.

49. Agrawal M, Emanuel AJ. Ethics of phase I oncology studies: reexamining the arguments and data. *JAMA* 2003;290:1075–1082.

50. Hawkins JS, Emanuel EJ. Clarifying confusions about coercion. *Hastings Cent Rep* 2005;35(5):16–19.

51. Horng S, Emanuel EJ, Wilfond B, Rackoff J, Martz K, Grady C. Descriptions of benefits and risks in consent forms for phase I oncology trials. *N Engl J Med* 2002;347:2134–2140.

52. Byock I, Miles SH. Hospice benefits and phase I cancer trials. *Ann Intern Med* 2003;138:335–337.

53. Kim SYH, Holloway RG, Frank S, et al. Volunteering for early phase gene transfer research in Parkinson disease. *Neurology* 2006;66:1010–1015.

54. The problems resulting from double agency are discussed in Shortell SM, Waters TM, Clarke KWB, Budetti PP. Physicians as double agents: maintaining trust in an era of multiple accountabilities. *JAMA* 1998;280:1102–1108.

55. Orentlicher D. Making research a requirement of treatment: why we should sometimes let doctors pressure patients to participate in research. *Hastings Cent Rep* 2005;35(5):20–28.

56. Guyatt GH, Keller JL, Jaeschke R, Rosenbloom D, Adachi JD, Newhouse MT. The n-of-1 randomized controlled trial: clinical usefulness. Our three-year experience. *Ann Intern Med* 1990;112:293–299 and Irwig L, Glasziou P, March L. Ethics of n-of-1 trials. *Lancet* 1995;345:469.

57. Lind SE. Innovative medical therapies: between practice and research. *Clin Res* 1988;36:546–551.

58. Ezekiel Emanuel and colleagues argue that participation in research in developing countries does not create undue inducement. See Emanuel EJ, Currie XE, Herman A. Undue inducement in clinical research in developing countries: is it a worry? *Lancet* 2005;366:336–340 and Pace CA, Emanuel EJ. The ethics of research in developing countries: assessing voluntariness. *Lancet* 2005;365:11–12.

59. McNeil P. Paying people to participate in research: why not? *Bioethics* 1997;11:390–396.

60. Dunn LB, Gordon NE. Improving informed consent and enhancing recruitment for research by understanding economic behavior. *JAMA* 2005;293:609–612.

61. Lemmens R, Elliott C. Guinea pigs on the payroll: the ethics of paying research subjects. *Accountability in Research* 1999;7:3–20 and Council for International Organizations of Medical Sciences. *International Ethical Guidelines for Biomedical Research Involving Human Subjects*. Geneva: World Health Organization, 2002, Guideline 7 and 45 CFR § 46.116.

62. Dickert N, Emanuel E, Grady C. Paying research subjects: an analysis of current policies. *Ann Intern Med* 2002;136:368–373.

63. Emanuel EJ. Ending concerns about undue inducement. *J Law Med Ethics* 2004;32:100–105 and Emanuel EJ. Undue inducement: nonsense on stilts. *Am J Bioethics* 2005;5(5):9–13.

64. Truog RD, Robinson W, Randolph A, Morris A. Is informed consent always necessary for randomized, controlled trials? *N Engl J Med* 1999;340:804–807.

65. Scott LD. Research-related injury: problems and solutions. *J Law Med Ethics* 2003;31:419–428.

66. Steinbrook R. Compensation for injured research subjects. *N Engl J Med* 2006;354:1871–1873.

67. Levine C, Faden R, Grady C, Hammerschmidt D, Eckenwiler L, Sugarman J. The limitations of "vulnerability" as a protection for human research participants. *Am J Bioethics* 2004;4(3):44–49.

68. Fost N. Waived consent for emergency research. *Am J Law Med* 1998;24:163–183.

69. McCarthy CR. To be or not to be: waiving informed consent in emergency research. *Kennedy Inst Ethics J* 1995;5:155–162.

70. Biros MH, Lewis RJ, Olson CM, Runge JW, Cummins RO, Fost N. Informed consent in emergency research: consensus statement from the Coalition Conference of Acute Resuscitation and Critical Care Researchers. *JAMA* 1995;273:1283–1287.

71. These regulations are discussed in Wichman A, Sandler AL. Research involving critically ill subjects in emergency circumstances: new regulations, new challenges. *Neurology* 1997;48:1151–1155.

72. 21 *CFR* § 50.24

73. Protection of human subjects: informed consent and waiver of informed consent in emergency research; final rule. *Federal Register* 1996;61:51498–51531.

74. 45 *CFR* § 46.116{d}

75. Waiver of informed consent requirements in certain emergency research. *Federal Register* 1996; 61:51531–51533.

76. Wichman A, Sandler AL. Research involving critically ill subjects in emergency circumstances: new regulations, new challenges. *Neurology* 1997;48:1151–1155.

77. Adams JG, Wegener J. Acting without asking: an ethical analysis of the Food and Drug Administration waiver of informed consent for emergency research. *Ann Emerg Med* 1999;33:218–223.

78. 45 *Code of Federal Regulations* § 46. Department of Health and Human Services Regulations for the Protection of Human Subjects. Revised June 18, 1991.

79. Wendler D. Protecting subjects who cannot give consent: toward a better standard for "minimal" risks. *Hastings Cent Rep* 2005;35(5):37–43.

80. Levine RL. Research in emergency situations: the role of deferred consent. *JAMA* 1995;273:1300–1302 and Katz J. Blurring the lines: research, therapy, and IRBs. *Hastings Cent Rep* 1997;27(1):9–11.

81. For a comprehensive account of the ethics of using children as clinical research subjects, see Ross LF. *Children in Medical Research: Access versus Protection*. New York: Oxford University Press, 2006.

82. For shorter reviews of the ethical and legal issues that arise in conducting research on children, see Glantz LH. Research with children. *Am J Law Med* 1998;24:213–244 and Kopelman LM. Children as research subjects: a dilemma. *J Med Philosophy* 2000;25:745–764.

83. American Academy of Pediatrics Committee on Bioethics. Informed consent, parental permission, and assent in pediatric practice. *Pediatrics* 1995;95:314–317. Obtaining assent for the treatment of children in a clinical context is discussed in chapter 2.

84. Ondrusek N, Abramovitch R, Pencharz P, Koren G. Empirical examination of the ability of children to consent to clinical research. *J Med Ethics* 1998;24:158–165.

85. See discussion in Woodward B. Challenges to human subjects protections in US medical research. *JAMA* 1999;282:1947–1952.

86. 45 *CFR* § 46:102(i) 1994.

87. Weijer C. The ethical analysis of risk. *J Law Med Ethics* 2000;28:344–361.

88. Freedman B, Fuks A, Weijer C. In loco parentis: minimal risk as an ethical threshold for research upon children. *Hastings Cent Rep* 1993;23(2):13–19.

89. Shah S, Whittle A, Wilfond B, Gensler G, Wendler D. How do institutional review boards apply the federal risk and benefit standards for pediatric research? *JAMA* 2004;291;476–482.

90. Wendler D, Belsky L, Thompson KM, Emanuel EJ. Quantifying the federal minimum risk standard: implications for pediatric research without a prospect of direct benefit. *JAMA* 2005;294:826–832.

91. Kopelman LM. What conditions justify risky nontherapeutic or "no benefit" pediatric studies: a sliding scale analysis. *J Law Med Ethics* 2004;32:749–758.

92. Fisher CB, Kornetsky SZ, Prentice ED. Determining risk in pediatric research with no prospect of direct benefit: time for a national consensus on the interpretation of federal regulations. *Am J Bioethics* 2007;7(3): 5–10.

93. These cases are cited in Woodward B. Challenges to human subjects protections in US medical research. *JAMA* 1999;282:1947–1952.

94. For an account of the history of HIPAA and a legal summary of its application to human subjects research, see Annas GJ. Medical privacy and medical research—judging the new federal regulations. *N Engl J Med* 2002;346:216–220 and Rothstein MA. Research privacy under HIPAA and the Common Rule. *J Law Med Ethics* 2005;31:154–159.

95. Shalowitz D, Wendler D. Informed consent for research and authorization under the Health Insurance Portability and Accountability Privacy Rule: an integrated approach. *Ann Intern Med* 2006;144:685–688.

96. Kulynych J, Korn D. The effect of the new federal medical-privacy rule on research. *N Engl J Med* 2002;346:201–204.

97. Portions of this section have been adapted from Bernat JL. Ethical issues in neurological treatment and clinical trials. In Noseworthy J (ed). *Neurological Therapeutics: Principles and Practice*, 2nd ed. Oxford, UK: Informa Healthcare, 2006:73–83.

98. Shimm DS, Spece RG. Ethical issues and clinical trials. *Drugs* 1993;46:579–584.

99. Kodish E, Lantos JD, Siegler M. Ethical considerations in randomized controlled clinical trials. *Cancer* 1990;65(Suppl):2400–2404.

100. The argument that physicians have an ethical imperative to participate in RCTs was made in Lindley RI, Warlow CP. Why, and how, should clinical trials be conducted? In Zeman A, Emanuel LL (eds). *Ethical Dilemmas in Neurology.* London: W. B. Saunders, 2000:73–86.

101. Claessens MT, Bernat JL, Baron JA. Ethical issues in clinical trials. *Br J Urol* 1995;76(Suppl 2):29–36. I have adapted some of this discussion in the section on RCTs from this article.

102. Illstrup DM. Randomized clinical trials: potential cost savings due to identification of ineffective medical therapies. *Mayo Clin Proc* 1995;70:707–710.

103. Stiller CA. Centralised treatment, entry to trial, and survival. *Br J Cancer* 1994;70:352–362.

104. Schultz KF. Subverting randomization in clinical trials. *JAMA* 1995;274:1456–1458.

105. Levine RJ. Ethics of clinical trials: do they help the patient? *Cancer* 1993;72(Suppl):2805–2810.

106. Sacks HS, Chalmers TC, Smith H Jr. Randomized versus historical controls for clinical trials. *Am J Med* 1982;72:233–240.

107. Fried C. *Medical Experimentation: Personal Integrity and Social Policy: Clinical Studies.* Vol. 5. New York: American Elsevier, 1974:47–48.

108. Freedman B. Equipoise and the ethics of clinical research. *N Engl J Med* 1987;317:141–145.

109. Karlawish JHT, Lantos J. Community equipoise and the architecture of clinical research. *Cambridge Q Healthc Ethics* 1997;6:385–396.

110. Johnson N, Lilford RJ, Brazier W. At what level of collective equipoise does a clinical trial become ethical? *J Med Ethics* 1991;17:30–34.

111. Morse MA, Califf RM, Sugarman J. Monitoring and ensuring safety during clinical research. *JAMA* 2001;285:1201–1205.

112. Mueller PS, Montori VM, Bassler D, Koenig BA, Guyatt GH. Ethical issues in stopping randomized trials early because of apparent benefit. *Ann Intern Med* 2007;146:878–881.

113. Djulbegovic B, Clarke M. Scientific and ethical issues in equivalence trials. *JAMA* 2001;285:1206–1208.

114. Claessens MT, Bernat JL, Baron JA. Ethical issues in clinical trials. *Br J Urol* 1995;76(Suppl 2):29–36.

115. Marquis D. How to resolve an ethical dilemma concerning randomized clinical trials. *N Engl J Med* 1999;341:691–693.

116. Kodish E, Lantos JD, Siegler M. *Cancer* 1990:2400–2404.

117. Kodish E, Lantos JD, Siegler M. *Cancer* 1990:2400–2404.

118. Silverman WA, Altman DG. Patients' preferences and randomized trials. *Lancet* 1996;347:171–174.

119. Gallo C, Perrone F, De Placido S, et al. Informed versus randomized consent to clinical trials. *Lancet* 1995;346:1060–1064.

120. Hellman S, Hellman DS. Of mice but not men: problems of the randomized clinical trial. *N Engl J Med* 1991;22:1585–1589.

121. Hellman D. Evidence, belief, and action: the failure of equipoise to resolve the ethical tension in the randomized clinical trial. *J Law Med Ethics* 2002;30:375–380.

122. Miller FG, Brody H. A critique of clinical equipoise: therapeutic misconception in the ethics of clinical trials. *Hastings Cent Rep* 2003;33(3):19–28.

123. Jansen LA. A closer look at the bad trial deal: beyond clinical equipoise. *Hastings Cent Rep* 2005; 35(5):29–36.

124. Chiong W. The real problem with equipoise. *Am J Bioethics* 2006;6(4):37–47.

125. Glass KC. Toward a duty to report clinical trials accurately: the clinical alert and beyond. *J Law Med Ethics* 1994;22:327–338 and Rennie D. Fair conduct and fair reporting of clinical trials. *JAMA* 1999;282:1766–1768.

126. Begg C, Cho M, Eastwood S, et al. Improving the quality of reporting randomized controlled trials: the CONSORT statement. *JAMA* 1996;276:637–639; Schulz KF. The quest for unbiased research: randomized clinical trials and the CONSORT reporting guidelines. *Ann Neurol* 1997;41:569–573; Moher D, Schulz KF, Altman DG. The CONSORT statement: revised recommendations for improving the quality of reports of parallel-group randomized trials. *JAMA* 2001;285:1987–1991; and Altman DG, Schulz KF, Moher D, et al. The revised CONSORT statement for reporting randomized trials: explanation and elaboration. *Ann Intern Med* 2001;134:663–694.

127. Drazen JM, Wood AJJ. Trial registration report card. *N Engl J Med* 2005;353:2809–2911.

128. De Angelis CD, Drazen JM, Frizelle FA, et al. Clinical trial registration: a statement from the International Committee of Medical Journal Editors. *N Engl J Med* 2004;352:1250–1251.

129. Zarin DA, Tse T, Ide NC. Trial registration at ClinicalTrials.gov between May and October 2005. *N Engl J Med* 2005;353:2779–2787.

130. See, for example, the discussion on this point in Freedman B. Placebo-controlled trials and the logic of clinical purpose. *IRB* 1990;12(6):1–6.

131. Freedman B. Equipoise and the ethics of clinical research. *N Engl J Med* 1987;317:141–145.

132. Miller FG, Brody H. What makes placebo-controlled trials unethical? *Am J Bioethics* 2002;2(2):3–9.

133. Rothman KJ, Michels KB. The continuing unethical use of placebo controls. *N Engl J Med* 1994;331:394–398. For related arguments, see Freedman B, Weijer C, Glass KC. Placebo orthodoxy in clinical research. I. Empirical and methodological myths. *J Law Med Ethics* 1996;24:243–251 and Freedman B, Weijer C, Glass KC. Placebo orthodoxy in clinical research. II. Ethical, legal, and regulatory myths. *J Law Med Ethics* 1996;24:252–259.

134. Declaration of Helsinki IV. World Medical Association, 41st World Medical Assembly, Hong Kong, September, 1989, as quoted in Rothman KJ, Michels KB. *N Engl J Med* 1994:394.

135. Temple R, Ellenberg SS. Placebo-controlled trials and active-control trials in the evaluation of new treatments. Part 1. Ethical and scientific issues. *Ann Intern Med* 2000;133:455–463 and Ellenberg SS, Temple R. Placebo-controlled trials and active-control trials in the evaluation of new treatments. Part 2. Practical issues and specific cases. *Ann Intern Med* 2000;133:464–470. An international task force of clinicians, statisticians, ethicists, and regulators similarly concluded that placebo-controlled trials in multiple sclerosis were ethical (despite the availability of partially effective therapies) if the patient-subjects were properly educated and provided informed consent. See Lublin FD, Reingold SC. Placebo-controlled clinical trials in multiple sclerosis: ethical considerations. *Ann Neurol* 2001;49:677–681.

136. Brody BA. When are placebo-controlled trials no longer appropriate? *Control Clin Trials* 1997;18:602–612. Physicians commonly appeal to altruism when they offer parents the opportunity to enroll their children with cancer in treatment trials. See Simon C, Eder M, Kodish E, Siminoff L. Altruistic discourse in the informed consent process for childhood cancer trials. *Am J Bioethics* 2006;6(5):40–47.

137. Chadwick D, Privitera M. Placebo-controlled studies in neurology: where do they stop? *Neurology* 1999;52:682–685. For a more general discussion of ethical issues in drug trials in neurology, see Alves WA, Macciocchi SN. Ethical considerations in clinical neuroscience: current concepts in neuroclinical trials. *Stroke* 1996;27:1903–1909.

138. Clark PI, Leaverton PE. Scientific and ethical issues in the use of placebo controls in clinical trials. *Ann Rev Public Health* 1994;15:19–28.

139. Johnson AG. Surgery as a placebo. *Lancet* 1994;344:1140–1142.

140. Reeves B. Health-technology assessment in surgery. *Lancet* 1999;253(Suppl I):S16–S18.

141. Freed CR, Greene PE, Breeze RE, et al. Transplantation of embryonic dopamine neurons for severe Parkinson's disease. *N Engl J Med* 2001;344:710–719.

142. Indeed, the procedure produced severe, irreversible, and unexpected dystonias and dyskinesias in 15% of the treated group. See Freed CR, Greene PE, Breeze RE, et al. *N Engl J Med* 2001:716. Cost savings is another benefit of identifying ineffective therapies. See Ilstrup DM. Randomized clinical trials: potential cost savings due to the identification of ineffective medical therapies. *Mayo Clin Proc* 1995;70:707–710.

143. Freeman TB, Vawter DE, Leaverton PE, et al. Use of placebo surgery in controlled trials of a cellular-based therapy for Parkinson's disease. *N Engl J Med* 1999;341:988–992.

144. Macklin R. The ethical problems with sham surgery in clinical research. *N Engl J Med* 1999;341:992–996.

145. Macklin R. *N Engl J Med* 1999:994–995.

146. Miller FG. Sham surgery: an ethical analysis. *Am J Bioethics* 2003;3(4):41–48.

147. Angell M. The ethics of clinical research in the third world. *N Engl J Med* 1997;337:847–849 and Lurie P, Wolfe SM. Unethical trials of interventions to reduce perinatal transmission of the human immunodeficiency virus in developing countries. *N Engl J Med* 1997;337:853–856. Some ethicists have compared the purposeful non-treatment of treatable HIV infections in these studies to the Tuskegee syphilis study discussed previously. For a comprehensive analysis of the ethical issues of conducting research in the developing world, see Lavery JV, Grady C, Wahl ER, Emanuel EJ (eds). *Ethical Issues in International Biomedical Research: A Casebook*. New York: Oxford University Press, 2007.

148. Varmus H, Satcher D. Ethical complexities of conducting research in developing countries. *N Engl J Med* 1997;337:1003–1005.

149. World Medical Association Declaration of Helsinki (2004). http://www.wma.net/e/policy/b3.htm (Accessed April 7, 2007). For a discussion of the tension these rules have caused in developing countries, and how the research establishment in the United States has responded to it, see Lurie P, Greco DB. U.S. exceptionalism comes to research ethics. *Lancet* 2005;356:1117–1119.

150. Levine RJ. The need to revise the Declaration of Helsinki. *N Engl J Med* 1999;341:531–534. The concept of the highest attainable and sustainable therapy standard is discussed in Bloom BR. The highest attainable standard: ethical issues in AIDS vaccines. *Science* 1998;279:186–188.

151. This concept is discussed further in Perinatal HIV Intervention Research in Developing Countries Workshop Participants. Science, ethics, and the future of research into maternal-infant transmission of HIV-1. *Lancet* 1999;353:832–835.

152. Brennan TA. Proposed revisions to the Declaration of Helsinki—will they weaken the ethical principles underlying human research? *N Engl J Med* 1999;341:527–531.

153. Loue S, Okello D. Research bioethics in the Ugandan context II: procedural and substantive reform. *J Law Med Ethics* 2000;28:165–173. The regulatory situation in Uganda and elsewhere in the world are analyzed in National Bioethics Advisory Commission. *Ethical and Policy Issues in International Research*. Bethesda, MD: National Bioethics Advisory Commission, 2000. See http://www.georgetown.edu/research/nrcbl/nbac/pubs.html (Accessed May 9, 2007).

154. Phanuphak P. Ethical issues in studies in Thailand of the vertical transmission of HIV. *N Engl J Med* 1998;338:834–835.

155. Shapiro HT, Meslin EM. Ethical issues in the design and conduct of clinical trials in developing countries. *N Engl J Med* 2001;345:139–142.

156. Participants in the 2001 conference on ethical aspects of research in developing countries. Moral standards of research in developing countries: from "reasonable availability" to "fair benefits." *Hastings Cent Rep* 2004;34(3):17–27. See also Lo B, Bayer R. Establishing ethical trials for treatment and prevention of AIDS in developing countries. *BMJ* 2003;327:337–339.

157. UNAIDS. Creating effective partnerships for HIV prevention trials: report of a UNAIDS consultation, Geneva 20–21 June 2005. *AIDS* 2006;20(6)W1–W11.

158. Portions of this section have been adapted from Bernat JL. Ethical issues in neurological treatment and clinical trials. In Noseworthy J (ed). *Neurological Therapeutics: Principles and Practice*, 2nd ed. Oxford, UK: Informa Healthcare, 2006:73–83.

159. Bodenheimer T. Uneasy alliance—clinical investigators and the pharmaceutical industry. *N Engl J Med* 2000;342:1539–1544. Most clinical trials sponsored by pharmaceutical companies now are conducted by contract research organizations (CRO). See Shuchman M. Commercializing clinical trials—risks and benefits of the CRO boom. *N Engl J Med* 2007;357:1365–1368.

160. Moses H, Dorsey ER, Matheson DHM, Their SO. Financial anatomy of biomedical research. *JAMA* 2005;294:1333–1342.

161. Shimm DS, Spece RG Jr. Industry reimbursement for entering patients into clinical trials: legal and ethical issues. *Ann Intern Med* 1991;115:148–151.

162. Miller FG, Rosenstein DL, DeRenzo EG. Professional integrity in clinical research. *JAMA* 1998;280:1449–1454.

163. Toulmin S. Divided loyalties and ambiguous relationships. *Soc Sci Med* 1986;23:783–787.

164. Klein JE, Fleischman AR. The private practicing physician-investigator: ethical implications of clinical research in the office setting. *Hastings Cent Rep* 2002;32(4):22–26.

165. Jonas H. Philosophical reflections on experimenting with human subjects. *Daedalus* 1969;98(2):219–247.

166. See the further discussion of these measures in Bernat JL, Goldstein ML, Ringel SP. Conflicts of interest in neurology. *Neurology* 1998;50:327–331.

167. Lind SE. Finder's fees for research subjects. *N Engl J Med* 1990;323:192–195. The legal issues in finder's fees are discussed in Lemmens T, Miller PB. The human subjects trade: ethical and legal issues surrounding recruitment incentives. *J Law Med Ethics* 2005;31:398–418.

168. Rodwin MA. Physicians' conflicts of interest: the limitations of disclosure. *N Engl J Med* 1989;321:1405–1408 and Morin K, Rakatansky H, Riddick FA Jr, et al. Managing conflicts of interest in the conduct of clinical trials. *JAMA* 2002;287:78–84.

169. Shimm DS, Spece RG Jr. *Ann Intern Med* 1991:148–151.

170. Dickert N, Grady C. What's the price of a research subject? Approaches to payment for research participation. *N Engl J Med* 1999;341:198–203.

171. Portions of this section were adapted from Bernat JL, Goldstein ML, Ringel SP. Conflicts of interest in neurology. *Neurology* 1998;50:327–331.

172. Blumenthal D, Causino N, Campbell E, Louis KS. Relationships between academic institutions and industry in the life sciences—an industry survey. *N Engl J Med* 1996;334:368–373.

173. Blumenthal D. Academic-industry relationships in the life sciences: extent, consequences, and management. *JAMA* 1992;268:3344–3349.

174. Rosenberg SA. Secrecy in medical research. *N Engl J Med* 1996;334:392–394.

175. Blumenthal D. *JAMA* 1992:3344–3349.

176. The magnitude of the joint profit-making ventures between academia and industry and the apparent control of academic prerogatives by wealthy corporate sponsors led Marcia Angell, the acting editor of the *New England Journal of Medicine*, to ask, not entirely rhetorically, if academic medicine was for sale. See Angell M. Is academic medicine for sale? *N Engl J Med* 2000;342:1516–1518.

177. See discussion in American Medical Association Council on Scientific Affairs and Council on Ethical and Judicial Affairs. Conflicts of interest in medical center/industry research relationships. *JAMA* 1990;263:2790–2793.

178. Blumenthal D. Academic-industrial relationships in the life sciences. *N Engl J Med* 2003;349:2452–2459.

179. American Medical Association Council on Scientific Affairs and Council on Ethical and Judicial Affairs. *JAMA* 1990:2790–2793.

180. Blumenthal D, Campbell EG, Anderson MS, Causino N, Louis KS. Withholding research results in academic life science: evidence from a national survey of faculty. *JAMA* 1997;277:1224–1228.

181. Mello MM, Clarridge BR, Studdert DM. Academic medical centers' standards for clinical-trial agreements with industry. *N Engl J Med* 2005;352:2202–2210.

182. Bekelman JE, Li Y, Gross CP. Scope and impact of financial conflicts of interest in biomedical research: a systematic review. *JAMA* 2003;289:454–465.

183. Emanuel EJ, Steiner D. Institutional conflict of interest. *N Engl J Med* 1995;332:262–267 and DuVal G. Institutional conflicts of interest: protecting human subjects, scientific integrity, and institutional accountability. *J Law Med Ethics* 2004;22:613–625.

184. Barnes M, Florencio PS. Financial conflicts of interest in human subjects research: the problem of institutional conflicts. *J Law Med Ethics* 2002;30:390–402.

185. Campbell EG, Weissman JS, Vogeli C, et al. Financial relationships between institutional review board members and industry. *N Engl J Med* 2006;355:2321–2329.

186. Johns MME, Barnes M, Florencio PS. Restoring balance to industry-academia relationships in an era of institutional financial conflicts of interest: promoting research while maintaining trust. *JAMA* 2003;289:741–746.

187. Moses H III, Braunwald E, Martin JB, Their SO. Collaborating with industry—choices for the academic medical center. *N Engl J Med* 2002;347:1371–1375 and Gelijns AC, Their SO. Medical innovation and institutional interdependence: rethinking university-industry connections. *JAMA* 2002;287:72–77.

188. Kassirer JP, Angell M. Financial conflicts of interest in biomedical research. *N Engl J Med* 1993:329:570–571.

189. Rodwin MA. Physicians' conflicts of interest: the limitations of disclosure. *N Engl J Med* 1989;321:1405–1408.

190. Goldner JA. Dealing with conflicts of interest in biomedical research: IRB oversight as the next best solution to the abolitionist approach. *J Law Med Ethics* 2000;28:379–404.

191. Witt MD, Gostin LO. Conflict of interest dilemmas in biomedical research. *JAMA* 1994;271:546–551.

192. McCrary SV, Anderson CB, Jakovljevic J, et al. A national survey of policies on disclosure of conflicts of interest in biomedical research. *N Engl J Med* 2000;343:1621–1626.

193. Schulman KA, Seils D, Timbie JW, et al. A national survey of provisions in clinical-trial agreements between medical schools and industry sponsors. *N Engl J Med* 2002;347:1335–1341.

194. Lo B, Wolf LE, Berkeley A. Conflict-of-interest policies for investigators in clinical trials. *N Engl J Med* 2000;343:1616–1620.

195. Martin JB, Kasper DL. In whose best interest? Breaching the academic-industrial wall. *N Engl J Med* 2000;343:1646–1649.

196. Moses H III, Martin JB. Academic relationships with industry: a new model for biomedical research. *JAMA* 2001;285:933–935.

197. Association of American Medical Colleges Task Force on Financial Conflicts of Interest in Clinical Research. *Protecting Subjects, Preserving Trust, Promoting Progress: Policy and Guidelines for the Oversight of Individual Financial Interests in Human Subjects Research.* Washington, DC: Association of American Medical Colleges, 2001.

198. For an example of an institution that formulated a conflict of interest policy in accordance with the AAMC guidelines, see Camilleri M, Gamble GL, Kopecky SL, Wood MB, Hockema ML. Principles and process in the development of the Mayo Clinic's individual and institutional conflict of interest policy. *Mayo Clin Proc* 2005;80:1340–1346.

199. For a review of the recent strict and controversial NIH professional staff conflict of interest guidelines, see Stossel TP. Regulating academic-industrial research relationships—solving problems or stifling progress? *N Engl J Med* 2005;353:1060–1065.

200. The details of some of these cases are described in Dingell JD. Shattuck Lecture—Misconduct in medical research. *N Engl J Med* 1993;328:1610–1615.

201. These definitions are cited and discussed in Dresser R. Defining scientific misconduct: the relevance of mental state. *JAMA* 1993;269:895–897.

202. As cited in Dresser R. *JAMA* 1993:895.

203. Dresser R. *JAMA* 1993:895–896.

204. Korenman SG, Berk R, Wenger NS, Lew V. Evaluation of the research norms of scientists and administrators responsible for academic integrity. *JAMA* 1998;279:41047.

205. Mishkin B. Responding to scientific misconduct: due process and prevention. *JAMA* 1988;260:1932–1936.

206. Improvements in the process of disciplinary action for scientific misconduct are offered in Parrish DM. Improving the scientific misconduct hearing process. JAMA 1997;277:1315–1319 and Youngner SJ. The scientific misconduct process: a scientist's view from the inside. *JAMA* 1998;279:62–64.

207. Mishkin B. Urgently needed: policies on access to data by erstwhile collaborators. *Science* 1995;270:927–928.

208. Poon P. Legal protections for the scientific misconduct whistleblower. *J Law Med Ethics* 1995;23:88–95.

209. Goldner JA. The unending saga of legal controls over scientific misconduct: a clash of cultures needing resolution. *Am J Law Med* 1998;24:293–343.

210. Some of these educational programs are described in Alberts B, Shine K. Scientists and the integrity of research. *Science* 1994;266:1660–1661 and Benditt J (ed). The culture of credit. *Science* 1995;268:1706–1718.

211. Mello MM, Brennan TA. Due process in investigations of research misconduct. *N Engl J Med* 2003;349:1280–1286.

212. For the policy of *Neurology*, see Daroff RB, Griggs RC. Scientific misconduct and breach of publication ethics. *Neurology* 2004;62:352–353. For the policy of the *Annals of Internal Medicine*, see Sox HC, Rennie D. Research misconduct, retraction, and cleansing the medical literature: lessons from the Poehlman case. *Ann Intern Med* 2006;144:609–613.

Neuroethics

20

Research in normal and abnormal brain function raises challenging ethical issues that have spawned a field of scholarship called "neuroethics."[1] Although this classification is of recent vintage, ethical problems have been discussed since the early days of neuroscience research. How will studies of brain function that reveal personality traits affect a person's privacy? How will knowledge of brain function contribute to answering age-old philosophical questions of whether humans have free will and what factors comprise personal identity? Is the mind simply the brain? Is morality an evolutionarily produced brain function? Newer ethical questions have been introduced by advances in neuroimaging and neurotherapeutics. How will researchers handle incidental findings discovered on functional magnetic resonance imaging (fMRI) scans when healthy people volunteer as controls in research studies? Should fMRI be used for criminal justice purposes such as lie detection or prediction of violent behavior? Can neuroimaging abnormalities mitigate personal responsibility for antisocial acts? How will neural prostheses and neural transplantation affect personal identity and human nature? Should treatments be offered by physicians to enhance normal cognitive, affective, or neuromuscular function? I briefly address these ethical and philosophical questions in this chapter.

The definition of the word "neuroethics" is evolving. At a conference held in San Francisco in May 2002, sponsored by the Dana Foundation and co-hosted by Stanford University and the University of California San Francisco, speakers and commentators attempted to map the boundaries of the emerging field of neuroethics.[2] William Safire, the *New York Times* journalist and Chairman of the Dana Foundation, delivered the opening address. Safire defined neuroethics as the branch of bioethics that raises unique questions because it deals with human consciousness, the centerpiece of human nature. He predicted that human personality and behavior will be changed with future advances in neuroscience, a fact that raises essential ethical issues that demand attention now. Safire suggested that it is these issues that comprise the proper focus of neuroethics.[3] In an influential book published in 2005, the cognitive neuroscientist Michael Gazzaniga defined neuroethics more broadly as "the examination of how we want to deal with the social issues of disease, normality, mortality, lifestyle, and the philosophy of living *informed by our understanding of underlying brain mechanisms.*"[4]

Adina Roskies observed that the word "neuroethics" could refer either to the ethical issues raised by neuroscience research or to the neurobiological basis of human ethical behavior.[5] Nearly all scholars currently using the term, however, intend the former meaning. In a recent article, Antonio Damasio addressed the latter meaning and summarized the evidence for the neural mechanisms underpinning moral behavior.[6] Damasio cited natural human experiments, beginning with the celebrated 19th century case of Phineas Gage, who survived a massive penetrating injury to both frontal lobes, but developed an "immoral" personality.[7]

Damasio then discussed more recent experimental paradigms that used fMRI to assess brain areas that are activated in normal persons during moral reflection and forming judgments.[8]

The question of who coined the term "neuroethics" remains a subject of debate. In his welcoming address at the 2002 San Francisco conference on neuroethics, Zach Hall of the University of California San Francisco attributed the word to William Safire, explaining that Safire had used it in a conversation with him in 2000 or 2001.[9] However, the word "neuroethics" was used earlier. In a 1989 article in *Neurologic Clinics*, the neurologist-ethicist Ronald Cranford used the term "neuroethical" to describe the unique clinical-ethical problems encountered by neurologists in practice, such as those involving patients with brain death, the vegetative state, dementia, paralysis, or respiratory dependency. Cranford also used the term "neuroethicist" to describe neurologists who are trained in clinical ethics and who, therefore, can make a dual contribution when they serve as members of hospital ethics committees. Cranford argued that neurologists can help analyze neuroethical dilemmas from their unique perspective bridging the gap between clinical neurology and clinical ethics.[10] I heard Cranford use the term "neuroethics" in this clinical context during the 1980s.

Most scholars who have used the term "neuroethics" since 2002 restrict it to the ethical issues raised by neuroscience research.[11] Although there is no reason for categorically limiting "neuroethics" to research issues (and some recent neuroethics textbook editors also have included clinical topics[12]), in this chapter I use the term in the conventional sense to describe the unique ethical problems introduced by neuroscience research. The most logical rhetorical solution would be to permit its usage for both research and clinical ethics topics by describing the former as "research neuroethics" and the latter as "clinical neuroethics." Thus, this chapter considers research neuroethics whereas chapters 11 to 18 consider clinical neuroethics.

Although a young discipline, the emerging field of neuroethics has generated a new professional society that conducts scholarly meetings[13] and a new dedicated professional journal.[14]

The Society for Neuroscience, the premier scientific organization dedicated to neuroscience research, now includes the study of ethical issues in its mission statement.[15] The scholars engaged in all these neuroethics activities generally restrict their purview to the ethical and philosophical issues raised by neuroscience research. The Dana Foundation in New York remains a leading sponsor of scholars working in this area.

NEURO-ENHANCEMENT

One of the earliest and most enduring neuroethics issues centers on the propriety of using neuropharmacology and other neurotechnologies to improve normal human function: the so-called enhancement debate. The traditional focus of medical practice has been to treat disease and disability with a goal of cure or at least re-establishment of normal functioning. The enhancement debate is controversial because it takes individuals who have normal functioning and asks if it is desirable or justified to use medical means to improve their functioning to levels above normal. Of course, people have used drugs such as alcohol, nicotine, and caffeine for this purpose for centuries. The ethical issue centers on whether providing requested enhancements for the healthy is a proper activity of the profession of medicine.

It is helpful to conceptualize the ethical issues inherent in enhancement by inspecting a few prototypic cases: (1) A normal student asks a physician to write a prescription for amphetamine for the purpose of improving his concentration and attention so that he can score higher on a standardized test; (2) A young mother follows the advice of the psychiatrist Peter Kramer: it is desirable for everyone to optimize mood by taking an antidepressant drug such as Prozac.[16] She requests a prescription although she is not depressed; or (3) A competitive amateur swimmer asks a physician to prescribe erythropoietin to improve his exercise endurance. These cases clearly would be classified as enhancement and not therapy.

There are other cases, however, in which the distinction between enhancement and therapy is less clear. People with short stature, in some studies, are not as successful in life as people of normal stature. Many parents of children with short stature wish them to receive growth hormone treatments to achieve normal stature to improve their appearance and confidence because they believe it will add to their overall health and well-being.[17] Whether one considers the prescription of growth hormone in this setting as treatment or enhancement is ambiguous and will be answered differently by physicians with different values.[18]

In a review of the enhancement debate as it pertains to neurologists, Anjan Chatterjee pointed out that there are three general areas in which enhancement technologies could be used in clinical neurology: (1) improving normal motor skills and movement; (2) improving normal cognitive function, concentration, attention and memory; and (3) improving normal mood and affect.[19] Chatterjee chose the infelicitous term "cosmetic neurology" to refer to these enhancement categories. I believe that the adjective "cosmetic" is misleading in this context because it erroneously suggests that the enhancements in question are intended to improve appearance or beauty whereas, in reality, they are prescribed with the intent to improve function. (The use of biotechnology for truly cosmetic purposes raises its own set of ethical problems, but they are different from those under consideration here.[20]) Chatterjee pointed out that although the ethical problems of enhancement technologies are serious, the "hand-wringing of ethicists" over them is unlikely to restrain their development, which he regards as inevitable. He therefore warned neurologists to become aware of these technologies and consider their position regarding prescribing them because they will soon find themselves being asked to prescribe one or more of these enhancement agents by normal persons seeking "better brains."

Enhancement of motor activity can be accomplished with anabolic steroids, amphetamines, erythropoietin, and other agents. Enhancement of cognitive activity can be produced by amphetamines and other stimulants, cholinesterase inhibitors, donepezil, and newer agents affecting cyclic AMP, glutamate receptors, and NMDA receptors. Mood and affect can be enhanced with selective serotonin reuptake inhibitors, corticotrophin releasing factor, neuropeptide agonists and antagonists, and other agents.[21] Non-pharmaceutical enhancement technologies could include transcranial magnetic stimulation.

The ethical issues of enhancement have been debated extensively.[22] In a critical review, Erik Parens pointed out that much of the problem results from a lack of clarity in the distinction between enhancement and treatment. He argues that the distinction is justified in some cases but not in others.[23] In a more recent analysis, he commented that the differences between supporters and critics of the enhancement-treatment distinction have been overblown and they have more in common than they think.[24] Those claiming an important distinction point out that the purpose of the medical profession is to treat disease and disability with the goal of improving deficient function to normal levels. Critics assert that enhancement is not an appropriate use of medical services. Those criticizing the importance of any distinction between enhancement and therapy generally embrace a broader vision of health and disease in which technologically induced improvement of function is considered therapeutic, irrespective of the starting point.

Martha Farah classified the ethical issues of brain enhancement into three general categories: (1) health issues involving safety, side effects, and unintended consequences; (2) social effects on those who do and do not choose enhancement and how one group affects the other; and (3) philosophical issues in which brain enhancement "challenges our understanding of personal effort and accomplishment, autonomy, and the value of people as opposed to things."[25] The safety issue is especially important given that it would be difficult to justify a serious side effect of a brain enhancement treatment given that the person taking it had no illness in the first place. Although some have argued that the doctrine of informed consent can dispose of this concern, that claim is not true when parents permit enhancement treatments of their children. Even scholars who advocated that society should permit the widespread availability of brain enhancement to consenting adults become protective when it comes to administering such treatment to children.[26]

The question of social effects centers on concerns about fairness. From a public policy and distributive justice perspective, how can we justify improving the lives of certain normal people and not others, because the induced improvement will provide them with an unfair advantage in a competitive society. The unfairness is magnified when the enhancement technologies are expensive and only wealthy people can afford them, thereby promoting or securing their privileged status.[27] For example, in some American communities, the threshold for diagnosing attention deficit hyperactivity disorder (ADHD) and prescribing stimulant treatment has been lowered to include normal children.[28] In one report, over 30% of boys in some schools took Ritalin or other stimulant drugs for alleged ADHD.[29] These data raise social questions: are we witnessing direct or indirect coercion of healthy people into treatment and widespread physician prescribing for brain enhancement rather than for disease?

The philosophical criticisms center on the nature of human beings and how, eventually, they might be ineluctably altered if the concept of enhancement were accepted unconditionally. Have people who have received brain enhancement had their humanness changed in some fundamental way? Some bioethics scholars worry that with repeated rounds of increasing enhancements over many generations, the very characteristics that make people human eventually will be lost.[30] Supporters counter that if cognitive enhancement drugs were safe and effective, "they would produce significant societal gains" and "competent adults should be free to decide whether or not to use [them]."[31] The most zealous advocates of enhancement, "transhumanists," hope enhancement technology will achieve a "posthuman" future of enhanced intellect, freedom from disease, immunity to aging, increased pleasure, and novel states of consciousness.[32]

NEUROIMAGING: INCIDENTAL RESEARCH FINDINGS

The development of increasingly sophisticated functional neuroimaging techniques, particularly fMRI, has introduced a set of interesting neuroethical problems. One of the earliest questions involved how researchers should handle incidental findings disclosed on research fMRIs of normal volunteers who serve as control subjects.[33] Consider the following two prototypic cases. (1) A normal person volunteered to serve as a control in a fMRI study of normal language function and his fMRI disclosed what might be a mass lesion in the brain. Should the researcher disclose this finding to him? How? Who is responsible for notification? What should the subject be told? Who arranges further assessment or treatment? (2) A young woman suffered a subarachnoid hemorrhage from a giant aneurysm. A year earlier she had served as a normal volunteer in a fMRI study of handedness and cerebral dominance. She now asks the researcher if her aneurysm could or should have been detected a year earlier on her research fMRI. What is the responsibility of researchers or a research scan to screen for clinical abnormalities? Should research scans always be interpreted by qualified radiologists or is the researcher's review sufficient? What MRI sequences are necessary for a researcher to declare a scan normal or not worthy of comment? What is the extent of the clinical duty, if any, that researchers owe their normal volunteer subjects?

It is helpful first to know if this is a common problem. Judy Illes and colleagues measured the frequency and severity of incidental findings on brain MRIs of research volunteers who were believed to be neurologically healthy. They classified incidental findings into four categories of seriousness: no referral, routine, urgent, or immediate. They found the overall incidence of incidental findings to be 6.6%. Older patients and men were more likely to show abnormalities. All of the findings in the older cohort were classified as routine but 75% (3 out of 4) of the incidental findings in the younger cohort were classified as urgent.[34] In a study seeking the preferences for notification of healthy control subjects who had participated in neuroimaging studies, Matthew Kirschen and colleagues found that 97% of these subjects wished to have incidentally discovered findings communicated to them irrespective of their potential clinical significance and 59% preferred that the communication be conducted by a physician affiliated with the research team.[35]

In an editorial, Robert Grossman and I offered several comments about the study by Illes et al.[36] We observed that because fMRI research is performed by psychologists and other neuroscientists who are not skilled in clinical image interpretation and because the research scan sequences often are not thorough, many potential incidental findings will not even be discovered using the study protocol. If all research scans required clinical standards to be met for completeness of sequences performed and required trained radiologists to interpret them, the added costs to the research protocol would be large and would create an impediment to research. If a scan abnormality is seen in a research protocol, who should receive the result and in what setting? To what extent should researchers receive training about those incidental findings that are present normally and therefore create no reason for concern or further assessment? We suggested that however these questions ultimately are answered, the process of consent and disclosure should follow established ethical guidelines for research. The informed consent process and form should itemize all the risks of participating including: (1) increased anxiety resulting from learning an abnormality may be present; (2) financial costs resulting from additional testing that may become necessary to better define the purported abnormality; and (3) health risks resulting from additional tests to further clarify the purported abnormality. The consent form also should clarify if the scan sequences are adequate for clinical purposes, whether the scan will be interpreted by a trained clinician, who would notify the patient of a possible abnormality and how, and who would be responsible for paying for further medical care that was required because of the finding.

The Working Group on Incidental Findings in Brain Imaging Research published a consensus statement in an article in *Science* in 2006.[37] They indicated that their findings and conclusions did not represent the official position of any agency and were intended simply to further the ongoing discussion. They concluded: (1) it is ethically desirable for suspicious incidental findings to be disclosed to the research subject because of the subject's right to know despite the lack of professional guidelines addressing whether incidental findings should be disclosed, how, and by whom; (2) the potentially harmful consequences of false-positive reports on normal volunteers has not been adequately studied; (3) wide variability exists about when and how incidental findings are reported to human subjects; (4) vulnerable subjects may require special assistance in arranging follow-up medical consultations; (5) it is desirable, when possible, to have a physician validate the presence of a suspected incidental finding; (6) it is desirable to have a physician communicate the incidental finding to the subject, when possible; (7) institutional review boards should require clarification of the complete process for handling the incidental findings; (8) there is no ethical requirement for the researcher to obtain clinical scans on the subject; and (9) research needs to be performed to study the costs and benefits of identifying incidental findings and referring subjects for appropriate medical follow-up.

NEUROIMAGING: THOUGHTS AND PREFERENCES

The widespread use of new and accessible noninvasive neuroimaging techniques, such as fMRI, raises social and legal neuroethical issues including privacy of thought, prediction of violence or disease, lie detection, and personal responsibility for behavior.[38] As discussed in chapter 17, there now are extra layers of confidentiality and privacy protection required for genetic test results because of their potential for abuse and unjustified discrimination if unauthorized persons were to gain access to them. A similar risk potential exists for fMRI data that might represent private human thoughts. Data on how a person thinks could influence how that person is treated by society, raising the potential for unjustified discrimination. Early experiments in the cognitive neuroscience of morality attempted to localize the brain regions activated during moral reflection and deliberation.[39] More recent studies by Michael Koenigs and colleagues showed that previous damage to the ventromedial prefrontal cortex (an area necessary to generate normal social emotions) leads to an overuse of utilitarian reasoning and difficulty in distinguishing right from wrong actions.[40] It is conceivable that once normal patterns of activation for moral capacity have been established, a person having an abnormal pattern may be subject to sanctions or discrimination in employment, education, housing, insurance, or the criminal justice system.

Psychologists have used functional neuroimaging to assess social attitudes and preferences. In a much discussed study of racial attitudes, Elizabeth Phelps and colleagues used fMRI to study the level of amygdala activation (thought to represent fear) in white volunteers who viewed photographs of unfamiliar black men's faces and unfamiliar white men's faces. They also performed two psychological tests indirectly measuring subjects' racial attitudes. They found a moderately strong correlation between the degree of amygdala activation on fMRI when the subjects viewed the black men's faces and high negative (prejudicial) scores on the subjects' tests of racial attitudes.[41]

Personal interests and desires may be inferred by findings on functional neuroimaging when tested in certain paradigms. In one PET scan study, detoxified cocaine addicts showed robust activation of limbic structures, including the amygdala and anterior cingulate cortex, when shown a cocaine-related videotape. This activation was not present in cocaine-naïve controls and was believed to represent drug craving by the detoxified addicts that was evoked by seeing the video.[42] A subsequent fMRI study using a similar paradigm confirmed these findings and showed that an identical pattern of limbic activation occurs in normal subjects when they view sexually explicit videos.[43] These findings have profound implications for our understanding of the neurobiology of addiction, particularly concerning how desire and craving may impact the voluntary control of behavior.[44]

Marketers have used fMRI results to test consumers' preferences for commercial items, an emerging business application called "neuromarketing."[45] In one fMRI study, consumers' brain responses to tasting Coca-Cola and Pepsi in both brand-cued and anonymous delivery paradigms were measured and compared to behavioral preference findings on taste tests. They found a strong correlation between behavioral preferences on taste tests and activation of the ventromedial prefrontal cortex on fMRI. This activation was more robust after brand-cued than anonymous delivery of the beverage, suggesting that the subjects' pleasure from tasting the beverages may have been enhanced by expectation.[46]

NEUROIMAGING: VIOLENCE AND ANTISOCIAL BEHAVIOR

Certain patterns of fMRI activation have been associated with violence, antisocial behavior, and personality disorders. Antonio Damasio and colleagues showed that damage to the orbitofrontal cortex and its connections before the age of 16 months was associated with later-life poor impulse control and antisocial behavior as evidenced by insensitivity to future consequences of decisions, defective autonomic responses to punishment contingencies, failure to respond to behavioral interventions, and defective social and moral reasoning.[47] Adrian Raine and colleagues showed an association between antisocial, psychopathic behavior and MRI evidence of volume reduction of the prefrontal cortex suggesting prior damage.[48] In a fMRI study of affective memory tasks, Kent Kiel and colleagues found that criminal psychopaths showed reduced affect-related activity in the amygdala-hippocampal formation, parahippocampal gyrus, ventral striatum, and in the anterior and posterior cingulate gyri with increased activity in the bilateral frontotemporal cortex.[49] Once such patterns of fMRI findings have become linked conclusively to violent or antisocial personality types, these scans could be sought by law enforcement agencies, schools, or employers.[50] The potential for abuse of these techniques is enormous. To minimize harms, neuroscientists must clearly state the accuracy and positive and negative predictive values of such scan findings on personality characteristics.[51]

An emerging forensic application of fMRI and other neurodiagnostic techniques is lie detection.[52] Lawrence Farwell and Sharon

Smith identified patterns of EEG spectra (which they called "brain fingerprinting") using memory and encoding-related multi-faceted electroencephalographic responses ("MERMER") and applied them to determine if a suspect had knowledge of the details of a crime. They believed that their results accurately discriminated truth-telling from lying.[53] Similarly, fMRI has been applied to identify the particular patterns associated with deception and purposeful lying. Using the "Guilty Knowledge Test," Daniel Langleben and colleagues identified characteristic patterns of fMRI activation in volunteer subjects who were asked to lie in comparison to others who were asked to tell the truth.[54] The presence of more widespread patterns of cortical activation, including activation of the anterior cingulate cortex, suggested deliberate deception. The areas activated during intentional deception are similar to those observed in normal subjects who are experiencing intense emotions that have a social context.[55]

Tatia Lee and colleagues found that subjects who feigned memory impairment (malingered) demonstrated distinct patterns of neural activation in a prefrontal-parietal-subcortical circuit when compared with normal controls.[56] Giorgio Ganis and colleagues performed fMRI to distinguish well-rehearsed lies from spontaneous lies. They showed that well-rehearsed lies elicited more activation in the right anterior frontal cortex than spontaneous lies whereas the opposite pattern occurred in the anterior cingulate and in posterior visual cortex. Both types of lies elicited more activation than telling the truth in anterior prefrontal cortex and the parahippocampal gyrus bilaterally, the right precuneus, and the left cerebellum.[57] Using these functional neuroimaging techniques for "mind reading" is no longer in the realm of science fiction.

As exciting and potentially important as these functional neuroimaging studies are, it is wise to insert a caveat about their interpretation. The activation of specific brain areas during the performance of a task or in response to a stimulus may indicate that these areas represent necessary neural pathways for performing the task or interpreting the stimulus but should not imply that they alone are sufficient.

Undoubtedly, the underlying neural networks are more widely distributed and the mechanisms more complex than the activation patterns seen on fMRI. The neurologist-neuroimaging scientist Marcus Raichle warned prudently that contemporary cognitive scientists should not repeat the mistake made by 19th century phrenologists by simply correlating examination findings with mental faculties. He suggested that neuroimaging scientists should continue to make correlations between the cognitive tasks that have been performed and the networks of brain activation that result. The more challenging effort, however, will be to "identify the elementary operations performed within such a network and relate these operations to the task of interest."[58]

Legal questions remain unanswered regarding how and by whom fMRI and similar technologies may be used in the contexts of criminal justice and civil litigation. It is possible that their use for forensic purposes violates federal statutory or constitutional protections.[59] The federal Employee Polygraph Protection Act that prohibits employers from requiring employees to undergo testing with a polygraph or "any other similar devices . . . used . . . for the purpose of rendering a diagnostic opinion regarding the honesty or dishonesty of an individual" may also ban using fMRI for employee lie detection.[60] In the criminal context, it is unclear if the penetrating character of fMRI violates the Fourth Amendment's protection against search of a criminal suspect.[61] Similarly, fMRI findings could violate a defendant's Fifth Amendment protection against compulsory self-incrimination. The continued use of these neuroimaging techniques will force courts to rule whether all citizens have a right to individual "cognitive privacy" to think their own thoughts and, if so, whether the information gleaned from these techniques violates that right.[62]

NEUROIMAGING: DISEASE PREDICTION

The use of structural and functional neuroimaging for disease prediction raises several neuroethical questions.[63] The evaluation of a patient for Alzheimer's disease (AD) includes anatomic brain imaging by MR or CT scan primarily to exclude alternative causes of dementia[64] and secondarily to look for findings believed to distinguish AD from other conditions.[65] Several provocative reports have claimed that the presence of specific findings on fMRI,[66] MRI,[67] and PET scans[68] also can predict which patients who currently have mild cognitive dysfunction or who are at risk for developing AD because of genetic factors will progress to AD. A predictive test with high positive and negative predictive values obviously would be helpful to physicians and patients. Among other benefits, it would permit the timely prescription of a neuroprotective intervention to attempt to retard disease progression. It also would afford an opportunity for patients to execute specific advance directives that would apply later when they developed progressive dementia.

In a recent workshop at Stanford University, Judy Illes and colleagues performed an ethical analysis of predictive neuroimaging tests to diagnose AD. They pointed out that, in addition to the tangible benefits, a positive test could have unintended negative consequences. A patient who tested positive might: (1) be made permanently ineligible for health insurance; (2) be stigmatized with the diagnosis of AD at an earlier stage, with consequent discrimination in areas such as permission to drive or eligibility to receive an organ transplant; (3) require psychological counseling for the same reason that patients undergoing predictive genetic testing for HD (see chapter 17) require pretest and posttest counseling; and (4) require genetic counseling if the AD is hereditary. Illes et al. considered the benefits and harms of screening populations, the elements of informed consent for testing, and research questions including the policy for handling incidental findings.[69]

The ethical issues in predictive testing and research on AD using structural and functional neuroimaging are being included in the ongoing Alzheimer's Disease Neuroimaging Initiative (ADNI). The ADNI is a 5-year public-private partnership (funded by the NIH, FDA, pharmaceutical manufacturers, and others) to test whether serial MRI, PET, other biological markers, and clinical and neuropsychological assessment can be combined to measure the progression of mild cognitive impairment and early AD.[70]

NEUROPROSTHETICS AND NEUROTRANSPLANTATION

Continuing developments in neuroprosthetics and neurotransplantation raise different ethical questions. Does personal identity or personality change after a person receives a neuroprosthesis or a neural transplant? Can neuroprostheses be used for mind control or other questionable practices? What is the liability for abuse of neural prostheses? Although both neuroprosthetics and neurotransplantation are in their infancy, it is desirable to anticipate and discuss the ethical problems that might arise once they become more fully developed.

A neuroprosthesis is an interface between a computer and a brain, spinal cord, or peripheral nerve.[71] The earliest neuroprosthesis in widespread use is the cochlear implant to treat deafness. The technology and success rates of cochlear implantation have improved dramatically.[72] Now, with consent of their parents, cochlear implants are routinely inserted in children to treat congenital or childhood-onset deafness. An interesting and surprising resistance to this practice has been generated by the deaf community, particularly from families with hereditary deafness for whom lifelong hearing loss is a valued part of their personal identity. Some of these people object to classifying their deafness as a disease or disability that requires cure.[73] Rather, they see deafness as "a life to be lived," value the unique features of "deaf life," and take pride in deaf culture.[74] Whereas normally hearing parents generally wish their deaf children to undergo cochlear implants to restore their hearing, parents who are deaf from hereditary disorders often do not. The ethical issue of how physicians should respond to parental consent or refusal for a cochlear implant for a child in this circumstance is complex.[75]

One of the most exciting applications is the development of neuromotor prostheses that provide voluntary control of movement for paralyzed patients.[76] Leigh Hochberg and colleagues created a successful brain-computer interface neuromotor prosthesis that permitted a paralyzed patient to activate computers and other devices by ideational patterns. They implanted a 96-micorelectrode array in the primary motor cortex of a man rendered quadriplegic three years earlier by a cervical spinal cord injury and recorded his neuronal ensemble activity. They found that his wish to move his hand modulated cortical spiking patterns. They used this reproducible electroencephalographic response to develop a "neural cursor," which the subject was able to learn to control by thinking about moving his hand. Following a period of practice, he became able to move the cursor on a computer monitor that he could see, simply by thinking about moving his hand. This system permitted him to open simulated e-mail and operate devices such as a television, even while conversing. He also was able to voluntarily open and close a prosthetic hand and perform rudimentary actions with a multi-jointed robotic arm.[77] The same issue of *Nature* reported a successful neuromotor prosthetics experiment in monkeys.[78]

Commentators pointed out that these devices have made reality of the formerly science-fiction concept of mechanically converting thoughts into actions.[79] Neuromotor prostheses provide paralyzed patients the opportunity to activate their environment to help them achieve more independent function. With future advances in electrical engineering and computing technology, the processing speed and efficiency will increase and paralyzed patients will be able to execute additional actions. Some futurists have advocated the placement of neuroprostheses in normal persons to enhance their function. The ethical problems resulting from this use of technology are similar to those that arise in other neuro-enhancement efforts.[80]

Neurotransplantation is also a field that is only beginning to be developed. It is now impossible to successfully transplant spinal cords or brains; whether it ever will be possible is unknown. Cellular neurotransplantation to repair the central nervous system has been attempted with neural stem cells and cells from other tissues. Recent reviews summarize the progress made in using neural stem cells to attempt to cure brain[81] and spinal cord diseases and the scientific questions that remain unanswered.[82] Neural stem cell transplantation remains a promising technique but before its future can be realized much more basic scientific work must be accomplished to better understand the biology of cell development, differentiation, and function. The problem of oncogene regulation, in particular, must be solved to assure that the infused stem cells do not produce a clone of malignant cells. Although human embryonic stem cells are theoretically the most promising stem cell to transplant because of their pluripotentiality, they have provoked scientific, ethical, religious, and political controversy because using them requires the destruction of an early-stage human embryo. Whether it is justified to use human embryos that have been already discarded from in vitro fertilization programs for research, cloning, or as a source of human embryonic stem cells remains a source of intense dispute.[83]

NEUROPHILOSOPHY

The final neuroethics subject I briefly consider is the most abstract: the neurophilosophical concepts of consciousness, mind, personhood, personal identity, and free will. Once the exclusive domain of philosophers and theologians, these topics have come under increasing neuroscientific scrutiny over the past few decades through the contributions of cognitive neuroscientists and experimental psychologists who study brain function using functional and structural neuroimaging, sophisticated electrical signal analysis, computational biology, and other analytic techniques. Philosophers who are knowledgeable about these neurobiological advances and have integrated them into their conceptual constructs also have made important contributions.[84] These exceedingly complex topics will continue to fascinate scholars and researchers but likely will remain elusive and speculative for many years to come.

In the introduction to an enlightening anthology of essays on the philosophy of consciousness, Güven Güzeldere observed, "There is perhaps no other phenomenon besides consciousness that is so familiar to each of us and yet has been so elusive to any systematic study, philosophical or scientific."[85] Consciousness has been studied from several perspectives: philosophy, experimental psychology, neurobiology, computational science, and (the synthesis of them all) cognitive neuroscience. Despite intense scrutiny by brilliant scientists and scholars[86] and noteworthy advances in our understanding of brain physiology, we still lack even the most rudimentary understanding of how the brain generates the exquisite property of self-awareness. We cannot even define the unique phenomenon of conscious awareness without being self-referential and circular. Cognitive neuroscientists have provided the most promising approach to analyzing consciousness but, despite this prodigious effort, they have barely scratched the surface of understanding.[87] At least some biologically sophisticated philosophers remain skeptical that humans possess the cognitive capacity to ever fully understand the mechanism of conscious awareness.[88]

The vast majority of neuroscientists and most philosophers now accept the premise that the mind is a direct product of the human brain and its operations. A corollary to this premise is that the human brain is both necessary and sufficient for generating the mind. The psychologist Steven Pinker said it most succinctly: "the mind is what the brain does." The Cartesian dualism of mind and body, accepted by scholars for so many years, has been crushed under the weight of accumulated research in experimental neuropsychology and cognitive neuroscience. All emotion, reason, feeling, perception, sentience, memory, thought, and behavior are functions solely of the brain.[89]

Personhood and personal identity have unique neuroethical appeal because of the critical importance of the brain in the composition of the person. As discussed in chapter 11, personhood is a psychosocial and legal concept but not a biological one. It refers to the presence of certain characteristics and capacities of a human organism that confer social or legal standing. Scholars differ on their opinions of the necessary components of

personhood but nearly all include self-awareness as an essential factor. Cognitive neuroscientists point out that the self-awareness dimension of personhood is generated (somehow) by the human cerebral cortex and its thalamic connections. Attempts to precisely define personhood and to delineate its boundaries, however, generally have failed.[90]

Personal identity is a concept related to personhood: it encompasses those attributes of the organism that define which person this is. Using a brain-transplantation thought experiment, the philosopher Bernard Gert argued that personal identity is most closely related to brain function, specifically to that of the cerebral hemispheres. He proposed the following thought experiment involving two persons who undergo reciprocal brain transplantation, assuming this science fiction scenario to be possible and successful. Person A's brain was transplanted into person B's head and person B's brain placed in person A's head. The body of person B containing the brain of person A would exhibit all the behaviors and have the memories, self-awareness, and other personal characteristics that identified him as person A; the reciprocal facts would also be true for the body of person A with person B's brain. Gert argued that we all would be more likely now to say that the body of person A was really person B and vice versa because the essential characteristics of personal identity depend only on brain function, not that of the remainder of the body.[91]

The free will argument dates back to Epicurus and the Greek philosophers. In its classical form, the debate is between those advocating determinism and those advocating indeterminism.[92] The determinists hold that free will is illusory and actions are predetermined because every act or action is an inevitable consequence of the hard-wiring and programming of the human organism through genetic and other biological factors. More sophisticated determinists emphasize that instinctual and affective motives for behavior have been genetically programmed into the organism and have been modified environmentally through the organism's development. Indeterminists, by contrast, hold that free will exists despite the genetically-environmentally programmed nature of the nervous system and that, as a result, people should be held accountable for their acts. Indeterminists believe that the sophisticated human system of morality is contingent on our capacity and responsibility to make reasoned and free choices in light of the social rules of behavior. Moreover, they hold that the human brain provides the capacity for these choices.

As moral agents, humans have a personal responsibility for the consequences of their actions.[93] Our criminal justice system is founded on a default mode in which we all are expected to have personal responsibility and accountability for our acts. In a criminal proceeding, we require defendants trying to absolve themselves of guilt to prove that they no longer have responsibility for their acts because of a severe physical or psychological illness that has incapacitated their moral agency. Society is better served by strictly limiting those instances in which courts adjudicate persons to be unaccountable for their actions. Neuroscientists should refrain from making tendentious assertions that accused criminals are "innocent on the grounds of insanity" merely because of the presence of neuroimaging findings of speculative significance.[94] Moreover, it is an abuse of neuroscience for "experts" to proffer these data in court as exculpatory evidence without unequivocal proof that they demonstrate loss of moral agency.

Developments in cognitive neuroscience inform the free-will debate. In a famous series of experiments, Benjamin Libet showed the existence of premotor potentials.[95] These potentials can be recorded from the premotor cortex 500 to 1,000 msec prior to a volitional movement. They appear to be "readiness potentials" that indicate the time we actually decide to make an action. Libet found that the time interval between the onset of the readiness potential and the point of conscious decision making was 300 msec. He further showed that there is approximately a 100 msec interval for the conscious self to decide whether to follow through with execution of an intended movement or to stop it, and argued that this interval provided humans the capacity to exercise free will.[96]

More recent studies of volitional movement by Mark Hallett's group provide a somewhat different interpretation. Hallett found that volitional movement was initiated in the mesial frontal lobe. The innate sense of volition was represented by a corollary discharge involving multiple areas with reciprocal connections in the parietal lobe and insular cortex. Hallett summarized his findings and their significance: "Free will is not a driving force for movement but a conscious awareness concerning the nature of the movement. Movement initiation and the perception of willing the movement can be separately manipulated. Movement is generated subconsciously, and the conscious sense of volition comes later, but the exact time of this event is difficult to assess because of the potentially illusory nature of introspection."[97]

The future promises a continued synthesis of further refinements in neurophilosophy that are informed by neuroscientific developments. The cognitive-neuroscience approach to the philosophical problems of consciousness, mind, personhood, personal identity, and free will appears to be the most fruitful pathway to further understanding. The 21st century will continue to be an exciting time for all observers to follow the fascinating developments in these areas. Neurologists can make an essential contribution as informed clinicians if they understand both neuroscience and neuroethics.

NOTES

1. Dozens of papers and a few texts have been published on "neuroethics." For recent reviews, see Farah MJ. Social, legal, and ethical implications of cognitive neuroscience: "neuroethics" for short. *J Cogn Neurosci* 2007;19:363–364; Illes J, Bird SJ. Neuroethics: a modern context for ethics in neuroscience. *Trends Neurosci* 2006;29:511–517; Glannon W. Neuroethics. *Bioethics* 2006;20:37–52; Farah MJ. Neuroethics: the practical and philosophical. *Trends Cogn Sci* 2005;9:34–40; Illes J (ed). *Neuroethics: Defining the Issues in Theory, Practice and*

Policy. New York: Oxford University Press, 2005; Glannon W (ed). *Defining Right and Wrong in Brain Science: Essential Readings in Neuroethics.* New York: Dana Press, 2007; and Glannon W. *Bioethics and the Brain.* New York: Oxford University Press, 2007.

2. Marcus SJ (ed). *Neuroethics: Mapping the Field. Conference Proceedings.* New York: Dana Press, 2002.

3. Safire W. Visions for a new field of "neuroethics." In Marcus SJ (ed). *Neuroethics: Mapping the Field. Conference Proceedings.* New York: Dana Press, 2002:3–9.

4. Gazzaniga MS. *The Ethical Brain.* New York: Dana Press, 2005.

5. Roskies A. Neuroethics for the new millennium. *Neuron* 2002;35:21–23.

6. Damasio A. Neuroscience and ethics: intersections. *Am J Bioethics* 2007;7(1):3–7.

7. Damasio H, Grabowski R, Frank A, Galaburda AM, Damasio AR. The return of Phineas Gage: clues about the brain from the skull of a famous patient. *Science* 1994;264:1102–1105.

8. Greene JD, Sommerville RB, Nystrom LE, et al. An fMRI investigation of emotional engagement in moral judgment. *Science* 2001;293:2105–2108 and De Martino B, Kumaran D, Seymour B, Dolan RJ. Frames, biases, and rational decision-making in the human brain. *Science* 2006;313:684–687.

9. Hall ZW. Welcome. In Marcus SJ (ed). *Neuroethics: Mapping the Field. Conference Proceedings.* New York: Dana Press, 2002:1–2.

10. Cranford RE. The neurologist as ethics consultant and as a member of the institutional ethics committee: the neuroethicist. *Neurol Clin* 1989;7:697–713.

11. For example, see Illes J (ed). *Neuroethics: Defining the Issues in Theory, Practice, and Policy.* New York: Oxford University Press, 2006 and Special Issue: Neuroethics. *Cerebrum* 2004;6(4):1–118. New York: Dana Press. This definition also applies to the prominent scholarly website on neuroethics maintained by Martha Farah of the University of Pennsylvania Center for Cognitive Neuroscience http://www.neuroethics.upenn.edu/ (Accessed May 12, 2007).

12. For example, see Giordano J, Gordijn B (eds). *The Silent Revolution in Neuroscience: Scientific, Philosophical and Ethical Perspectives.* New York: Cambridge University Press, 2008 (in preparation) and Illes J, Fins JJ (eds). Ethics, neuroimaging & limited states of consciousness. *Am J Bioethics* 2008 (in preparation).

13. The Neuroethics Society. http://www.neuroethicssociety.org/index.html (Accessed May 12, 2007).

14. *The American Journal of Bioethics—Neuroscience* began publication in 2007. For the justification of publishing a journal dedicated solely to neuroethics, see Illes J. Ipsa scientia potestas est (knowledge is power). *Am J Bioethics* 2007;7(1):1–2.

15. Society for Neuroscience, Washington, DC. Society Mission. http://www.sfn.org/index.cfm?pagename= mission&section=about_SfN (Accessed May 12, 2007).

16. Kramer P. *Listening to Prozac.* New York: Penguin Books, 1993.

17. This issue is analyzed critically in Gill DG. "Anything you can do, I can do bigger?": the ethics and equity of growth hormone for small normal children. *Arch Dis Child* 2006;270–272. For prevailing practices, see Cuttler L, Silvers JB, Singh J, et al. Short stature and growth hormone therapy: a national study of physician recommendation patterns. *JAMA* 1996;276:531–537.

18. Daniel N. Normal functioning and the treatment-enhancement distinction. *Camb Q Healthc Ethics* 2000; 9:309–322.

19. Chatterjee A. Cosmetic neurology: the controversy over enhancing movement, mentation, and mood. *Neurology* 2004;63:968–974.

20. For a discussion of cosmetic ethics, see Frank AW. Emily's scars: surgical shapings, technoluxe, and bioethics. *Hastings Cent Rep* 2004;34(2):18–29. Anjan Chatterjee recently defended his choice of the term "cosmetic neurology" by comparing it to cosmetic surgery. See Chatterjee A. Cosmetic neurology and cosmetic surgery: parallels, predictions, and challenges. *Camb Q Healthc Ethics* 2007;16:129–137.

21. The data to support these effects are summarized in Chatterjee A. Cosmetic neurology: the controversy over enhancing movement, mentation, and mood. *Neurology* 2004;63:968–974. The medications used in enhancement are reviewed in Mehlman MJ. Cognition-enhancing drugs. *Milbank Q* 2004; 82:483–506.

22. See Wolpe PR. Treatment, enhancement, and the ethics of neurotherapeutics. *Brain Cogn* 2002;50:387–395; Farah MJ. Emerging ethical issues in neuroscience. *Nature Neurosci* 2002;5:1123–1129; Sandel M. The case against perfection. *Atlantic Monthly* 2004;293(3):51–62; Kamm FM. Is there are problem with enhancement? *Am J Bioethics* 2005;5(3):5–14; and Cheshire WP Jr. Drugs for enhancing cognition and their ethical implications: a hot new cup of tea. *Expert Rev Neurotherapeutics* 2006;6(3):263–266.

23. Parens E. Is better always good? The Enhancement Project. *Hastings Cent Rep* 1998;28(1) Special Supplement:S1–S17.

24. Parens E. Authenticity and ambivalence: toward understanding the enhancement debate. *Hastings Cent Rep* 2005;35(3):34–41.

25. Farah MJ. Neuroethics: the practical and philosophical. *Trends Cogn Sci* 2005;9:34–40.

26. Mehlman MJ. Cognition-enhancing drugs. *Milbank Q* 2004;82:483–506.

27. President's Council on Bioethics. *Beyond Therapy: Biotechnology and the Pursuit of Happiness.* New York: Dana Press, 2003.

28. Liliefeld SO. Scientifically unsupported and supported interventions for childhood psychopathology: a summary. *Pediatrics* 2005;115:761–764.

29. Diller LH. The run on Ritalin: attention deficit disorder and stimulant treatment in the 1990s. *Hastings Cent Rep* 1996;26(2):12–14. For the current criteria for using stimulants in children with ADHD, see Brown RT, Amler RW, Freeman WS, et al. Treatment of attention-deficit/hyperactivity disorder: overview of the evidence. *Pediatrics* 2005;115:e749–e757.

30. The bioethicist Leon Kass and the futurist Francis Fukuyama have written eloquently on this thesis. See Kass L. *Life, Liberty and the Defense of Dignity: The Challenge for Bioethics.* San Francisco: Encounter Books, 2002 and Fukuyama F. *Our Posthuman Future: Consequences of the Biotechnology Revolution.* New York: Farrar, Strauss and Giroux, 2002. Kass developed this position is developed in its fullest form in President's Council on Bioethics. *Beyond Therapy: Biotechnology and the Pursuit of Happiness.* New York: Dana Press, 2003. The philosopher Michael Sandel recently constructed a similar argument against the desirability of humans trying to achieve perfection through genetic engineering. See Sandel MJ. *The Case Against Perfection: Ethics in the Age of Genetic Engineering.* Cambridge, MA: Harvard University Press, 2007.

31. Mehlman MJ. Cognition-enhancing drugs. *Milbank Q* 2004;82:483–506.

32. For a primer on transhumanist philosophy, see Agar N. Whereto transhumanism? The literature reaches a critical mass. *Hastings Cent Rep* 2007;37(3):12–17.

33. For an early analysis of this subject, see Illes J, Desmond J, Huang LF, et al. Ethical and practical considerations in managing incidental neurologic findings in fMRI. *Brain Cogn* 2002;50:358–365.

34. Illes J, Rosen AC, Huang L, et al. Ethical consideration of incidental findings on adult brain MRI in research. *Neurology* 2004;62:888–890. Similar data were reported in Katzman GL, Dagher AP, Patronas NJ. Incidental findings on brain magnetic resonance imaging from 1000 asymptomatic volunteers. *JAMA* 1999;282;36–39.

35. Kirschen MP, Jaworska A, Illes J. Subjects' expectations in neuroimaging research. *J Magn Reson Imaging* 2006;23:205–209.

36. Grossman RI, Bernat JL. Incidental research imaging findings: Pandora's costly box. *Neurology* 2004;62:849–850.

37. Illes J, Kirschen MP, Edwards E, et al. Incidental findings in brain imaging research. *Science* 2006; 311:783–784.

38. These social and ethical issues in neuroimaging were reviewed in Illes J, Racine E. Imaging or imagining? A neuroethics challenge informed by genetics. *Am J Bioethics* 2005;5(2):5–18. Portions of this section were abstracted from this article.

39. Greene JD, Sommerville RB, Nystrom LE, et al. An fMRI investigation of emotional engagement in moral judgment. *Science* 2001;293:2105–2108. For a review of these studies, see Greene JD. From neural "is" to moral "ought": What are the moral implications of neuroscientific moral psychology? *Nature Rev Neurosci* 2003;4:847–850.

40. Koenigs M, Young L, Adolphs R, et al. Damage to the prefrontal cortex increases utilitarian moral judgments. *Nature* 2007;446:865–866.

41. Phelps EA, O'Connor KJ, Cunningham WA, et al. Performance on indirect measures of race evaluation predicts amygdala activation. *J Cogn Neurosci* 2000;12:729–738.

42. Childress AR, Mozley PD, McElgin W, Fitzgerald J, Reivich M, O'Brien CP. Limbic activation during cue-induced cocaine craving. *Am J Psychiatry* 1999;156:11–18.

43. Garavan H, Pankiewicz H, Bloom A, et al. Cue-induced cocaine craving: neuroanatomical specificity for drug users and drug stimuli. *Am J Psychiatry* 2000;157:1789–1798.

44. These data are reviewed in Hyman SE. The neurobiology of addiction: implications for voluntary control of behavior. *Am J Bioethics* 2007;7(1):8–11.

45. Lee N, Broderick AJ, Chamberlain L. What is "neuromarketing"? A discussion and agenda for future research. *Int J Psychophysiol* 2007;63:199–204.

46. McClure SM, Li J, Tomlin D, Cypert KS, Montague LM, Montague PR. Neural correlates of behavioral preference for culturally familiar drinks. *Neuron* 2004;44:379–387.

47. Anderson SW, Bechara A, Damasio H, Tranel D, Damasio AR. Impairment of social and moral behavior related to early damage in human prefrontal cortex. *Nature Neurosci* 1999;2:1032–1037.

48. Raine A, Lencz T, Bihrle S, LaCasse L, Colletti P. Reduced prefrontal gray matter volume and reduced autonomic activity in antisocial personality disorder. *Arch Gen Psychiatry* 2000;57:119–127.

49. Kiehl KA, Smith AM, Hare RD, et al. Limbic abnormalities in affective processing by criminal psychopaths as revealed by functional magnetic resonance imaging. *Biol Psychiatry* 2001;50:677–684.

50. Canli T, Amin Z. Neuroimaging of emotion and personality: scientific evidence and ethical considerations. *Brain Cogn* 2002;50:431–444.

51. idem. Scanning the social brain. *Nature Neurosci* 2003;6:1239.

52. Greely HT. Prediction, litigation, privacy, and property: some possible legal and social implications of advances in neuroscience. In Garland B (ed). *Neuroscience and the Law: Brain, Mind, and the Scales of Justice.* New York: Dana Press, 2004:114–156.

53. Farwell LA, Smith SS. Using brain MERMER testing to detect concealed knowledge despite efforts to conceal. *J Forensic Sci* 2001;46:135–143. The use of this technique in criminal cases is discussed in Gazzaniga MS. *The Ethical Brain.* New York: Dana Press, 2005:111–113. Two commercial firms, Cephos Corporation and No Lie MRI, have announced that they plan to offer commercial lie detection technology based on fMRI technology. See Greely HT. Knowing sin: making sure good science does not go bad. In Read CA (ed). *Cerebrum 2007: Emerging Ideas in Brain Science.* New York: Dana Press, 2007:85–94.

54. Langleben DD, Schroeder L, Maldjian JA,et al. Brain activity during simulated deception: an event-related functional magnetic resonance study. *Neuroimage* 2002;15:727–732.

55. Moll JR, de Oliviera-Souza R, Eslinger PJ. Morals and the human brain: a working model. *Neuroreport* 2003; 14:229–305.

56. Lee TM, Liu HL, Tan LH, et al. Lie detection by functional magnetic resonance imaging. *Hum Brain Mapp* 2002;15:157–164.

57. Ganis G, Kosslyn SM, Stose S, Thompson WL, Yurgelun-Todd DA. Neural correlates of different types of deception: an fMRI investigation. *Cereb Cortex* 2003:13:830–836.

58. Raichle M. Neuroimaging. In Dana Alliance for Brain Initiatives. *The 2006 Progress Report on Brain Research.* New York: Dana Press, 2006:5–10. Raichle objects to the term "activation" that is used commonly among the functional neuroimaging scientific community to describe brain areas that show increased metabolic activity in response to stimuli because it misleadingly implies a specific mechanism. Personal communication, September 12, 2006.

59. Tovino SA. Currents in contemporary ethics. The confidentiality and privacy implications of functional magnetic resonance imaging. *J Law Med Ethics* 2005;33:844–850. Each of the examples in this paragraph was provided in this article.

60. 29 U.S.C. § 2002(1) (2005); § 2001(3) (2005).

61. Boire RG. Searching the brain: the Fourth Amendment implications of brain-based deception detection devices. *Am J Bioethics* 2005;5(2):62–63.

62. Boire RG. On cognitive liberty. *J Cognitive Liberties* 1999/2000;1(1):7–13. For a review of the legal aspects of functional neuroimaging, see Tovino SA. Functional neuroimaging and the law: trends and directions for future scholarship. *Am J Bioethics* 2007;7(9):44–56.

63. Rosen AC, Bokde AL, Pearl A, Yesavage JA. Ethical and practical issues in applying brain functional imaging to the clinical management of Alzheimer's disease. *Brain Cogn* 2002;50:498–519.

64. Knopman DS, DeKosky ST, Cummings JL, et al. Practice parameter: diagnosis of dementia (an evidence-based review). Report of the Quality Standards Subcommittee of the American Academy of Neurology. *Neurology* 2001;56:1143–1153.

65. For example, see Galton CJ. Patterson K, Graham K, et al. Differing patterns of temporal atrophy in Alzheimer's disease and semantic dementia. *Neurology* 2001;57:216–225 and Valenzuela MJ, Sachdev P. Magnetic resonance spectroscopy in AD. *Neurology* 2001;56:592–598.

66. Smith CD, Andersen AH, Kryscio RJ, et al. Altered brain activation in cognitively intact individuals at high risk for Alzheimer's disease. *Neurology* 1999;53:1391–1396.

67. Killiany RJ, Gomez-Isla T, Moss M, et al. Use of structural magnetic resonance imaging to predict who will get Alzheimer's disease. *Ann Neurol* 2000;47:430–439.

68. Silverman DHS, Small GW, Chang CY, et al. Positron emission tomography in evaluation of dementia: regional brain metabolism and long-term outcome. *JAMA* 2001;286:2120–2177. A later critical review cast doubt on these findings. See Gill SS, Rochon PA, Guttman M, Laupacis A. The value of positron emission tomography in the clinical evaluation of dementia. *J Am Geriatr Soc* 2003;51:258–264.

69. Illes J, Rosen A, Grecius M, Racine E. Prospects for prediction: ethics analysis of neuroimaging in Alzheimer's disease. *Ann NY Acad Sci* 2007;1097;278–295.

70. See Mueller SG, Weiner MW, Thal LJ, et al. The Alzheimer's Disease Neuroimaging Initiative. *Neuroimaging Clin N Am* 2005;15:869–877. http://www.loni.ucla.edu/ADNI/ (Accessed May 17, 2007).

71. See Wickelgren I. Neuroprosthetics: brain-computer interface adds a new dimension. *Science* 2004; 306:1878–1879 and Abbott A. Neuroprosthetics: in search of the sixth sense. *Nature* 2006;442:125–127.

72. Waltzman SB. Cochlear implants: current status. *Expert Rev Med Devices* 2006;3:647–655.

73. Hintermair M. Albertini JA. Ethics, deafness, and new medical technologies. *J Deaf Stud Deaf Educ* 2005; 10:184–192.

74. Hyde M, Power D. Some ethical dimensions of cochlear implantation for deaf children and their families. *J Deaf Stud Deaf Educ* 2006;11:102–111.

75. Berg AL, Herb A, Hurst M. Cochlear implants in children: ethics, informed consent, and parental decision making. *J Clin Ethics* 2005;16:239–250.

76. Leuthardt EC, Schalk G, Moran D, Ojemann JG. The emerging world of neuroprosthetics. *Neurosurgery* 2006;59:1–14.

77. Hochberg L, Serruya MD, Friehs GM, et al. Neuronal ensemble control of prosthetic devices by a human with tetraplegia. *Nature* 2006;442:164–171.

78. Santhanam G, Ryu SI, Yu BM, Afshar A, Shenoy KV. A high-performance brain-computer interface. *Nature* 2006;442:195–198.

79. Scott SH. Neuroscience: converting thoughts into action. *Nature* 2006;442:141–142.

80. For a scholarly discussion of the issue of neuroprostheses for enhancement and other ethical issues of neuroprostheses, see Chase VD. *Shattered Nerves: How Science is Solving Modern Medicine's Most Perplexing Problem*. Baltimore: Johns Hopkins University Press, 2006.

81. See Kornblum HI. Introduction to neural stem cells. *Stroke* 2007;38(2 Suppl):810–816; Kim SU. Genetically engineered human neural stem cells for brain repair in neurological diseases. *Brain Dev* 2007;29(4):193–201; and Martino G, Pluchino S. The therapeutic potential of neural stem cells. *Nat Rev Neurosci* 2006;7:395–406.

82. Garbossa D, Fontanella M, Fronda C, et al. New strategies for repairing the injured spinal cord: the role of stem cells. *Neurol Res* 2006;28:500–504 and Belegu V, Oudega M, Gary DS, McDonald JW. Restoring function after spinal cord injury: promoting spontaneous regeneration with stem cells and activity-based therapies. *Neurosurg Clin N Am* 2007;18:143–168.

83. There is an enormous literature on human embryonic stem cell research and cloning. For a balanced scientific and ethical analysis, see Guenin LM. The morality of unenabled embryo use—arguments that work and arguments that don't. *Mayo Clin Proc* 2004;79:801–808. For a dialectic of moral arguments to permit or ban this research see Green RM. Determining moral status. *Am J Bioethics* 2002;2(1):20–30 and Meilander G. The point of a ban: or, how to think about stem cell research. *Hastings Cent Rep* 2001; 31(1):9–16. For a political history of stem cell research in the United States, see Okie S. Stem-cell research—signposts and roadblocks. *N Engl J Med* 2005;353:1–5. For the positions of the American Academy of Neurology and the American Neurological Association, see American Academy of Neurology and the American Neurological Association. Position statement regarding the use of embryonic and adult human stem cells in biomedical research. *Neurology* 2005;64:1679–1680.

84. For noteworthy examples, see Churchland PS. *Brain-Wise: Studies in Neurophilosophy*. Cambridge, MA: MIT Press, 2003, Dennett D. *Brainstorms: Philosophical Essays on Mind and Psychology*. Cambridge, MA: MIT Press, 1978; and Searle JD. *Mind: A Brief Introduction*. New York: Oxford University Press, 2004.

85. Block N, Flanagan O, Güzeldere G. *The Nature of Consciousness: Philosophical Debates*. Cambridge, MA: MIT Press, 1997:1.

86. Notable books attacking the problem include Dennett DC. *Consciousness Explained*. Boston: Little Brown, 1991; Damasio AR. *The Feeling of What Happens*. New York: Harcourt Brace, 1999; and Hobson JA. *Consciousness*. New York: Scientific American Library, 1999. For a unique approach to understanding consciousness that

creatively applies the ideas of the mathematician Kurt Gödel, see Hofstadter D. *I Am a Strange Loop*. New York: Basic Books, 2007.

87. The cognitive neuroscientist Christof Koch made a valiant attempt to identify the fundamental "neural correlate of consciousness" in Koch C. *The Quest for Consciousness*. Englewood, CO: Roberts and Co. Publishers, 2004.

88. For the best example, see McGinn C. *The Problem of Consciousness*. Oxford: Blackwell Publishers, 1991.

89. For three elegant defenses of this thesis, see Damasio AR. *Descartes' Error: Emotion, Reason and the Human Brain*. New York: G.P. Putnam's Sons, 1994; Crick F. *The Astonishing Hypothesis: The Scientific Search for the Soul*. New York: Scribners, 1994; and Pinker S. *How the Mind Works*. New York: Norton, 1997.

90. Farah MJ, Heberlein AS. Personhood and neuroscience: naturalizing or nihilating? *Am J Bioethics* 2007;7(1):37–48.

91. Gert B. Personal identity and the body. *Dialogue* 1971;10(3):458–478. Other philosophers have proposed even more bizarre thought experiments to clarify the relationship between the brain/mind and personal identity. For example, see the imaginative thought experiments of Derek Parfit in Parfit D. *Reasons and Persons*. New York: Oxford University Press, 1984.

92. I rely on the discussions of free will in Gazzaniga MS, Steven MS. Free will in the twenty-first century: a discussion of neuroscience and the law. In Garland B (ed). *Neuroscience and the Law: Brain, Mind, and the Scales of Justice*. New York: Dana Press, 2004:51–70 and Churchland PS. *Brain-Wise: Studies in Neurophilosophy*. Cambridge, MA: MIT Press, 2003:201–237.

93. See discussion in Tancredi LR. The neuroscience of free will. *Behav Sci Law* 2007;25:295–308.

94. Neuroimaging findings such as fMRI now are being introduced into criminal trials as exculpating evidence of guilt. See the discussion of new legal issues raised by functional neuroimaging data in, Morse SJ. New neuroscience, old problems. In Garland B (ed). *Neuroscience and the Law: Brain, Mind, and the Scales of Justice*. New York: Dana Press, 2004:157–198.

95. Libet B. Conscious vs neural time. *Nature* 1991;352:27–28.

96. Libet discusses the free will philosophical implications of his series of experiments in Libet B. *Mind Time: The Temporal Factor in Consciousness*. Cambridge, MA: Harvard University Press, 2004.

97. Hallett M. Volitional control of movement: The physiology of free will. *Clin Neurophysiol* 2007; 118:1179–1192.

Index